Mosby's
CRITICAL CARE
NURSING CONSULTANT

Mosby's
CRITICAL CARE
NURSING CONSULTANT

Edited by

JANET HICKS KEEN, RN, MS(N), CCRN, CEN

Consultant in Emergency, Trauma, and Critical Care Nursing
Staff Nurse, Level II
St. Joseph's Hospital of Atlanta
Atlanta, Georgia

PAMELA L. SWEARINGEN, RN

Special Project Editor

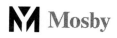 Mosby

St. Louis Baltimore Boston
Carlsbad Chicago Naples New York Philadelphia Portland
London Madrid Mexico City Singapore Sydney Tokyo Toronto Wiesbaden

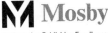

Mosby

Dedicated to Publishing Excellence

A Times Mirror
Company

Vice President and Publisher: Nancy Coon
Editor: Barry Bowlus
Associate Developmental Editor: Cynthia Anderson
Project Manager: Patricia Tannian
Production Editor: Heidi Fite-Crowley
Book Design Manager: Gail Morey Hudson
Manufacturing Manager: Dave Graybill
Cover Design: Teresa Breckwoldt

Printed in the United States of America
Composition by The Clarinda Company
Printing/binding by Maple-Vail Book Mfg. Group

Mosby–Year Book Inc.
11830 Westline Industrial Drive
St. Louis, Missouri 63146

International Standard Book Number 0-8151-3178-X

97 98 99 00 01/9 8 7 6 5 4 3 2 1

CONTRIBUTORS

LOLITA ADRIEN, RN, MS, CETN, CGRN

Clinical Nurse Specialist
Enterostomal Therapy/Ostomy Services
John Muir Medical Center
Walnut Creek, California

ROBERT AUCKER, PharmD

Clinical Pharmacist
St. Joseph's Hospital of Atlanta
Adjunct Professor, Mercer Southern School of Pharmacy
Adjunct Assistant Professor
Kennesaw State College School of Nursing
Atlanta, Georgia

LINDA S. BAAS, RN, PhD, CCRN

Assistant Professor, College of Nursing and Health
University of Cincinnati Medical Center
Cincinnati, Ohio

MARIANNE SAUNORUS BAIRD, RN, MN, CCRN

Case Manager/Clinical Nurse Specialist
Department of Nursing
St. Joseph's Hospital of Atlanta
Atlanta, Georgia

CAROL BARCH, RN, MN, CCRN, CNRN, CFNP

Program Director
Department of Neurology, UPMC Stroke Institute
University of Pittsburgh
Pittsburgh, Pennsylvania

CHERYL L. BITTEL, RN, MSN, CCRN

Clinical Nurse Specialist, Cardiovascular Services
Department of Nursing
Saint Joseph's Hospital of Atlanta
Atlanta, Georgia

MIMI CALLANAN, RN, MSN

Epilepsy Clinical Specialist
Stanford Comprehensive Epilepsy Center
Department of Neurology and Neurological Sciences
Stanford University Medical Center
Stanford, California

ALICE DAVIS, RN, PhD, CNRN, CCRN

Post Doctoral Fellow
University of Michigan School of Nursing
Ann Arbor, Michigan

CHERI A. GOLL, RN, MSN

Assistant Program Director
Nursing and Patient Care Services
Indiana University Medical Center
Indianapolis, Indiana

PATRICIA HALL, RN, PhD, CCRN

Clinical Nurse Specialist, Cardiac Services
Department of Patient Services
Promina Kennestone Hospital
Marietta, Georgia

URSULA HEITZ, RN, MSN

Nursing Consultant
Nashville, Tennessee

MIMA M. HORNE, RN, MS, CDE

Diabetes Clinical Nurse Specialist
Coastal Diabetes Center
New Hanover Regional Medical Center
Adjunct Lecturer, School of Nursing
University of North Carolina—Wilmington
Wilmington, North Carolina

MARGUERITE McMILLAN JACKSON, RN, PhD, CIC, FAAN

Administrative Director, Epidemiology Unit
Assistant Clinical Professor of Family & Preventive Medicine
Division of Epidemiology
University of California—San Diego Medical Center
San Diego, California

PATRICIA R. JANSEN, RN, MSN, CS

Geriatric Clinical Nurse Specialist/Clinical Consultant
San Jose, California

JOYCE YOUNG JOHNSON, RN, PhD, CCRN

Assistant Professor
School of Nursing
Georgia State University, College of Health Sciences
Atlanta, Georgia

JANET HICKS KEEN, RN, MS(N), CCRN, CEN

Consultant in Emergency, Trauma, and Critical Care Nursing
Staff Nurse, Level II
St. Joseph's Hospital of Atlanta
Atlanta, Georgia

MARGUERITE J. MURPHY, RN, MSN, CCRN

Nursing Consultant, Clinical Faculty
Gordon College
Barnesville, GA

DENNIS G. ROSS, RN, MAE, PhD

Professor of Nursing
Castleton State College
Castleton, Vermont

MARILYN SAWYER SOMMERS, RN, PhD, CCRN

Associate Professor, College of Nursing and Health
Staff Nurse, Surgical ICU/Trauma
University of Cincinnati Medical Center
Cincinnati, Ohio

JANICE SPEAS, RN, MSN, CIC

Infection Control Specialist
Patient Care Management
St. Joseph's Hospital of Atlanta
Atlanta, Georgia

BARBARA TUELLER STEUBLE, RN, MS

Staff Nurse, Operating Room
Sutter Amador Hospital
Jackson, California

JOHANNA K. STIESMEYER, RN, MS, CCRN

Consultant, Nursing Education Services
Placitas, New Mexico

NANCY STOTTS, RN, MN, EdD

Professor
Department of Physiological Nursing
University of California—San Francisco
San Francisco, California

ANN COGHLAN STOWE, RN, MSN

Chairperson and Assistant Professor
Department of Nursing
West Chester University
West Chester, Pennsylvania

KAREN S. WEBBER, RN, MN

Assistant Professor, School of Nursing
Memorial University of Newfoundland
St. John's, Newfoundland, Canada

PATRICIA D. WEISKITTEL, RN, MSN, CNN

Renal Clinical Nurse Specialist
Department of Nursing
University Hospital
Cincinnati, Ohio

CONSULTANTS

ROBIN DONOHOE DENNISON, RN, MSN, CCRN, CS

Critical Care Consultant
Lexington, Kentucky

KATHLEEN M. STACY, RN, MS, CCRN

Critical Care Clinical Nurse Specialist
Tri-City Medical Center
Oceanside, California

MARY E. LOUGH, MS, RN, CCRN

Critical Care Cardiovascular Clinical Nurse Specialist
Sequoia Hospital
Redwood City, California
Assistant Clinical Professor
University of California—San Francisco
San Francisco, California

REVIEWERS

JODY GRAHN, RN, BSN

Clinical Educator
Oconee Memorial Hospital

SUSAN KAISER, RN, BSN, CCRN

PRN Nurse
Georgetown University Hospital
Washington, District of Columbia

PREFACE

Mosby's Critical Care Nursing Consultant is a uniquely designed quick reference for nurses who manage the care of critically ill or injured patients. The carefully considered writing style and layout make the reference easy to read and use—important since the nurse's valuable time is often limited. The reference includes over 200 topics organized alphabetically and within the Appendix. Each topic has been researched and written by authors with expertise in their fields. Important topics that apply to many critical conditions are included within the Appendix.

A two-page, chart-like format covers major aspects of each condition or procedure. Icons are used to visually direct the reader to subheadings within a given section. Pathophysiology, history, and initial presentation are discussed in the "Overview" column. Next, assessment findings and diagnostic tests are outlined. The "Collaborative Management" column includes interdisciplinary referrals and patient education.

In the "Nursing Diagnosis/Interventions" column, there are a number of interventions for each critical disorder. Not all interventions are appropriate for each patient; it is the authors' intent that the interventions that do apply to the individual patient be used in the development of a personalized plan of care. Because of the collaborative nature of critical care nursing, interdisciplinary interventions may be included along with nursing interventions. It is assumed that the nurse will consult the physician or use a designated care map or other previously approved directions before implementing interventions that require a prescription from the physician.

The "Miscellanea" column includes a quick check of findings that suggest the need for immediate physician consultation. In addition, the reader is referred to related topics also included in the text. For example, the section on "Cardiac Surgery: CABG" refers the reader to the closely related sections "Hemodynamic Monitoring" and "Hemorrhagic Shock."

For clarity and consistency throughout the book, normal or generally anticipated values are given for hemodynamic monitoring and other measurements. However, all values should be individualized to correspond to the patient's normal or optimal range of measurements.

Our primary goal is to provide a quick reference for busy critical care nurses to use in their daily practice. The book can serve as a resource for clinicians as well as a supplemental text for nursing educators and students. Mosby's *Critical Care Nursing Consultant* was written to provide a quick reminder of previously learned concepts. It is assumed that the reader has a background in critical care pathophysiology and assessment parameters.

The authors are committed to providing the most relevant and accurate information in this rapidly changing field and welcome suggestions from users so that we can enhance the usefulness of future editions of the book.

Janet Hicks Keen
Pamela L. Swearingen

CONTENTS

APPENDIXES

Mosby's
CRITICAL CARE
NURSING CONSULTANT

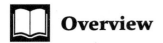

Overview

PATHOPHYSIOLOGY

Blunt abdominal trauma typically results in injury to solid viscera (eg, liver, spleen). Hollow organs (eg, stomach, intestines) tend to be compressible but may rupture, especially when full. *Penetrating* trauma typically results in injury to organs in the direct path of the instrument or missile, but high-velocity weapons may cause injury to adjacent organs as well. Pathophysiologic changes include massive fluid shifts; systemic inflammation and metabolic changes; coagulation problems; inflammation, infection, and abscess formation caused by release of GI secretions and bacteria into peritoneum; and nutritional and electrolyte alterations resulting from disruption of GI tract integrity.

COMMON INJURIES

Liver: Most frequently involved in penetrating trauma but also affected by blunt injury. Control of bleeding and bile drainage major concerns.

Spleen: Frequently injured after blunt trauma. Massive hemorrhage common.

Stomach: Because stomach flexible and readily displaced, usually not injured with blunt trauma, but may be injured by direct penetration.

Small Intestine and Mesentery: Penetrating or nonpenetrating forces may result in injury. Perforations or contusions can cause release of bacteria and intestinal contents into abdominal cavity, resulting in serious infection.

Colon: Injury most frequently caused by penetrating forces; may be caused by blunt forces. Because of its high bacterial content, infection even greater concern than with small bowel injury.

Major Vessels: Include abdominal aorta, inferior vena cava, hepatic vein; associated with rapid hemorrhage.

Retroperitoneal Vessels: Tears can cause significant bleeding into retroperitoneal space; detection is difficult.

HISTORY/RISK FACTORS

- Vehicular collision
- Fall
- Victim of violent act (stabbing, physical altercation)

CLINICAL PRESENTATION

- Mild tenderness to severe abdominal pain; pain localized to site of injury or diffuse.
- Involuntary guarding, rigidity, rebound tenderness (peritoneal signs) caused by intraperitoneal blood or fluid collection.
- Referred shoulder pain caused by fluid or air under diaphragm. Kehr's sign may be noted, especially when patient is recumbent.

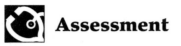

Assessment

PHYSICAL ASSESSMENT

Abdominal assessment highly subjective; serial evaluations by same examiner strongly recommended to detect subtle changes.

Inspection: Ecchymosis over LUQ suggests splenic rupture; erythema and ecchymosis across lower portion of abdomen suggest intestinal injury caused by lap belts. Grey Turner's sign may indicate retroperitoneal bleeding from pancreas, duodenum, vena cava, aorta, or kidneys. Cullen's sign may be present as a result of intraperitoneal bleeding from liver or spleen. Entrance and exit (if present) wounds should be identified. *Note:* Outward signs of injury absent in up to 36% of patients with abdominal trauma (Beachly, 1993).

Auscultation: Bowel sounds likely to be ↓/absent. Presence of bowel sounds, however, does not exclude significant abdominal injury.

Palpation: Tenderness to light palpation suggests pain from superficial or abdominal wall lesions. Deep palpation may reveal mass in area of hematoma. Measurements of abdominal girth helpful in identifying ↑ girth attributable to gas, blood, or fluid. Visual evaluation unreliable.

Percussion: Unusually large areas of dullness percussed over ruptured blood-filled organs. Fixed area of dullness in LUQ suggests ruptured spleen. Absence/↓ in size of liver dullness may be caused by free air below diaphragm, a consequence of hollow viscus perforation, or, in unusual cases, liver displacement through a ruptured diaphragm. Presence of tympany suggests gas; dullness suggests enlargement caused by blood or fluid.

VITAL SIGNS/HEMODYNAMICS

RR: ↑

HR: ↑

BP: Nl initially; then ↓ with massive blood loss

Temp: ↑ from inflammation/infection

CVP/PAP: ↓ as a result of hemorrhage

SVR: ↑ because of catecholamine release; may ↓ if SIRS, sepsis ensues

CO: ↓ as a result of volume loss

LABORATORY STUDIES

Hct: If measured immediately after injury may be nl, but serial levels will reveal ↓ during resuscitation and as extravascular fluid mobilizes during recovery phase.

WBCs: Leukocytosis expected immediately after injury. A later ↑ or left shift reflects ↑ in neutrophils and signals inflammatory response and possible intraabdominal infection.

Glucose: Initially ↑ because catecholamine release and insulin resistance associated with major trauma. Glucose metabolism abnormal after major hepatic injury; patients should be monitored for severe hypoglycemia.

Electrolytes: Sodium, potassium, and chloride levels may ↓ because of gastric suctioning or vomiting.

BUN: ↑ associated with shock, dehydration, GI bleeding, infection, and impaired kidney function.

Amylase: ↑ levels associated with pancreatic or upper small bowel injury.

Liver Enzymes: ↑ AST, ALT, and ALP reflect hepatic dysfunction caused by liver ischemia during prolonged hypotensive episodes or direct traumatic damage.

Bilirubin: ↑ direct (conjugated) indicates liver's inability to excrete bilirubin. ↑ indirect (unconjugated) signals rapid destruction of RBCs or possible retroperitoneal hematoma.

Occult Blood: Gastric contents and stool tested for blood in initial and recovery periods because GI bleeding can occur as a result of direct injury or later complications, including gastric erosion.

IMAGING

X-rays: Flat and upright chest x-rays done to exclude chest injuries. Chest, abdominal, and pelvic x-rays may reveal fractures, missiles, free intraperitoneal air, hematoma, hemorrhage.

CT Scan: Can detect intraperitoneal and retroperitoneal bleeding and free air (associated with rupture of hollow viscera).

Angiography: Performed selectively to evaluate injury to spleen, liver, pancreas, duodenum, and retroperitoneal vessels when other diagnostic findings equivocal.

DIAGNOSTIC PROCEDURES

DPL: Insertion of large, flexible catheter into peritoneum to check for intraabdominal bleeding. Indicated for blunt trauma when S&S of injury obscured by intoxication, CNS injury, or depression, or if prolonged general anesthesia to be used for other injuries. Unnecessary for obvious intraabdominal injury. If gross blood recovered, immediate laparotomy indicated. If blood not recovered, 1 L NS or LR rapidly infused and then drained into sterile bedside drainage device. If drained lavage bloody, intraperitoneal bleeding confirmed. *Note:* Indwelling urinary catheter inserted preprocedure to prevent inadvertent puncture of full bladder. Stomach decompressed with gastric tube to avoid vomiting.

Collaborative Management

Oxygen: High-flow supplemental O_2 indicated initially and then titrated according to ABGs.

Fluid Management: Immediate volume resuscitation critical. Initially LR, NS, or similar solution given. Colloid solutions such as albumin helpful postop if hypoalbuminemia occurs as a result of hepatic injury or ischemia. Typed and cross-matched fresh blood optimal for replacing large blood losses, but since it is rarely available, combination of PRBCs and FFP often used.

Gastric Intubation: Enables gastric decompression. Aspirated contents checked for blood to aid in diagnosis of lower esophageal, gastric, duodenal injury.

Urinary Drainage: *Via* Foley catheter to monitor UO, assess for hematuria.

Pharmacotherapy

Antibiotics: Abdominal trauma associated with high incidence of intraabdominal abscess, sepsis, and wound infection, particularly with injury to terminal ileum and colon. Persons with suspected intestinal injury started on parenteral antibiotic therapy immediately. Broad-spectrum antibiotics continued postop.

Analgesics: Opiates alter the sensorium, making assessment difficult, thus seldom used in early stages of trauma. Analgesics used immediately postop to relieve pain and promote ventilatory excursion.

Nutrition: Complex nutritional needs often present because of hypermetabolic state and traumatic or surgical disruption of nl GI function. Prompt initiation of parenteral feedings (if enteric feedings contraindicated) and supplemental calories, proteins, vitamins, minerals essential for healing.

Surgical Considerations for Penetrating Injuries: Removing penetrating objects can result in additional injury; removal attempts made only under controlled situations with surgeon and OR immediately available. There is a trend toward observation of patients without obvious injury or peritoneal signs.

Indications for laparotomy: Positive peritoneal signs, shock, GI hemorrhage, free air in peritoneal cavity as seen on x-ray, evisceration, massive hematuria, positive findings on DPL.

Surgical Considerations for Nonpenetrating Injuries: Physical examination usually reliable in determining necessity for surgery in alert, cooperative, unintoxicated patients. Additional diagnostic tests such as DPL or CT scan necessary to evaluate need for surgery in other cases (eg, intoxication, CNS injury).

Indications for immediate laparotomy: Clear signs of peritoneal irritation, free air in peritoneum, hypotension caused by suspected abdominal injury or persistent and unexplained hypotension, positive DPL findings, GI aspirate or rectal smear positive for blood, or other positive findings in diagnostic tests such as CT scan or arteriogram. Carefully evaluated, stable patients with blunt abdominal trauma may be admitted to critical care for observation. Vigilant serial observations necessary to detect subtle changes suggesting internal bleeding.

PATIENT-FAMILY TEACHING

- Importance of seeking medical attention if indicators of infection or bowel obstruction occur (eg, fever, severe or unusual abdominal pain, nausea and vomiting, unusual drainage from wounds or incisions, change in bowel habits)
- Injury prevention education: instructions regarding seat belt application, firearm safety, injury prevention strategies suitable for persons involved
- Referral to trauma support groups
- Alcohol/substance abuse rehabilitation program

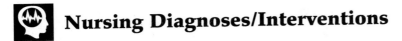 **Nursing Diagnoses/Interventions**

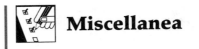 **Miscellanea**

Fluid volume deficit r/t active loss secondary to physical injury
Desired outcomes: Within 12 h of this diagnosis, patient normovolemic: MAP $\geq$70 mm Hg, HR 60-100 bpm, NSR on ECG, CVP 2-6 mm Hg, PAWP 6-12 mm Hg, CI $\geq$2.5 L/min/m^2, SVR 900-1200 dynes/sec/cm^{-5}, UO $\geq$0.5 ml/kg/h, warm extremities, brisk capillary refill (<2 sec), distal pulses >2+ on 0-4+ scale.

- Monitor BP q15min. Be alert to changes in MAP >10 mm Hg. A small but sudden ↓ in BP could signal decompensation.
- Monitor HR, ECG, and CV status q15min until volume restored and VS stable. Check ECG to note HR ↑ and myocardial ischemic changes (ie, ventricular dysrhythmias and ST-segment changes), which can occur as a result of dilutional anemia in susceptible individuals.
- If there is evidence of volume depletion or active blood loss, administer pressurized fluids rapidly through several large-caliber (16-gauge or larger) catheters. Use short, large-bore IV (trauma) tubing to maximize flow rate. Avoid stopcocks, which slow infusion rate. Warm fluids to prevent hypothermia.
- Measure central pressures and thermodilution CO q1-2h or more frequently if there is ongoing blood loss. Be alert to low/↓ CVP and PAWP. ↑ HR, along with ↓ PAWP, ↓ CO/CI, and ↑ SVR, suggests hypovolemia. Anticipate slightly ↑ HR and CO resulting from hyperdynamic CV state in some patients undergoing volume resuscitation. Also anticipate mild to moderate pulmonary hypertension, especially with concurrent thoracic injury.
- Measure UO q1-2h. Be alert to output <0.5 ml/kg/h for 2 consecutive h, which usually reflects inadequate intravascular volume.
- Monitor for hypovolemia, including cool extremities, capillary refill >2 sec, and absent/↓ amplitude of distal pulses.
- Estimate ongoing blood loss. Measure all bloody drainage from tubes or catheters, noting color. Note frequency of dressing changes because of blood saturation.

Pain r/t physical injury secondary to external trauma or surgery
Desired outcomes: Within 2 h of this diagnosis, patient's subjective evaluation of pain improves, as documented by pain scale. Nonverbal indicators of discomfort, such as grimacing, absent.

- Evaluate preop and postop pain using pain scale. Preop pain is anticipated and a vital diagnostic aid. Intense or prolonged pain postop, especially when accompanied by other peritoneal signs, can signal bleeding, bowel infarction, infection, or other complications.
- Recognize that opiate analgesics can ↓ GI motility, causing nausea, vomiting, and delay of bowel activity. These factors are especially significant if patient has had a recent laparotomy.

CONSULT MD FOR

- Abnormal VS: RR >20 breaths/min, HR >100 bpm, SBP <90 mm Hg
- Abnormal hemodynamics: CVP <2 mm Hg, PAWP <6 mm Hg, CI <2.5 L/min/m^2
- SpO_2 <90%
- UO <0.5 ml/kg/h $\times$ 2 h
- Altered mentation
- Occult blood in vomitus, blood-tinged stool/urine
- New-onset peritoneal signs
- ↑ postop abdominal pain
- Abnormal or purulent wound drainage
- S&S of complications: bowel ischemia, mesenteric infarction

RELATED TOPICS

- Antimicrobial therapy
- Fecal ostomies/diversions
- Multisystem injury
- Nutritional support, enteral and parenteral
- Pain
- Shock, septic
- Systemic inflammatory response syndrome

ABBREVIATIONS

DPL: Diagnostic peritoneal lavage
FFP: Fresh frozen plasma
PRBCs: Packed red blood cells
SIRS: Systemic inflammatory response syndrome
Td: Combined tetanus diphtheria toxoid

Risk for infection r/t inadequate primary/secondary defenses, tissue destruction, environmental exposure, multiple invasive procedures

Desired outcome: Patient infection free: core/rectal temp ≤37.8°C, HR ≤100 bpm, orientation × 3, and no unusual redness, warmth, drainage at incisions/drain sites.

- Monitor VS for infection: ↑ temp, RR, HR. ↑ CO and ↓ SVR suggest sepsis. Consult physician if these are new findings.
- Keep all surgically placed tubes or drains patent by irrigating or attaching to low-pressure suction. Promptly report unrelieved loss of tube patency.
- Check incisions/wound sites for infection: redness, warmth, delayed healing, purulent or unusual drainage.
- Give parenteral antibiotics in a timely fashion. Reschedule if dose delayed ≥1 h. Recognize that failure to administer antibiotics on schedule may result in inadequate blood levels and treatment failure.
- Give tetanus immunoglobulin and Td as necessary. Ensure that patient receives a wallet card to document immunization if given.
- Change dressings q24h or more often if wet or soiled. Prevent cross-contamination from various wounds by changing one dressing at a time.

Altered gastrointestinal tract tissue perfusion r/t interruption of arterial or venous blood flow or hypovolemia secondary to abdominal trauma

Desired outcome: By time of hospital discharge, patient has adequate GI tract tissue perfusion: normoactive bowel sounds; soft, nondistended abdomen; and return of bowel elimination.

- Auscultate for bowel sounds qh during acute phase of trauma and q4-8h during recovery phase. Confer with physician for prolonged absence of bowel sounds during postop period, which may signal bowel ischemia or mesenteric infarction.
- Evaluate for peritoneal signs (abdominal pain, tenderness; involuntary abdominal guarding; abdominal wall rigidity; rebound tenderness; abdominal pain with movement or coughing; ↓/absent bowel sounds), which may occur initially as a result of injury or may not develop until days or wks later if complications attributable to slow bleeding or other mechanisms occur.
- Ensure adequate intravascular volume.
- Evaluate laboratory data for evidence of bleeding (eg, serial Hct) or organ ischemia (eg, AST, ALT, LDH).
- Document amount and character of GI secretions, drainage, and excretions. Note changes that suggest bleeding (presence of frank or occult blood) or obstruction (eg, failure to eliminate flatus or stool within 3-4 days of surgery).

REFERENCES

Beachly M, Farrar J: Abdominal trauma: putting the pieces together, *Am J Nurs* 93(11): 26-34, 1993.

Lawrence DM: Gastrointestinal trauma, *Crit Care Nurs Clin North Am* 5(1): 127-140, 1993.

Neff JA, Kidd PS: *Trauma nursing: the art and science,* St Louis, 1993, Mosby.

Van Rueden K, Dunham CM: Sequelae of massive fluid resuscitation in trauma patients, *Crit Care Nurs Clin North Am* 6(3): 463-472, 1994.

Author: **Janet Hicks Keen**

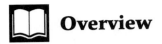 **Overview**

PATHOPHYSIOLOGY
Occurs most often after exposure to a nephrotoxic agent. Injury to epithelial layer of the renal tubule impairs the kidneys' ability to concentrate urine. Na^+ excretion remains close to nl, but K^+, urea, and creatinine excretion ↓, resulting in ↑ serum levels. Usually lasts 5-14 days; renal function gradually returns to nl.

MORTALITY
Patient easier to stabilize, has faster recovery, and has up to 50% ↓ in mortality rate compared to patients with oliguric ATN.

HISTORY/RISK FACTORS
• Exposure to nephrotoxic agent
  Antibiotics: eg, aminoglycosides, cephalosporins, tetracycline
  Anesthetics: eg, methoxyflurane
  Heavy metals: eg, lead, mercury, gold
  Organic solvents: eg, carbon tetrachloride
  Others: Diuretics, NSAIDs, acetaminophen, radiologic contrast media, ethylene glycol, fungicides and pesticides
• Preexisting renal disease, renal ischemia
• Septicemia: resulting from toxins released by microorganisms
• Advanced age
• DM, hypovolemia, rhabdomyolysis
• Exposure to nephrotoxin concurrent with ischemic event

CLINICAL PRESENTATION
• UO >400 ml/24 h up to 2 L/h
• Postural hypotension, dry mucous membranes
• ↑ BUN, creatinine, K^+

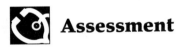 **Assessment**

PHYSICAL ASSESSMENT
Variable, depending on extent of fluid/electrolyte imbalance
Neuro: Dizziness, personality changes, seizures, coma
Resp: Tachypnea, Kussmaul's respirations
CV: Tachycardia, postural hypotension, dysrhythmias

MS: Weakness, flaccidity, paresthesias
Integ: Poor skin turgor, flushed skin, dry oral mucous membranes

VITAL SIGNS/HEMODYNAMICS
RR: ↑
HR: ↑
BP: Postural changes; may be ↓
Temp: May be ↑
MAP/CVP/PAP/PAWP: ↓ if hypovolemic
ECG: Sinus tachycardia; tall peaked T waves; loss of P waves; prolonged PR interval; progressive widening of QRS, possibly leading to cardiac arrest
Other: May progress to oliguric ATN; hemodynamics would then reflect fluid volume excess

LABORATORY STUDIES
Urinalysis: May reveal ↓ specific gravity; ↓ osmolality; ↑ protein; presence of brown granular casts, crystals, epithelial cells; creatinine clearance ↓ to 2-15 ml/min.
Chemistries: May show ↑ BUN, creatinine; BUN/creatinine ratio ≥10:1; ↑ K^+, PO_4^{3-}, and osmolality; ↓ Ca^{2+}.
Hematology: Hct ↑ as a result of hemoconcentration; Hct and Hgb may be ↓ as a result of ↓ renal function.
Myoglobin: ↑ if cause of ATN is rhabdomyolysis.
ABGs: May show metabolic acidosis.

IMAGING
KUB, Renal Ultrasonogram: To r/o other causes of ↓ renal function

DIAGNOSTIC PROCEDURE
Percutaneous Renal Biopsy: To r/o other cause of ↓ renal function

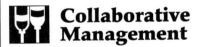 **Collaborative Management**

Early recognition and treatment of underlying cause essential to minimize progression to oliguric ATN.
Supplemental O_2: May be necessary because of Kussmaul's respirations secondary to metabolic acidosis.
Fluid Management: Maintains RBF and UO.
IV hydration: Crystalloid or colloid fluids used; NS, D_5W, LR typically prescribed.
Diuretics: Mannitol used to ↓ tubular swelling, facilitate clearance of cellular debris, and ↑ RBF, GFR. Furosemide and

ethacrynic acid ↓ tubular obstruction by removing cellular debris. Low-dose dopamine (1-3 μg/kg/min) may be used to promote RBF, ↑ GFR, and ↑ effects of furosemide.

Treatment of Electrolyte/Acid-Base Imbalances
Hyperkalemia: $NaHCO_3$ or rapid infusion of D_5W and regular insulin to provide rapid-acting, short-term ↓ in K^+ level. Oral or rectal sodium polystyrene sulfonate (Kayexalate) is slower, but longer acting. Calcium gluconate blocks effects of K^+ on myocardium and may be used when hyperkalemic ECG changes present.
Hyperphosphatemia/hypocalcemia: Phosphate binders (eg, calcium carbonate [Tums]) bind phosphate in the gut and enable absorption of calcium.
Hyponatremia: May occur with rapid diuresis. Hypertonic (3%-5%) NaCl used to correct it.
Acidosis: $NaHCO_3$ given if HCO_3^- <12-15 mEq/L.
Nutrition: Diet modification based on degree of renal function. High-calorie (2000-3000 cal/day), low-protein (40-60 g/day or 0.6 g/kg/day) diet ↓ accumulation of protein byproducts. Low-potassium (2 g or less) and low-sodium (2 g or less) diet also may be indicated. TPN may be prescribed.
Dialysis: Usually not required unless there are continued ↑ in BUN (>100 mg/dl), creatinine (>10 mg/dl), and K^+. Hemodialysis, PD, or continuous hemofiltration may be used.
Pharmacotherapy: The following are considered before administration of medication: method of excretion, effect on BUN level, and fluid/electrolyte status. Certain drugs must be avoided or administered in ↓ dosage or frequency. If patient being dialyzed, timing of drug administration should be considered to maintain therapeutic serum levels. Consult pharmacist.

PATIENT-FAMILY TEACHING
• Current level of renal function and prognosis for recovery
• Diet modifications
• Purpose, expected results, anticipated sensations of nursing/medical interventions
• Medications: drug name, purpose, dosage, schedule, precautions, drug-drug and food-drug interactions, potential side effects
• Importance/means of avoiding infections
• How to identify changes in renal function: monitoring weight, BP, I&O qd

Nursing Diagnoses/Interventions

Risk for fluid volume deficit r/t compromised renal regulatory mechanisms or diuretic therapy
Desired outcome: Patient maintains normovolemia: HR 60-100 bpm, RR 12-20 breaths/min, BP wnl for patient without postural changes, MAP 70-105 mm Hg, CVP 2-6 mm Hg, PAP 20-30/8-15 mm Hg, PAWP 6-12 mm Hg, UO $\geq$0.5 ml/kg/h, and 24-h I = O + 500 ml (for insensible loss).

- Monitor I&O qh. $\downarrow$ UO may signal hypovolemia. An adequate intake but $\downarrow$ UO may signal development of oliguric ATN.
- Monitor for weight loss of 1 kg/24 h or continued loss over consecutive days.
- Assess for other potential causes of fluid volume deficit: vomiting, diarrhea, gastric suction, fistula drainage.
- Check VS qh. Monitor for $\uparrow$ HR and $\downarrow$ BP. Note postural changes in VS: $\downarrow$ SBP >15 mm Hg, $\downarrow$ DBP >10 mm Hg, and $\uparrow$ in HR >20 bpm.
- Assess hemodynamic pressures qh. Be alert to $\downarrow$ CVP, PAP, CO.
- Administer IV fluids as prescribed. Encourage PO fluids as allowed.
- Monitor response to diuretic therapy: fluid status, VS, and electrolyte values. Compare 24-h output to intake. Adjust fluid therapy as necessary.
- Assess for signs of hypovolemia: dry oral mucous membranes, poor skin turgor.
- Monitor Hgb and Hct. Steadily $\downarrow$ levels can occur with hemodialysis or blood loss from other sources (eg, GI tract). $\uparrow$ Hct may signal dehydration.

Risk for infection r/t multiple invasive monitoring devices and immunodeficiency secondary to protein-calorie malnourishment and $\downarrow$ renal function
Note: Infection is primary cause of death associated with ATN. Gram-negative sepsis, combined with hypovolemia, $\uparrow$ concentration of toxins from organisms in renal tubule, thereby $\uparrow$ renal damage.
Desired outcomes: Patient remains infection free: normothermia; absence of growth in urine, wound, sputum, or blood cultures; clear chest x-ray; and WBCs $\leq$11,000 μl.

- Check temp q2-4h. An $\uparrow$ of 0.5°-1.0° C (1°-2° F) can be significant.
- Monitor body secretions for signs of infection: change in color of sputum from clear; cloudy, foul-smelling urine; purulent drainage from or redness around wounds or catheter sites.
- Change all IVs, central lines at regular intervals according to agency protocol.
- Maintain aseptic technique when performing all procedures. Limit invasive procedures.
- Encourage nutritional intake that provides adequate essential amino acids and caloric intake.
- Monitor for signs of pneumonia: changes in breath sounds, productive cough, change in chest x-ray.
- Monitor WBC levels for $\uparrow$.

Decreased cardiac output r/t disruption of cardiac electrical conductivity secondary to hyperkalemia
Desired outcome: Within 24 h after treatment initiation, patient attains adequate CO: HR 60-100 bpm, BP wnl for patient, PAP 20-3-/8-15 mm Hg, CO 4-7 L/min, NSR on ECG (or no ectopy or other conduction defect).

- Monitor K$^+$ levels. K$^+$ may be $\uparrow$ with burn or multisystem injury.
- Monitor for S&S of hyperkalemia: irritability, anxiety, abdominal cramping, diarrhea, weakness, paresthesias.
- Monitor ECG for hyperkalemic changes: tall peaked T waves, loss of P waves, widening of QRS complexes.
- Administer bicarbonate, D$_5$W, Kayexalate as prescribed. If giving Kayexalate enema, mix to thick suspension; avoid paste, which $\downarrow$ exchange surface, thereby limiting effectiveness. Ensure 30-60 min retention.
- Administer calcium gluconate as prescribed to counteract effects of K$^+$ on the heart. Use limited to emergencies, since hypercalcemia can precipitate cardiac arrest.

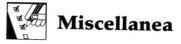 **Miscellanea**

CONSULT MD FOR
- Hyperkalemic ECG changes: loss of P waves, widening QRS complexes
- Marked $\uparrow$ in K$^+$ level (>5.5 mEq/L)
- UO <0.5 ml/kg/h for 2 consecutive h
- Hypovolemia: $\downarrow$ BP, $\downarrow$ CO, $\downarrow$ PAWP

RELATED TOPICS
- Acute tubular necrosis: oliguric
- Hemodialysis
- Hyperkalemia
- Hyperphosphatemia
- Hypocalcemia
- Metabolic acidosis, acute

ABBREVIATIONS
GFR: Glomerular filtration rate
PD: Peritoneal dialysis
RBF: Renal blood flow

REFERENCES

Blakely P, McDonald BR: Acute renal failure due to acetaminophen ingestion: a case report and review of the literature, *J Am Soc Nephrol* 6(1): 48-53, 1995.

Chew SL et al: Outcome in acute renal failure, *Nephrol Dial Transplant* 8: 101-107, 1993.

Douglas S: Acute tubular necrosis: diagnosis, treatment, and nursing implications, *AACN Clin Issues in Crit Care Nurs* 3(3): 688-687, 1992.

King BA: Detecting acute renal failure, *RN* 57(3): 35-39, 1994.

Mandal AK, Visweswaran RK, Kaldas NR: Treatment considerations in acute renal failure, *Drugs* 44(4): 565-577, 1992.

Stark JL: Acute renal failure in trauma: current perspectives, *Crit Care Nurs Q* 16(4): 49-60, 1994.

Stark JL: Acute tubular necrosis: difference between oliguria and nonoliguria, *Crit Care Nurs Q* 14(4): 22-27, 1992.

Author: **Marguerite J. Murphy**

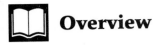 **Overview**

PATHOPHYSIOLOGY

Most common cause of ARF. Initially an ischemic event damages the tubular epithelium, followed by damage to the basement membrane if ischemia is prolonged. This results in urine leakage into renal interstitium, tubule obstruction as a result of swelling and accumulation of cellular debris, and ↓ GFR. Oliguria (UO <400 ml/24 h) occurs with high urine Na^+. Tubular function usually returns within 10-14 days, heralded by diuresis. However, the kidneys' ability to excrete electrolytes and urea remains impaired, with ↑ serum K^+, PO_4^{3-}, creatinine, and BUN. Diuresis lasts a few days to 6 wks, followed by gradual return to nl function.

MORTALITY

50%-70% among critically ill patients

HISTORY/RISK FACTORS

- Renal ischemia: caused by cardiogenic shock, hemorrhage, intraoperative hypotension, multiple trauma, hypovolemia, burns
- Exposure to nephrotoxic agents: eg, aminoglycoside antibiotics, NSAIDs, diuretics, radiologic contrast
- Advanced age
- Preexisting renal disease
- Heart failure, DM

CLINICAL PRESENTATION

Oliguric Phase: UO <400 ml/24 h, edema, pulmonary congestion, hyperkalemia, uremic syndrome (nausea, vomiting, anorexia, seizures)
Diuretic Phase: UO >400 ml/24 h (may be up to 4-5 L/24 h), postural hypotension, altered mental status

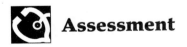 **Assessment**

PHYSICAL ASSESSMENT
OLIGURIC PHASE

Neuro: Personality changes, seizures, coma
Resp: Tachypnea, dyspnea, Kussmaul's respirations, orthopnea, crackles
CV: Tachycardia, hypertension, JVD, S_3 gallop, dysrhythmias
GI: Nausea, vomiting, anorexia
MS: Weakness, paresthesias, flaccidity (caused by hyperkalemia)
Integ: Edema, pruritus, pallor, delayed wound healing, uremic frost
DIURETIC PHASE

Neuro: Dizziness, personality changes, seizures, coma
Resp: Tachypnea
CV: Tachycardia, postural hypotension, dysrhythmias
Integ: Poor skin turgor, flushed skin, dry oral mucous membrane

VITAL SIGNS/HEMODYNAMICS
OLIGURIC PHASE

RR: ↑
HR: ↑
BP: ↑
CVP/PAWP: ↑
CO: NI or ↓ if fluid overload leads to heart failure
ECG: Sinus tachycardia; *with hyperkalemia:* tall peaked T waves, loss of P waves, prolonged PR interval, progressive widening of QRS

DIURETIC PHASE

RR: ↑
HR: ↑
BP: NI or ↓, postural changes
Temp: ↑ possible
CVP/PAWP: ↓ possible
ECG: Sinus tachycardia; *with hyperkalemia:* tall peaked T waves, loss of P waves, prolonged PR interval, progressive widening of QRS

LABORATORY STUDIES

Urinalysis (performed before diuretic therapy): May reveal Na^+ >40 mEq/L; fraction excretion of Na^+ >3%; ↓ specific gravity and osmolality; ↑ protein; presence of brown granular casts, crystals, epithelial cells; ↓ creatinine clearance to 1 ml/min.
Chemistries: May show ↑ BUN, creatinine; BUN/creatinine ratio ≥10:1; ↑ K^+, PO_4^{3-}, osmolarity; ↓ Ca^{2+}.
Hct/Hgb: Usually ↓; Hct may ↑ during diuresis because of hemoconcentration.
ABGs: Metabolic acidosis possible.

IMAGING

KUB, Renal Ultrasonogram: To evaluate cause of ATN.

DIAGNOSTIC PROCEDURE

Percutaneous Renal Biopsy: To evaluate cause of ↓ renal function. Postprocedure hematuria should clear over 24 h. Minimize activities that ↑ abdominal pressure (eg, coughing). Monitor for hemorrhage, bowel or liver puncture.

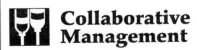 **Collaborative Management**

Early recognition and treatment of underlying cause essential to minimize tubular injury.

Supplemental O_2: May be necessary because of Kussmaul's respirations secondary to metabolic acidosis and pulmonary congestion.

Fluid Management

IV hydration: Improves RBF before extensive damage occurs. Crystalloid or colloid fluids administered with careful monitoring of PAP and CO, especially with CV disease. Typical fluid challenge: 1 L NS, D_5W, or LR infused over 2 h. UO should be >30 ml in first h after fluid administration.
Volume expanders, diuretics: Diuretics, eg, mannitol, furosemide, ethacrynic acid, controversial but frequently prescribed. These agents ↓ tubular obstruction by facilitating clearance of cellular debris and ↑ RBF, GFR. Low-dose dopamine (1-3 μg/kg/min) may be used to promote RBF and ↑ effects of furosemide. Prostaglandins may be used to promote renal vasodilatation (controversial).
Fluid intake restriction: Usually to 500-1000 ml/24 h or calculated by adding 500 ml (for insensible loss) to UO (for previous 24 h) to determine allowed 24-h fluid intake.

Treatment of Electrolyte/Acid-Base Imbalances

Hyperkalemia: $NaHCO_3$ or rapid infusion of D_5W and regular insulin to provide rapid-acting, short-term ↓ in K^+ level. Oral or rectal sodium polystyrene sulfonate (Kayexalate) is slower, but longer acting. Calcium gluconate blocks effects of K^+ on myocardium and may be used when hyperkalemic ECG changes present.
Hyperphosphatemia/hypocalcemia: Phosphate binders (eg, calcium carbonate [Tums]) enable absorption of calcium.
Hyponatremia: May occur with rapid diuresis. Hypertonic (3%-5%) NaCl used to correct it.
Acidosis: $NaHCO_3$ given if HCO_3^- <12-15 mEq/L.
Nutrition: High-calorie (2000-3000 cal/day), low-protein (40-60 g/day or 0.6 g/kg/day), low-potassium (2 g or less), and low-sodium (2 g or less) diet. TPN may be used.
Dialysis: Indicated for fluid volume excess, BUN >100 mg/dl, serum creatinine >10 mg/dl, hyperkalemia. Hemodialysis, PD, or continuous hemofiltration may be used.
Pharmacotherapy: Many drugs avoided or administered in ↓ dosage or frequency. During dialysis, timing of drug administration critical to maintain therapeutic serum levels. Consult pharmacist.

PATIENT-FAMILY TEACHING

- Current level of renal function and prognosis for recovery
- Diet modifications, fluid restrictions
- Importance/means of avoiding infections
- How to identify changes in renal function: monitoring weight, BP, I&O qd

Nursing Diagnoses/Interventions

Fluid volume excess r/t compromised renal regulatory mechanisms during oliguric phase secondary to renal tubular injury

Desired outcome: Within 24 h after treatment initiation, patient becomes normovolemic: HR 60-100 bpm, BP wnl for patient, MAP 70-105 mm Hg, CVP 2-6 mm Hg, PAP 20-30/8-15 mm Hg, PAWP 6-12 mm Hg, clear breath sounds, UO $\geq$0.5 ml/kg/h, and no peripheral edema.

- Monitor I&O qh. Subtle changes occur early and may be missed unless careful comparisons made continually.
- Monitor for weight gain of 0.5-1.5 kg/24 h.
- Administer diuretics and monitor response. Peak diuresis following furosemide administration occurs within 2 h. Mannitol should be administered rapidly to promote rapid $\uparrow$ in UO. If immediate diuresis does not occur, continued use of diuretics should be evaluated to prevent systemic complications or further renal damage.
- Maintain fluid restrictions.
- Monitor for pulmonary congestion: crackles, S_3 gallop, frothy sputum, $\downarrow$ SpO_2.
- Monitor VS and hemodynamic pressures qh. Be alert to $\uparrow$ HR, RR, BP, MAP, SVR, CVP, PAP, PAWP; and $\downarrow$ CO.

Decreased cardiac output r/t disruption of cardiac electrical conductivity secondary to hyperkalemia

Desired outcome: Within 24 h after treatment initiation, patient attains adequate cardiac output: HR 60-100 bpm, BP wnl for patient, PAP 20-30/8-15 mm Hg, CO 4-7 L/min, NSR on ECG (or no ectopy or other conduction defect).

- Monitor K^+ levels. K^+ may be $\uparrow$, especially with burn or multisystem injury.
- Monitor for S&S of hyperkalemia: irritability, anxiety, abdominal cramping, diarrhea, weakness, paresthesias.
- Monitor ECG for hyperkalemic changes: tall peaked T waves, loss of P waves, widening of QRS complexes.
- Administer bicarbonate, D_5W, Kayexalate as prescribed. If giving Kayexalate enema, mix to thick suspension; avoid paste, which $\downarrow$ exchange surface, thereby limiting effectiveness. Ensure 30-60 min retention.
- Administer calcium gluconate as prescribed to counteract effects of K^+ on the heart. Use limited to emergencies, since hypercalcemia can precipitate cardiac arrest.

Risk for infection r/t multiple invasive monitoring devices and immunodeficiency secondary to protein-calorie malnourishment and $\downarrow$ renal function

Note: Infection primary cause of death associated with ATN. Gram-negative sepsis, combined with hypovolemia, $\uparrow$ concentration of toxins from organisms in renal tubule, thereby $\uparrow$ renal damage.

Desired outcome: Patient remains infection free: normothermia; absence of growth in urine, wound, sputum, or blood cultures; clear chest x-ray; and WBCs $\leq$11,000 μl.

- Check temp q2-4h. An $\uparrow$ of 0.5°-1.0° C (1°-2° F) can be significant.
- Monitor body secretions for signs of infection: change in color of sputum from clear; cloudy, foul-smelling urine; purulent drainage from or redness around wounds or catheter sites.
- Change all IVs, central lines according to agency protocol.
- Maintain aseptic technique when performing all procedures. Limit invasive procedures.
- Encourage nutritional intake that provides adequate essential amino acids and caloric intake.
- Monitor for signs of pneumonia: changes in breath sounds, productive cough, change in chest x-ray.
- Monitor WBC levels for $\uparrow$.

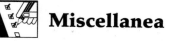 **Miscellanea**

CONSULT MD FOR

- Hyperkalemic ECG changes: tall peaked T waves, loss of P waves, widening of QRS
- UO $<$0.5 ml/kg/h for 2 consecutive h
- Patient receiving routine dose/frequency of medications excreted or metabolized by kidney
- $\uparrow$ pulmonary congestion: crackles, S_3 gallop, frothy sputum, SpO_2 $<$90%
- $\downarrow$ mentation
- $\downarrow$ CO
- Ineffective diuretic therapy

RELATED TOPICS

- Acute tubular necrosis: nonoliguric
- Continuous arteriovenous hemofiltration/ Continuous venovenous hemofiltration
- Hemodialysis
- Hyperkalemia
- Hyperphosphatemia
- Hypocalcemia
- Metabolic acidosis, acute
- Peritoneal dialysis

ABBREVIATIONS
GFR: Glomerular filtration rate
PD: Peritoneal dialysis
RBF: Renal blood flow

REFERENCES
Chew SL et al: Outcome in acute renal failure, *Nephrol Dial Transplant* 8: 101-107, 1993.
Douglas S: Acute tubular necrosis: diagnosis, treatment, and nursing implications, *AACN Clin Issues in Crit Care Nurs* 3(3): 688-687, 1992.
King BA: Detecting acute renal failure, *RN* 57(3): 35-39, 1994.
Mandal AK, Visweswaran RK, Kaldas NR: Treatment considerations in acute renal failure, *Drugs* 44(4): 565-577, 1992.
Stark JL: Acute renal failure in trauma: current perspectives, *Crit Care Nurs Q* 16(4): 49-60, 1994.
Stark JL: Acute tubular necrosis: difference between oliguria and nonoliguria, *Crit Care Nurs Q* 14(4): 22-27, 1992.

Author: **Marguerite J. Murphy**

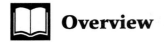 **Overview**

PATHOPHYSIOLOGY
Severe sudden depletion of adrenocortical hormones. ↓ mineralocorticoids (aldosterone) cause large urinary losses of Na^+ and water. Hyperkalemia and metabolic acidosis can develop because of ↓ urinary excretion of K^+ and H^+. Glucocorticoid (cortisol) deficiency intensifies hypovolemia as a result of ↓ vascular response to catecholamines (epinephrine, norepinephrine). Cortisol depletion also may cause hypoglycemia.

COMPLICATIONS
Severe hypotension, shock, and death without adequate parenteral adrenocortical hormone and fluid replacement.

HISTORY/RISK FACTORS
Primary: Autoimmune disease, infection, bilateral adrenal hemorrhage, bilateral adrenalectomy, tumor invasion
Secondary: Exogenous steroid administration; destruction of pituitary gland by tumors, infarcts, trauma, surgery, infection

PRECIPITATING FACTORS
- Extreme emotional or physiologic stress
- Abrupt withdrawal of exogenous steroids
- Adrenalectomy or hypophysectomy
- Sepsis, HIV disease

CLINICAL PRESENTATION
Hypotension (particularly postural), tachycardia, confusion, weakness, nausea, abdominal pain, hyperthermia, weight loss

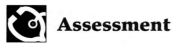 **Assessment**

PHYSICAL ASSESSMENT
Neuro: Weakness, lethargy
CV: Orthostasis, hypotension
GI: Nausea, vomiting, abdominal pain
Integ: Dehydration (eg, poor skin turgor, sunken and soft eyeballs), bronze hue to skin caused by excess ACTH

VITAL SIGNS/HEMODYNAMICS
RR: Nl
HR: ↑
BP: ↓
Temp: Possible ↑
CVP/PAWP: ↓
ECG: Hyperkalemic signs: peaked T waves, widening QRS complex, lengthened PR interval, and flattened-to-absent P wave. Severe hyperkalemia may result in asystole.

LABORATORY STUDIES
Serum Cortisol Levels: ↓
Plasma ACTH Levels: ↑ in primary adrenal failure
Serum Sodium Levels: ↓ to <137 mEq/L
Serum Aldosterone Levels: ↓ in primary Addison's disease
Serum Potassium Levels: ↑ to >5.0 mEq/L initially; may ↓ dramatically with treatment
Fasting Blood Glucose Levels: ↓ to <80 mg/dl
ACTH Stimulation Test: Minimal ↑ in plasma cortisol in response to ACTH analog

Collaborative Management

Glucocorticoid Replacement: Immediate IV bolus of hydrocortisone usually given, followed by repeat doses as needed q6-8h or by continuous infusion. Emergency mineralocorticoid replacement (fludrocortisone) usually unnecessary because of mineralocorticoid effects of hydrocortisone.
IV Fluids: Rapid volume restoration essential. Initially, D_5NS, usually 1 L in 1 h, followed by 1-2 L over next 6-8 h. Volume expanders used if hypotension persists. Saline solutions used to correct hyponatremia.
IV Glucose: Usually included in IV fluids to correct hypoglycemia.
Insertion of Flow-Directed PA Catheter: To assess volume status on a continuous basis.
Vasopressors: If no response to initial therapy. Because of ↓ response to catecholamines, vasopressors and inotropic agents less effective than they would be in nl individuals. See Appendix for table of inotropic and vasoactive agents.

Treatment of Underlying Cause/Precipitating Factor: Eg, antibiotics for infection, stabilization of physiologic status, stress reduction interventions.

PATIENT-FAMILY TEACHING
- Medications: purpose, dosage, route, precautions, drug-drug and food-drug interactions, potential side effects.

Glucocorticoids (eg, cortisone acetate, prednisone):
Take in diurnal pattern to mimic nl secretion (ie, ⅔ in AM and ⅓ in afternoon).
Take with food to ↓ gastric irritation.
Weigh regularly; report gains of >1 kg/wk to physician.
Avoid exposure to infection; be alert to S&S of infection (eg, fever, nausea, diarrhea, malaise).
S&S of overreplacement: moon face, truncal obesity, edema, striae, easy bruising, slow wound healing, chronic fatigue, emotional lability.
S&S of underreplacement: weight loss, hyperpigmentation, skin creases, anorexia, nausea, abdominal discomfort, chronic fatigue, depression, irritability.

Mineralocorticoids (eg, fludrocortisone, deoxycorticosterone acetate):
Typical dietary modification to include liberal amounts of sodium, protein, carbohydrates.
Weigh regularly; report sudden gains or losses >1 kg/wk.
S&S of overreplacement: edema, muscle weakness, hypertension.
S&S of underreplacement: excessive urination, weight loss, ↓ skin turgor.

- Importance of controlling emotional and physiologic stress, which ↑ adrenal demand. Drug dosages may need to be ↑ during times of stress.
- Procedure for obtaining Medic-Alert bracelet or card identifying diagnosis.
- Importance of contacting physician immediately for nausea or vomiting that would prevent oral intake of medications.

Nursing Diagnoses/Interventions

Fluid volume deficit r/t failure of regulatory mechanisms secondary to impaired secretion of aldosterone, causing ↑ sodium excretion with resultant diuresis

Desired outcome: Within 8 h of treatment initiation, patient becomes normovolemic: BP wnl for patient, HR 60-100 bpm, RR 12-20 breaths/min with eupnea, CVP 2-6 mm Hg, PAWP 6-12 mm Hg, NSR on ECG, and orientation × 3.

- Monitor VS and hemodynamic measurements q15min until stable. Be alert to BP <90/60 mm Hg, HR >120 bpm, CVP <2 mm Hg, and PAWP <6 mm Hg.
- Monitor for orthostatic hypotension at frequent intervals. Measure BP and HR with patient reclining, then sitting. ↓ ≥20 mm Hg or ↑ in HR >20 bpm >3 min after changing position indicates mild to moderate dehydration.
- Administer IV fluids as prescribed to replace ECF volume. Initially, rapid fluid replacement is essential.
- Maintain accurate I&O records. Weigh patient qd.
- Monitor patient continuously on cardiac monitor; observe for ECG changes typical of hyperkalemia.
- Observe for S&S of electrolyte imbalance:
    Hyperkalemia: Lethargy, nausea, hyperactive bowel sounds with diarrhea, numbness or tingling in extremities, muscle weakness.
    Hyponatremia: Headache, malaise, muscle weakness, abdominal cramps.
- Monitor laboratory results for abnormalities. With appropriate treatment, serum Na$^+$ levels should ↑ to nl and serum K$^+$ levels should ↓ to nl.
- Assess LOC and respiratory status at frequent intervals. Institute safety measures as indicated. Reorient and reassure patient as needed.
- Encourage oral fluid intake as condition stabilizes. Add sodium-rich foods as tolerated.

Risk for injury r/t potential for acute regulatory dysfunction (cortisol and aldosterone deficiency) secondary to ↑ psychologic, emotional, or physical stressors with ↑ hormonal demand and inadequate adrenal reserves

Desired outcome: Patient verbalizes orientation × 3 and has stable weight, UO <80-125 ml/h, HR 60-100 bpm, BP wnl for patient, and normothermia.

- Monitor for signs of ↑ crisis: ↑ UO, changes in LOC, orthostatic hypotension, nausea, vomiting, and tachycardia.
- Provide quiet environment to ↓ external stimuli and stress. Transfer to private room, if possible. Keep lights dim and minimize use of radios or other appliances.
- Monitor for hyperthermia. Maintain cool environmental temp. As prescribed, use tepid baths, antipyretics, and cooling blankets to ↓ body temp.
- Assist with care, and provide 90-min periods of uninterrupted rest as often as possible.
- Limit visitors and length of time spent with patient. Caution visitors not to discuss stress-provoking topics but rather to speak softly and reassuringly.
- Maintain strict environmental asepsis and monitor carefully for signs of infection. Avoid exposing patient to staff members or visitors with colds or infections.

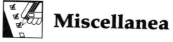

Miscellanea

CONSULT MD FOR

- Hypovolemia: BP <90/60 mm Hg, HR >120 bpm, CVP <2 mm Hg, PAWP <6 mm Hg
- Hyperkalemia: peaked T waves, widened QRS, lengthened PR, flat or absent P wave
- Worsening crisis: ↑ UO, change in LOC, orthostasis, nausea, vomiting

RELATED TOPICS

- Hemodynamic monitoring
- Hyperkalemia
- Hyponatremia
- Hypovolemia
- Shock, septic
- Transsphenoidal hypophysectomy

ABBREVIATIONS

ACTH: Adrenocorticotropic hormone
ECF: Extracellular fluid

REFERENCES

Epstein CD: Adrenocortical insufficiency in the critically ill patient, *AACN Clin Issues in Crit Care Nurs* 3(3): 705-713, 1992.

Horne MM: Endocrinologic dysfunctions. In Swearingen PL, Keen JH (eds): *Manual of critical care nursing,* ed 3, St Louis, 1995, Mosby.

Lee LM, Gumowski J: Adrenocortical insufficiency, a medical emergency, *AACN Clin Issues in Crit Care Nurs* 3(2): 319-330, 1992.

Peterson A, Drass J: How to keep adrenal insufficiency in check, *Am J Nurs* 93(10): 36-39, 1993.

Author: **Mima M. Horne**

Overview

PATHOPHYSIOLOGY
Occurs when ↑ permeability of alveolar-capillary membrane leads to leaks and accumulation of protein-rich fluid in interstitial and intraalveolar spaces. Surfactant activity ↓, and alveoli collapse and resist reexpansion. Eventually the interstitium, alveoli, and terminal airways fill with fluid, blood, and protein. Gas exchange no longer occurs, resulting in edema, hemorrhage, and focal atelectasis. V/Q mismatching occurs as lung areas are perfused but not ventilated. PaO_2 falls and there is an ↑ in shunt fraction (amount of blood returning to arterial system without passing through ventilated lung) and physiologic dead space. Fatigue occurs as WOB ↑, and respiratory failure ensues.

MORTALITY RATE
High, approaching 60% despite aggressive treatment

HISTORY/RISK FACTORS
- Trauma, massive blood transfusion
- Inhalation of toxic substances, aspiration of gastric contents
- Severe pneumonia, acute pancreatitis
- Near drowning
- Air or fat embolus
- Drug overdose
- Neurologic injury
- Gram-negative sepsis; sepsis with DIC
- Hemorrhagic or other shock
- Postperfusion cardiopulmonary bypass
- O_2 toxicity

CLINICAL PRESENTATION
Early: Dyspnea, hyperventilation, cough, ↑ WOB
Later: Rapid and shallow breathing, profound respiratory distress, diaphoresis, mental obtundation

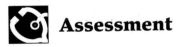 **Assessment**

PHYSICAL ASSESSMENT
Neuro: ↓ LOC, restlessness, confusion
Resp
Early: Clear breath sounds, tachypnea, dyspnea with exertion

Later: Crackles, wheezing, rhonchi, ↓ breath sounds, intercostal-suprasternal retractions, pallor, cyanosis, grunting respirations
CV: Tachycardia, dysrhythmias

VITAL SIGNS/HEMODYNAMICS
RR: ↑
HR: ↑
BP: ↓ with underlying shock, sepsis
Temp: NI; ↑ with infection
PAWP: NI in ARDS; ↑ with pulmonary edema caused by LV failure, an important factor in differential diagnosis
CO: Depends on underlying disease process
ECG: Sinus tachycardia; ventricular dysrhythmias possible because of hypoxemia

LABORATORY STUDIES
ABGs: Characterized by refractory hypoxemia (↓ PaO_2 unresponsive to ↑ FiO_2). Initially pH >7.45 because of hyperventilation. As ARDS worsens, pH falls to <7.35 because of respiratory acidosis. pH may ↓ further because of metabolic acidosis resulting from anaerobic metabolism.
Tracheal Protein/Plasma Protein Ratio: Differentiates between cardiogenic and noncardiogenic pulmonary edema (ARDS). Compares total protein in tracheal aspirate with total protein in plasma. Ratio in cardiogenic pulmonary edema <0.5, whereas ratio in ARDS generally >0.7.
Lactic Acid Level: Byproduct of anaerobic metabolism; accumulates in serum in presence of hypoxemia.

IMAGING
Serial Chest X-ray: May be nl in early stages. As ARDS progresses, lungs show bilateral diffuse infiltrates. In later stages few air spaces may be left, resulting in completely white appearance on x-ray.

DIAGNOSTIC PROCEDURES
SpO_2: For continuous monitoring of oxygenation.
SvO_2: Sensitive indicator of O_2 available for tissue oxygenation. Value <50% associated with impaired tissue oxygenation.
$P(A-a)O_2$: Alveolar-arterial oxygen tension difference. ↑ in ARDS and reflects intrapulmonary shunting.
QS/QT: Ratio of shunt to cardiac output. Measures intrapulmonary shunting. NI physiologic shunt 3%-4%; may ↑ to 15%-20% with ARDS.
Pulmonary Function Tests: Lung compliance ↓. Lung volumes also ↓, particularly FRC.

Collaborative Management

Goals: maintenance of adequate arterial oxygenation and pulmonary ventilation and treatment of underlying condition.
O_2: To provide PaO_2 levels >60 mm Hg with FiO_2 ≤0.50.
Mechanical Ventilation: Nearly always indicated because ↓ in lung compliance significantly ↑ WOB, and ↑ in physiologic dead space causes compensatory ↑ in ventilatory requirements.
PEEP: Allows for better PaO_2 with administration of lower levels of FiO_2. Also ↑ FRC by maintaining open alveoli that are otherwise collapsed.
Corticosteroids: Controversial. Short-term, high-dose may be useful in stabilizing alveolar-capillary membrane.
Fluid Therapy: Goal: to maintain minimum PAWP to provide adequate CO. Fluid volume kept slightly depleted to minimize fluid leakage through damaged capillary membrane. Use of crystalloid vs colloid fluids is controversial. Generally, colloids reserved for hypoalbuminemia and crystalloids for all other conditions.
Sedation: Extreme agitation may require sedation with benzodiazepines (eg, lorazepam [Ativan] or propofol [Diprivan]). Morphine sulfate ↓ pain, relieves anxiety, and causes mild vasodilatation. Paralysis with NMBA, such as vecuronium bromide (Norcuron), may be necessary if mechanical ventilation not tolerated despite sedation. Appropriate sedation (eg, with lorazepam) and analgesia (eg, morphine) necessary.
Nutritional Support: Energy outlay with respiratory failure is high. If patient unable to consume adequate calories with enteral feedings, TPN *via* peripheral or central access instituted.

PATIENT-FAMILY TEACHING
- Need for frequent ABG analysis
- Medications: drug name, purpose, dosage, schedule, precautions, drug-drug and food-drug interactions, potential side effects
- Purpose, expected results, anticipated sensations of medical/nursing interventions

Nursing Diagnoses/Interventions

Impaired gas exchange r/t alveolar-capillary membrane changes secondary to ↑ permeability with alveolar injury and collapse

Desired outcome: Within 12-24 h of initiation of therapy, patient has adequate gas exchange: PaO_2 >60 mm Hg, $PaCO_2$ <45 mm Hg, and pH 7.35-7.45. Within 4-6 days of initiation of therapy, RR 12-20 breaths/min with eupnea and there are no adventitious breath sounds.

- Assess respiratory rate, depth, rhythm, and use of accessory muscles and for respiratory distress: restlessness, anxiety, confusion, tachypnea.
- Assess breath sounds with each VS check to ascertain their presence and character. Adventitious sounds, usually present in later stages of ARDS, are not as likely to occur during early stage.
- Monitor serial ABGs; compare ABG saturation with pulse oximetry saturation for accuracy.
- Administer O_2; monitor FiO_2 to ensure patient is receiving prescribed concentrations.
- Monitor pulmonary function tests, especially tidal volume and minute ventilation. Expect ↓ tidal volume and ↑ minute ventilation with respiratory distress.
- Position to promote adequate gas exchange. Usually semi- to high-Fowler's position is optimal.
- Keep oral airway, manual ventilating bag, and emergency intubation equipment at bedside for use should condition deteriorate.

Activity intolerance r/t imbalance between O_2 supply and demand secondary to ↓ alveolar O_2 supply and ↑ metabolic O_2 demands as a result of ↓ WOB

Desired outcome: Within 24-48 h of treatment initiation, patient verbalizes ↓ in fatigue and associated symptoms.

- Group procedures and activities to provide frequent rest periods (optimally, at least 90-120 min).
- ↓ metabolic demands for O_2 by limiting or pacing activities and procedures.
- If patient is restless, which causes ↑ O_2 demand, determine cause of restlessness, eg, hypoxemia or anxiety.
- Schedule rest times after meals to avoid competition for O_2 supply during digestion.
- Monitor SpO_2 during activity to evaluate limits of activity; recommend optimal positions for oxygenation.
- Assess temp q2-4h. Provide treatment as indicated to ↓ temp and thus O_2 demands.

Risk for infection r/t ↑ environmental exposure, tissue destruction (during intubation or suctioning), and invasive procedures

Desired outcome: Patient infection free: normothermia, WBCs <11,000 μl, clear sputum, negative sputum culture.

- Assess for infection: temp >38° C (100.4° F), tachycardia, change in character of sputum.
- To minimize risk of cross-contamination, wash hands before/after contact with respiratory secretions of any patient and before/after contact with patient undergoing intubation.
- Recognize that bacteria and spores are introduced easily during suctioning. Follow standard techniques:
    Use sterile technique.
    Suction tracheobronchial tree before oropharynx.
    Consider use of closed system for suctioning.
    Change suction cannisters and tubing q24h or according to agency policy.
    Use single-use saline for suctioning. If not available, tightly recap bottle; dispose of unused portion within established time frame.
- Suction as needed rather than routinely.
- Provide oral hygiene at least q4-8h to prevent overgrowth of nl flora and aerobic gram-negative bacilli.

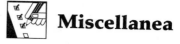 # Miscellanea

CONSULT MD FOR
- Refractory hypoxemia: inability to maintain PaO_2 >60 mm Hg with FiO_2 ≤.05
- SpO_2 <90%
- New-onset temp >38.33° C (101° F)
- Change in character of sputum (eg, clear, thin→yellow, thick)
- New-onset crackles, wheezes, rhonchi, especially associated with ↓ PaO_2

RELATED TOPICS
- Agitation syndrome
- Anxiety
- Mechanical ventilation
- Multiple organ dysfunction syndrome
- Multisystem injury
- Paralytic therapy
- Pneumonia, hospital-associated
- Shock, septic

ABBREVIATIONS
FRC: Functional residual capacity
NMBA: Neuromuscular blocking agent
P(A-a)O_2: Alveolar-arterial oxygen tension difference
Svo$_2$: Mixed venous oxygen saturation

REFERENCES
Atkins P: Respiratory consequences of multi-system crisis: the adult respiratory distress syndrome, *Crit Care Nurs Q* 16(4): 27-38, 1994.

Howard C: Respiratory dysfunctions. In Swearingen PL, Keen, JH (eds): *Manual of critical care nursing,* ed 3, St Louis, 1995, Mosby.

Juarez P: Mechanical ventilation for the patient with severe ARDS, PC-IRV, *Crit Care Nurse* 12(4): 34-39, 1992.

O'Hanlon-Nichols T: Adult respiratory distress syndrome following thoracic trauma, *Crit Care Nurs Clin North Am* 5(4): 723-734, 1993.

Vollman KM: Adult respiratory distress syndrome: mediators on the run, *Crit Care Nurs Clin North Am* 6(2): 341-358, 1994.

Author: **Cheri A. Goll**

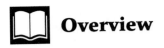 **Overview**

PATHOPHYSIOLOGY

Extreme anxiety, outwardly expressed as agitation, restlessness, and ↑ random motor movement. May be prompted by emotional, pathophysiologic, or environmental factors. Persistent agitation contributes to unrelieved stress, which can retard healing and ↑ mortality.

This section focuses on use of sedatives when nonpharmacologic interventions are ineffective in relieving agitation. A variety of factors—major organ dysfunction, use of multiple medications, tissue catabolism— render the critically ill vulnerable to toxic effects of many sedatives. Sedatives are withdrawn periodically (usually qd) to enable evaluation of underlying mental status.

HISTORY/RISK FACTORS

- Neurologic, sensory/perceptual impairment
- Prolonged critical illness
- Psychiatric disorder
- Alcohol, opioid, drug addiction
- Sleep deprivation
- Altered glucose metabolism
- Electrolyte imbalance
- ↓ cerebral perfusion pressure
- Infective process, especially of neurologic system
- Hepatic/renal impairment
- Multiple medications

CLINICAL PRESENTATION

Subjective: Fear, uncertainty, helplessness, distorted perceptual and cognitive function
Objective: Restlessness, ↑ motor movement, poor eye contact

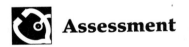 **Assessment**

PHYSICAL ASSESSMENT

Neuro: Shaking, tremors, ↑ muscle tension, pupil dilatation
Resp: Tachypnea, hyperventilation
CV: Superficial vasoconstriction, tachycardia
Other: ↑ perspiration, guarding

VITAL SIGNS/HEMODYNAMICS

RR: ↑
HR: ↑
BP: slightly ↑
Temp: NI

ICP: May ↑ if impaired cerebral perfusion a contributing factor
Other: PAP/CO depend on underlying condition
ECG: Sinus tachycardia; ↑ endogenous catecholamines may contribute to ectopy in susceptible individuals

LABORATORY STUDIES

ABGs: R/o hypoxemia as cause; may show respiratory alkalosis caused by tachypnea
Chemistries: Detect electrolyte, glucose abnormalities that contribute to agitation and monitor for ↑ BUN/creatinine or ↑ liver enzymes, reflecting metabolic toxicity
Alcohol, Toxicology Screen: Checks for intoxicants
C&S: Of suspected material (eg, blood, CSF) to check for infective process

IMAGING

Chest X-ray: Detects pneumonia, other conditions that can interfere with oxygenation
Head CT Scan: To r/o cerebral thrombosis, other intracranial processes

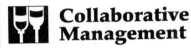 **Collaborative Management**

After organic causes addressed, a variety of therapeutic options are available to produce sedation. Alleviation of pain essential.
Opiate Analgesics: IV morphine widely used in intermittent bolus doses and as a continuous infusion. Other common opiates include meperidine (Demerol) and fentanyl citrate (Sublimaze).
Benzodiazepines: Relieve anxiety, promote sleep, and produce sedation by specific depressant effect on γ-aminobutyric acid (GABA). Also produce muscle relaxation and promote amnesia. Safety, ease of use, lack of paradoxical agitation, lack of recall, and reversibility with flumazenil (Romazicon) are favorable characteristics of benzodiazepines.
Lorazepam (Ativan): Has no active drug metabolites; less likely to accumulate in elders or in patients with hepatic failure. Frequently used for DT prophylaxis.
Diazepam (Valium): Inexpensive. Has long half-life, which causes prolonged sedation and may ↑ length of stay in ICU. An active metabolite may result in sedative effects for up to 200 h after a given dose. Avoided with liver dysfunction or severe heart failure.
Midazolam (Versed): Short-acting and rapidly metabolized, thus useful for short

procedures, eg, bronchoscopies and endoscopies. Strong amnesic effects. Continuous infusions required to maintain sedation for prolonged use; may lead to extended sedation and difficulty with extubation, particularly with sepsis or hepatic impairment.
Chlordiazepoxide (Librium): Sometimes used to manage agitation associated with alcohol withdrawal. However, because it has several long-lived active metabolites, it is a poor choice for sedation and DT prophylaxis when compared to newer benzodiazepines. Lorazepam generally preferred.
Anesthetic Agents: Forms of anesthesia increasingly employed in ICU. Many anesthetics restricted to use by or with direct supervision of an anesthesiologist.
Propofol: Lipid suspension; administered as titrated, continuous infusion to provide desired level of sedation to intubated, mechanically ventilated patients. Extubation time predictable because recovery time generally <10 min. Recovery time after prolonged infusion not ↑, which contrasts with some benzodiazepines. Hemodynamic changes (eg, vasodilatation, ↓ MAP) minimized by adequate hydration and gradual changes in infusion rate.
Neuroleptics: Used to ↓ agitation in disoriented and agitated patients. Keep well hydrated to avoid hypotension associated with parenteral use of these drugs.
Haloperidol lactate (Haldol): Especially helpful in DT, acute confusional states, and during withdrawal of sedatives. IV route considered investigational but widely used in the critically ill because onset of action rapid and extrapyramidal side effects occur less frequently than with IM route.
Chlorpromazine (Thorazine): Sometimes used as a sedative, particularly for psychosis. Produces α-receptor blockade; hypotension likely.

PATIENT-FAMILY TEACHING

- Recall of unpleasant procedures (eg, cardioversion, endoscopy) ↓; this is a desired effect of the benzodiazepines.
- Reinforce necessary information, such as NPO instructions, need to call for assistance when changing positions, and need for deep breathing at frequent intervals until comprehension demonstrated.
- Review outcome or findings of procedure as necessary until patient expresses satisfactory understanding.

Nursing Diagnoses/Interventions

Anxiety r/t actual or perceived threat of death, change in health status, unfamiliar people or environment, the unknown, or to self-concept or role

Desired outcome: Within 4-6 h of initiating therapy, anxiety ↓ as evidenced by verbalization of same, HR ≤100 bpm, RR ≤20 breaths/min, and ↓ restlessness and extraneous motor movement.

- Carefully assess for and correct pathophysiologic factors contributing to anxiety.
- Evaluate adequacy of pain control. Administer opiate or other analgesics in small doses at frequent intervals.
- Initiate nonpharmacologic measures to ↓ anxiety.

  Massage: To relax muscular tension and ↑ local circulation. Back and foot massage particularly relaxing.

  ROM exercises: To relax muscles, improve circulation, and prevent pain r/t stiffness and immobility.

  Progressive relaxation: To ↓ muscle tension.

  Controlled breathing: To relieve hyperventilation.

  Promoting self-control: Feelings of helplessness and lack of control contribute to anxiety. Techniques such as PCA and promoting self-helping behaviors contribute to feelings of self-control.

  Preparatory information: Eg, preop teaching.

  Distraction: Encourage focusing on something unrelated to pain or source of anxiety. Examples include conversing, reading, watching TV or videos, listening to music.

  Humor: Can be excellent distraction and may help patient cope with stress.

- Administer short-acting benzodiazepine in small doses at frequent intervals. Monitor for excessive sedation and respiratory depression. Have flumazenil (Romazicon) immediately available for reversal of drug effects.
- If anxiety profound and associated with sensory/perceptual alterations (eg, hallucinations), consider use of antipsychotic agent. Ensure adequate hydration before use; monitor closely for hypotension.

Impaired gas exchange (or risk for same) r/t ↓ O_2 supply secondary to ↓ ventilatory drive occurring with sedative use and CNS depression

Desired outcome: Within 1 h of intervention, patient has adequate gas exchange: orientation × 3; Pao_2 ≥80 mm Hg; $Paco_2$ 35-45 mm Hg; Spo_2 ≥90; RR 12-20 breaths/min with eupnea.

- Assess respiratory rate, depth, and rhythm at least qh when patient heavily sedated. Fully sedated patients require continuous direct monitoring until VS stable and protective reflexes (eg, gag reflexes) present.
- In heavily sedated patients, continuously monitor Spo_2 *via* pulse oximetry. Alternatively, monitor chest wall movement *via* apnea monitor. Have appropriate antidote (eg, naloxone for opiates, flumazenil for benzodiazepines) and airway management equipment immediately available.
- Position to promote full lung expansion. Encourage deep breathing at frequent intervals.

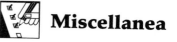 # Miscellanea

CONSULT MD FOR

- Agitation caused by hypoxemia, substance withdrawal
- Persistent or unrelieved pain
- Excessive sedation, hypoventilation

RELATED TOPICS

- Anxiety
- Delirium
- Head injury
- Mechanical ventilation
- Psychosocial needs, patient

REFERENCES

Bird R, Makela E: Alcohol withdrawal: what is the benzodiazepine of choice? *Ann Pharmacother* 28: 67-71, 1994.

Carrasco G et al: Propofol vs midazolam in short-, medium-, and long-term sedation of critically ill patients, *Chest* 103(2): 557-564, 1993.

Clark S, Fontaine D, Simpson T: Recognition, assessment, and treatment of anxiety in the critical care setting, *Crit Care Nurse* (Suppl): 2-14, Aug 1994.

Inaba-Roland K, Maricle R: Assessing delirium in the acute care setting, *Heart Lung* 21(2): 48-55, 1992.

Snider BS: Use of muscle relaxants in the ICU: nursing implications, *Crit Care Nurse* 13(6): 55-60, 1993.

Author: **Janet Hicks Keen**

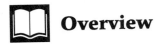 **Overview**

PATHOPHYSIOLOGY
Commonly ingested intoxicant, often coingested with other drugs. Complications include altered mental status, dehydration, vomiting with aspiration, hypoglycemia, and ↑ risk of injury. Chronic alcohol ingestion may result in severe withdrawal symptoms: CV instability, hallucinations, seizures.

HISTORY/RISK FACTORS
Coingestion with other agents ↑ likelihood of toxicity.

CLINICAL PRESENTATION
Depends on individual's alcohol tolerance, but may include odor of alcohol on breath; confusion, aggressive behavior, irritability, which may progress to stupor, coma.

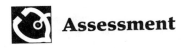 **Assessment**

PHYSICAL ASSESSMENT
Neuro: Memory loss, stupor, loss of DTRs, coma, seizures r/t hypoglycemia; *with withdrawal:* tremens, hallucinations (especially auditory)
Resp: Hypoventilation, respiratory failure; rhonchi and wheezing if aspiration has occurred
CV: Tachycardia, A-fib, cardiac arrest (if intoxication severe)
Renal: Significant UO initially; later, dehydration results in oliguria
Assoc Findings: Dry oral mucosa, hypoglycemia, hypothermia, lactic acidosis, hypokalemia

VITAL SIGNS/HEMODYNAMICS
RR: ↓ in severe intoxication
HR: ↑
BP: ↓
Temp: ↓

CVP/PAWP: ↓ as a result of dehydration
CO: ↓
ECG: Ventricular or bradycardic dysrhythmias

LABORATORY STUDIES
Blood Alcohol: Legal intoxication is 250 mg/dl. Nontolerant individuals can show symptoms at 150 mg/dl, coma at 250 mg/dl, and death at 450 mg/dl.
Toxicology Screen: Checks for presence of other drugs.
Chemistries: Serum glucose often ↓; may be dangerously low. Electrolyte disturbances include ↓ K^+, Na^+, Mg^{2+}. BUN/creatinine levels checked for impaired renal function. ↑ bilirubin and liver enzymes suggest liver damage resulting from chronic (eg, cirrhosis) or acute (eg, alcoholic hepatitis) liver failure.
CBC: To establish baseline; later to check for ↑ WBCs attributable to pneumonia, other infection.
ABGs: To monitor respiratory status.

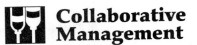 **Collaborative Management**

Support of Resp Systems: O_2 supplementation.
Fluid Replacement: Mild to severe hypovolemia usually present. Replacement fluids depend on type of fluid lost and severity of deficit, serum electrolytes, and acid-base status.
Treatment of Hypokalemia: IV potassium, 40-80 mEq/L, according to serum electrolytes/patient's condition.
Alcohol Removal: Usually alcohol removed *via* endogenous metabolic processes. In life-threatening intoxication, liver and kidneys may not be able to break down and excrete the alcohol, and thus hemodialysis can be of substantial benefit.
Prevention of Emesis: Antiemetics given for nausea and vomiting; gastric tube inserted and maintained at low continuous suction.
Treatment of Hypoglycemia: D_{50} bolus; then continuous infusion of D_5W, based on serum

glucose results. Thiamine deficiency common with chronic alcohol ingestion. IV thiamine given before D_{50} to avoid sudden precipitation of heart failure and worsening neurologic impairment.
Anticipation/Treatment of Withdrawal: Usually with short-acting benzodiazepines such as lorazepam (Ativan). Amount of medication corresponds to usual 24-h alcohol intake: eg, 60 ml (2 oz) 80% liquor = 10 mg diazepam (Valium), 25 mg chlordiazepoxide (Librium), and 2 mg lorazepam. Patients drinking 1 qt vodka a day may need as much as 400 mg chlordiazepoxide or 160 mg diazepam. Cautious use of benzodiazepines with long half-lives (diazepam, flurazepam, clonazepam) with chronic alcohol consumption is important because of ↓ metabolism caused by cirrhosis.
Treatment of DTs: Most severe progression of withdrawal; can result in death. S&S usually develop 72-96 h after cessation of drinking and can include disorientation, psychosis, agitation, severe diaphoresis, tachycardia, CV collapse, and fever. Sedation with benzodiazepines enables rest and sleep.
Treatment/Prevention of Seizures: Because alcohol-withdrawal seizures may occur during first 6-48 h after abstinence, benzodiazepines given to raise seizure threshold during withdrawal period. IV diazepam is the drug of choice to achieve control over active seizure(s).
Vitamin/Mineral Supplements: Thiamine given to prevent Wernicke-Korsakoff syndrome; multivitamins and multiminerals given because of potential for malnutrition r/t inadequate food intake and malabsorption caused by alcohol's irritating effect on GI tract. C, B-complex, zinc, and magnesium especially important to replace.

PATIENT-FAMILY TEACHING
- Purpose, expected results, anticipated sensations of all nursing/medical interventions
- Alcoholics Anonymous (consult local phone book)

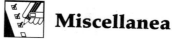

Nursing Diagnoses/Interventions

Ineffective airway clearance r/t presence of tracheobronchial secretions; obstruction; ↓ sensorium

Desired outcome: Within 2-24 h of intervention/treatment, patient has clear airway: clear breath sounds over upper airways and lung fields, RR 12-20 breaths/min with eupnea, Pao_2 ≥80 mm Hg, $Paco_2$ 35-45 mm Hg, pH 7.35-7.45, and Spo_2 ≥92%.

- Assess respiratory function frequently. Be alert to respiratory distress, restlessness and confusion, and cyanosis.
- Suction oropharynx or *via* ET tube prn.
- Monitor ABG values for hypoxia (Pao_2 <80 mm Hg) and respiratory acidosis ($Paco_2$ >45 mm Hg, pH <7.35).
- Monitor respiratory patterns; provide continuous apnea monitoring if available.
- Monitor O_2 saturation continuously. Be alert to values <92%, depending on baseline and clinical presentation.
- Administer and evaluate effects of antiemetics.
- Place patient in side-lying position during vomiting to ↓ aspiration risk.

Risk for fluid volume deficit r/t excessive losses secondary to vomiting, diaphoresis, and diuretic effects of ETOH

Desired outcome: Normovolemia maintained/restored: UO ≥0.5 ml/kg/h, moist mucous membranes, balanced I&O, BP wnl for patient, HR ≤100 bpm, stable weight, urine specific gravity 1.010-1.020, CVP 2-6 mm Hg, and PAWP 6-12 mm Hg.

- Monitor hydration status on an ongoing basis. Be alert to continuing dehydration. Maintain adequate fluid intake to ensure positive fluid state (eg, 50-100 ml > all hourly losses).
- Assess for electrolyte imbalance, in particular hypokalemia: irregular pulse, cardiac dysrhythmias, and serum K^+ <3.5 mEq/L. Administer K^+ supplements at rate not >10-20 mEq/L.
- Monitor I&O qh; assess for output ↑ out of proportion to intake, bearing in mind insensible losses.
- Monitor laboratory values, including serum electrolytes and serum and urine osmolality. Be alert to BUN ↑ out of proportion to creatinine (indicator of dehydration), high urine specific gravity, low urine Na^+, and ↑ Hct and serum protein concentration.

Sensory/Perceptual alterations r/t chemical alterations secondary to ingestion of alcohol or alcohol withdrawal

Desired outcome: Within 48 h of intervention, patient verbalizes orientation to time, place, and person.

- Establish and maintain calm, quiet environment to minimize sensory overload. Dim lights when possible.
- At frequent intervals, assess orientation to time, place, and person. Reorient as necessary.
- Orient to the unit, and explain all procedures before performing them. Include significant others in orientation process.
- Monitor for alcohol withdrawal/DTs: disorientation with loss of touch with reality, delirium, agitation, severe diaphoresis, tachycardia, CV collapse, and fever.
- Administer short-acting benzodiazepines (eg, oxazepam, lorazepam) if S&S of alcohol withdrawal occur.
- Do not leave patient alone if he or she is agitated or confused.
- If patient hallucinating, intervene in the following ways:
    Be reassuring. Explain that hallucinations may be very real to the patient but that they are not real; they are caused by the consumed substance, and they will go away eventually.
    As appropriate, try to involve family/significant others because patient may have more trust in them.
    Tell patient you will check on him or her at frequent intervals (eg, q5-10min) or that you will stay at patient's side.

Miscellanea

CONSULT MD FOR
- Onset of DTs
- ↓ LOC
- UO <0.5 ml/kg/h × 2 h
- Complications: dysrhythmias, hypokalemia, S&S of aspiration pneumonia, ↓ LOC

RELATED TOPICS
- Agitation syndrome
- Cirrhosis
- Delirium
- Hypovolemia
- Pneumonia, aspiration

ABBREVIATION
DTR: Deep tendon reflex

REFERENCES

Berk WA, Henderson W. Alcohols. In Tintinalli JE, Ruiz E, Krome RL (eds): *Emergency medicine: a comprehensive study guide,* ed 4, New York, 1996, McGraw-Hill.

Ford M: Alcohols and glycols. In Rippe J et al (eds): *Intensive care medicine,* ed 3, Boston, 1996, Little, Brown.

Keen JH, Baird MS, Allen JH: *Mosby's critical care and emergency drug reference,* ed 2, St Louis, 1996, Mosby.

Stiesmeyer JK: Drug overdose. In Swearingen PL, Keen JH (eds): *Manual of critical care nursing,* ed 3, St Louis, 1995, Mosby.

Author: **Johanna K. Stiesmeyer**

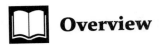 **Overview**

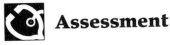 **Assessment**

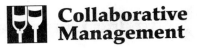 **Collaborative Management**

PATHOPHYSIOLOGY

Consciousness, the state of awareness of self and environment, consists of two components: content (cognition and affect) and arousal (appearance of wakefulness). Alterations in consciousness occur because of physiologic, psychologic, or environmental factors.

HISTORY/RISK FACTORS

- Cardiovascular disorders: result in ↓ CO or ↓ perfusion
- Pulmonary disorders: result in hypoxia, hypoxemia
- Cerebral ischemia/injury
- Advanced age
- Sensory/perceptual factors: deprivation, overload; impaired sensation, perception
- Metabolic factors: hypoglycemia, hyperglycemia, hypermetabolism, hypometabolism
- Fluid and electrolyte disturbances: Na^+ and K^+ imbalances, hypovolemia

CLINICAL PRESENTATION

Delirium: Transient clouding of consciousness progressing from confusion and global cognitive impairment to psychosis. Characterized by disorientation to time, place, person; alternating periods of hyperirritability and drowsiness. Daytime drowsiness contrasted with nighttime agitation.

Stupor: Responsiveness only to vigorous and repeated stimuli. Usually r/t diffuse organic cerebral dysfunction.

Coma: Nl responses to external stimuli or inner need not consistently elicited. Occurs when CNS function disrupted by cerebral structural changes, cerebrovascular impairment, or metabolic conditions.

Vegetative State: Chronic condition following brain injury; characterized by return of wakefulness (eyes open and sleep patterns may be observed) but without observable signs of cognitive function. Usually permanent.

Locked-In Syndrome: Characterized by paralysis of all four extremities and lower cranial nerves but with preservation of cognition/consciousness. Occurs because of disruption of pathways of brainstem motor neurons. Prevents communication by word or body movement; lateral eye movement and eye blinking communication possible.

PHYSICAL ASSESSMENT

Mini Mental Status Examination: Measures orientation, recall, attention, calculation, language. Scores <23 indicate cognitive dysfunction (see Appendix).

Glasgow Coma Scale: Assesses best eye opening, motor, verbal responses. Scores range from 3-15, with 3 being unresponsive and 15 being awake, alert, and oriented (see Appendix).

Rancho Los Amigos (RLA) Cognitive Functioning Scale: Eight-level scale describing levels of cognitive functioning from unresponsive to sensory stimuli to purposeful/appropriate actions (see Appendix).

VITAL SIGNS/HEMODYNAMICS

Nl or variable, according to underlying condition

NEURODIAGNOSTIC TESTING

CT Scan: Can diagnose cerebral hemorrhage, infarction, hydrocephalus, cerebral edema, structural shifts.

MRI: Identifies type, location, extent of injury; can follow metabolic processes and detect structural changes.

EEG: Measures spontaneous brain electrical activity *via* surface electrodes. Detects areas of abnormal brain activity (irritability) r/t drug overdose, coma, or suspected brain death. Document use of anticonvulsants if they cannot be withheld 24-48 h before EEG testing.

Evoked Responses: Evaluation of brain response to external stimulus (ie, auditory, visual, somatosensory); can determine extent of CNS damage in uncooperative, confused, or comatose patients.

NEUROPSYCHOLOGIC TESTING

Establishes baseline for rehabilitation by evaluating higher cortical function, such as memory and language.

Delirium: Correct physiologic imbalances, drug interactions, and sensory/perceptual impairment. Eliminate sensory/perceptual deficits *via* use of hearing aid, eyeglasses. Reorient to self and environment; initiate appropriate neuropsychiatric therapy.

Coma: Low-level cognitive function requires initiation of sensory stimulation program. If confused/agitated, requires structured program that minimizes stimulation. Rehabilitation consultation includes physical, occupational, speech therapy.

Locked-In Syndrome: Establish means of communication. Obtain mental health and rehabilitation consultation. Minimize sleep-wake cycle disturbances.

Vegetative State: Long-term prognosis not optimistic. Supportive care to minimize such complications as pressure ulcers and aspiration. Stimulation program for low-level cognitive function may be initiated.

PATIENT-FAMILY TEACHING

- Reorientation techniques
- Sensory stimulation strategies
- Methods of communication

Nursing Diagnoses/Interventions

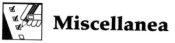

Miscellanea

Sensory/Perceptual alterations r/t physiologic changes, psychologic changes, environmental changes, sensory deprivation, sensory overload, and drug interactions

Desired outcome: Within 48 h of diagnosis, arousal and cognition levels improve and patient responds consistently and appropriately to stimuli.

- Assess for causes of sensory/perceptual deficits. Wearing eye glasses or hearing aids ↓ misinterpretation of visual and auditory stimuli.
- Assess environment for causes of disorientation and confusion. Maintain day/night environment. Keep clocks and calendars within patient's visual field.
- Assess for sensory deprivation/overload. ↓ or ↑ stimulation based on need. Agitation and confusion necessitate structure and reorientation interventions, eg, quiet, controlled environment; reorientation; gentle repetition. Comatose or stuporous patients require stimulation techniques, eg, photos of significant others; tactile, olfactory, oral stimulation.
- Orient to time, place, and person during all interactions. Explain procedures in understandable terms.
- Provide liberal visitation to facilitate significant others' assistance with reorientation, sensory stimulation.
- Assess underlying cause of confusion or delirium before using sedation, anxiolytic, analgesic, or antipsychotic drug therapy.

Impaired verbal communication r/t neurologic deficits

Desired outcome: Within 24 h of this diagnosis, patient communicates needs and feelings and exhibits ↓ frustration and fear r/t communication barriers.

- Evaluate factors impairing communication: physiologic (cortical, brainstem, cranial nerve injury) or psychologic (depression, fear, anger).
- During communication use patient's name, face patient, use eye contact if patient awake, speak clearly, and use a nl tone of voice.
- Be alert to nonverbal messages, especially eye movement, blinking, facial expressions, and head and hand movements. Attempt to validate these signals with patient.
- Reassure patient you are attempting to find methods of communication.
- Continue communication attempts, even if patient does not respond to or acknowledge verbal stimulation.
- Encourage significant others to continue attempts at communication.
- Brainstem-evoked potentials and hearing tests help evaluate ability to receive and process auditory stimuli. Treatment of otitis media in patients who have ET tubes will improve hearing.
- Obtain a speech therapy consultation to assess nature and severity of communication impairment and assist in developing a communication plan.
- Obtain a mental health consultation to assist patient who is angry, frustrated, and fearful owing to communication impairment.

Impaired physical mobility r/t perceptual or cognitive impairment or imposed restrictions of movement

Desired outcome: By time of discharge from ICU, patient demonstrates ROM and muscle strength within 10% of baseline parameters.

- Assess muscle strength and tone. Consult PT and OT for evaluation and treatment plan.
- Manage ↓ muscle tone (flaccidity).
  Maintain body alignment and positioning.
  Perform passive ROM and stretching exercises.
  Avoid prolonged periods of limb flexion.
  Apply splints and other devices to maintain functional position of the extremities.
  Turn patient q2h; consider allowing patient to sit in chair as he or she stabilizes.
- Manage ↑ muscle tone (spasticity).
  Avoid supine position; use side-lying, semiprone, prone, high-Fowler's positions.
  Position limbs opposite flexion posture.
  Use skeletal muscle relaxant, such as baclofen (Lioresal) to ↓ tone.
- Monitor calcium and alkaline phosphatase levels. ↑ levels can lead to heterogenous ossification, which is seen with states of impaired mobility.
- Assess and maintain skin integrity.
- Prevent pulmonary complications:
  Encourage coughing and deep breathing, or suction as needed.
  Assess swallowing ability before initiating oral feedings. Obtain dysphagia consultation if swallowing reflexes impaired.
  Initiate enteral feeding protocol for patients with feeding tubes to prevent aspiration.

CONSULT MD FOR

- Deterioration in LOC
- Temp ≥38.33 ° C (101° F)
- Complications such as contractures, pressure ulcer, pneumonia, hypercalcemia, hyperphosphatemia

RELATED TOPICS

- Agitation syndrome
- Head injury
- Nutritional support, enteral and parenteral
- Pneumonia, aspiration
- Pneumonia, hospital-associated
- Pressure ulcers

REFERENCES

Ackerman LL: Alteration in level of responsiveness, *Nurs Clin North Am* 28(4): 729-745, 1993.

Davis A: Alterations in consciousness. In Swearingen PL, Keen JH (eds): *Manual of critical care nursing,* ed 3, St Louis, 1995, Mosby.

Geary SM: Intensive care unit psychosis revisited: understanding and managing delirium in the critical care setting, *Crit Care Q* 17(1): 51-63, 1994.

Lipowski ZJ: Update on delirium, *Psychiatr Clin North Am* 15(2): 335-346, 1992.

Minarik PA: Cognitive assessment of the cardiovascular patient in the acute care setting, *J Cardiovasc Nurs* 9(4): 36-52, 1995.

Author: **Alice Davis**

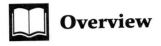 **Overview**

PATHOPHYSIOLOGY

Exaggerated or hypersensitivity response to an antigen (or allergen) in a sensitized person, usually occurring 1-20 min after exposure. Histamine released from the cells stimulates H_1 receptors causing vasodilatation, ↑ capillary permeability, bronchiole and other smooth muscle dilatation, and copious mucus production. Systemic effects occur, including respiratory distress and obstruction, fluid loss from vascular spaces, distributive shock, and end-organ dysfunction.

HISTORY/RISK FACTORS

- Recent exposure to antigenic agent: eg, antibiotic, anesthetic, iodized contrast medium, latex
- Blood transfusion
- Insect bites/stings

CLINICAL PRESENTATION

Early (immediate): Uneasiness, lightheadedness, pruritus, flushing

Late (usually within min): Rapid progression from lightheadedness to syncope; urticaria; respiratory distress; abdominal cramps, diarrhea, vomiting; angioedema (tissue swelling), especially of eyes, lips, tongue, hands, feet, genitalia

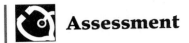 **Assessment**

PHYSICAL ASSESSMENT

Neuro: ↓ LOC, coma

Resp: Dyspnea, stridor, coughing productive for clear or "whitish" mucus, wheezes, crackles, rhonchi, ↓ breath sounds, cyanosis, pulmonary edema, respiratory arrest

CV: ↓ peripheral pulses, palpitations, tachycardia, dysrhythmias, shock

GU: ↓ UO, incontinence

GI: Nausea, vomiting, diarrhea, abdominal cramping

VITAL SIGNS/HEMODYNAMICS

RR: ↑

HR: ↑

BP: ↓

Temp: Nl or slight ↑

CVP/PAWP: ↓

MAP: ↓

CO: ↓

SVR: ↓

ECG: Dysrhythmias common, including A-tach, PACs, PVCs progressing to VT or VF

LABORATORY STUDIES

ABGs: Evaluate status of oxygenation and acid-base balance. Initially, Pao_2 nl, but levels ↓ as ↑ bronchoconstriction, ↑ lung water, and hypotension cause profound V/Q mismatch. ↑ $Paco_2$ (>50 mm Hg) heralds imminent respiratory arrest. If shock state persists, metabolic acidosis develops.

Spo₂: For continuous monitoring of Sao_2 and to evaluate effectiveness of supplemental O_2, other therapies.

IMAGING

Chest X-ray: If pulmonary edema suspected.

Collaborative Management

GENERAL

Limit Exposure: *If caused by insect:* remove stinger. *If caused by IV drug:* remove container and tubing from catheter. Aspirate blood from catheter to remove all traces of medication—especially important with central line or long IV catheter.

Airway/Oxygenation: Administer humidified O_2; may require ET intubation. Tracheostomy or cricothyroidotomy may be necessary if severe laryngeal edema present.

Fluid Resuscitation: Rapid administration of crystalloids (eg, NS, LR) or colloids to ↑ intravascular volume.

MAST, PSAG: ↑ SVR and may improve BP.

PHARMACOTHERAPY

Epinephrine: Counteracts effects of anaphylaxis by neutralizing histamine and inhibiting further release. *Standard dose:* 0.3-0.5 mg (0.3-0.5 ml of 1:1000 solution) SC. If SBP <70-80 mm Hg, may be given IV: 1-3 ml of 1:10,000 solution diluted in 10 ml NS. Also given endotracheally if no IV access. Continuous infusion of 1-4 μg/min may be used as necessary.

Antihistamines: H_1 blocker, diphenhydramine (Benadryl) 25-50 mg IV or IM. In addition, H_2 blockade *via* cimetidine or ranitidine may be used in some cases.

Corticosteroids: To ↓ capillary permeability and release of chemical mediators. Effect not immediate but will help prevent late reactions.

IV Aminophylline, Inhaled Bronchodilators (eg, albuterol, terbutaline): For continued bronchospasm.

Vasopressors: Necessary if fluid replacement does not reverse shock. Dopamine, norepinephrine, or epinephrine titrated for desired response. See "Inotropic and Vasoactive Agents" in Appendix.

PATIENT-FAMILY TEACHING

- Information about antigen that caused anaphylaxis, including how to avoid it in the future
- Purpose, necessity of wearing Medic-Alert tag or bracelet identifying allergy
- Information about anaphylaxis emergency treatment kits
- Importance of reporting immediately S&S of allergy: flushing, warmth, itching, anxiety, hives
- Importance of identifying and checking all OTC medications for potential allergens

Nursing Diagnoses/Interventions

Ineffective airway clearance r/t tracheobronchial obstruction secondary to bronchoconstriction and ↑ secretions associated with histamine response
Desired outcome: Within 2 h of treatment/intervention, patient has adequate airway clearance: eupnea with nl breath sounds in all lung fields.
- Assess airway patency continuously. Be alert to ↓ air movement, expiratory wheezing, SOB, dyspnea. Keep suction equipment readily available.
- Administer epinephrine as indicated. If patient not in shock, give SC. Patients taking β-blocking drugs, such as propranolol, may not respond to epinephrine. Glucagon may be tried if epinephrine ineffective.
- Auscultate lung fields for wheezes and air movement. As bronchoconstriction and obstruction progress, wheezing may ↓; therefore it is important to listen for air movement as well.
- Prepare for ET intubation if SOB and respiratory distress continue. If laryngeal edema present, an oral airway will be ineffective because the obstruction is lower than the posterior pharynx.
- If laryngeal edema prevents intubation, prepare for tracheostomy or cricothyroidotomy.
- Administer inhaled or IV bronchodilators as indicated. Monitor for tachycardia and other dysrhythmias, especially if aminophylline used.
- Monitor ABGs for improving/worsening condition. Be alert to ↑ $Paco_2$ (>50 mm Hg) and ↓ Pao_2 (<60 mm Hg).

Impaired gas exchange r/t alveolar-capillary membrane changes secondary to ↑ capillary permeability associated with histamine response
Desired outcome: Within 2 h of treatment/intervention, patient has adequate gas exchange: eupnea, Pao_2 ≥80 mm Hg, Spo_2 ≥90.
- Administer humidified supplemental O_2. Monitor Spo_2, being alert to levels <90%.
- Antihistamines (eg, diphenhydramine, cimetidine) may be given to compete with histamine at receptor sites and control lung edema.
- As prescribed, administer glucocorticoids (eg, hydrocortisone) for their antiinflammatory effects. Be aware that glucocorticoid effects may not be apparent for several h.
- If BP stable, assist to sitting position to promote gas exchange.
- Remain with patient; encourage slow, deep breathing if possible. Alleviate anxiety by responding calmly and explaining procedures before performing them.

Decreased cardiac output r/t ↓ preload and afterload secondary to release of vasoactive chemical mediators and associated vasodilatation and ↓ capillary permeability
Desired outcome: Within 4 h of treatment initiation, patient has adequate cardiac output: BP ≥90/60 mm Hg, peripheral pulses >2+ on 0-4+ scale, CO ≥4.0 L/min, CI ≥2.5 L/min/m^2, SVR ≥900 dynes/sec/cm^{-5}; UO ≥0.5 ml/kg/h; and NSR on ECG.
- Assess for physical and hemodynamic indicators of ↓ CO: ↓ amplitude of peripheral pulses, ↓ MAP, ↓ SVR (↓ afterload caused by vasodilatation). As available, monitor CO/CI.
- Monitor for dysrhythmias, such as A-tach, PVCs, VT, and VF, which may signal hypoxemia or occur as a side effect of drug therapy.
- Administer fluid replacement therapy. Up to 2-3 L may be required. Volume expanders may be given with crystalloids to ↑ vascular volume. During fluid resuscitation, assess for S&S of fluid volume excess: crackles, JVD, and ↑ PAP, PAWP, RAP.
- Administer epinephrine. Observe for therapeutic effects as evidenced by ↑ SVR, CO/CI, arterial BP and MAP, and UO; stronger peripheral pulses; warming of extremities.
- Prepare for possible vasopressor infusion if hypotension persists after fluid resuscitation and epinephrine administration.
- If prescribed, apply PASG to ↑ SVR. PASG must be released gradually when no longer needed to prevent precipitous ↓ in BP.

Impaired skin integrity r/t urticaria and angioedema secondary to allergic response
Desired outcomes: Within 4 h of treatment initiation, patient states that urticaria is controlled. Skin remains intact.
- Assess for urticaria and itching of hands, feet, neck, genitalia.
- Administer antihistamines as prescribed to relieve itching.
- Discourage scratching. If it is unavoidable, teach patient to use pads of fingertips rather than nails.
- Apply cool washcloths or ice packs as a soothing measure to irritated and edematous areas.

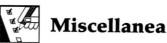

Miscellanea

CONSULT MD FOR
- Signs of airway compromise: ↑ SOB, dyspnea, ↓ air movement, ↓ Pao_2, ↓ Sao_2, ↑ $Paco_2$
- CV instability: SBP <90 mm Hg, SVR <900 dynes/sec/cm^{-5}, CI <2.5 L/min/m^2, serious dysrhythmias, inadequate response to fluid replacement therapy
- Complications: oliguria; ↓ LOC caused by hypoxia or cerebral edema occurring with interstitial fluid shifts
- Rebound hypersensitivity response occurring 8-12 h after initial event as medications wear off but slow-acting chemical mediators are still in circulation

RELATED TOPICS
- Increased intracranial pressure
- Mechanical ventilation
- Multiple organ dysfunction syndrome
- Respiratory failure, acute
- Vasopressor therapy

REFERENCES
Boxer MB: Anaphylaxis without cause, *Emerg Med* 25(1): 20-30, 1993.
Carroll P: Speed—the essential response to anaphylaxis, *RN* 57(6): 26-36, 1994.
Goodfellow L: Adverse reaction to Benadryl, *Nursing* 26(7): 39, 1996.
Hollingsworth HM: Anaphylaxis, *Emerg Med* 24(12): 142-148, 1992.
Keen JH, Baird MS, Allen JH: *Mosby's critical care and emergency drug reference*, ed 2, St Louis, 1996, Mosby.
Steuble BT: Septic and anaphylactic shock. In Swearingen PL, Keen JH (eds): *Manual of critical care nursing*, ed 3, St Louis, 1995, Mosby.
Tribett D: Mechanisms for immunological injury. In Kinney M, Packa D, Dunbar S: *AACN's clinical reference for critical care nursing*, ed 3, St Louis, 1993, Mosby.

Author: **Janet Hicks Keen**

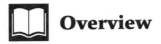

Overview

PATHOPHYSIOLOGY
Reduction in total body Hgb concentration. As Hgb ↓, O_2-carrying capacity of blood ↓, resulting in tissue hypoxia. Originate from one of three main problems:

Acute/Chronic Blood Loss: GI bleeding, trauma, ruptured blood vessel(s)

↓ Erythrocyte Production: Iron deficiency, lead poisoning, thalassemias, renal failure

↑ Erythrocyte Destruction: Hemolytic anemias caused by abnormal Hgb, RBC membrane anomalies (spherocytosis, hemolytic uremic syndrome), physical trauma to blood (extracorporeal "bypass" circulation, balloon counterpulsation, prosthetic heart valve), bacterial endotoxins (malaria, clostridia)

HISTORY/RISK FACTORS
- Hemoglobinopathies
- Hemolytic anemias: hereditary spherocytosis, G6PD deficiency, thalassemias (Cooley's, Mediterranean), erythroblastosis fetalis
- Renal failure
- Malignancy
- Bone marrow suppression
- Vitamin B_{12} deficiency: blood loss, hemorrhage, menorrhagia, folic acid or iron deficiency

CLINICAL PRESENTATION
Chronic: Pallor, melena, fatigue, weight loss, dyspnea on exertion, uremia, sensitivity to cold, intermittent dizziness, paresthesias

Chronic hemolytic anemia: Jaundice, renal failure, hematuria, arthritis, ↑ gallstone incidence, skin ulcers

Acute: Fever, chest pain, heart failure, confusion, irritability, tachycardia, orthostatic hypotension, dyspnea, tachypnea, frank bleeding

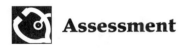

Assessment

PHYSICAL ASSESSMENT
Neuro: Altered mental status, weakness
Resp: Tachypnea, orthopnea, crackles

CV: Tachycardia, S_3/S_4 gallops, orthostasis, pallor
GI: Hepatosplenomegaly
Other: Weight loss, spider angiomas, smooth tongue, skin ulcers

VITAL SIGNS/HEMODYNAMICS
RR: ↑
HR: ↑
BP: Orthostatic changes if bleeding acute
Temp: Nl
CVP/PAWP: ↓ if bleeding acute; ↑ if LV failure attributable to profound anemia
CO: Initial compensatory ↑; later ↓ if profound anemia impairs myocardial O_2
SVR: Initial ↓ caused by ↓ viscosity and compensatory hyperdynamic state; ↑ if fluid volume deficit or profound anemia and impaired tissue perfusion present
ECG: Sinus or other tachycardia; dysrhythmias with ↑ ventricular irritability caused by impaired myocardial oxygenation

LABORATORY STUDIES
CBC: ↓ RBCs, ↑ reticulocytes (RBC precursors) as a result of ↑ bone marrow production of RBCs, ↓ Hgb/Hct
RBC Morphology
  Normocytic: MCV 80-100 μ_3
  Macrocytic: MCV >100 μ_3
  Microcytic: MCV <80 μ_3
Sickle Cell Test: Checks for Hgb S, a sign of sickle cell anemia
Hgb Electrophoresis: Checks for abnormal Hgb
ESR: ↑ in hemolytic anemia more often than in other anemias
C3 Proactivator: ↑ in hemolytic anemia
Total Iron-Binding Capacity: Nl or ↓, depending on anemia type
Unconjugated Bilirubin: ↑ in hemolytic anemia because of liver's inability to process ↑ bilirubin released during hemolysis
Peripheral Blood Smear: May reveal abnormally shaped RBCs
Coombs' Test: Positive in antibody-mediated/immunologic hemolysis

IMAGING
X-rays, Bone Scans: May reveal ↑ bone density or aseptic necrosis.
Liver/Spleen Scans: May reveal disease or dysfunction of either organ contributing to anemia.

DIAGNOSTIC PROCEDURES
Bone Marrow Aspiration: May reveal abnormal size, shape, or amount of erythrocytes or reticulocytes in various anemias.

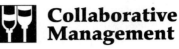

Collaborative Management

ALL ANEMIAS
Volume Replacement: If hypovolemic, aggressive fluid/blood replacement mandatory to prevent profound hypotension and shock. Also assists in preventing deposition of hemolyzed RBCs in microvasculature.

Transfusions/Blood Component Replacement: PRBCs necessary to ↑ O_2-carrying capacity of blood.

O_2 Therapy: To relieve dyspnea and ↑ O_2 available for tissue use.

SELECTED ANEMIAS
Vitamin B_{12}: Injections or IV infusion necessary for pernicious anemia.

Iron: If iron deficiency present.

Folic Acid: Supplements of 1 mg/day used to treat megaloblastic anemia help prevent hemolytic crisis.

Epoetin Alfa; Recombinant Erythropoietin (Epogen/Procrit): Stimulates RBC production in bone marrow for patients with hypofunction/lack of RBC production, particularly when related to renal failure.

Bone Marrow Transplantation: Recommended for some sickle cell disease or aplastic anemia to provide mechanism for regenerating nl RBC production.

Elimination of Causative Factor: Certain drugs (eg, phenytoin and barbiturates) and chemicals, cold temps, and stress can worsen many anemias, especially hemolytic and aplastic anemias. Identification and removal can prevent life-threatening crisis.

PATIENT-FAMILY TEACHING
- Etiology of patient's specific anemia
- Purpose of blood product transfusion therapy, expected results, anticipated sensations
- Importance of avoiding physically and psychologically stressful situations, which can exacerbate symptoms/precipitate hemolytic crisis
- S&S of impending hypoxemia: altered mental status, activity intolerance, SOB, chest pain, weakness

Nursing Diagnoses/Interventions

Impaired gas exchange r/t lack of RBCs or hemoglobin abnormalities

Desired outcome: Within 48-96 h of treatment initiation, patient has adequate gas exchange: HR and RR within 10% of baseline (or HR 60-100 bpm and RR 12-20 breaths/min), Hgb and Hct returned to baseline (or Hgb >12 mg/dl and Hct >37%), O_2 saturation >90%, and SBP returned to baseline (or >90 mm Hg within 24 h of treatment initiation).

- Administer supplemental O_2.
- Monitor O_2 saturation using pulse oximeter. Be alert to values <90% or, if chronically ↓, a sustained drop of >10% of baseline.
- Maintain large-bore (18 gauge) IV catheter(s) in case transfusion or rapid volume expansion necessary.
- Transfuse with PRBCs as prescribed to facilitate O_2 delivery and assist in volume expansion.
- Carefully evaluate dyspnea and chest pain in sickle cell patients because of possibility of pulmonary infarction.
- Monitor ECG for dysrhythmias, ischemic changes (ST-segment elevation), which can signal impaired myocardial oxygenation associated with profound anemia.

Activity intolerance r/t anemia/lack of O_2-carrying capacity of blood

Desired outcomes: Within 48 h of treatment initiation, patient's activity tolerance improves: HR and RR return to within 10% of baseline (or HR 60-100 bpm and RR 12-20 breaths/min) and SBP returns to within 10% baseline (or >90% mm Hg). Within 24 h of treatment initiation patient is able to assist minimally with self-care activities.

- Alternate periods of rest and activity to avoid physically stressing patient and ↑ O_2 demand.
- Reposition slowly to evaluate effects of position change on myocardial and cerebral perfusion.
- Reduce fear, pain, and anxiety to ↓ O_2 demand.

Miscellanea

CONSULT MD FOR
- Spo_2 <90%
- SBP <90 mm Hg
- Hgb <9 or Hct <27
- Dysrhythmias, ischemic ECG changes

RELATED TOPICS
- Blood and blood products (see Appendix)
- GI bleeding: lower
- GI bleeding: upper
- Multisystem injury
- Shock, hemorrhagic

ABBREVIATIONS
MCV: Mean corpuscular volume
PRBCs: Packed red blood cells

REFERENCES
Baird MS: Hematologic dysfunctions. In Swearingen PL, Keen JH (eds): *Manual of critical care nursing,* ed 3, St Louis, 1995, Mosby.

Eisenstaedt RS: Transfusion therapy: blood components and transfusion complications. In Rippe JM et al (eds): *Intensive care medicine,* ed 3, Boston, 1996, Little, Brown.

Koda-Kimble MA, Young LY: *Applied therapeutics: the clinical use of drugs,* Vancouver, Wash, 1992, Applied Therapeutics.

Lottman MS, Thompson KS: Assessment of the hematologic system. In Phipps WJ et al (eds): *Medical-surgical nursing: concepts & clinical practice,* ed 5, St Louis, 1995, Mosby.

Williams WJ: Approach to the patient. In Bentler E et al (eds): *Williams' hematology,* ed 5, New York, 1995, McGraw-Hill.

Author: **Marianne Saunorus Baird**

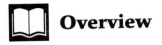 **Overview**

PATHOPHYSIOLOGY

Chest discomfort or pain associated with myocardial ischemia. Can occur at rest or with exercise and may result from sudden ↓ in coronary blood flow caused by coronary thrombosis, spasm, or blood flow that is insufficient to meet myocardial O_2 demands (eg, during exercise). Acute chest pain caused by ischemia may occur when coronary perfusion pressure is low, eg, sudden hypotension, or when O_2 demands greatly ↑, eg, with aortic stenosis.

FORMS OF ANGINA

Stable: No ↑ in frequency or severity over several mos.

Unstable: Quality of pain changed or ↑ in frequency, duration, or severity; can occur with exertion or at rest.

Prinzmetal's (variant): May occur at rest, long after exercise, and during sleep; usually caused by coronary vasospasm.

HISTORY/RISK FACTORS

- Family hx of CAD
- Hyperlipidemia, hypercholesterolemia
- Hypertension, DM, obesity
- Age >65 yr
- Male; postmenopausal female
- Cigarette smoking
- Anemia, thyrotoxicosis
- ↑ stress
- Sedentary life-style

CLINICAL PRESENTATION

- Substernal discomfort described as deep, visceral, squeezing, choking, burning, heavy, tight, aching. Many deny presence of chest "pain" but admit to severe "discomfort" or "pressure."
- Lasts 1-4 min but usually not >30 min.
- Relieved by NTG, usually within 45-90 sec.

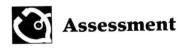 **Assessment**

PHYSICAL ASSESSMENT

Neuro: Anxiety
Resp: Mild tachypnea, SOB, crackles if heart failure present
CV: Irregular pulse with dysrhythmias; S_4 gallop during ischemic episodes

VITAL SIGNS/HEMODYNAMICS

RR: Nl or ↑
HR: ↑
BP: ↑ or ↓
Temp: Nl

CO: Nl or ↓
PAWP: Nl or ↑
Other: BP, HR ↑ in response to ↑ sympathetic tone. With myocardial ischemia, CO and BP ↓. Advanced heart failure causes ↑ PAWP.

12/18-Lead ECG: In absence of pain and with patient at rest, may be nl; therefore must be obtained during chest pain episode. ST-segment and T-wave changes, which occur during chest pain and disappear with relief of pain, are significant. Most characteristic is ST-segment depression with or without T-wave inversion. In variant or Prinzmetal's, ST segments may be elevated during episode. 18-lead ECG better reflects RV electrical activity.

LABORATORY STUDIES

Serum Enzymes: CK-MB level >10% total CK suggests myocardial muscle damage. Cardiac troponin I levels ≥3.1 ng/ml specific for myocardial injury.

IMAGING

Chest X-ray: May reveal cardiomegaly, which signals myocardial ischemia and ↓ contractility.

DIAGNOSTIC PROCEDURES

Cardiac Catheterization: To visualize patency of coronary arteries and show extent of CAD.

Stress Test: Patient exercises to elicit chest pain while being monitored by ECG; any associated ECG changes documented. Positive stress test results: (1) ≥1.0 mm depression or downsloping ST segment that lasts 0.08 sec and (2) frequent PVCs or runs of VT.

Thallium Treadmill: Patient exercises after thallium injection. Scans obtained immediately after exercise and 4 h later determine if infarcted or ischemic areas with ↓ uptake fill in after 4 h. Ischemic areas that fill in are considered to have viable tissue and reversible damage.

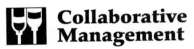 **Collaborative Management**

Oxygen: 2-4 L/min by nasal cannula or as indicated by ABGs.

Pharmacotherapy

Nitroglycerin (sublingual and spray): For short-term therapy.

Nitroglycerin IV: For unstable angina; titrated until relief obtained.

IV morphine sulfate: Given in small increments (ie, 2 mg) until relief obtained. Usually not necessary unless MI is occurring.

Calcium blockers (eg, nifedipine): Cause vasodilatation of coronary and peripheral arteries to relieve chest pain caused by coronary artery spasm; ↓ contraction and O_2 demand.

β Blockers (eg, propranolol): ↓ cardiac workload and thus O_2 demand.

Anticoagulants: Eg, heparin and antiplatelet drugs (eg, aspirin), to prevent thrombus formation.

Limit Activities: Complete rest during acute episode and other restrictions based on activity tolerance.

PTCA: With *angioplasty,* balloon-tipped catheter inserted into coronary arterial lesion. Balloon inflated to compress plaque material against vessel wall, thereby opening narrowed lumen. With *atherectomy,* catheter similarly placed and plaque mechanically removed. Ideal candidate has single vessel disease with discrete, proximal, noncalcified lesion.

Complications after PTCA: Acute coronary artery occlusion, AMI, coronary artery spasm or rupture, bleeding, renal hypersensitivity to contrast material, hypokalemia, vasovagal reaction, dysrhythmias, and hypotension. Restenosis can occur 6 wks to 6 mos after PTCA, although patient may not experience angina.

Excimer Laser Coronary Angioplasty: Enables treatment of distal coronary lesions in tortuous arteries. Laser ablates only the tissue it contacts.

Intracoronary Stent Placement: Stents are metal-mesh tubes that keep arteries open. Balloon-expanded stents most commonly used; inserted during procedure similar to PTCA.

PATIENT-FAMILY TEACHING

- Importance of activity limitation and its rationale: to minimize O_2 requirements and thus ↓ chest pain
- Necessity of reporting any further episodes of chest pain
- Measures that prevent complications of ↓ mobility, eg, active ROM exercises
- Risk factor modification: diet low in cholesterol and saturated fat, smoking cessation, stress management
- Actions to take if chest pain unrelieved or ↑ in intensity:

  Stop and rest. Take one NTG while lying or sitting down; wait 5 min. If pain not relieved, take second NTG; wait 5 min. If pain not relieved, take third NTG. Lie down if headache occurs. Vasodilatation effect of NTG causes ↓ in BP and transient headache.

  If pain not relieved after 3 NTGs taken over 15-min period, call physician or dial 911 or local emergency number.
- Phone number for American Heart Association: 1-800-242-8721

Nursing Diagnoses/Interventions

Pain (chest) r/t biophysiologic injury secondary to ↓ myocardial O₂ supply

Desired outcomes: Within 1 h of intervention, patient's subjective evaluation of discomfort improves, as documented by pain scale.

- Assess and document character of chest pain, including location, duration, quality, intensity, precipitating and alleviating factors, presence/absence of radiation, and associated symptoms. Have patient rate discomfort from 0 (no pain) to 10 (severe pain).
- Measure BP and HR with each episode. ↑ possible because of sympathetic stimulation resulting from pain. Alternately, if chest pain is caused by ischemia, cardiac output may ↓, resulting in low BP.
- Obtain 12/18-lead ECG during chest pain. Ischemia is usually demonstrated by ST-segment depression and T-wave inversion.
- Administer O₂ per nasal cannula at 2-4 L/min.
- Provide only light meals to prevent O₂ supply and demand mismatch.
- Position patient according to comfort level. Keep patients on IV NTG on complete bed rest until condition stabilizes. Profound orthostatic hypotension possible.
- Provide care in calm and efficient manner; provide reassurance and support during chest pain episodes.
- Maintain quiet environment and group care activities to enable periods of uninterrupted rest.
- Administer nitrates, titrating IV NTG so that chest pain is relieved, yet SBP remains >90 mm Hg. Titrate by gradual incremental ↑ q5min.
- If hypotension occurs (SBP 80-90 mm Hg), ↓ flow rate to ½ or less of infusing dose and administer small fluid challenge (eg, 250-500 ml) unless contraindicated by overt heart failure. If severe hypotension (<80 SBP mm Hg) occurs, stop infusion and contact physician, who may prescribe a low-dose positive inotropic agent (eg, dopamine or dobutamine).
- Monitor for side effects of NTG: headache, hypotension, syncope, facial flushing, and nausea. If side effects occur, place in a supine position and consult physician.
- Administer β blockers and calcium channel blockers, which relieve chest pain by diminishing coronary artery spasm, causing coronary and peripheral vasodilatation and ↓ myocardial contractility and O₂ demand. Monitor for side effects, eg, bradycardia and hypotension. Be alert to indicators of heart failure, eg, fatigue, SOB, weight gain, and edema, and to evidence of heart block, eg, syncope and dizziness.
- Administer heparin and aspirin as prescribed. Monitor for excessive anticoagulation. Monitor PTT.

Activity intolerance r/t imbalance between O₂ supply and demand secondary to ↓ cardiac output associated with CAD

Desired outcome: Within 12-24 h before discharge from CCU, patient exhibits cardiac tolerance to ↑ levels of activity: RR <24 breaths/min, NSR on ECG, BP within 20 mm Hg of nl for patient, HR <120 bpm (or within 20 bpm of resting HR if on β-blocker therapy), and absence of chest pain.

- Assist with identifying activities that precipitate chest pain; teach use of NTG prophylactically before activities.
- Assist in progressive activity program from Levels I-IV:

I Bed rest	Flexion/extension of extremities qid, 15 × each extremity; deep breathing qid, 15 breaths; position change from side to side q2h
II OOB to chair	As tolerated, tid for 20-30 min
III Ambulate in room	As tolerated, tid for 20-30 min
IV Ambulate in hall	Initially, 50-200 ft bid; progressing to 50-200 ft qid

- Assess response to activity progression. Be alert to chest pain, SOB, excessive fatigue, and dysrhythmias. Monitor for ↓ in BP >20 mm Hg and ↑ in HR to >120 bpm (>20 bpm above resting HR in patients receiving β-blocker therapy).

 # Miscellanea

CONSULT MD FOR
- Symptomatic or significant hypotension: SBP ≤80 mm Hg or associated with chest pain, dysrhythmias, SOB
- Persistent or worsening chest pain, especially if associated with nausea, vomiting, diaphoresis, or SOB
- ECG evidence of injury, infarction: ST-segment elevation, T-wave inversion, new Q waves
- Serious or symptomatic dysrhythmias

RELATED TOPICS
- Cardiac surgery: CABG
- Coronary artery disease
- Myocardial infarction, acute
- Percutaneous transluminal coronary angioplasty/atherectomy
- Vasopressor therapy

REFERENCES

Adams J et al: Cardiac troponin I: a marker with high specificity for cardiac injury, *Circulation* 88(1): 101-106, 1993.

Callahan LL, Frohlich GC: Understanding nonsurgical coronary revascularization procedures, *Am J Nurs* 95(3): 52 H-I, 52 L, 1995.

Engler MB, Engler MM: Assessment of the cardiovascular effects of stress, *J Cardiovasc Nurs* 10(1): 51-63, 1995.

Futterman LG, Lemberg L: Cardiology case book. Angina, linked angina, chest pain: an enigma within a dilemma, *Am J Crit Care* 4(4): 325-331, 1995.

Hofgren C, Karlson BW, Herlitz J: Prodromal symptoms in subsets of patients hospitalized for suspected acute myocardial infarction, *Heart Lung* 24(1): 3-10, 1995.

Author: **Barbara Tueller Steuble**

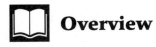

Overview

DESCRIPTION
Visualization of artery or vein *via* direct injection of contrast medium. Contrast agents usually ionized and characterized as LOCA or HOCA. HOCA in large volumes (eg, with aortograms, mesenteric arteriograms with brisk GI bleeding) ↑ risk of renal and systemic complications.

COMPLICATIONS
Hematoma: If small (diameter <5 cm), usually not significant; but if larger, can compress surrounding vessels and nerves, causing neurovascular damage.
Thrombus: Occurs when platelets and fibrin continue to collect at puncture site after hemostasis has occurred. Vessel wall injury, sluggish blood flow, and ↑ coagulation contribute. Large thrombus may occlude blood flow and result in tissue ischemia.
Pseudoaneurysm: Occurs when blood leaks into surrounding tissue and coagulates, forming a pouch around the vessel. Can close spontaneously, but may rupture, causing massive blood loss.
Renal: Contrast medium, especially in high concentrations, can damage glomeruli and renal tubules, resulting in ARF or ATN. Hypertonicity of contrast medium causes osmotic diuresis, leading to ↓ blood volume and further ↑ in concentration.
Hypersensitivity Reaction: Usually mild. Typically occurs immediately after contrast injection, but may be delayed several h.
Nausea, Vomiting, Pain, Warmth: R/t hypertonicity of contrast medium.
Vasovagal Reaction: Results in bradycardia and hypotension; usually resolved by raising patient's legs. May be prolonged or result in cardiac arrest.
Thromboemboli: Several possible etiologies: clots from catheter or guide wire, debris in contrast medium, air, disruption of intimal plaques by catheter or injection.

RISK FACTORS (for complications)
Hematoma Formation, Bleeding, Pseudoaneurysm: Obesity, advanced age, hypertension, coagulopathies, use of sheaths, access *via* brachial or axillary arteries.
Neurovascular Compromise: Use of brachial or axillary artery. Even small hematoma at these sites fills adjacent compartment, compressing radial and medial nerves.
Pain, Warmth, Nausea, Vomiting: ↑ in intensity with use of HOCA.

Renal Damage: Preexisting renal disease, DM, advanced age, dehydration, heart failure, large volume of contrast, repeated contrast exposure, HOCA. Combination of two or more factors significantly ↑ risk of ATN.
Hypersensitivity Reaction: Asthma, allergies, serious health problems (eg, COPD).
Vasovagal Response: Pain or full bladder with femoral artery access.

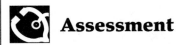

Assessment

PHYSICAL ASSESSMENT (findings suggestive of complications)
Neuromusc: ↓ LOC (attributable to renal complications, hypersensitivity reaction, ↑ K^+); numbness, tingling, paresthesias, muscle weakness (attributable to thromboemboli, ↑ K^+)
Resp: ↓ rate/depth (caused by sedatives, analgesics); laryngospasm, bronchospasm (as a result of systemic reaction)
CV: ↓/absent peripheral pulses; delayed capillary refill (with hematoma, thrombosis); bruit/thrill or pulsating mass (with pseudoaneurysm), bradycardia and hypotension (with vasovagal response), tachycardia and hypotension (with hemorrhage)
GU: Initial UO ↑ caused by osmotic diuresis; then nl or ↓
Integ: Urticaria; hematoma, bruising, oozing of blood at puncture site; coolness and pallor with compromised circulation; poor skin turgor, dry oral mucous membrane with dehydration

VITAL SIGNS/HEMODYNAMICS
RR: Nl or ↑
HR: ↑ with hypovolemia; ↓ with vasovagal response
BP: ↓ with vasovagal response or hypovolemia
Temp: Nl or ↑
CVP/PAP/CO: ↓ with hypovolemia
ECG: Hyperkalemic changes associated with ↓ renal function: tall peaked T waves, loss of P waves, widening of QRS

LABORATORY STUDIES
Serum Creatinine/BUN: To evaluate renal function preprocedure. Postprocedure may show ↑ values with ↓ renal function.
Coagulation Studies: To evaluate hemostasis.
Hct, Hgb: To provide baseline preprocedure. Postprocedure may reveal ↓ with blood loss, ↑ Hct with dehydration.

IMAGING
Color Flow Doppler Ultrasonography: To diagnose and evaluate thrombosis and pseudoaneurysm; may be used to treat pseudoaneurysm.

Collaborative Management

Supplemental O_2: May be necessary if O_2 saturation <90% because of sedation-related respiratory depression or blood loss. Continuous SpO_2 recommended until patient fully alert.
Fluid Management: IV fluids necessary to maintain or ↑ hydration before, during, after procedure.
Furosemide or low-dose dopamine: May be used to augment RBF and promote excretion of contrast medium. Furosemide used only with adequate hydration.
NS: Administered rapidly to treat hypotension r/t blood loss or vasovagal response.
Colloids or blood products: Used if major blood loss occurs.
Pharmacotherapy: Borderline or ↓ renal function necessitates identifying medications that are contraindicated or that require dose adjustment.
Diphenhydramine, H_2 blockers, hydroxyzine: May be used to prevent or treat contrast media reaction.
Analgesics: For postprocedure pain.
Surgical Intervention: May be necessary to treat hematoma, thrombosis, or pseudoaneurysm if conservative measures inadequate or condition deteriorates.

PATIENT-FAMILY TEACHING
Preprocedure
- Fasting, need for additional IV fluids
- Purpose, duration, expected results, anticipated sensations
- Identification of allergies to iodine, shellfish, IVP dye
- Postprocedure activity limitations and assessments (frequent VS, site, pulse checks)

Postprocedure
- Importance of adequate hydration
- S&S of complications
- How to apply manual pressure to groin (if femoral site) when coughing, sneezing, vomiting

Nursing Diagnoses/Interventions

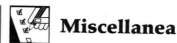 ## Miscellanea

Risk for fluid volume deficit r/t osmotic diuresis secondary to administration of contrast medium; r/t blood loss secondary to procedure

Desired outcome: Patient remains normovolemic: UO ≥0.5 ml/kg/h, HR 60-100 bpm, BP wnl, CVP 2-6 mm Hg, PAP 20-30/8-15 mm Hg, CO 4-7 L/min.

- Encourage fluid intake preprocedure and postprocedure unless contraindicated. Adequate hydration essential. Maintain UO of 50-100 ml/h for 6-8 h or until contrast excreted.
- Monitor I&O qh. If output > intake, ↑ fluid intake unless contraindicated. UO <0.5 ml/kg/h may signal hypovolemia or ↓ renal function.
- Keep large-bore, patent IV access available to facilitate rapid infusion of crystalloid or colloid fluids if needed.
- Monitor weight qd. Be alert to loss >1 kg/day or continued loss over consecutive days.
- Monitor VS q15min postprocedure until stable, then q1-2h. Be alert to ↓ BP and ↑ HR, RR.
- Check hemodynamic pressures qh. Monitor for and correct ↓ CVP/PAP.
- Maintain compression over puncture site per agency protocol, using pressure dressing (may mask hematoma), manual pressure, sandbag, or mechanical compression device.
- Assess puncture site per agency protocol. Apply manual compression to puncture site for ↑ hematoma or continued oozing. Bleeding commonly recurs 2-3 h postprocedure.
- If sheath in place, follow agency protocol for removing and applying pressure. Assess puncture site and distal pulses after compression to ensure bleeding has stopped and large hematoma/thrombus does not cause vascular compromise.
- Maintain activity restrictions per agency protocol. Usually, puncture site immobilized for 4-6 h. If femoral artery accessed, HOB should not be elevated >30-45 degrees for several h postprocedure.

Altered peripheral tissue perfusion (or risk for same) r/t interruption of arterial blood flow secondary to vessel obstruction by thrombi or hematoma

Desired outcome: Peripheral tissue perfusion maintained postangiography: distal pulses palpated or identified by Doppler, warm skin, brisk capillary refill (<2 sec), and absence of peripheral neurovascular deficits.

- Assess pulses distal to puncture site per agency protocol. Be alert to continued ↓ strength or absence of pulse.
- Perform neurovascular assessment distal to puncture site per agency protocol: note skin color, capillary refill, weakness, numbness, tingling, and pain. Compare examined extremity to its opposite.
- Do not measure BP in affected extremity.
- Monitor puncture site for new or ↑ hematoma. Apply compression if it occurs. Monitor distal pulse during compression. Compression should not totally occlude vessel and thus eliminate pulse.

CONSULT MD FOR

- UO <0.5 ml/kg/h × 2 h
- Neurovascular changes distal to puncture site
- Bleeding at puncture site not stopped by continued compression
- Large or enlarging hematoma at puncture site
- S&S of hypovolemia
- Changes in LOC
- ECG changes associated with hyperkalemia or marked bradycardia

RELATED TOPICS

- Acute tubular necrosis: oliguric and non-oliguric
- Anaphylaxis
- Bradycardia
- Compartment syndrome
- Hyperkalemia
- Shock, hemorrhagic

ABBREVIATIONS

HOCA: High-osmolality contrast agent
LOCA: Low-osmolality contrast agent
RBF: Renal blood flow

REFERENCES

Barbiere CC: A new device for control of bleeding after transfemoral catheterization, *Crit Care Nurse* 15(1): 51-53, 1995.

Barth KH: Patient care aspects of vascular and non-vascular interventional radiology procedures, *Semin Interventional Radiog* 11(2): 83-88, 1994.

Bettman MA: Complications of angiographic contrast agents, *Semin Interventional Radiog* 11(2): 89-92, 1994.

Borgart MA: Time to hemostasis: a comparison of manual versus mechanical compression of the femoral artery, *Am J Crit Care* 4(2):149-156, 1995.

Jones C, Holcomb E, Rohrer T: Femoral artery pseudoaneurysm after invasive procedures, *Crit Care Nurse* 15(4): 47-51, 1995.

Spies JB: Complications of diagnostic arteriography, *Semin Interventional Radiog* 11(2): 93-101, 1994.

Author: **Marguerite J. Murphy**

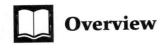 **Overview**

DESCRIPTION

Performed to compress coronary atherosclerotic plaque material against the vessel wall (angioplasty) or mechanically remove it (atherectomy). Indicated for surgical candidates whose angina is refractory to medical treatment. Also performed for postinfarction, postbypass, and chronic stable anginas. Ideal candidate has single vessel disease with discrete, proximal, noncalcified lesion.

POST-PTCA COMPLICATIONS

Acute coronary artery occlusion, AMI, coronary artery spasm, bleeding, circulatory insufficiency, renal hypersensitivity to contrast material, hypokalemia, vasovagal reaction, dysrhythmias, hypotension. Restenosis can occur 6 wks to 6 mos after PTCA, although angina may not be experienced.

HISTORY/RISK FACTORS (for CAD)

- Family hx of CAD
- Hypercholesterolemia, hyperlipidemia
- Hypertension, DM, obesity
- Age >65 yrs
- Male; postmenopausal female
- Cigarette smoking
- ↑ stress
- Sedentary life-style

CLINICAL PRESENTATION

Unstable or preinfarction angina, requiring emergency PTCA. Elective PTCA may be scheduled for stable but refractory angina.

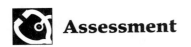 **Assessment**

PHYSICAL ASSESSMENT (in presence of acute angina)

Neuro: Anxiety
Resp: Mild tachypnea, SOB, crackles if heart failure present
CV: Irregular pulse with dysrhythmias; S_4 gallop during ischemic episodes

VITAL SIGNS/HEMODYNAMICS

RR: Nl or ↑
HR: ↑
BP: ↑ or ↓
Temp: Nl
CO: Nl or ↓
PAWP: Nl or ↑

Other: BP, HR ↑ in response to ↑ sympathetic tone. With myocardial ischemia, CO and BP ↓. Advanced heart failure causes ↑ PAWP.

12/18-Lead ECG: In absence of pain and at rest may be nl; therefore obtain during chest pain. ST-segment and T-wave changes, which occur during spontaneous chest pain and disappear with relief of pain, are significant. Most characteristic is ST-segment depression with or without T-wave inversion. In variant or Prinzmetal's angina, ST segments may be elevated. 18-lead ECG better reflects RV electrical activity.

LABORATORY STUDIES

Serum Enzymes: CK-MB level >10% total CK suggests myocardial muscle damage and can occur post-PTCA. ↑ troponin or ↑ myoglobin level is a strong indicator of myocardial damage and assists in diagnosis of AMI. Mg^{2+}, K^+: Often ↓ in AMI; low levels associated with ↑ dysrhythmias.
CBC: Establishes baseline levels in case of bleeding complications if surgery necessary.
Clotting Studies: Establish baseline if intracoronary thrombolytics used or surgery becomes necessary.

IMAGING

Chest X-ray: May reveal cardiomegaly, which signals myocardial ischemia and ↓ contractility.

DIAGNOSTIC PROCEDURES

ECG: Q waves signal MI and meet one of two criteria. They are either wide (>.04 sec) or deep (>25% of total voltage of QRS).
Cardiac Catheterization: Determines presence/extent of CAD; establishes exact location and size of affected coronary arteries. Discrete, proximal narrowings amenable to PTCA intervention.

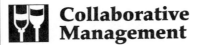 **Collaborative Management**

Pharmacotherapy

Nitrates and morphine sulfate: May be administered and titrated to ↓ or eliminate acute chest pain.
Anticoagulant/antiplatelet drugs: Eg, ASA, heparin, Coumadin, dextran, ticlopidine (Ticlid) to prevent thrombus formation, extension.
Midazolam (Versed)/other benzodiazepines: Used during procedure for light sedation.

PTCA (angioplasty): PA catheter passed through vena cava and right atrium into the heart to measure pressure. Introducer sheath inserted into femoral artery, guidewire passed into aorta and coronary artery, and balloon catheter passed over guidewire to stenotic site. Balloon inflated repeatedly for 60-90 sec at 4-15 atm pressure. Subsequently, radiopaque dye injected to determine whether goal has been met: stenosis <50% of vessel diameter. Introducer sheath left in femoral artery for up to 12 h after PTCA for heparin infusion or in event of need for repeat angiography.
Intracoronary stents: Follows angioplasty procedure. Scaffold device inserted into coronary artery to secure flaps of media and intima against arterial wall, thereby promoting vascular patency. Used in patients at risk for abrupt vessel closure.
PTCA (atherectomy): Catheter similarly placed and plaque mechanically removed.
Post-PTCA Procedure: Complete bed rest for 6-12 h; patient must not move affected leg until sheath removed. Heparin may be continued for 6-12 h postprocedure.

PATIENT-FAMILY TEACHING

- Discussion of CAD and purpose of angioplasty/atherectomy:
    Location of CAD, using heart model or drawing
    Use of local anesthetic and sedation during procedure
    Insertion site of catheter: groin or arm
    Sensations that may occur: mild chest discomfort; feeling of heat as dye injected
    Use of fluoroscopy during procedure; hx of sensitivity to contrast material
    Ongoing observations made by nurse during procedure: BP, HR, ECG, leg or arm pulses, blood tests
    Importance of lying flat in bed 6-12 h after procedure
    Necessity of nursing assistance with eating, drinking, and toileting after procedure
    Need for ↑ fluid intake after procedure to wash dye out of system
- Discharge instructions: importance of taking antiplatelet drugs to prevent restenosis, avoidance of strenuous activity during first few wks at home, S&S to report to MD (GI upset, repeat of angina, fainting)
- If anxiety experienced preprocedure, arrangement for meeting with patient who has had successful angioplasty/atherectomy

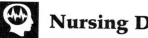 # Nursing Diagnoses/Interventions

Decreased cardiac output r/t negative inotropic changes secondary to vessel occlusion, infarction, coronary artery spasm, and cardiac tamponade; and r/t electrical factors secondary to PTCA-induced dysrhythmias

Desired outcomes: Within 24 h of this diagnosis, patient has adequate cardiac output: BP wnl, HR 60-100 bpm, NSR on ECG, peripheral pulses >2+ on 0-4+ scale, warm and dry skin, UO ≥0.5 ml/kg/h, CO 4-7 L/min, RAP 4-6 mm Hg, PAP 20-30/8-15 mm Hg, PAWP 6-12 mm Hg, patient oriented × 3 and free from anginal pain.

- Monitor BP, RAP, and PAP continuously; monitor PAWP and CO qh. The following signal ↓ cardiac output: ↓ BP, measured CO, and RAP; ↑ HR, PAP, and PAWP.
- Monitor ECG for dysrhythmias and ST-segment and T-wave changes. Observe for bradydysrhythmias during sheath removal. Have atropine, emergency resuscitation equipment immediately available. Run 12/18-lead ECGs qd.
- Monitor UO qh for first 4 h and thereafter according to agency protocol.
- Measure CK-MB band immediately post-PTCA, then q8h for 24 h; report elevations. Optimally, CK-MB will be 0%-5% of total CK.
- Monitor responses to antianginal and coronary vasodilatory medications; report BP < desired range. Hypotension can also occur as a result of vessel occlusion. Treat hypotension immediately. Usually, fluids given and patient placed supine.
- When patient first sits up, ensure that it is done in stages to minimize likelihood of postural hypotension. Monitor VS at frequent intervals during this stage.
- Monitor continuously for bleeding at sheath insertion site. Check Hct level for ↓ from baseline.
- Monitor for cardiac tamponade: hypotension, tachycardia, pulsus paradoxus, JVD, muffled heart sounds, elevation and plateau pressuring of PAWP and RAP and, possibly, enlarged heart silhouette on chest x-ray.
- When heparin and antiplatelet drugs discontinued, monitor closely for indicators of coronary occlusion: ST-segment elevation on ECG, angina, hypotension, tachycardia, dysrhythmias, diaphoresis.
- Monitor peripheral pulses (radial or pedal) and color and temp of extremities q4h for first 24 h.
- Monitor mental alertness on an ongoing basis.

Altered peripheral tissue perfusion (or risk for same): Involved limb, r/t interruption of arterial blood flow secondary to presence of angioplasty sheath or risk of clot formation in vessel after sheath removal

Desired outcome: On admission to CCU and continuously thereafter, patient has adequate tissue in involved limb: warm skin, peripheral pulses >2+ on 0-4+ scale, nl skin color, ability to move toes, and complete sensation.

- Monitor circulation to affected limb q30min for 2 h and then q2h thereafter. Assess pulses, temp, color, sensation, and mobility of toes. Be alert to weak or thready pulses, coolness and pallor of extremity, and complaints of numbness and tingling.
- Inspect sheath site for external or subcutaneous bleeding.
- Keep sandbag at insertion site until discontinued.
- Maintain immobilization of limb at least 6 h or until discontinued.
- Keep HOB ≤15 degrees to prevent kinking of sheath.
- Monitor sheath patency by evaluating for continuous IV infusion into involved vessel.
- Instruct patient to notify staff immediately if numbness, tingling, or pain occurs at affected extremity.

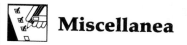 # Miscellanea

CONSULT MD FOR
- UO ≤0.5 ml/kg/h × 2 h
- Significant ↓ in Hct from baseline: indicative of bleeding, possibly retroperitoneal bleeding
- ↓/absent pulses distal to catheter insertion site or other evidence of altered peripheral tissue perfusion; significant hematoma or ecchymosis at insertion site
- Evidence of cardiac tamponade: ↓ BP, ↑ HR, JVD, paradoxical pulse, muffled heart sounds
- Evidence of cardiogenic shock, pulmonary edema
- Symptomatic or significant hypotension: SBP ≤80 mm Hg or associated with chest pain, dysrhythmias, SOB
- Serious or symptomatic dysrhythmias (eg, runs of VT, advancing heart block)
- Significant changes in ECG: presence of Q waves, ST-segment elevation/depression

RELATED TOPICS
- Angina pectoris
- Cardiac catheterization
- Cardiac surgery: CABG
- Cardiac tamponade
- Coronary artery disease
- Hemodynamic monitoring
- Myocardial infarction, acute

REFERENCES
Gardner E et al: Intracoronary stent update: focus on patient education, *Crit Care Nurse* 16(2): 65-75, 1996.

Kern LS: Pulling femoral sheaths, *Crit Care Nurse* 12(4): 76, 1992.

McKenna M: Management of the patient undergoing myocardial revascularization: percutaneous transluminal coronary angioplasty, *Crit Care Nurs Clin North Am* 4(2): 231-242, 1992.

Author: **Marianne Saunorus Baird**

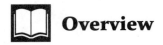

Overview

DESCRIPTION
Medications/devices that manage symptomatic cardiac dysrhythmias or control abnormal rhythms resulting from dysfunctional pacing (automaticity), problems with conduction velocity (too fast or too slow), or conduction pathway/direction (reentry or accessory pathway). Dysrhythmias may involve atria (sinus node or accessory pacemakers), AV node/AV junction, right or left bundle branches, bundle of His/His-Purkinje system, and ventricles.

HISTORY/RISK FACTORS
- CAD (and its risk factors), cardiomyopathy, valvular heart disease, MI
- Electrolyte imbalances, especially ↓ K^+ and Mg^{2+}
- Use of catecholamines or positive inotropes
- Use of cardiac medications by renal or liver-impaired patients
- Malnutrition; prolonged vomiting or diarrhea
- Thyroid or adrenal disease

CLINICAL PRESENTATION
Varies from no reported symptoms to cardiopulmonary arrest, depending on dysrhythmia type and patient's ability to compensate for perfusion deficits resulting from ↓ CO

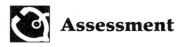

Assessment

PHYSICAL ASSESSMENT
Varies with each dysrhythmia
Neuro: Altered LOC, syncope, weakness, fainting, vertigo, anxiety, restlessness
Resp: SOB, dyspnea on exertion
CV: Chest pain, activity intolerance, palpitations, sense of "skipped beats"
GI: Nausea, vomiting, epigastric pressure
GU: ↓ UO
Integ: Diaphoresis, pallor, cyanosis

VITAL SIGNS/HEMODYNAMICS
Vary with each dysrhythmia

RR: ↑
HR: ↑ or ↓
BP: Possibly ↓
Temp: Nl
CVP/PAWP: Nl, ↑, or ↓
SVR: ↑
CO: ↓
12/18-Lead ECG
May exhibit one of the following *rhythms:*
- Pacemaker other than SA node: in atria, AV junction, or ventricles with faster or slower pacing than SA node
- SA node pacing >140 bpm or <50 bpm
- Faster or slower conduction velocity (ie, heart block)
- Alternate conduction pathway (ie, accessory pathways such as WPW or LGL syndromes)

Dysrhythmias may be *continuous or intermittent,* including:
- Atrial: PACs, A-tach, A-flutter, A-fib, SVT
- AV junction: heart block (first, second, third degree), junctional tachycardia, PJCs, junctional escape rhythm, SVTs
- Ventricle: PVCs, VT, VF, torsades de pointes

Ambulatory Monitoring/Cardiac Event Recording/24-h Holter Monitoring: Identify subtle dysrhythmias and symptoms associated with dysrhythmias. Patient records symptoms as ECG is monitored and stored.

LABORATORY STUDIES
Electrolytes: To identify abnormal values (eg, K^+ and Mg^{2+} anomalies) that may precipitate dysrhythmias.
Therapeutic Drug Levels: May reflect underdosage/overdosage of cardiac medications. Antihypertensives and bronchodilators may interfere with action of certain antidysrhythmics.
Drug/Toxicology Screening: To identify overdose on cardiotoxic drug (eg, cyclic antidepressant) or use of cocaine, other dysrhythmogenic agents.
ABGs: Possible hypoxemia or pH abnormality that may precipitate electrolyte imbalance.

IMAGING
Chest X-ray: Possible enlarged cardiac silhouette reflective of heart disease.

Echocardiography: To evaluate ventricular pumping action, including estimation of ventricular EF.
Cardiac Catheterization: To assess for CAD.

DIAGNOSTIC PROCEDURES
EP Study: Pacing stimuli given at varying sites and voltages to determine dysrhythmia's point of origin, inducibility, and effectiveness of drug therapy in its suppression.
Exercise Stress Testing: Can be used with 24-h Holter monitoring to detect various dysrhythmias, including advanced grades of PVCs (caused by ischemia), and to guide therapy. ECG and BP monitored while patient walks on treadmill or pedals stationary bike. Test continues until patient reaches target HR, becomes symptomatic (ie, chest pain, dysrhythmias, abnormal BP, severe fatigue), or has significant ECG changes from physical stress of exercise.
Atrial ECGs: Use of temporary epicardial pacing wires or special skin electrodes to record atrial electrical activity, including pacing and conduction information.

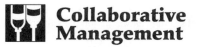

Collaborative Management

GENERAL
Supplemental O_2: To support O_2 delivery to tissues.
Continuous ECG Monitoring: To detect all dysrhythmias, observing onset, duration, and termination of intermittent dysrhythmias.
Spo_2: To detect ↓ O_2 saturation associated with potentially lethal dysrhythmias.
Cardiac Pacing: Transcutaneous, transvenous, or epicardial methods to ↑ or ↓ HR.
Management of Other Dysrhythmia Causes: Including hypoxia, K^+ or Mg^{2+} imbalance, preexisting acidosis, hypothermia, neuroendocrine disorders, or drug overdosage/toxicity.
Initiation of Synchronized Cardioversion or Defibrillation: For tachydysrhythmias resulting in altered mentation, chest pain, hypotension, or cardiac arrest.
CPR: Necessary for all pulseless rhythms (asystole, PEA, pulseless VT and VF). ACLS guidelines used to guide resuscitation.
Dietary Guidelines: Low-fat, low-cholesterol, ↓-caffeine diet may be prescribed.

PHARMACOTHERAPY

Management depends on dysrhythmia's site of origin and cause. Asymptomatic dysrhythmias may not be treated. Dysrhythmias treated with lowest possible dose of antidysrhythmic that successfully terminates the rhythm while avoiding toxicity. Toxicity/overdosage may lead to more pathologic or lethal dysrhythmias.

SVTS

Include atrial, AV junctional tachycardias, A-flutter, and A-fib. Conduction may not be 1:1 from site of origin to ventricle.

β Blockers: Vaughan-Williams Class II agents that slow sinus automaticity, slow AV conduction velocity, control ventricular response to SVTs, and shorten action potential of Purkinje fibers.

Atenolol (Tenormin): 5 mg IV push, not to exceed 1 mg/min. Wait 10 min and repeat dose.

Metoprolol (Lopressor): 5 mg slow IV, repeated q5min to total of 15 mg.

Propranolol (Inderal): 1-3 mg IV push slowly over 1 min. Assess response throughout bolus, since BP may ↓ rapidly.

Calcium Channel Blockers: Vaughan-Williams Class IV drugs that depress automaticity in SA and AV nodes, block slow calcium current in AV junctional tissue, slow AV nodal conduction velocity, and may terminate reentrant pathways involved in AV junctional tachycardias.

Verapamil (Calan): 5 mg IV push very slowly over 2-3 min. Does not suppress accessory pathway conduction.

Diltiazem (Cardizem): 15-20 mg slow IV push over 2 min. May repeat if needed at 20-25 mg slow IV push. Maintenance infusion: 5-15 mg/h titrated to control HR.

Other Agents

Adenosine (Adenocard): For emergency management of symptomatic SVT. Dosage: 6 mg rapid IV push followed immediately with 3-5 ml flush solution. May cause transient pause of 1-3 sec. Can double dose and repeat × 2 if ineffective.

Digoxin (Lanoxin): Cardiac glycoside that slows conduction; used in nonemergency management of A-fib with a rapid ventricular

response. Loading dose: 10 μg/kg total dose divided into four doses.

VT/VF

Pacing site(s) located on ventricle; atria do not contract in synchrony with ventricles during these dysrhythmias.

Class I Agents: Local anesthetics and other drugs that ↓ automaticity of ventricular conduction, delay ventricular repolarization, ↓ conduction velocity, ↑ AV node conduction, and suppress ventricular automaticity.

Procainamide: To control supraventricular and ventricular dysrhythmias. Not recommended for first line treatment of VF because of vasodilatory effects. Loading dose not to exceed 17 mg/kg IV infusion. Maintenance infusion: 1-4 mg/min.

Lidocaine: First line medication for VT and VF. Loading dose: 1.0-1.5 mg/kg IV bolus. Maintenance infusion: 1-4 mg/min.

Class III Agents: ↑ action potential and refractory period of Purkinje fibers, ↑ VF threshold, restore injured myocardial cell electrophysiology toward nl, and suppress reentrant dysrhythmias.

Amiodarone: For unresponsiveness to other antidysrhythmics. Loading dose: 5 mg/kg IV over 2 h *via* central line. Do not exceed 1.2 g in 24 h.

Bretylium: For unresponsiveness to lidocaine, primarily for VF. Loading dose: 5 mg/kg IV push. Do not exceed 30 mg/kg if dosage repeated. Maintenance infusion: 1-4 mg/min.

Sotalol HCl: For unresponsiveness to most other ventricular antidysrhythmic agents. Initial dose: 80 mg PO q12h; may ↑ to a total of 640 mg qd for life-threatening, refractory dysrhythmias.

BRADYCARDIA/ASYSTOLE

HR 0-59 bpm. Generally, unless HR <50 bpm, no treatment required unless symptoms are present. Causes of bradycardia include sinus node dysfunction, AV junctional or ventricular rhythms, AV heart block (usually second or third degree).

Atropine: Blocks slowing action of vagus nerve on the heart, resulting in ↑ HR. Dosage: 0.5-1.0 mg repeated q3-5min up to 0.04 mg/kg for bradycardia. Use 1 mg IV push q3-5min up to 0.04 mg/kg for asystole.

Catecholamines: Stimulate receptors of SNS, resulting in ↑ HR.

Epinephrine: For bradycardia, 2-10 μg/min.

Dopamine: For bradycardia, 5-20 μg/kg/min.

Isoproterenol: For bradycardia, 2-10 μg/min. Use cautiously in patients at high risk for MI.

Epinephrine bolus: For asystole, 1 mg q3-5 min until pulse restored, along with CPR.

SURGERY

ICD: Programmed to deliver synchronized cardioversion or defibrillation when HR > programmed rate or abnormal ECG morphology present. New devices also act as cardiac pacemakers.

Myocardial Revascularization: Performed alone or in conjunction with EP mapping studies, with excision or cryoablation of dysrhythmia focus.

OTHER PROCEDURES

Radiofrequency Catheter Ablation: Small catheter placed in heart *via* cardiac catheterization, wherein electrically generated heat stimulus is applied to dysrhythmia's point of origin. The heat "burns" the heart in a small, localized area, resulting in necrosis of abnormal tissue generating the dysrhythmia.

PATIENT-FAMILY TEACHING

- Importance of promptly reporting adverse symptoms, eg, chest pain, lightheadedness, SOB, activity intolerance, prolonged "palpitations," fainting
- Self-measuring of pulse rate/rhythm
- Causes of dysrhythmia; electrical devices used to treat it
- At-home dietary guidelines, especially regarding ↓-caffeine, low-cholesterol, low-fat diet
- Importance of smoking cessation
- Relaxation techniques that help control environmental stress
- Altered sexuality if ICD in place
- Medications: purpose, dosage, schedule, precautions, drug-drug and food-drug interactions, and potential side effects
- Follow-up instructions per physician protocol
- Support groups

Nursing Diagnoses/Interventions

Decreased cardiac output r/t altered rate, rhythm, conduction; r/t negative inotropic cardiac changes secondary to cardiac disease
Desired outcome: Within 15 min of dysrhythmia onset, patient has adequate cardiac output: SBP >90 mm Hg, HR 60-100 bpm with NSR on ECG, PAP 20-30/8-15 mm Hg, PAWP 6-12 mm Hg, CVP 2-6 mm Hg, CO 4-7 L/min, CI 2.5-4.0 L/min/m^2, or all within 10% of baseline parameters.
- Monitor continuous ECG, noting onset, duration, pattern, termination of dysrhythmias, and response to antidysrhythmic drugs.
- Monitor VS for baseline status and prn for changes in cardiac rhythm, including PAP, PAWP, and CVP if PA catheter in place.
- Document dysrhythmias by saving rhythm strips. Use 12/18-lead ECG to diagnose new, symptomatic dysrhythmias.
- Note changes in Spo$_2$ with symptomatic dysrhythmias.
- Provide supplemental O$_2$ for symptomatic dysrhythmias.
- Monitor laboratory data to assess cause of dysrhythmias, particularly K$^+$, Mg^{2+}, and drug levels outside therapeutic range, as these may precipitate dysrhythmias.
- Initiate ACLS algorithms or institutional protocols for emergency.
- ↓ as many environmental stressors as possible, including noise and unpleasant interactions with others.

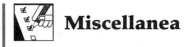 **Miscellanea**

CONSULT MD FOR
- Failure of dysrhythmia to respond to prescribed treatments
- Inappropriate "firing" of ICD device
- Failure to attain or exceeding of therapeutic antidysrhythmic drug level
- Worsening symptoms: chest pain, SOB, ↓ BP, altered mental status, Spo$_2$ <90%, and ↑ PAP, PAWP, or CVP
- Possible complications: heart failure, cardiac arrest, hypoxemia, new or worsening dysrhythmias, antidysrhythmic drug toxicity

RELATED TOPICS
- Cardiac surgery: CABG
- Cardiac surgery: valvular disorders
- Cardiomyopathy
- Coronary artery disease
- Drug overdose: cocaine
- Drug overdose: cyclic antidepressant
- Heart failure, left ventricular
- Hypokalemia
- Hypomagnesemia
- Myocardial infarction, acute

ABBREVIATIONS
EF: Ejection fraction
EP: Electrophysiologic
ICD: Implantable cardioverter/defibrillator
LGL: Lown-Ganong-Levine
PEA: Pulseless electrical activity
SNS: Sympathetic nervous system
WPW: Wolff-Parkinson-White

- If patient has chest pain, initiate appropriate management protocol.
- Remain with patient if new dysrhythmias or deterioration occurs; treat as prescribed, monitor response, and reassure patient.
- Administer medications that support CO and BP if antidysrhythmics and cardioversion are ineffective. Consider electrical therapies per ACLS algorithms.

Altered cerebral, renal, peripheral, and cardiopulmonary tissue perfusion r/t interrupted arterial blood flow to vital organs secondary to inadequate arterial pressure

Desired outcomes: Within 24 h of resuscitation, patient has adequate tissue perfusion: all vital parameters returned to within 10% of baseline or HR 60-100 bpm, SBP >90 mm Hg, RR 12-20 breaths/min, UO ≥0.5 ml/kg/h, oriented × 3, peripheral pulses ≥2+ on 0-4+ scale, brisk capillary refill (<2 sec), skin warm and dry.

- Check neurologic status q1-2h to assess cerebral perfusion.
- Monitor I&O qh to assess renal perfusion.
- Monitor ABGs as needed/prescribed to check pH for normalization postcode.
- Check serum lactate level to monitor for improvement of perfusion/tissue oxygenation.
- Monitor peripheral pulses, capillary refill, and skin q2h.
- Titrate vasoactive drugs, if needed, to maintain SBP >90 mm Hg.

REFERENCES

American Heart Association: *Textbook of advanced cardiac life support,* Dallas, 1994, The Association.

Collins MA: When your patient has an implantable cardioverter/defibrillator, *Am J Nurs* 94(3): 34-39, 1994.

Dunnington CS: Sotalol hydrochloride (Betapace): a new antidysrhythmic drug, *Am J Crit Care* 2(5): 397-406, 1993.

Dziadulewicz L: The use of atrial electrograms in the diagnosis of supraventricular dysrhythmias, *AACN Clin Issues in Crit Care Nurs* 3(1): 203-208, 1992.

Goodrich CA: Management of tachyarrhythmias in the CCU: *Curr Issues in Crit Care Nurs (Suppl):* 7-11, November 1995.

Keen J, Baird M, Allen J: *Mosby's critical care and emergency drug reference,* ed 2, St Louis, 1996, Mosby.

Porterfield LM: The cutting edge in arrhythmias, *Crit Care Nurse (Suppl):* June 1993.

Author: **Marianne Saunorus Baird**

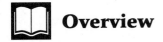 **Overview**

DESCRIPTION
Often required for suspected or confirmed infectious processes, which are a leading cause of death. Recently, ↑ in organisms resistant to antimicrobials has led to more conservative and restrictive use.

INAPPROPRIATE ANTIMICROBIAL USE
- Administration before culture collected (alters result)
- Prescription of multi-antibiotics or potent broad-spectrum antibiotics without considering appropriateness for specific infection site
- Failure to consult with infectious disease experts in choosing appropriate therapy
- Incomplete assessment of culture sensitivity/resistance panels that indicate need for change in therapy
- Not discontinuing antimicrobial as indicated by clinical findings
- Lack of understanding of appropriate blood concentration to limit development of resistance
- Failure to note toxic or side effects that are clouded by use of multiple antibiotics
- Failure to change to oral route when indicated

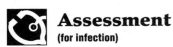 **Assessment**
(for infection)

PHYSICAL ASSESSMENT
Variable, depending on infection site
Neuro: Confusion, change in LOC
Resp: Thick, purulent sputum; coughing; adventitious breath sounds
GU: Cloudy, foul-smelling urine; frequent urination, burning
Integ: Incision or open wound with erythema, edema, tenderness, pain, warmth, irritation, presence of drainage

VITAL SIGNS/HEMODYNAMICS
RR: ↑
HR: ↑
BP: NI; ↓ if septicemic
Temp: ↑
CVP/PAWP: Usually ↓ because of insensible fluid loss or SIRS
CO: ↑ early; ↓ later if septicemic
SVR/MAP: ↓ if septicemic
ECG: NI or sinus tachycardia

LABORATORY STUDIES
C&S: Of sites suspected of infection/colonization
WBCs: ↑ with ↑ in number of band neutrophils on differential (shift to left)

IMAGING
X-ray: To r/o abscess, collection of purulent material
CT: To r/o abscess

DIAGNOSTIC PROCEDURE
Needle Aspiration of Fluid Collection, Abscess: Aspirate sent for culture

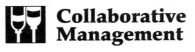 **Collaborative Management**

GENERAL
- Monitor incidence of antibiotic utilization (usually *via* pharmacy)
- Institute system of flagging/tracking susceptibility patterns of organisms (antibiogram) of the agency or of particular units (usually done by microbiology laboratory)

PHARMACOTHERAPY
Initiate after culture specimens obtained. Treatment options may be limited as a result of development of resistance to antimicrobials. Empirical treatment depends on suspected site of infection or acquisition.
Community-Acquired Infections: Usually gram-positive cocci or gram-negative bacilli. Eg, cefazolin or oxacillin and an aminoglycoside may be selected. Ciprofloxacin plus an antipseudomonal penicillin, such as piperacillin, is another frequently used combination.
Hospital-Associated Infections, Including Possible *Pseudomonas* Disorders: Usually managed with combination antibiotic therapy, an aminoglycoside and antipseudomonal penicillin.
Anaerobes: Clindamycin, penicillin, chloramphenicol, or metronidazole (Flagyl, mainly used for fungal infections), or imipenem/cilastatin (Primaxin).

SPECIFIC ANTIMICROBIAL AGENTS
Selected according to several criteria:
- Appropriateness for specific infection site
- Assessment of C&S panel
- Adverse effects in specific clients (eg, hypersensitivity, renal/hepatic insufficiency)
- Cost-savings, ease of use; compliance with prescribed regimen

Aminoglycosides: Amikacin, gentamicin, tobramycin. Potentially nephrotoxic, especially in patients with borderline renal function or if used concomitantly with cephalosporins. Qd administration will ↑ peak concentration for greater antimicrobial effectiveness.
Antipseudomonal Penicillins: Ticarcillin, azlocillin, mezlocillin, piperacillin. Piperacillin often chosen for its broader spectrum.
Antistaphylococcal Penicillins: Neutropenia and ↑ liver enzymes can result with high doses of oxacillin.
β-Lactamase Inhibiting Compounds: Clavulanate and sulbactam. Enhance activity of many antibiotics.
Cephalosporins: Cefazolin, cefoxitin, cefotetan, cefotaxime, ceftriaxone. Initial drug may be changed to less costly and more narrow spectrum cephalosporin after carefully evaluating susceptibility results.
Fluroquinolones: Ciprofloxacin, ofloxacin. Potent; may be administered orally.
Folate Synthesis Inhibitors:
Trimethoprim/sulfamethoxazole: inexpensive.
Glycopeptides: Vancomycin, teicoplanin. Vancomycin has been used inappropriately by providers. Now generally used only for serious infections with β-lactamase resistance and methicillin resistance. Its use may require approval according to preestablished guidelines or by infectious disease physician.

ANTIBIOTIC PROPHYLAXIS
May be indicated before/after invasive procedures, surgery, or trauma. Hospital guidelines should incorporate current recommendations of CDC, American College of Surgeons, and other authorities.

PATIENT-FAMILY TEACHING
- Purpose, need for appropriate use of antimicrobials; importance of compliance with prescribed administration details; reporting of side effects
- Importance of refraining from requesting antimicrobials when they are of questionable/no value (eg, ineffective for viral infections)
- Risk of development of resistance by organisms with overuse
- Major side effects that can occur with antimicrobial use and importance of reporting them (eg, phlebitis with IV administration, allergic reaction)
- CDC phone number: 404-329-1819; 404-329-3286

◼ Nursing Diagnoses/Interventions

Risk for infection r/t inadequate primary defenses secondary to interruption in skin integrity; invasive lines, drains, catheters; immunocompromised status
Desired outcome: Patient remains infection free: normothermia, WBCs <11,000 μl, negative C&S results, and no S&S of infection.
- Review susceptibility panels of culture reports. As needed, call microbiology laboratory for verbal report before posting computer/printed copy to chart.
- Review clinical findings of C&S reports with physician in relation to prescribed antimicrobials.
- Administer antimicrobials at prescribed intervals and over recommended duration of time to ensure maximal peak levels and consistent blood levels.
- Carefully monitor IV site and patient for allergic/adverse reactions during administration.
- Be aware of the potential for toxicity with impaired renal and hepatic function and that antimicrobial therapeutic regimens may be individualized in relation to renal or hepatic function.

 Miscellanea

CONSULT MD FOR
- Results of C&S studies, especially if antibiotic resistance present or infectious organism not sensitive to prescribed antibiotic
- New-onset S&S of infection while taking antibiotics: erythema, tenderness, induration, purulent drainage of wounds; change in color, appearance of sputum; temp >38.33° C (101° F); WBCs >11,000 μl

RELATED TOPICS
- Methicillin-resistant *Staphylococcus aureus*
- Pneumonia, hospital-associated
- Recomendations for isolation precautions in hospitals (see Appendix)
- Shock, septic
- Vancomycin-resistant enterococci

ABBREVIATION
SIRS: Systemic inflammatory response syndrome

REFERENCES
Garner JS, Hospital infection control practices advisory committee: Guidelines for isolation precautions in hospitals, *Infect Control Hosp Epidemiol* 17: 53-80, 1996.
US DHHR/CDC: Recommendations for preventing the spread of vancomycin resistance: recommendations of the Hospital Infection Control Practices Advisory Committee (HICPAC), *MMWR*, September 22, 1995.
Wenzel RP: *Prevention and control of nosocomial infections,* ed 2, Baltimore, 1993, Williams & Wilkins.

Author: **Janice Speas**

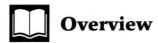 **Overview**

PATHOPHYSIOLOGY
Common psychologic reaction to stress in which feelings of uneasiness, apprehension, or dread occur in response to actual or perceived threat. Manifested on four levels: mild, moderate, severe, and panic. Mild and moderate anxiety may be effective coping strategies for stress.

HISTORY/RISK FACTORS
- Change in health status
- Actual or perceived threat of death, loss of loved one, loss of material possessions
- Neuropsychiatric disorders (phobias): eg, manic depression
- Unfamiliar people, change in environment
- Change in socioeconomic status
- Sensory overload/deprivation
- Threat to self-concept, roles, values
- Developmental transition
- Loss of body part

CLINICAL PRESENTATION
- Restlessness, irritability
- Tachypnea
- Rapid speech
- Tremors

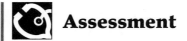 **Assessment**

PHYSICAL ASSESSMENT
Mild: Restlessness, irritability, ↑ questions, focusing on the environment
Moderate: Inattentiveness, expressions of concern, narrowed perceptions, insomnia, ↑ HR
Severe: Expression of feelings of doom; rapid speech, tremors, poor eye contact; preoccupation with the past; inability to understand the present; tachycardia, palpitations, nausea, clammy hands and skin, diaphoresis, hyperventilation
Panic: Inability to concentrate or communicate, distortion of reality, ↑ motor activity, vomiting, tachypnea

VITAL SIGNS/HEMODYNAMICS
RR: ↑
HR: ↑
BP: Slight ↑
Temp: NI
CVP/PAWP: NI
CO: Slight ↑
Other: CV response r/t endogenous catecholamine release

LABORATORY STUDY
ABGs: To exclude hypoxemia as contributing factor

Collaborative Management

Consultation: Psychologist, psychiatric clinical nurse specialist, chaplain, or OT, according to individual needs.
Pharmacotherapy: Sedatives/anxiolytics should not be used exclusively, but rather with appropriate nursing, mental health interventions.
Anxiolytics: Benzodiazepines relieve anxiety and produce sedation and sleep. Short-acting agents commonly used in ICU include lorazepam (Ativan) or midazolam (Versed).
Analgesics: Opiates and other analgesics used when pain a contributing factor.
Affective Touch: Expressive, personal, caring, comforting. May be positively or negatively perceived; influenced by cultural patterns.
Therapeutic Touch: Includes massage, acupressure, use of space around individual to mobilize energy fields.

PATIENT-FAMILY TEACHING
- Relaxation and imagery techniques
- Identification of adaptive coping behavior
- Purpose, expected results, anticipated sensations of nursing/medical interventions
- Medications: drug name, purpose, dosage, schedule, precautions, food-drug and drug-drug interactions, potential side effects

Nursing Diagnoses/Interventions

Anxiety r/t actual or perceived threat of death; change in health status; threat to self-concept, roles, values; unfamiliar people and environment; the unknown

Desired outcomes: Within 2 h of intervention, anxiety absent/↓ as evidenced by verbalization of same; HR ≤100 bpm; RR ≤20 breaths/min; absence of/↓ in irritability, restlessness.

- Engage in honest communication; provide empathetic understanding. Actively listen and establish an atmosphere that enables free expression.
- Assess level of anxiety. Be alert to verbal and nonverbal cues. For severe anxiety or panic state, refer to mental health team members as appropriate.
- If hyperventilation occurs, encourage slow, deep breathing by having patient mimic your own breathing pattern.
- Validate assessment of anxiety. ("You seem distressed; are you uncomfortable now?")
- After anxiety episode, review and discuss thoughts and feelings that led to the episode.
- Identify coping behaviors currently being used, eg, denial, anger, repression, withdrawal, daydreaming, or drug or alcohol dependence. Review coping behaviors used in the past. Assist in using adaptive coping to manage anxiety.
- Encourage expression of fears, concerns, questions.
- Introduce self, other team members; explain each individual's role as it relates to care map.

Sensory/Perceptual alterations r/t therapeutically or socially restricted environment; psychologic stress; altered sensory reception, transmission, integration; chemical alteration

Desired outcomes: At time of intervention, patient verbalizes orientation × 3, relates ability to concentrate, expresses satisfaction with sensory stimulation received.

- Assess factors contributing to sensory/perceptual alteration:
  Environmental: Excessive, constant, monotonous noise; restricted environment (immobility, traction, isolation); social isolation (restricted visitors, impaired communication); therapies
  Physiologic: Altered organ function, sleep or rest pattern disturbance, medication, previous hx of altered sensory perception
- Determine appropriate sensory stimulation needed; plan care accordingly.
- Control factors that contribute to environmental overload: eg, avoid constant lighting (maintain day-night patterns); ↓ noise whenever possible (eg, ↓ alarm volumes, avoid loud talking, keep room door closed, provide earplugs).
- Provide meaningful sensory stimulation:
  Display clocks, large calendars, and meaningful photographs and objects from home.
  Provide radio, music, reading materials. Earphones help block out external stimuli.
  Position patient toward window when possible.
  Discuss current events, time of day, topics of interest during patient care activities.
  As needed, orient to surroundings. Direct patient to reality as necessary.
  Establish personal contact by touch to promote, maintain contact with real environment.
  Encourage significant others to communicate with patient often, using nl tone of voice.
  Convey concern and respect. Introduce self, and call patient by name.
  Stimulate vision with mirrors, colored decorations, and pictures.
  Stimulate sense of taste with sweet, salty, and sour substances if appropriate.
  Encourage use of eyeglasses and hearing aids.
- Inform patient before initiating interventions and using equipment.
- Encourage participation in decision making; provide choice when possible.
- Assess sleep-rest pattern to evaluate its contribution to the sensory/perceptual disorder. Ensure that patient attains at least 90 min of uninterrupted sleep as frequently as possible.

Health-seeking behaviors: Relaxation technique effective for stress reduction and facilitation of ↓ sympathetic tone

Desired outcome: Within the 24 h after instruction, patient demonstrates relaxation technique.

- Explain that to ↓ sympathetic tone and anxiety, patient can practice relaxation response.
  1. Sit quietly in a comfortable position. Close your eyes.
  2. Relax all muscles, starting at feet and progressing to facial muscles.
  3. Breathe through your nose. As you breathe out, say the word "one" silently to yourself. Become aware of your breathing and continue for ≈ 20 min.
  4. Do not worry whether you are achieving a deep level of relaxation. Maintain a passive attitude and permit relaxation to occur at its own pace. Expect distractions to occur, but just ignore them. Continue breathing and repeating the word "one."
- Encourage this technique once or twice a day.

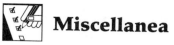 # Miscellanea

CONSULT MD FOR
- Severe or panic state

RELATED TOPICS
- Agitation syndrome
- Alterations in consciousness
- Psychosocial needs, family/significant others
- Psychosocial needs, patient

REFERENCES

Hall P: Critical care nursing: psychosocial aspects of care. In Burrell L (ed): *Adult nursing in hospital and community settings,* Norwalk, Conn, 1992, Appleton & Lange.

Kozier B et al: *Fundamentals of nursing: concepts, process, and practice,* ed 5, Redwood City, Calif, 1995, Addison-Wesley.

Lazarus R, Folkman S: *Stress: appraisal and coping,* New York, 1984, Springer.

Author: **Patricia Hall**

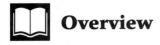 **Overview**

PATHOPHYSIOLOGY
Aneurysm: Most often develops at sites of atherosclerotic lesions. As lesions worsen, hemorrhage occurs, which weakens and dilates arterial wall. Tension ↑, producing even more dilatation. Acute hypertension may ↓ flow, leading to ischemia.

Dissection: Sudden and very serious threat to life because vessel disruption may continue along any arterial branch of the aorta, compromising the heart, brain, or kidneys. Likelihood of dissection ↑ dramatically when aneurysm size exceeds 6 cm.

INCIDENCE/MORTALITY
Approximately 2000 episodes occur annually, with mortality rate approaching 100% if dissection left untreated.

HISTORY/RISK FACTORS
- Hypertension, coarctation or medial necrosis of aorta
- Connective tissue disorders: eg, Marfan's or Ehlers-Danlos syndromes
- Blunt chest trauma
- Pregnancy
- Family hx of aortic aneurysm

CLINICAL PRESENTATION
- Sudden onset of severe, tearing chest or abdominal pain unrelieved by position or respiratory change. May radiate to back or neck.
- Vasovagal responses, S&S of heart failure, neurologic deficits may occur depending on involved arterial branches.

Assessment

PHYSICAL ASSESSMENT
Neuro: Confusion, lethargy, sensorimotor changes
Resp: Crackles, dyspnea if aortic valve/coronary arteries involved
CV: Pulse deficits or BP differences between extremities help identify site of dissection. If bleeding extends to pericardium, cardiac tamponade possible.
GI: ↓/absent bowel sounds, distention
GU: ↓ UO if dissection involves renal arteries

VITAL SIGNS/HEMODYNAMICS
RR: ↑
HR: ↑
BP: ↑, which may precipitate dissection; ↓ if trauma or rupture has occurred.
CO: Usually ↓; marked ↓ if trauma or rupture present.
CVP/PAWP: ↓ if hemorrhagic. PAWP ↑ if LV heart failure present as a result of very proximal dissection into coronary arteries/aortic valve.
SVR: Often ↑ as a result of hypertension.
Other: ↓ BP and pulses in one or both upper extremities signals involvement of subclavian arteries. ↓ BP, pulses in lower extremities suggest dissection into aortic bifurcation.

LABORATORY STUDIES
Hct/Hgb: To check for acute blood loss.
Chemistries/Cardiac Enzymes: Establishes baseline in event of compromise to heart, brain, kidneys.

IMAGING
Chest/Abdominal X-ray: Widening of aortic arch or descending aorta. Upright position necessary to demonstrate widening of mediastinum.
Echocardiography: Locates general site of dissection.
Aortogram or Digital Subtraction Angiogram: Locates actual site of tear and dissection *via* use of contrast material.
CT Scan: Often as useful as aortogram in locating dissection.

Collaborative Management

Antihypertensive Therapy: Initiated as soon as possible to prevent further aortic dissection. Usually nitroprusside started. After pressure control achieved, oral antihypertensive therapy begun.
Propranolol Therapy: To ↓ velocity of LV ejection, HR, and BP. Usually administered IV in increments of 1 mg at 5-min intervals until HR ↓ to 60-80 bpm.
Absolute Bed Rest: To prevent further dissection.
Pain Relief: IV morphine sulfate, 2-10 mg.
Sedation: To prevent sympathetic stimulation, which can ↑ BP.
Surgical Treatment: Recommended for proximal dissection, distal dissection when vital organ compromise occurs, impending rupture, or when pain and BP are refractory to medications. Involves removal of dissected vessel sections and replacement with Teflon grafts.

PATIENT-FAMILY TEACHING
- Relaxation techniques such as guided imagery or meditation to ↓ BP; avoidance of techniques that involve exercise, eg, progressive muscle relaxation
- Purpose, expected results, anticipated sensations of all nursing/medical interventions
- Importance of reporting immediately any ↑ or change in character or location of pain

Nursing Diagnoses/Interventions

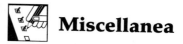 # Miscellanea

Altered peripheral, cardiopulmonary, renal, and cerebral tissue perfusion r/t interruption of arterial blood flow secondary to narrowed aortic lumen

Desired outcome: Within 48 h of this diagnosis, patient has adequate tissue perfusion: distal pulses bilaterally equal and >2+ on 0-4+ scale; brisk capillary refill (<2 sec); warm skin; bilaterally equal sensations in extremities; bilaterally equal SBP; BP wnl for patient; UO ≥0.5 ml/kg/h; equal and normoreactive pupils; and orientation × 3.

- Perform bilateral assessment of BP and distal pulses (particularly radial, femoral, and dorsalis pedis) qh during initial phase of dissection, and then q4h as condition stabilizes. Note changes in strength or symmetry of distal pulses. Correlate cuff pressures with arterial monitor recordings. Be alert to any change in color, capillary refill, and temp of each extremity.
- A difference in SBP between extremities >10 mm Hg could be a result of rupture or extension of the dissection.
- Monitor for paresthesias of the extremities, a sign of ↓ peripheral perfusion.
- Assess for signs of pericardial tamponade: JVD, muffled heart sounds, ↓ SBP (<90 mm Hg or >20 mm Hg drop in systolic trend), and paradoxical pulse.
- Assess CV status by monitoring heart rate and rhythm, ECG, and cardiac enzyme levels. Be alert for ST-segment changes and ↑ cardiac enzymes.
- Monitor UO qh. Be alert to sudden ↓, which could be caused by extension of the dissection.
- Assess neurologic status qh. Report restlessness and changes in LOC, pupil size, or reaction to light.

Pain r/t biophysical injury secondary to necrosis at aortic media and distal tissue hypoperfusion

Desired outcomes: Within 24-48 h of this diagnosis, subjective evaluation of pain improves, as documented by pain scale. Nonverbal indicators, such as grimacing, are ↓/absent.

- Monitor at frequent intervals for discomfort, rating discomfort from 0 (no pain) to 10 (severe pain). Medicate with analgesics.
- Teach relaxation techniques to use in conjunction with analgesics. Examples include guided imagery and meditation. Avoid progressive muscle relaxation, which may ↑ cardiac and aortic workload.
- During episodes of pain, assess for change in peripheral pulses or altered hemodynamics (ie, BP, PAP, PAWP, CO, SVR) because such changes often are associated with ↑ in aortic dissection.
- Control BP during episodes of pain by titrating nitroprusside, other vasodilators.
- Be alert to any ↑ in pain severity or change in location, which may signal need for emergency surgery.

CONSULT MD FOR

- ↓/absent femoral, radial, dorsal is pedal pulse, which could be caused by extension of dissection
- >10 mm Hg difference in SBP between extremities
- Signs of pericardial tamponade: JVD, muffled heart sounds, ↓ SBP (<90 mm Hg or >20 mm Hg drop in systolic trend), and paradoxical pulse
- UO <0.5 ml/kg/h × 2 h
- Altered mental status, pupillary response
- ↑ in severity or change in location of pain

RELATED TOPICS

- Aortic regurgitation
- Cardiac trauma
- Hemodynamic monitoring
- Hypertensive crisis
- Immobility, prolonged
- Pain

REFERENCES

Baas LS, Steuble, BT: Cardiovascular dysfunctions. In Swearingen PL, Keen JH (eds): *Manual of critical care nursing*, ed 3, St Louis, 1995, Mosby.

Gaudio C et al: Magnetic resonance imaging of aortic disease in the elderly, *Cardiol in the Elderly* 2(1): 9-13, 1994.

Hill EM: Perioperative management of patients with vascular disease, *AACN Clin Issues in Crit Care* 6(4): 547-561, 1995.

Kinney MR et al: *Comprehensive cardiac care*, ed 7, St Louis, 1996, Mosby.

Author: **Linda S. Baas**

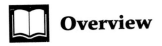 **Overview**

PATHOPHYSIOLOGY

Aortic valve insufficiency, allowing backward flow (regurgitation) and causing retrograde blood leakage into the left ventricle during diastole. LVEDV and LVEDP ↑, causing ventricular dilatation and, ultimately, LV failure. When chronic, EDV ↑, but pressure is not markedly ↑ because LV dilatation and hypertrophy are gradual. If acute, there is a dramatic ↑ in LVEDP with only a minor ↑ in LVEDV.

HISTORY/RISK FACTORS

- Rheumatic fever
- Rheumatoid arthritis
- Idiopathic valve calcification
- Infective endocarditis
- Marfan's syndrome
- Hypertension
- Thoracic aneurysm, aortic aneurysm/dissection
- Advanced age
- Trauma

CLINICAL PRESENTATION

May be asymptomatic for yrs and then present with chest pain, dyspnea on exertion, fatigue, exertional syncope. If acute, onset presentation will be severe LV failure with dyspnea at rest, anxiety, restlessness, pulmonary edema (coughing, frothy sputum, pallor, cyanosis).

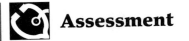 **Assessment**

PHYSICAL ASSESSMENT

Neuro: Weakness, fatigue, ↓ mental acuity
Resp: Tachypnea, dyspnea, crackles
CV: Diastolic blowing murmur at second ICS, RSB, beginning immediately with S_2; S_1 ↓/absent; presence of S_3; water hammer pulse (forceful, with rapidly collapsing peak)

VITAL SIGNS/HEMODYNAMICS

RR: ↑
HR: ↑
BP: ↑ SBP with widened pulse pressure; ↓ if failure severe
Temp: N/a
LVEDP: ↑
PAWP: ↑
CO: ↓
ECG: LV hypertrophy, especially in precordial leads; sinus tachycardia; conduction disturbances

IMAGING

Chest X-ray: If chronic, reveals boot-shaped cardiac silhouette resulting from LV dilation; if acute or decompensated, pulmonary congestion.
Echocardiography: Will show aortic valve incompetence; may reveal aortic valve calcification, ↑ LVEDV.

DIAGNOSTIC PROCEDURE

Cardiac Catheterization: To show extent of aortic regurgitation, LV function.

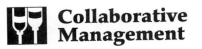 **Collaborative Management**

O₂: *Via* nasal cannula or other device; titrated to maintain SpO_2 ≥92%-96%. Mechanical ventilation may be necessary.
Low-Calorie Diet (if weight control necessary) and Low-Sodium Diet: Sodium limited to ↓ fluid retention. Fluids may be limited to 1500 ml/day.
Pharmacotherapy
Digitalis glycosides: When symptoms of LV failure ensue.
Diuretics: To ↓ intravascular volume and ↓ preload.
Vasodilators: Oral or parenteral agents to ↓ afterload.
Inotropic agents: Dobutamine, milrinone, amrinone to improve myocardial contractility.
Antibiotic prophylaxis: Penicillin or other antibiotic taken before dental, surgical, other invasive procedure to prevent valvular infection, endocarditis, septicemia.
Valve Replacement: Performed for moderate to severe disease; mortality rate ≈ 6%. Heterograft (pig, cow tissue) or mechanical valve used. Valve surgery ↑ risk for thrombosis and embolism (particularly with mechanical mitral valves and A-fib) and for valvular endocarditis.

PATIENT-FAMILY TEACHING

- Physiologic process of LV heart failure; how fluid volume ↑ because of poor heart functioning
- Importance of low-sodium diet and medications to help ↓ volume overload; how to read and evaluate food labels
- S&S of fluid volume excess that necessitate medical attention: irregular or slow pulse, ↑ SOB, orthopnea, ↓ exercise tolerance, steady weight gain (≥1 kg/day for 2 successive days with nl eating)
- Purpose/procedure/expected results for valve replacement surgery
- Warning signals to stop activity and rest: chest pain, SOB, dizziness or faintness, unusual weakness
- Importance of antibiotic prophylaxis
- Need for Medic-Alert bracelet
- Phone number for American Heart Association: 1-800-242-8721

Nursing Diagnoses/Interventions

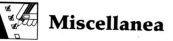 ## Miscellanea

Decreased cardiac output r/t negative inotropic changes in the heart secondary to myocardial cellular destruction and dilatation

Desired outcomes: Within the 24-h period before discharge from CCU, patient has adequate cardiac output: SBP ≥90 mm Hg; CO 4-7 L/min; CI 2.5-4 L/min/m²; RR 12-20 breaths/min; HR ≤100 bpm; UO ≥0.5 ml/kg/h; I = O + insensible losses; warm and dry skin; orientation × 3; PAWP ≤18 mm Hg; and RAP 4-6 mm Hg.

- Assess for the following factors associated with ↓ CO and LV congestion: JVD, dependent edema, hepatomegaly, fatigue, weakness, ↓ activity level, SOB with activity. Additional S&S include:

  Mental status: Restlessness, ↓ responsiveness
  Lung sounds: Crackles, rhonchi, wheezes
  Heart sounds: Gallop, murmur, and ↑ HR
  Urinary output: UO <0.5 ml.kg/h × 2 consecutive h
  Skin: Pallor, mottling, cyanosis, coolness, diaphoresis
  Vital signs: SBP <90 mm Hg, HR >100 bpm, RR >20 breaths/min, ↑ temp

- Be alert to PAWP >18 mm Hg and RAP >6 mm Hg. Although nl PAWP is 6-12 mm Hg, these patients usually need ↑ filling pressures for adequate preload, with PAWP at 15-18 mm Hg.
- Measure CO/CI q2-4h and prn. Adjust therapy to maintain CO within 4-7 L/min and CI at 2.5-4 L/min/m².
- Monitor I&O and weigh patient qd, noting trends. Strict fluid restriction (eg, 1000 ml/day) often prescribed.
- Minimize cardiac workload by assisting with ADL when necessary.
- Monitor for compensatory mechanisms, including ↑ HR and BP caused by sodium and water retention.
- Administer medications as prescribed. Observe for the following desired effects:

  Vasodilators: ↓ BP, ↓ SVR, ↑ CO/CI
  Diuretics: ↓ PAWP
  Inotropes: ↑ CO/CI, ↑ BP

- Be alert to the following undesirable effects:

  Vasodilators: Hypotension, headache, nausea, vomiting, dizziness
  Diuretics: Weakness, hypokalemia
  Inotropes: Dysrhythmias, headache, angina

- Position according to comfort level.

Activity intolerance r/t imbalance between O_2 supply and demand secondary to ↓ myocardial contractility

Desired outcome: Within 12-24 h before discharge from CCU, patient exhibits cardiac tolerance to ↑ levels of activity: RR <24 breaths/min, NSR on ECG, BP within 20 mm Hg of nl for patient, HR within 20 bpm of patient's resting HR, peripheral pulses >2+ on 0-4+ scale, and absence of chest pain.

- Plan nursing care to enable extended (at least 90 min) periods of rest.
- Monitor physiologic response to activity, reporting any symptoms of chest pain, new or ↑ SOB, ↑ in HR >20 bpm above resting HR, and ↑ or ↓ in SBP >20 mm Hg.
- To prevent complications of immobility, perform or teach patient and significant others active, passive, and assistive ROM exercises.

CONSULT MD FOR

- Inability to maintain Spo_2 ≥92% despite supplemental O_2
- Deteriorating cardiac performance: new onset S_3 or summation gallop, murmur, dysrhythmias, frothy sputum, crackles, sustained hypotension
- Unacceptable hemodynamics: CO <4 L/min, PAWP >18 mm Hg, SVR >1200 dynes/sec/cm^{-5}, MAP <70 mm Hg
- UO <0.5 mg/kg/h × 2 consecutive h
- Complications: pulmonary edema, cardiogenic shock, unrelieved chest pain, ECG evidence of ischemia

RELATED TOPICS

- Cardiac surgery: valvular disorders
- Endocarditis, infective
- Heart failure, left ventricular

ABBREVIATIONS

EDV: End-diastolic volume
ICS: Intercostal space
LVEDP: Left ventricular end-diastolic pressure
LVEDV: Left ventricular end-diastolic volume
RSB: Right sternal border

REFERENCES

Dracub K, Dunbar SB, Baker DW: Rethinking heart failure, *Am J Nurs* 95(7): 22-28, 1995.

Roelandt JRT, Meeter K: Diagnosis and management of valvular heart disease in the elderly, *Cardiol in the Elderly* 1(3): 235-243, 1993.

Steuble BT: Valvular heart disease. In Swearingen PL, Keen JH (eds): *Manual of critical care nursing*, ed 3, St Louis, 1995, Mosby.

Treasure T: The pulmonary autograft as an aortic valve replacement, *Lancet:* 343, May 28, 1994.

Vitello-Cicciu J, Lapsley D: Valvular heart disease. In Kinney M, Packa D, Dunbar S: *AACN's clinical reference for critical care nursing*, ed 3, 1993, St Louis, Mosby.

Author: **Barbara Tueller Steuble**

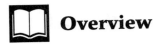

Overview

PATHOPHYSIOLOGY
Obstruction to forward flow (stenosis) from left ventricle across the aortic valve, usually caused by congenital factors. As ventricular blood flow is obstructed by the stenotic valve, intramyocardial wall tension ↑ to enable heart to pump blood through the highly resistant valve opening. If unrelieved, stenosis results in LV failure and pulmonary congestion/edema. Ventricular hypertrophy and high intramyocardial wall tension result in ↓ endocardial blood flow, often triggering angina and ventricular dysrhythmias.

HISTORY/RISK FACTORS
- Congenital heart disease
- Degenerative sclerosing, thickening, calcification of valve leaflets
- Atherosclerotic heart disease
- Male gender
- Advanced age

CLINICAL PRESENTATION
Chest pain, syncope, dyspnea, exertional angina, dizziness, palpitations, anxiety

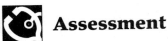

Assessment

PHYSICAL ASSESSMENT
Neuro: Weakness, fatigue, ↓ mental acuity
Resp: Tachypnea, dyspnea with exertion, crackles
CV: Systolic, blowing murmur at second ICS, RSB; may radiate to neck; thrill, paradoxical splitting of S_2, slow carotid arterial uptake
Integ: Skin over shins shiny and hairless

VITAL SIGNS/HEMODYNAMICS
RR: ↑
HR: ↑
BP: *If nl DBP:* widened pulse pressure. *If decompensated:* narrow pulse pressure, ↓ MAP.
PAWP: ↑
LVEDP: ↑
Other: Decompensation produces ↓ LV stroke volume with narrow pulse pressure and markedly ↓ CO

ECG: NSR with LV hypertrophy; if severe, LA hypertrophy; conduction abnormalities: first degree AV block, bundle branch block

IMAGING
Chest X-ray: Identifies LV hypertrophy, calcification of aortic valve cusps, and possibly cardiomegaly.
Echocardiography: Reveals LV wall thickening, dilatation; impaired movement of aortic valve.

DIAGNOSTIC PROCEDURE
Cardiac Catheterization: Determines severity of obstruction; assesses LV function, coronary arterial filling. Pressure gradient between left ventricle and aorta >50 mm Hg.

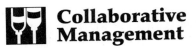

Collaborative Management

O₂: *Via* nasal cannula or other device; titrated to maintain SpO_2 ≥92%-96%. Mechanical ventilation may be necessary.

PHARMACOTHERAPY
Digitalis Glycosides: Used if patient has ↑ LV volume or ↓ EF.
Diuretics: Used cautiously, since hypovolemia may ↓ elevated LVEDP and then ↓ CO, causing orthostatic hypotension.
Antidysrhythmics: Usually not necessary. May be used for A-fib, which requires treatment, since loss of atrial contraction further ↓ CO. β Blockers and other myocardial depressants avoided.
Vasodilators: Nitroprusside may be used cautiously for afterload reduction.
Antibiotic Prophylaxis: Penicillin or other antibiotic taken before dental, surgical, other invasive procedure to prevent endocarditis.

SURGICAL PROCEDURES
IABP: For severe LV failure; augments diastolic coronary arterial filling.
Valve Replacement: For moderate to severe disease; mortality rate ≈6%. Heterograft (pig, cow tissue) or mechanical valve used. Valve surgery ↑ risk for thrombosis and embolism (particularly with mechanical mitral valves and in A-fib) and for valvular endocarditis.

PBV: For dilatation of stenotic heart valves when surgery an unacceptable alternative. Catheter passed into femoral artery to measure supravalvular and LV pressures before valvuloplasty. Balloon valvuloplasty catheter is then passed over guidewire into left ventricle and then inflated 3 times for 12-30 sec. If successful, results in significant improvement in valve gradient and blood flow across the valve.
Complications: Cerebral embolization, disruption of valve ring, acute valve regurgitation, valvular restenosis, hemorrhage at catheter insertion site, guidewire perforation of left ventricle, dysrhythmias.
Commissurotomy: Stenotic valve opened by a dilating instrument. When performed early in disease course, chances of success good; however, may result in valve regurgitation and recurrent stenosis.

PATIENT-FAMILY TEACHING
- Physiologic process of LV heart failure; how fluid volume ↑ because of poor heart functioning
- Importance of low-sodium diet and medications to help ↓ volume overload; how to read and evaluate food labels
- S&S of fluid volume excess necessitating medical attention: irregular or slow pulse, ↑ SOB, orthopnea, ↓ exercise tolerance, steady weight gain (≥1 kg/day for 2 successive days)
- If taking digitalis, technique for measuring HR; parameters for holding digitalis (usually for HR <60/min) and notifying physician
- Purpose/procedure/expected results for valve replacement surgery, PBV, commissurotomy as applicable
- Importance of avoiding activities that require straining; use of stool softeners, bulk-forming agents, laxatives as needed
- Warning signals to stop activity and rest: chest pain, SOB, dizziness or faintness, unusual weakness; use of prophylactic NTG
- Importance of antibiotic prophylaxis
- Phone number for American Heart Association: 1-800-242-8721

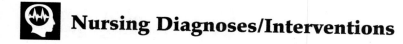 **Nursing Diagnoses/Interventions**

Decreased cardiac output r/t negative inotropic changes in the heart secondary to myocardial cellular destruction and dilatation

Desired outcomes: Within the 24-h period before discharge from CCU, patient has adequate cardiac output: SBP ≥90 mm Hg; CO 4-7 L/min; CI 2.5-4 L/min/m^2; RR 12-20 breaths/min; HR ≤100 bpm; UO ≥0.5 ml/kg/h; I = O + insensible losses; warm and dry skin; orientation × 3; PAWP ≤18 mm Hg; and RAP 4-6 mm Hg.

- Assess for these factors associated with ↓ CO: JVD, dependent edema, hepatomegaly, fatigue, weakness, ↓ activity level, SOB with activity. Additional S&S include:
  Mental status: Restlessness, ↓ responsiveness
  Lung sounds: Crackles, rhonchi, wheezes
  Heart sounds: Gallop, murmur, ↑ HR
  Urinary output: UO <0.5 ml/kg/h × 2 consecutive h
  Skin: Pallor, mottling, cyanosis, coolness, diaphoresis
  Vital signs: SBP <90 mm Hg, HR >100 bpm, RR >20 breaths/min, ↑ temp
- Be alert to PAWP >18 mm Hg and RAP >6 mm Hg. Although nl PAWP is 6-12 mm Hg, these patients usually need ↑ filling pressures for adequate preload, with PAWP at 15-18 mm Hg.
- Measure CO/CI q2-4h and prn. Adjust therapy to maintain CO within 4-7 L/min and CI at 2.5-4 L/min/m^2.
- Monitor I&O and weigh patient qd, noting trends. Strict fluid restriction (eg, 1000 ml/day) often prescribed.
- Minimize cardiac workload by assisting with ADL when necessary.
- Monitor for compensatory mechanisms, including ↑ HR and BP caused by sodium and water retention.
- Administer medications as prescribed. Observe for the following desired effects:
  Vasodilators: ↓ BP, ↓ SVR, ↑ CO/CI
  Diuretics: ↓ PAWP
  Inotropes: ↑ CO/CI, ↑ BP
- Be alert to the following undesirable effects:
  Vasodilators: Hypotension, headache, nausea, vomiting, dizziness
  Diuretics: Weakness, hypokalemia
  Inotropes: Dysrhythmias, headache, angina
- Position according to comfort level.

Activity intolerance r/t imbalance between O$_2$ supply and demand secondary to ↓ myocardial contractility

Desired outcome: Within 12-24 h before discharge from CCU, patient exhibits cardiac tolerance to ↑ levels of activity: RR <24 breaths/min, NSR on ECG, BP within 20 mm Hg of nl for patient, HR within 20 bpm of patient's resting HR, peripheral pulses >2+ on 0-4+ scale, and absence of chest pain.

- Plan nursing care to enable extended (at least 90 min) periods of rest.
- Monitor physiologic response to activity, reporting any symptoms of chest pain, new or ↑ SOB, ↑ in HR >20 bpm above resting HR, and ↑ or ↓ in SBP >20 mm Hg.
- To prevent complications of immobility, perform or teach patient and significant others active, passive, and assistive ROM exercises.

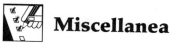 **Miscellanea**

CONSULT MD FOR
- LV failure: crackles, dyspnea, S$_3$ gallop, fatigue
- ↓ CO: dizziness, syncope, angina, UO <0.5 ml/kg/h, which suggests cardiac decompensation
- Narrowing pulse pressure (widened pulse pressure expected)
- New-onset dysrhythmias, conduction abnormalities

RELATED TOPICS
- Cardiac surgery: valvular disorders
- Endocarditis, infective
- Heart failure, left ventricular
- Hemodynamic monitoring
- Percutaneous balloon valvuloplasty

ABBREVIATIONS
EF: Ejection fraction
IABP: Intraaortic balloon pump
ICS: Intercostal space
LVEDP: Left ventricular end-diastolic pressure
LVEDV: Left ventricular end-diastolic volume
PBV: Percutaneous balloon valvuloplasty
RSB: Right sternal border

REFERENCES
Davis JS, Small BM: Advances in the treatment of aortic stenosis across the lifespan, *Nurs Clin North Am* 30(2): 317-332, 1995.

Lindroos M: Clinical signs of aortic valve stenosis in old age, *Cardiol in the Elderly* 1(4): 295-301, 1993.

Roelandt JRT, Meeter K: Diagnosis and management of valvular heart disease in the elderly, *Cardiol in the Elderly* 1(3): 235-243, 1993.

Steuble BT: Valvular heart disease. In Swearingen PL, Keen JH (eds): *Manual of critical care nursing,* ed 3, St Louis, 1995, Mosby.

Vitello-Cicciu J, Lapsley D: Valvular heart disease. In Kinney M, Packa D, Dunbar S: *AACN's clinical reference for critical care nursing,* ed 3, 1993, St Louis, Mosby.

Author: **Barbara Tueller Steuble**

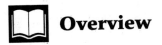 **Overview**

PATHOPHYSIOLOGY

Hyperreactive bronchial airways respond to irritants with diffuse narrowing and bronchial inflammation causing mucosal edema, ↑ mucus production, and plugging. If bronchospasms not reversed after 24-h maximum doses of β-agonist and theophylline therapy, SA is diagnosed. V/Q mismatch occurs as poorly ventilated alveoli continue to be perfused. Shunting of blood from nonventilated alveoli to other alveoli cannot compensate for ↓ ventilation, and hypoxia occurs. Tachypnea and tachycardia associated with ↑ O_2 requirements and ↑ WOB.

COMPLICATIONS

Respiratory collapse, death by asphyxiation

HISTORY/RISK FACTORS

- Asthma
- Reactive airways
- Respiratory infection
- Allergens (airborne or ingested)
- Chemical irritants (smoke, air pollution)
- Physical irritants (cold air, exercise)
- Emotional stress
- Dehydration

CLINICAL PRESENTATION

- Onset usually gradual
- ↑ sputum production, coughing, wheezing, dyspnea over several days
- ↑ WOB: ↑ insensible water loss *via* exhaled water vapor, diaphoresis ↓ oral intake (contributes to hypovolemia)
- Mucosal edema, tenacious secretions
- Insomnia, anorexia, restlessness

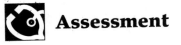 **Assessment**

PHYSICAL ASSESSMENT

Neuro: ↓ LOC, confusion, disorientation, agitation
Resp: Tachypnea, use of accessory muscles, chest retractions, nasal flaring, ↓ tactile fremitus, hyperresonance, dullness over areas of atelectasis, expiratory wheezing, prolonged expiratory phase, coarse rhonchi, cyanosis (late sign). Absence of wheezing may result from severe bronchial constriction. When air volume moved through airways so minimal that it does not cause a sound, respiratory collapse imminent.
CV: Tachycardia, hypotension, paradoxical pulse (>10 mm Hg)
Integ: Diaphoresis

VITAL SIGNS/HEMODYNAMICS

RR: ↑
HR: ↑
BP: ↓
Temp: Nl; or ↑ with infection
CVP/PAWP: ↓ with dehydration; ↑ with pulmonary hypertension
CO: ↓, nl, or ↑ depending on catecholamine stimulation, hydration
SVR: ↑ in response to hypovolemia (eg, with chronic lung disease)

LABORATORY STUDIES

ABGs: Initially Pao_2 nl, then ↓. Usually $Paco_2$ ↓ in early stages. When $Paco_2$ nl or > nl, respiratory failure may be imminent because of relative hypoventilation.
Spo_2: Optimal values ≥90%.
Sputum: Gross examination shows ↑ viscosity or actual mucous plugs. C&S may show microorganisms with infection.
CBC: ↑ eosinophils in patients not receiving corticosteroids. Hct may be ↓ because of hypovolemia.
Serum Theophylline Level: Therapeutic range is 10-20 mg/ml.

DIAGNOSTIC PROCEDURES

Pulmonary Function Testing: FEV, peak flow ↓ during acute episodes.
ECG: Usually tachycardia; bronchodilators (eg, metaproterenol) produce dysrhythmias.

IMAGING

Chest X-ray: Usually shows lung hyperinflation; may r/o other causes of respiratory failure.

Collaborative Management

O_2 Therapy: High doses indicated unless chronic CO_2 retention present. Titrate to maintain Spo_2 90%-94%. Use nasal cannula if possible; progress to Venturi or nonrebreathing mask if necessary to maintain adequate Spo_2. Humidify O_2 to help liquefy secretions.

Intubation and Mechanical Ventilation:
Elected if $Paco_2$ continues to ↑, if Pao_2 ↓ to <60 mm Hg, or if intolerable respiratory distress occurs.

Pharmacotherapy

Bronchodilators: Dilate smooth muscles of the airways. Given IV, eg, aminophylline, magnesium sulfate; or SC, eg, terbutaline, epinephrine. Aerosolized medications, eg, albuterol (Proventil), isoetharine (Bronkosol), not used until parenteral medications promote sufficient bronchodilation to enable gas flow and thus distribution of inhaled bronchodilators.

Corticosteroids: Given IV to ↓ inflammatory response. Dosage varies according to severity of episode and whether steroids being taken. Acute adrenal insufficiency can develop if steroids routinely taken at home but not during hospitalization.

Sedatives and tranquilizers: Avoided unless patient extremely agitated and unable to cooperate with therapy. These agents depress CNS response to hypoxia, hypercapnia, and airway obstruction.

Antibiotics: Given if infectious pulmonary process suspected.

Fluid Replacement: Crystalloids used to replace insensible losses.

PATIENT-FAMILY TEACHING

- Pursed-lip breathing technique:
    Inhale through nose.
    Form lips in "O" shape as if whistling.
    Exhale slowly through pursed lips.
- Effective cough (see **Ineffective airway clearance**)
- Medications: drug name, purpose, dosage, schedule, precautions, food-drug and drug-drug interactions, potential side effects
- Progressive relaxation, other stress reduction techniques
- Purpose, expected results, anticipated sensations of nursing/medical interventions

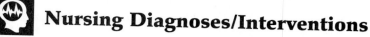

Nursing Diagnoses/Interventions

Impaired gas exchange r/t altered O_2 supply secondary to ↓ alveolar ventilation present with narrowed airways

Desired outcome: Within 2-4 h of treatment initiation, patient has adequate gas exchange: Pao_2 >60 mm Hg, $Paco_2$ 35-45 mm Hg, and pH 7.35-7.45. Within 24-48 h of treatment initiation, RR 12-20 breaths/min with eupnea, and breath sounds clear and bilaterally equal.

- Monitor for hypoxia: restlessness, agitation, changes in LOC. Remember that cyanosis is a late sign.
- Position to promote optimal gas exchange, usually high-Fowler's position with patient leaning forward and elbows propped on over-the-bed table.
- Monitor for ↓ breath sounds, wheezes, rhonchi. Progression to ↓ breath sounds/absence of wheezing may signal severe bronchoconstriction and minimal air flow.
- Administer humidified O_2 as prescribed. Monitor ABGs, Spo_2. Be alert to ↓ Pao_2, ↑ $Paco_2$, and ↓ saturation levels, which are signals of respiratory compromise.

Ineffective airway clearance r/t presence of ↑ tracheobronchial secretions and ↓ ability to expectorate secondary to fatigue

Desired outcome: Within 24-48 h of treatment initiation, patient's airway free of excess secretions: presence of eupnea and absence of adventitious breath sounds and excessive coughing.

- Assess ability to clear secretions. Keep emergency suction equipment at bedside.
- Encourage oral fluid intake to help ↓ secretion viscosity.
- Encourage effective cough:
    Take several deep breaths.
    After last inhalation, cough 3-4 times on same exhalation until most of air expelled.
    Repeat several times until cough becomes productive.
- After crisis phase is resolved, implement chest physiotherapy with postural drainage.

Anxiety r/t actual or perceived threat of death, hypoxemia, fear of unknown

Desired outcomes: Within 1-2 h of intervention, anxiety absent or ↓ as evidenced by patient's verbalization of same, HR ≤100 bpm, RR ≤20 breaths/min, absence of/↓ irritability and restlessness.

- Assess level of anxiety. Be alert to verbal and nonverbal cues.
    Mild: Restlessness, irritability
    Moderate: Narrowed perceptions, insomnia, ↑ HR
    Severe: Rapid speech, tremors, palpitations, hyperventilation
    Panic: Inability to concentrate or communicate, distortion of reality, increased motor activity, vomiting, tachypnea
- Encourage expression of fears, concerns, and questions.
- Reduce sensory overload by providing an organized, quiet environment.
- Enable support persons to be in attendance whenever possible.
- For severe anxiety, refer to psychiatric clinical nurse specialist, case manager, or other health-team members as appropriate.
- Review coping behaviors used in past. Assist in using adaptive coping to manage anxiety.

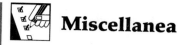

Miscellanea

CONSULT MD FOR

- ↓ breath sounds, especially with progression from loud to soft/absent wheezing
- Failure to maintain Spo_2 of 90%-92%
- Imminent respiratory collapse: cyanosis of lips, nail beds; Pao_2 <60 mm Hg with 100% Fio_2; ↑ $Paco_2$ despite therapy

RELATED TOPICS

- Mechanical ventilation
- Pneumonia, community-acquired and hospital-associated
- Respiratory failure, acute

ABBREVIATION

FEV: Forced expiratory volume

REFERENCES

Borkgren MW, Gronkiewicz GA: Update your asthma care from hospital to home, *Am J Nurs* 95(1): 26-35, 1995.

Busse WW: The effect of treatment with corticosteroids on asthma airway structure and function, *Chest* 107(3): 1365-1385, 1995.

Eisenbeis C: Full partner in care: teaching your patient how to manage her asthma, *Nursing* 26(1): 48-51, 1996.

Howard C: Respiratory dysfunctions. In Swearingen PL, Keen JH (eds): *Manual of critical care nursing*, ed 3, St Louis, 1995, Mosby.

Thompson J, Grathwohn K: Misuse of metered-dose inhalers in hospitalized patients, *Chest* 105(3): 715-717, 1994.

Author: **Cheri A. Goll**

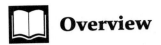 **Overview**

PATHOPHYSIOLOGY

Cardiac dysrhythmia wherein chaotic "firing" of numerous atrial pacing sites generates atrial quivering rather than contraction. Ventricular rate response varies from bradycardia to tachycardia or a controlled rate of 60-100 bpm. Without atrial contraction, VEDV may ↓ 10%-40%, resulting in ↓ CO. Lack of atrial contraction results in blood stasis and possibly atrial clot formation, potentially leading to embolization. A-fib may become chronic, necessitating measures to ↓ atrial clot formation.

HISTORY/RISK FACTORS

- CAD (and its risk factors), MI
- Angina, myocardial ischemia
- Atrial enlargement, valvular disease
- Frequent PACs or A-flutter
- Use of caffeine/other stimulants
- Use of quinidine

CLINICAL PRESENTATION

Activity intolerance/unusual fatigue, SOB, chest pain, nausea, syncope, or diaphoresis if CO ↓ >10%. Often asymptomatic with controlled ventricular response.

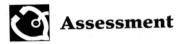 **Assessment**

PHYSICAL ASSESSMENT

Neuro: Altered LOC, syncope, weakness, fainting, vertigo, anxiety, restlessness
Resp: Dyspnea, SOB
CV: Chest discomfort, activity intolerance, sense of "pounding" in chest, hypotension
GI: Nausea, vomiting, epigastric pressure
GU: Possible ↓ UO
Integ: Diaphoresis, pallor, cyanosis

VITAL SIGNS/HEMODYNAMICS

RR: NI or ↑
HR: ↑
BP: NI, ↑, or ↓
Temp: NI
CVP/PAWP: NI, ↑, or ↓
SVR: ↑
CO: ↓
12/18-Lead ECG: Rhythm irregularly irregular, atrial rate >350 bpm, ventricular rate variable, P waves "f" (fibrillatory) and manifested as wavy baseline, PR interval and P:QRS cannot be determined, QRS of nl duration (unless bundle branch block present).

Ambulatory/24-h Holter Monitoring: May reveal onset of rhythm (if new onset) and changes in ventricular rate/response with activity and over time.

LABORATORY STUDIES

Serum Electrolytes: To identify abnormalities (eg, ↓ K$^+$, Mg^{2+}) that could precipitate atrial dysrhythmias.
Therapeutic Drug Levels: Monitoring of antidysrhythmic levels to control rhythm and prevent toxicity. Other medications, eg, those used for hypertension and respiratory disorders, also may precipitate A-fib.
Drug/Toxicology Screening: Amphetamines, cocaine, other stimulants can precipitate A-fib.
ABGs: Checks for hypoxemia and pH abnormalities that may interfere with electrolyte balance.

IMAGING

Chest X-ray: May reflect enlarged cardiac silhouette reflective of heart disease.
Echocardiography: Evaluates CO and myocardial contractility/pumping, with calculation of ventricular EF.
Cardiac Catheterization: To assess for CAD.

DIAGNOSTIC PROCEDURES

EP Study: Administers pacing stimuli at multiple sites with varying voltages to discern appropriate drug therapy to manage dysrhythmia.
Atrial Electrogram: Uses temporary epicardial pacing wires or skin electrodes to record atrial electrical activity, including pacing and conduction.

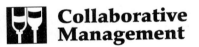 **Collaborative Management**

GENERAL

Supplemental O$_2$: To support tissue oxygenation.
Spo$_2$: To monitor O$_2$ saturation changes resulting from dysrhythmia.
Rapid Atrial/Antitachycardia Pacing: Specialized pulse generator (pacemaker) used to exceed HR, attain capture, and then slowly ↓ HR. When successful, fibrillatory sites overridden by pacer and HR is controlled.
Diet: Recurrent dysrhythmias may necessitate low-fat, low-cholesterol, ↓-caffeine diet.
Synchronized Cardioversion: May be used to convert A-fib back to sinus rhythm in unstable patients or in those who cannot be converted with drug therapy alone.

PHARMACOTHERAPY

Toxicity/overdose of antidysrhythmics may lead to lethal dysrhythmias; therefore lowest dose should be used. Goal: to stabilize atrial pacing to one site to facilitate nl cardiac cycle with adequate CO and BP.

β Blockers: To ↓ rapid ventricular HR and ↓ cardiac irritability associated with A-fib.
Metoprolol (Lopressor): 5 mg slowly IV, repeated q5min to total of 15 mg.
Propranolol (Inderal): 1-3 mg IV push at ≤1 mg/min. May repeat × 1 after 2 min as needed.
Atenolol (Tenormin): 5 mg IV push at ≤1 mg/min. Wait 10 min. Repeat dose if needed.
Calcium Blockers: To alter cardiac action potential to ↓ rapid ventricular HR associated with A-fib. These drugs avoided in accessory conduction pathways (ie, WPW).
Diltiazem (Cardizem): 15-20 mg slow IV push over 2 min. May repeat at 20-25 mg slow IV push if needed. Begin infusion at 5-15 mg/h and titrate to control HR.
Other Antidysrhythmics
Digoxin: To slow conduction through AV node for nonemergency management of A-fib, thus ↓ HR and ↑ contractility. *Loading dose:* total of 10 μg/kg divided into four doses over 24 h. Cardioversion avoided if patient is receiving digitalis therapy.
Procainamide (Pronestyl): 20-30 mg IV infusion until dysrhythmia suppressed, BP ↓, QRS widens >50%, or a total of 17 mg/kg given.
Anticoagulants: May be used for chronic A-fib to prevent clot formation in atria.

SURGERY

ICD: Programmed to deliver synchronized cardioversion or defibrillation when HR > programmed rate or abnormal ECG morphology present. Newer devices include cardiac pacing. May not be effective in controlling A-fib.

PATIENT-FAMILY TEACHING

- Importance of reporting all adverse symptoms
- Cause of and electrical devices used to treat rhythm
- Relaxation techniques for controlling environmental stress
- Prescribed diet, particularly caffeine reduction
- Altered sexuality and support groups if patient has ICD placed
- Medications: drug name, dosage, purpose, schedule, precautions, drug-drug and food-drug interactions, and potential side effects

Nursing Diagnoses/Interventions

Decreased cardiac output r/t altered rate, rhythm, conduction, or negative inotropic changes
Desired outcomes: Within 15 min of onset of A-fib with resultant instability of VS, patient is converted to a rhythm with adequate CO. VS return to within 10% of baseline.

- Implement continuous ECG monitoring, noting onset, duration, and pattern of A-fib, including response to medication.
- Monitor VS q5-15min when patient unstable and per routine if patient stable. Include hemodynamic parameters if PA catheter in use.
- Document dysrhythmias *via* rhythm strips.
- Provide supplemental O_2 for symptomatic dysrhythmias, noting SpO_2.
- Initiate ACLS algorithms or institutional protocols for emergencies.
- Remain with patient and treat new symptomatic dysrhythmias as prescribed/per protocol, using ACLS guidelines.
- ↓ as many stressors as possible in patient's environment.
- Administer medications to support CO and BP if antidysrhythmics and cardioversion ineffective.

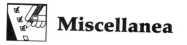 # Miscellanea

CONSULT MD FOR
- Failure of dysrhythmia to respond to prescribed treatments
- Inappropriate "firing" of ICD device
- Failure to attain/exceeding of therapeutic drug level
- Chest pain, SOB, ↓ BP, altered mental status
- SpO_2 <90% and ↑ PAP, CVP, PAWP
- Potential complications: hypoxemia, cardiac arrest, heart failure, new/worsened dysrhythmias, antidysrhythmic drug toxicity

RELATED TOPICS
- Antidysrhythmic therapy
- Coronary artery disease
- Heart failure, left and right ventricular
- Hypokalemia
- Hypomagnesemia
- Pulmonary embolus, thrombotic
- Supraventricular tachycardia

ABBREVIATIONS
EF: Ejection fraction
EP: Electrophysiologic
ICD: Implantable cardioversion/defibrillator
MODS: Multiple organ dysfunction syndrome
VEDV: Ventricular end-diastolic volume
WPW: Wolff-Parkinson-White

REFERENCES
American Heart Association: *Textbook of advanced cardiac life support,* Dallas, 1994, The Association.

Dracup K: *Meltzer's intensive coronary care: a manual for nurses,* ed 5, Norwalk, CT, 1995, Appleton & Lange.

Finkelmeier BA: Ablative therapy in the treatment of tachyarrhythmias, *Crit Care Nurs Clin North Am* 6(1): 103-110, 1994.

Goodrich CA: Management of tachyarrhythmias in the CCU, *Curr Issues in Critical Care Nurs (Suppl):* 7-11, November 1995.

Jacobsen C: Arrhythmias and conduction disturbances. In Woods SL: *Cardiac nursing,* ed 3, Philadelphia, 1995, Lippincott.

Keen J, Baird M, Allen J: *Mosby's critical care and emergency drug reference,* ed 2, St Louis, 1996, Mosby.

Kellen JC, Ramadan D: The patient with recurrent atrioventricular nodal reentrant tachycardia or chronic atrial fibrillation or flutter, *Crit Care Nurs Clin North Am* 6(1): 41-54, 1994.

Porterfield LM: The cutting edge in arrhythmias, *Crit Care Nurse (Suppl):* June 1993.

Authors: **Marianne Saunorus Baird and Barbara Tueller Steuble**

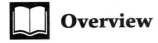 **Overview**

PATHOPHYSIOLOGY

Life-threatening response of ANS to external stimuli; occurs after SCI, particularly cervical and high thoracic (above T6) lesions. Can occur during acute phase of SCI or not until several yrs after injury. If AD not identified promptly, treated, and reversed, potential consequences include seizures, SAH, and fatal stroke.

Possible Stimuli

Bladder: Most common; distention, infection, calculi, cystoscopy

Bowel: Fecal impaction, rectal examination, suppository insertion

Skin: Tight clothing or sheets, temp extremes, sores, areas of broken skin

INCIDENCE

Experienced by most patients with C-spine or some degree of high T-spine SCI

HISTORY/RISK FACTORS

- C-spine SCI, T-spine SCI above T6
- Urinary retention, UTI
- Constipation
- Impaired skin integrity

CLINICAL PRESENTATION

Severe and throbbing headache, hypertension, nasal congestion, bradycardia; cutaneous vasodilatation, flushed skin, sweating above level of injury; gooseflesh, pallor, vasoconstriction below injury level

Assessment

PHYSICAL ASSESSMENT

Neuro: Headache, blurred vision

Resp: Nasal congestion

CV: Vasodilatation above level of injury; vasoconstriction below; profound hypertension ($\geq$300/150 mm Hg); bradycardia

GI: Nausea

Integ: *Above injury level:* sweating, flushed skin; *below injury level:* pilomotor erection (gooseflesh), pallor, chills

VITAL SIGNS/HEMODYNAMICS

RR: ↑ or nl

HR: ↓ or nl

BP: Profound ↑ ($\geq$300/150 possible)

Temp: Nl

CVP/PAWP: ↓

CO: ↓

SVR: Profound ↓

IMAGING

Spinal X-rays: A-P/lateral films detect fractures or dislocations of vertebral bodies, narrowing of spinal canal, hematomas. Additional views (odontoid, bilateral oblique, flexion-extension) may be necessary, particularly in the obese and heavily muscled.

CT Scan: Reveals soft tissue injury or subtle fractures.

MRI: Defines internal organ structures, detects tissue changes such as edema or infarction, and evaluates vascular integrity.

Collaborative Management

Immobilization of Injured Site: With or without surgical intervention.

C-spine injury: Skeletal traction to immobilize and reduce fracture or dislocation. Achieved *via* Gardner-Wells, Cone, or Crutchfield tongs, or a halo device and plaster or fiberglass jacket for skeletal fixation of head and neck. Surgery in immediate postinjury phase controversial but may include decompression laminectomy, closed or open fracture reduction, or spinal fusion for stabilization.

T-spine injury: May require surgical stabilization *via* Harrington rods or laminectomy with spinal fusion, using bone taken from iliac crest.

Special Frame or Bed: Eg, Roto Rest kinetic treatment table.

Urinary Catheterization: Indwelling or intermittent to decompress atonic bladder in immediate postinjury phase. Intermittent catheterization may be necessary if a reflex neurogenic bladder that fills and empties automatically fails to develop.

Pharmacotherapy

Stool softeners (eg, docusate sodium): To begin bowel-training program and prevent fecal impaction with bowel distention, which could stimulate AD.

Hyperosmolar laxatives (eg, glycerine suppository): To prevent fecal impaction and facilitate bowel movements on a regular basis (part of a bowel-training program).

Irritant or stimulant laxatives (eg, bisacodyl): To stimulate bowel movements as part of a bowel-training program.

Antihypertensives (eg, hydralazine HCl [Apresoline], sublingual nifedipine [Procardia], phentolamine [Regitine]): To treat severe hypertension that occurs with AD.

PATIENT-FAMILY TEACHING

- AD: causes, S&S, methods of treatment
- Medications: drug name, purpose, dosage, schedule, precautions, food-drug and drug-drug interactions, potential side effects
- Purpose, expected results, anticipated sensations of all nursing/medical interventions
- Address and phone numbers of National Spinal Cord Injury Association: 545 Concord Ave., Cambridge, MA 02138; 617-441-8500, 800-962-9629

Nursing Diagnoses/Interventions

Dysreflexia (or risk for same) r/t abnormal response of ANS to a stimulus
Desired outcomes: Patient has no symptoms of AD: dry skin above injury level, BP wnl for patient, HR ≥60 bpm, and absence of headache. ECG shows NSR.
- Assess for AD: severe, throbbing headache; cutaneous vasodilatation, flushed skin, sweating above injury level. Also assess for profoundly ↑ BP, nasal stuffiness, blurred vision, nausea, bradycardia. Be alert to signs occuring below injury level: gooseflesh, pallor, vasoconstriction.
- Assess for cardiac dysrhythmias *via* cardiac monitor during initial postinjury stage (2 wks).
- Avoid stimuli that cause AD: *bladder stimuli* (distention, calculi, infection, cystoscopy); *bowel stimuli* (fecal impaction, rectal examination, suppository insertion); *skin stimuli* (pressure from tight clothing or sheets, temp extremes, sores, areas of broken skin).
- If AD occurs, implement the following:
  Elevate HOB or place in sitting position to ↓ BP by inducing postural hypotension.
  Monitor BP and HR q3-5min until stable.
  Remove offending stimulus.
  Catheterize distended bladder using lubricant containing local anesthetic.
  Check for urinary catheter obstruction. As indicated, irrigate catheter using ≤30 ml NS.
  If UTI suspected, obtain urine for C&S.
  Gently check for fecal impaction, using local anesthetic ointment.
  Check for sensory stimuli, and loosen clothing, bed covers, other constricting fabric.
- Consult physician for severe or prolonged hypertension or symptoms that do not abate. Establish baseline neurologic status and reevaluate frequently until BP stable. Observe for indicators of subarachnoid or intracerebral hemorrhage: headache, altered LOC, nuchal rigidity, ↑ temp, change in pupil size/reaction.
- Be prepared to administer antihypertensive agent.
- Remain calm and supportive during these episodes.

Risk for impaired skin integrity r/t immobility secondary to immobilization device or paralysis
Desired outcome: Patient's skin remains intact during hospital course.
- Impaired skin integrity or cutaneous stimulation can trigger AD. Perform skin assessments at least q8h. Pay close attention to skin over bony prominences, around halo vest edges.
- Turn and reposition patient after spinal cord has been stabilized. Massage susceptible skin at least q2h. If turning allowed before immobilization with tongs, halo, surgery, use logrolling.
- Keep skin clean and dry.
- Pad halo jacket edges (eg, with sheepskin) to minimize irritation and friction.
- Provide pressure-relief mattress most appropriate for patient's injury.

Urinary retention r/t inhibition of spinal reflex arc secondary to spinal shock after SCI
Desired outcome: Within 24 h, UO ≥0.5 ml/kg/h with output comparable to intake.
- Be aware that urinary retention with stretching of bladder muscle may trigger AD.
- Assess for urinary retention: suprapubic distention and intake > output.
- Catheterize on admission. Patients usually have an indwelling catheter for first 48-96 h after injury, followed by intermittent catheterization to retrain bladder.
- Ensure continuous patency of drainage system to prevent blockage of flow, urinary reflux.
- Maintain fluid intake of at least 2.5-3 L/day to prevent early stone formation.
- Tape catheter over pubis in both male and female to prevent traction on catheter, which can lead to ulcer formation in urethra and erosion of urethral meatus.
- If catheterized >14 days, C&S recommended with use of a sulfonamide to prevent bacteremia.
- If AD triggered, catheterize using anesthetic jelly.
  If catheter obstructed, gently instill ≤30 ml NS in attempt to open catheter.
  If catheter remains obstructed, remove it and insert another, using anesthetic lubricant.
  If UTI is the suspected trigger, obtain urine specimen for C&S testing.

Constipation or fecal impaction r/t neuromuscular impairment secondary to spinal shock
Desired outcome: Patient has bowel elimination of soft and formed stools q2-3 days.
- Monitor for constipation (nausea, abdominal distention, malaise) and fecal impaction (nausea, vomiting, ↑ abdominal distention, palpable colonic mass, presence of hard fecal mass).
- Until bowel sounds present and paralytic ileus resolved, maintain NPO gastric suction.
- Perform gentle digital examination to determine presence of fecal impaction and check for rectal reflexes. Be sure to use anesthetic lubricant.
- Before return of rectal reflex arc, it may be necessary to remove feces manually. If fecal impaction present in atonic bowel, a small-volume enema may be necessary. Use generous amounts of anesthetic lubricant when performing rectal examination or administering enema.

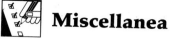

Miscellanea

CONSULT MD FOR
- Severe or prolonged hypertension
- Symptomatic bradycardia
- Absent bowel sounds
- Indicators of subarachnoid, intracerebral hemorrhage associated with severe hypertension

RELATED TOPICS
- Mechanical ventilation
- Multisystem injury
- Shock, neurogenic
- Spinal cord injury, cervical
- Spinal cord injury, thoracic

ABBREVIATIONS
AD: Autonomic dysreflexia
ANS: Autonomic nervous system
SAH: Subarachnoid hemorrhage
SNS: Sympathetic nervous system

REFERENCES
Adsit PA, Bishop C: Autonomic dysreflexia—don't let it be a surprise, *Orthop Nurs* 14(3): 17-20, 1995.
Huston CJ, Boelman R: Emergency! autonomic dysreflexia, *Am J Nurs* 95(6): 55, 1995.
Joseph AC, Juma S: Autonomic dysreflexia and video-urodynamics, *Urol Nurs* 14(2): 66-67, 1994.
Nolan S: Current trends in the management of acute spinal cord injury, *Crit Care Nurs Q* 17(1): 64-78, 1994.

Author: **Ann Coghlan Stowe**

Overview

PATHOPHYSIOLOGY
Causes are multiple, including imperfect surgical hemostasis, inadequate heparin reversal, platelet dysfunction, trauma to vascular endothelium or blood vessels, coagulation factor deficiencies, hyperfibrinolysis.

INCIDENCE
5%-20% of patients experience postop bleeding; 3%-15% require reexploration of surgical site.

HISTORY/RISK FACTORS
- Liver disease, VWf deficiency, pancreatitis
- DIC, fibrinogen/platelet disorder, thrombocytopenia, vitamin K deficiency
- Malignancy, pregnancy-induced hypertension, menorrhagia, uremia
- Anticoagulant or thrombolytic therapy
- Bleeding or bruising with minor injuries, nosebleeds, hemophilia
- Intraoperative hypothermia, hemodilution, or anticoagulation
- Clinical state or pharmacologic therapy (eg, chemotherapy) that inhibits removal of activated clotting factors, FDPs, and thromboplastin by reticuloendothelial system
- "Blood trauma" caused by extracorporeal "bypass" circulation
- Balloon counterpulsation (IABP)
- Shock/hypotension, anoxia
- Medications: quinidine, amrinone, penicillin, dipyridamole, aspirin, NSAIDs

CLINICAL PRESENTATION
- Bleeding from incision or drains/tubes in incisional area
- With DIC: bleeding from all invasive sites and mucous membranes
- With hypovolemia or hemorrhagic shock: hypotension, tachycardia, tachypnea, cool and clammy skin, restlessness or ↓ LOC

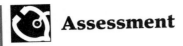 **Assessment**

PHYSICAL ASSESSMENT
Neuro: Restlessness, ↓ LOC
Resp: Nl to tachypneic
CV: Tachycardia, hypotension
MS: Hemarthrosis
GI: Jaundice, hepatomegaly, splenomegaly, GI bleeding
GU: Hematuria
Integ: Petechiae, ecchymosis, hematoma, purpura

VITAL SIGNS/HEMODYNAMICS
RR: ↑ or nl
HR: ↑ or nl
BP: Nl or ↓
Temp: Nl or ↓
CVP/PAWP: Nl or ↓
SVR: Nl or ↑
CO: Nl or ↓
12/18-Lead ECG: With ↓ BP, may reveal changes r/t myocardial ischemia: sinus tachycardia, PACs, and PVCs

LABORATORY STUDIES
Platelet Count: Possibly ↓
Bleeding Time: Possibly ↑, signaling platelet dysfunction, ↓ platelets, abnormal VWf, uremia, FDPs
PT: Possibly ↑, indicative of liver disease, Coumadin therapy, ↓ fibrinogen
PTT: Possibly ↑, indicative of clotting factor dysfunction/deficiency
Thrombin Time: ↑, indicative of ↓ fibrinogen or dysfunctional fibrinogen, heparin effect, circulating FDPs (helpful in diagnosing DIC)
Fibrinogen: ↓, indicative of fibrinolysis, DIC, liver disease
FDPs: ↑, indicative of abnormal amounts of fibrinolysis, possibly DIC
D-Dimer: ↑, indicative of ↑ thrombin and plasmin formation; may signal DIC
CBC: ↓ values reflect bleeding

IMAGING
CT Scan: Assesses affected surgical areas to diagnose internal bleeding

Collaborative Management

Differential Diagnosis: To determine whether cause is surgical or one of coagulation. If surgical, patient must be returned to OR for exploration.
Evaluation of Laboratory Data: To determine cause, whether vascular/platelet disorder, coagulation factor defect, hyperfibrinolysis.
Measurement/Estimation of Continued Blood Loss: To quantify loss to determine blood replacement therapy.
Application of Direct Pressure: If bleeding site close to surface or in a location that can be compressed adequately.
PEEP: Can ↓ mediastinal bleeding.
Fluid Replacement: To support BP through maintenance of cardiac output.
Blood/Blood Product Replacement: To support tissue oxygenation and hemostasis; includes platelet transfusions.
Coagulation Factor Replacement: To support blood coagulation and hemostasis if factors deficient or dysfunctional.
Pharmacotherapy
Antifibrinolytic therapy: ε-aminocaproic acid (Amicar) and tranexamic acid (TEA) to inhibit fibrinolysis for patients who are bleeding as a result of a variety of causes. In DIC these agents are used with extreme caution as they may convert a bleeding disorder into a thrombotic problem.
Vitamin K and folate: May be given for liver disease, DIC, or intestinal dysfunction to replace deficiencies of these substances.
Desmopressin acetate (DDAVP): Enhances platelet function by ↑ plasma levels of factor VIII, VWf, and plasminogen activator.
Vasoactive drugs: May be used to support BP/CO in conjunction with fluid volume replacement. Medication infusions include dopamine, epinephrine, and norepinephrine.
Surgery: If bleeding profuse and uncontrolled (eg, open heart surgery patients who lose >300 ml first h, >250 ml second h, and >150 ml for each subsequent h), patient is returned to OR for exploration and hemostasis.

PATIENT-FAMILY TEACHING
- Causes of bleeding and appropriate measures for management of underlying bleeding disorder if present
- Medications: drug name, purpose, dosage, schedule, precautions, drug-drug and food-drug interactions, and potential side effects; discussion of OTC medications that promote bleeding
- Purpose, expected results, anticipated sensations of all nursing/medical interventions

Nursing Diagnoses/Interventions

Altered protection r/t postop bleeding resulting from vascular and platelet disorders, coagulation factor defects, or hyperfibrinolysis

Desired outcome: Within 24-48 h of treatment initiation, bleeding controlled: markedly ↓/absent frank bleeding from invasive sites and mucosal surfaces, secretions/excretions negative for blood, absence of new/↑ ecchymoses, HR 60-100 bpm, RR 12-20 breaths/min, SBP >90 mm Hg, or all within 10% of baseline.

- Discuss bleeding hx with patient/significant others, including excessive bleeding from small wounds, bleeding gums, hematuria, tarry/bloody stools, vomiting of blood, nosebleeds, heavy menstruation, unusually "easy" bruising tendency.
- Question patient with no previous hx of bleeding about current medications, including OTC preparations.
- Monitor coagulation/clotting tests qd.
- Support tissue oxygenation *via* O_2 administration; monitor O_2 saturation with continuous SpO_2.
- Monitor closely for ↑ bleeding, bruising, petechiae, and purpura. Assess for internal bleeding by measuring all bloody drainage and testing suspicious secretions for blood.
- Observe for dysrhythmias *via* continuous ECG monitoring.
- Monitor neurologic status closely. ↓ LOC may indicate intracranial bleeding.
- ↓ risk of further bleeding by using alcohol-free mouthwash with swabsticks for oral hygiene and electric razor for shaving, avoiding unnecessary venipunctures and IM injections, holding pressure over invasive sites for 3-5 min or 10-15 min for arterial punctures.

Risk for fluid volume deficit r/t bleeding/hemorrhage

Desired outcome: Patient normovolemic: HR 60-100 bpm, RR 12-20 breaths/min, SBP >90 mm Hg (or these values within 10% of baseline), warm extremities, distal pulses >2+.

- Monitor VS at least q2h, noting ↑ in HR and RR and ↓ in BP or pulse pressure. With profuse bleeding, monitor VS at least q15min.
- Measure UO at least q2h.
- Monitor CBC qd for significant alterations in Hgb, Hct, and platelets.
- Assess for signs of impending shock.
- Maintain at least one 18-gauge or larger IV catheter for shock management.

Risk for injury r/t potential for blood transfusion reaction

Desired outcome: Throughout transfusion and ≤8 h after transfusion, patient has no fever, chills, flushing, rash, or lesions and exhibits baseline VS.

- Check blood to be transfused with another professional to ensure crossmatch report and requisition form match blood unit information.
- During infusion, check VS q15min for first h. Check frequently throughout first 15 min for hemolytic transfusion reaction.
- Observe for reaction throughout transfusion and for 8 h following it. If transfusion reaction occurs:

    Stop infusion immediately, maintaining IV with NS.
    Maintain BP using fluid volume resuscitation and vasopressors.
    Monitor HR and ECG for changes.
    Administer diuretics and fluids to promote diuresis.
    Obtain blood and urine for institutional protocol for transfusion workup.
    Perform blood cultures if patient exhibits signs of sepsis.

Miscellanea

CONSULT MD FOR
- Uncontrolled bleeding, hypotension, signs of impending shock
- SpO_2 <90%
- Presence of blood in secretions/excretions
- Possible complications: hemorrhagic shock, MODS, changes in sensorium, acute DIC, heparin rebound (reappearance of hypocoagulability following heparin neutralization with protamine)

RELATED TOPICS
- Anemias
- Aortic aneurysm/dissection
- Cardiac surgery: CABG
- Cardiac surgery: valvular disorders
- Disseminated intravascular coagulation
- Hemolytic crisis
- Multiple organ dysfunction syndrome
- Multisystem injury
- Shock, hemorrhagic

ABBREVIATIONS
FDPs: Fibrin degradation products
IAPB: Intraaortic balloon pump
MODS: Multiple organ dysfunction syndrome
VWf: von Willebrand's factor

REFERENCES
Atkins PJ: Postoperative coagulopathies, *Crit Care Nurs Clin North Am* 5(3): 459-471, 1993.

Baird M: Bleeding and thrombotic disorders. In Swearingen PL, Keen JH (eds): *Manual of critical care nursing,* ed 3, St Louis, Mosby, 1995.

Bell TN: Disseminated intravascular coagulation, *Crit Care Nurs Clin North Am* 5(3): 389-410, 1993.

Coffland FI, Shelton DM: Blood component replacement therapy, *Crit Care Nurs Clin North Am* 5(3): 543-556, 1993.

Whitman GR: Hypertension and hypothermia in the immediate postoperative period, *Crit Care Nurs Clin North Am* 3(7): 661-673, 1991.

Author: **Marianne Saunorus Baird**

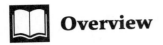 **Overview**

PATHOPHYSIOLOGY

Dysrhythmia in which HR ↓ to <60 bpm because of disturbance in automaticity (pacing), conduction pathway, or combination of both. May result from several dysrhythmias, including sinus bradycardia, AV heart block, "escape" rhythms (junctional or ventricular), and sick sinus syndrome (sinus arrest or pauses). May cause symptoms indicative of low cardiac output and perfusion deficits, eg, altered mental status, chest pain.

HISTORY/RISK FACTORS

- CAD (and its risk factors), MI
- ↑ ICP
- Hypoxemia, airway suctioning
- Drug overdose, antidysrhythmic drug toxicity, digoxin use
- Vagal stimulation: ie, vasovagal reaction
- Hypothyroidism
- Stokes-Adams syndrome
- Electrolyte imbalances, especially hyperkalemia, hypermagnesemia

CLINICAL PRESENTATION

- May be symptom free or may have lightheadedness, dizziness, weakness, unusual fatigue with ADLs, chest discomfort, SOB
- May appear pale, use short sentences

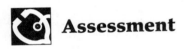 **Assessment**

PHYSICAL ASSESSMENT

Neuro: ↓ LOC, syncope, weakness, fainting, vertigo, anxiety, restlessness
Resp: Dyspnea, SOB, crackles in lung bases
CV: Chest discomfort, activity intolerance, sense of "skipped beats"
GI: Nausea, vomiting, feeling of epigastric pressure
GU: ↓ UO
Integ: Diaphoresis, pallor, cyanosis

VITAL SIGNS/HEMODYNAMICS

RR: ↑ or nl
HR: ↓
BP: ↓ or nl
Temp: Nl
CVP/PAWP: Nl, ↑, or ↓
SVR: ↑
CO: ↓
12/18-Lead ECG
Sinus bradycardia: Regular rhythm, atrial rate <60 bpm, ventricular rate <60 bpm, P waves before each QRS, QRS of nl duration with P:QRS 1:1, PR interval nl (0.12-0.20 sec).

Junctional escape rhythm: Regular rhythm. P waves may be absent (and thus atrial rate unable to be determined), inverted, or follow QRS. Ventricular rate 40-60 bpm with QRS of nl duration, PR interval with inverted P waves <0.12 sec. P rate usually > QRS, but can be 1:1.

Ventricular escape rhythm/idioventricular rhythm: Rhythm may be regular or irregular. No P waves, so atrial rate undetermined. Ventricular rate <40 bpm, QRS widened/sometimes bizarre, no PR interval or P:QRS.

Sick sinus syndrome (sinus arrest or sinus pauses): Rhythm irregular, atrial rate variable (sinus node "fires" inconsistently), ventricular rate <60 bpm when sinus node fails to fire, P waves usually before each QRS with P:QRS 1:1, PR interval 0.12-0.20 sec (nl).

AV heart block

> *Second degree Type II (Mobitz II):* Rhythm regular or irregular, atrial rate > ventricular rate (P:QRS = P > QRS) with ventricular rate <60 bpm, number of P waves preceding QRS may vary or be constant (2:1, 3:1, 4:1), QRS of nl duration, PR intervals on conducted beats may be nl or >0.20 sec.

> *Third degree (complete heart block):* Rhythm generally regular (R-R intervals all equal), atrial rate > ventricular rate, P waves regular (P-P intervals all equal), QRS of either nl duration (<0.12 sec) or prolonged (>0.20 sec), PR intervals vary tremendously, no relationship between P and QRS.

LABORATORY STUDIES

Serum Electrolytes: ↑ K^+ and Mg^{2+} precipitates ↓ HR and may significantly change rhythm, especially with antidysrhythmics.
Drug Levels: To check for/prevent toxicity. Digoxin, β blockers, calcium channel blockers may precipitate ↓ HR. In addition, opiates or cardiotoxic drugs, eg, cyclic antidepressants, can cause bradycardic dysrhythmias.
ABGs: May reflect hypoxemia or pH change that can alter electrolyte balance and precipitate dysrhythmias.

IMAGING

Chest X-ray: May reflect enlarged cardiac silhouette indicative of heart disease.
Echocardiography: Use of ultrasound to evaluate ventricular pumping action, including estimation of ventricular EF.
Cardiac Catheterization: Assesses for CAD.

DIAGNOSTIC PROCEDURES

24-h Holter/Cardiac Event Monitoring: Identifies subtle dysrhythmias during ambulation and throughout day. Abnormal rhythms correlated with symptoms; patient/health care provider records when symptoms occur.

Exercise Stress Testing: Used alone or with 24-h Holter monitoring to detect dysrhythmias. May not yield useful information regarding bradycardia as readily as tachycardias.

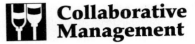 **Collaborative Management**

GENERAL

Supplemental O_2: Supports continuous O_2 delivery to tissues.
SpO_2: Detects ↓ O_2 saturation caused by ↓ HR.
Continuous ECG Monitoring: Detects all dysrhythmias, onset and duration, and termination for intermittent dysrhythmias.
Management of Other Causes of Dysrhythmias: Eg, hypoxia, hyperkalemia, hypermagnesemia, preexisting acidosis, hypothermia, hypothyroidism, hypoadrenalism, drug overdose/toxicity.
Cardiac Pacing: Transcutaneous, transvenous, or epicardial mode to treat dysrhythmias that fail to respond to drug therapy or as a bridge to permanent pacemaker.
Diet: Low-fat, low-cholesterol, ↓-caffeine diet for recurrent dysrhythmias.
CPR: If bradycardia deteriorates into PEA or asystole.

PHARMACOTHERAPY

Goal: to ↑ number of ventricular contractions enough to ↑ cardiac output and BP.
Atropine: Parasympatholytic/vagolytic drug that blocks vagus nerve action, resulting in ↑ HR. *Dosage:* Total of 0.04 mg/kg with doses averaging 0.5-1.0 mg IV push.
Catecholamine Infusions: Stimulate B_1 receptors of sympathetic nervous system, resulting in ↑ HR.
Epinephrine: 2-10 μg/min continuously.
Dopamine: 5-10 μg/kg/min continuously.
Isoproterenol: 2-10 μg/min continuously. Used cautiously in patients at high risk for myocardial ischemia.

SURGERY

Permanent Pacemaker: Small electrical pulse generator implanted SC to provide electrical impulse to heart when normal pacemakers (ie, SA node) fail to maintain HR.

PATIENT-FAMILY TEACHING

- Importance of promptly reporting chest pain, lightheadedness, SOB, activity intolerance, and syncope
- Self-measuring of pulse rate/rhythm
- Causes of bradycardia; pacing devices used during/after hospitalization; anticipated sensations
- At-home dietary guidelines
- Importance of smoking cessation

Nursing Diagnoses/Interventions

Decreased cardiac output r/t altered rate, rhythm, conduction; r/t negative inotropic cardiac changes secondary to cardiac disease
Desired outcome: Within 15 min of onset of serious dysrhythmias, patient has adequate cardiac output: SBP >90 mm Hg, HR 60-100 bpm, PAP 20-30/8-15 mm Hg, PAWP 6-12 mm Hg, CVP 2-6 mm Hg, CO 4-7 L/min, CI 2.5-4.0 L/min/m², or all within 10% of baseline.

- Monitor continuous ECG, noting response to antidysrhythmic agents.
- Monitor VS for baseline status and prn for changes in cardiac rhythm, including PA readings if PA catheter present.
- Document dysrhythmias by saving rhythm strips. Use 12/18-lead ECG to diagnose new dysrhythmias.
- Note changes in SpO_2 with symptomatic bradycardia.
- Manage life-threatening dysrhythmias using ACLS guidelines.
- Provide supplemental O_2 for symptomatic bradycardia.
- Monitor lab values to assess cause of bradycardia.
- Administer medications that support cardiac output and BP if antidysrhythmics or cardiac pacing insufficient to ↑ BP.
- Implement transcutaneous pacing as a "bridge" to other invasive pacing modes if indicated.
- If PVCs noted with bradycardia, administer medications to ↑ HR before treating PVCs. PVCs may disappear as HR ↑.

 # Miscellanea

CONSULT MD FOR

- Failure of bradycardia to respond to prescribed treatments
- Worsening symptoms: chest pain; SOB; dyspnea; ↓ BP; altered mental status; SpO_2 <90%; ↑ PAP, PAWP, or CVP; bradycardia
- Possible complications: heart failure, cardiac arrest (PEA, asystole), hypoxemia, new dysrhythmias

RELATED TOPICS

- Antidysrhythmic therapy
- Cardiomyopathy
- Coronary artery disease
- Heart block: AV conduction disturbance
- Hyperkalemia
- Hypermagnesemia

ABBREVIATIONS

EF: Ejection fraction
PEA: Pulseless electrical activity

REFERENCES

American Heart Association: *Textbook of advanced cardiac life support,* Dallas, 1994, The Association.

Baas LS, Meissner JE: Cardiovascular care. In *Illustrated manual of nursing practice,* ed 2, Springhouse, Pa, 1994, Springhouse.

Huszar RJ: *Basic dysrhythmias: interpretation and management,* ed 2, St Louis, 1994, Mosby Lifeline.

Keen J, Baird M, Allen J: *Mosby's critical care and emergency drug reference,* ed 2, St Louis, 1996, Mosby.

Moungey SJ: Patients with sinus node dysfunction or atrioventricular blocks, *Crit Care Nurs Clin North Am* 6(1): 55-68, 1994.

Porterfield LM: The cutting edge in arrhythmias, *Crit Care Nurse (Suppl):* June 1993.

Steuble BT: Dysrhythmias and conduction disturbances. In Swearingen PL, Keen JH (eds): *Manual of critical care nursing,* ed 3, St Louis, 1995, Mosby.

Authors: **Marianne Saunorus Baird and Barbara Tueller Steuble**

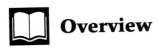 **Overview**

PATHOPHYSIOLOGY

Involves lung tissue changes, including airway inflammation, loss of ciliary action, mucosal gland hypertrophy, alveolar hyperinflation, and bronchial mucosal edema, all of which result in ↑ mucus production. Mucous plugs develop in the stretched alveoli, causing bronchiole obstruction. Recurrent URIs with *Streptococcus pneumoniae* and *Haemophilus influenzae* are common because of inability to clear bronchial tree of mucus. As disease progresses, acute exacerbations ↑ in severity and duration, ultimately causing respiratory failure. Pulmonary hypertension can lead to RV failure (cor pulmonale).

INCIDENCE

Most common respiratory disease in the US

HISTORY/RISK FACTORS

- Cigarette smoking
- Air pollution
- Occupational exposure to dusts/gases

CLINICAL PRESENTATION

Chronic: Morning cough, clear and copious secretions, anorexia, cyanosis, dependent edema

Acute (exacerbation): Fever, dyspnea, thick and tenacious sputum

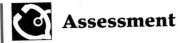 **Assessment**

PHYSICAL ASSESSMENT

Use of accessory muscles, prolonged expiratory phase, digital clubbing, ↓ thoracic expansion, dullness over areas of consolidation, adventitious breath sounds (especially coarse rhonchi and wheezing), ankle edema, JVD, bloated appearance

VITAL SIGNS/HEMODYNAMICS

RR: ↑
HR: ↑
BP: ↓ if heart failure present
Temp: ↑ if infection present
PAP: ↑ as a result of pulmonary hypertension
CVP: May be ↑ because of RV heart failure
PAWP: Necessary to reflect accurate hydration status with advanced disease
ECG: May reveal atrial and ventricular dysrhythmias. Most patients have atrial dysrhythmia because of atrial dilatation and RV hypertrophy caused by pulmonary hypertension.

LABORATORY STUDIES

ABGs: Will reveal hypoxemia (Pao_2 <60 mm Hg) and hypercapnia ($Paco_2$ >50-60 mm Hg). Baseline pH may be 7.35-7.38, but during acute exacerbation, as the $Paco_2$ ↑, pH may ↓ below 7.35.
Sputum Culture: May reveal infective organisms.
CBC: Will reveal chronically ↑ Hgb as a compensatory response to chronic hypoxemia and ↑ WBCs in the presence of acute bacterial infection.

IMAGING

Chest X-ray: Will reveal nl A-P diameter, nearly nl diaphragm position, and ↑ peripheral lung markings.

DIAGNOSTIC PROCEDURES

Pulmonary Function Tests: Will show ↓ VC, ↑ residual volume, and ↑ expiratory reserve volume.

Collaborative Management

O_2 Therapy: To treat hypoxemia. Used cautiously at low flow rate (1-2 L/min) with chronic CO_2 retention in which hypoxemia stimulates respiratory drive.
Intubation/Mechanical Ventilation: Intubation may be necessary if unable to maintain patent airway as a result of tenacious or copious secretions, ineffective cough, or fatigue. Mechanical ventilation required if unable to maintain adequate ABGs (Pao_2 >60 mm Hg) with supplemental O_2; decision for use made carefully, since weaning may be difficult.
Hydration: IV fluids may be necessary to replace fluids lost from insensible sources (eg, tachypnea, diaphoresis with fever).
Pharmacotherapy
Bronchodilators: To open airways by relaxing smooth muscles.
Steroids (ie, prednisone): To ↓ inflammation, thereby ↑ air flow. Acute adrenal insufficiency can develop if drugs discontinued abruptly (eg, during hospitalization).
Antibiotics: Based on sensitivity studies from sputum cultures.
Chest Physiotherapy: To help loosen and mobilize pulmonary secretions.
Diuretics/Na Restriction: To reduce fluid overload in heart failure.

PATIENT-FAMILY TEACHING

- Use of home O_2, including instructions for when to use it, importance of not ↑ prescribed flow rate, precautions, community resources for replacement.
- S&S of RV heart failure that necessitate medical attention: ↑ dyspnea, fatigue; ↑ coughing; changes in amount, color, consistency of sputum; swelling of ankles, legs; fever; sudden weight gain.
- Avoiding infectious individuals, especially those with URIs. Importance of yearly flu and pneumococcal vaccines.
- Review of Na-restricted diet; importance of good nutrition in treating this disorder.
- Importance of pacing activity level to conserve energy.
- "Double-cough" technique:
  Sit upright with upper body flexed forward slightly.
  Take 2-3 breaths and exhale passively.
  Inhale again, but only to mid-inspiratory point.
  Exhale by coughing quickly 2-3 times.

Nursing Diagnoses/Interventions

Ineffective airway clearance r/t ↓ energy, which results in ineffective cough; or r/t ↑ tracheobronchial secretions

Desired outcome: Patient coughs appropriately and has effective airway clearance as evidenced by absence of adventitious breath sounds.

- Auscultate breath sounds q2h and after coughing. Be alert to changes in adventitious breath sounds.
- Assess ability to clear secretions. Keep emergency suction equipment at bedside.
- Teach "double cough" technique, which prevents small airway collapse that can occur with forceful coughing (see **PATIENT-FAMILY TEACHING**).
- Ensure that O_2 is humidified to aid in liquefying tracheobronchial secretions.
- Administer chest physiotherapy to mobilize secretions.

Impaired gas exchange r/t altered O_2 supply secondary to ↓ alveolar ventilation present with stretched, destroyed, or blocked alveoli

Desired outcome: Within 1-2 h of treatment initiation, patient has adequate gas exchange: Pao_2 >60 mm Hg, $Paco_2$ 35-45 mm Hg, and pH 7.35-7.45. Within 24-48 h of treatment initiation, RR 12-20 breaths/min with eupnea, and breath sounds clear and bilaterally equal (or return to baseline).

- Monitor for hypoxia: restlessness, agitation, changes in LOC. Remember that cyanosis is a late sign.
- Position to promote optimal gas exchange, usually high-Fowler's position with patient leaning forward and elbows propped on over-the-bed table.
- Auscultate breath sounds at frequent intervals. Monitor for ↓/adventitious breath sounds. Acute progression to ↓ breath sounds/absence of wheezing may signal severe bronchoconstriction and minimal air flow.
- Deliver O_2 as prescribed. Monitor ABGs, Spo_2. Be alert to ↓ Pao_2, ↑ $Paco_2$, and ↓ saturation levels, which are signals of respiratory compromise.

Altered nutrition: Less than body requirements, r/t ↓ intake secondary to fatigue and anorexia

Desired outcome: At hospital discharge, patient is consuming adequate nutrition and exhibits stable weight, positive nitrogen (N) state on N studies, and serum albumin 3.5-5.5 μg/dl.

- Monitor food and fluid intake. If indicated, obtain dietary consultation for calorie counts, food preferences.
- Provide small, frequent meals that are nutritious and easy to consume.
- Unless otherwise indicated, provide more calories from unsaturated fat sources than from carbohydrate sources. During process of carbohydrate metabolism, the body uses O_2 and produces CO_2. Patients with COPD take in less O_2 and retain CO_2. A high-fat diet minimizes CO_2 production and retention.

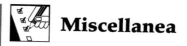 # Miscellanea

CONSULT MD FOR

- Respiratory decompensation: agitation, restlessness, ↓ LOC, use of accessory muscles, Spo_2 <90%
- URI: change in amount, color of sputum; respiratory distress; ↑ adventitious breath sounds
- Heart failure: ↑ PAWP associated with pulmonary crackles, JVD, S_3 gallop

RELATED TOPICS

- Emphysema
- Heart failure, right ventricular
- Immobility, prolonged
- Mechanical ventilation
- Pneumonia, community-acquired

ABBREVIATIONS

URI: Upper respiratory infection
VC: Vital capacity

REFERENCES

Garshick E, Schenker MB, Dosman JA: Occupational induced airways obstruction, *Med Clin North Am* 80(4): 851-878, 1996.

Howard C: Chronic bronchitis. In Swearingen PL (ed): *Manual of medical-surgical nursing care,* ed 3, St Louis, 1994, Mosby.

Johannsen JM: Chronic obstructive pulmonary disease: current comprehensive care for emphysema and bronchitis, *Nurse Pract* 19(1): 59-67, 1994.

Owens GR: Chronic obstructive pulmonary disease. In Bone RC (ed): *Pulmonary and critical care medicine,* St Louis, 1995, Mosby.

Small SP, Graydon JE: Perceived uncertainty, physical symptoms, and negative mood in hospitalized patients with COPD, *Heart Lung* 21(6): 568-574, 1992.

Weaver TE, Narsavage GL: Physiological and psychosocial variables related to functional status in chronic obstructive pulmonary disease, *Nurs Res* 41(5): 286-287, 1992.

Author: **Cheri A. Goll**

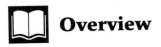 **Overview**

PATHOPHYSIOLOGY

Caused by thermal, electrical, chemical, or radiant agents. Outcome determined by agent, patient's age, intensity/duration of exposure, and burn location, depth, and percentage of body exposure. Categorized based on depth or magnitude. The longer and more intense the exposure, the greater the severity of depth and magnitude.

Superficial Partial-Thickness: "First-degree" burn; damages epidermis; heals within 24-72 h.

Deep Partial-Thickness: "Second-degree" burn; involves varying levels of the dermis; heals within 3-35 days.

Full-Thickness: "Third-degree" burn; exposes poorly vascularized fat layer. Wounds <4 cm in diameter allowed to heal by granulation; larger wounds closed by skin grafting.

Electrical Burn Injury: Often involves extensive damage to deep and underlying tissues, nerves, blood vessels, and muscles along conduction path and at electrical current exit site.

HISTORY

- Exposure to thermal, chemical, electrical, radiant agent
- Inhalation of smoke, chemicals, or CO or other product of combustion

RISK FACTORS (for complications)

- Entrapment in enclosed area
- Cardiopulmonary disease, diabetes mellitus
- Immunosuppression
- Malnutrition

CLINICAL PRESENTATION

Rule of Nines: Enables quick estimation of burn injury extent (Fig. 1).

Injury-Severity Grading System: Developed by ABA; categorizes burns as minor, moderate, and major. ABA advocates treatment of major burns in a burn center or facility with expertise in burn care. Moderate burns usually require hospitalization, not necessarily in a burn unit; minor burns often treated in emergency department or as outpatient.

	Partial-thickness	Full-thickness
Major:	>25%	>10%
Moderate:	15%-25%	<10%
Minor:	<15%	< 2%

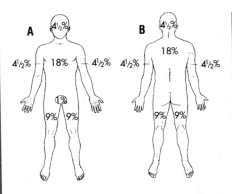

Fig. 1 Estimation of adult burn injury: rule of nines. **A,** Anterior view. **B,** Posterior view. (From Thompson JM et al: *Mosby's clinical nursing,* ed 4, St Louis, 1997, Mosby.)

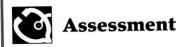 **Assessment**

PHYSICAL ASSESSMENT

Resp: Inflammation caused by inhalation of heat, smoke, or noxious chemicals usually causes airway obstruction within 6-72 h postburn. CO poisoning possible with exposure to products of combustion. Singed nasal hairs, burns in perioral area, or coughing up of soot suggests inhalation injury.

Clinical indicators: Stridor, hoarseness, cough, dyspnea, tachypnea, crackles, rhonchi; signs of CO poisoning: cherry-red skin coloring, headache, tinnitus, vertigo, convulsions

CV: Fluid shifts, direct damage to heart or blood vessels, obstruction of microcirculation, compression of blood vessels, and hemorrhage caused by clotting disorders all contribute to CV instability. ↑ capillary permeability caused by inflammatory response at burn site(s) results in shift of intravascular fluid into interstitial spaces, causing ↓ circulating volume and ↑ viscosity of remaining intravascular fluid; capillary sludging/thrombus formation result.

Clinical indicators: ↓ LOC, pallor, dry mucous membranes, cool skin temp, tachycardia, hypotension, ↓ peripheral pulses, delayed capillary refill; cardiac dysrhythmias possible with electrical burns and electrolyte imbalance

Renal: ↓ circulatory volumes result in ↓ RBF and low UO. Myoglobin or hemoglobin in urine reflected by dark, concentrated urine. Poor renal perfusion can result in ATN and ARF with buildup of metabolic waste products and electrolyte imbalances.

GI: Shunting of blood from GI tract/paralytic ileus may cause ↓/absent bowel sounds, nausea and vomiting, and abdominal distention. Occult or frank blood may be present in stools, vomitus with GI ulceration (Curling's ulcer).

Integ: Evaporative fluid loss, hypothermia, and infection. Scar formation can result in contractures. Circumferential burns can constrict underlying tissue, blood vessels, and muscles (ischemic myositis) with tissue necrosis.

Wound Sepsis: Primary cause of death in burn injury. The larger the wound, the higher the risk for infection.

Clinical indicators: Eschar separation, ↑ exudate, pockets of purulent material, poorly defined burn margins, edema, discoloration, superficial ulceration

Systemic/septic shock: Changes in LOC, tachycardia, tachypnea, ↓ BP with low SVR, hyperglycemia

VITAL SIGNS/HEMODYNAMICS

RR: ↑
HR: ↑
BP: ↓ or nl
Temp: ↓ with hypothermia; ↑ with sepsis
CVP/PAWP: ↓
CO: ↓ with hypovolemia; ↑ with sepsis
SVR: ↑ with hypovolemia; ↓ with sepsis
ECG: Sinus tachycardia, PVCs, ventricular dysrhythmias with hypokalemia; diffuse injury patterns, dysrhythmias possible with electrical burns

LABORATORY STUDIES

Baseline Blood Work

Hct: ↑ secondary to dehydration caused by fluid shifts from intravascular space

Hgb: ↓ secondary to hemolysis

Serum Na$^+$: ↓ secondary to massive fluid shifts

Serum K$^+$: ↑ caused by cell lysis and fluid shifts

BUN: ↑ secondary to hypovolemic status, ↑ protein catabolism

CK: Evaluated as an index of muscle damage; particularly important in electrical injuries. The higher the CK, the more extensive the muscle damage.

ABGs: Determine hypoxemia and acid-base abnormalities.

UA: Checks for myoglobinuria present with muscle injury resulting from burns. If greatly ↑, may cause ARF.

24-h Urine: Checks for catabolism and onset/resolution of ARF.

Carboxyhemoglobin: Checks for CO in blood secondary to smoke inhalation.

C&S Studies: Evaluate sputum, blood, urine, wound tissue for infection. Burn wound sepsis defined as 10^5 microorganisms per g burn wound tissue with active invasion of adjacent unburned skin. Common causative organisms include *Pseudomonas aeruginosa, Klebsiella, Serratia, Escherichia coli, Enterobacter cloacae.*

IMAGING

Chest X-rays: Usually nl on admission; changes 24-48 h postburn injury may reflect atelectasis, pulmonary edema.

DIAGNOSTIC PROCEDURES

Bronchoscopy: May be necessary in determining extramucosal carbonaceous material and state of mucosa in inhalation injuries.

VC, Tidal Volume, Inspiratory Force Measurements: May demonstrate ↓ values with inhalation injury.

12-Lead ECG: Checks myocardial damage secondary to electrical burn injury.

Collaborative Management

Humidified O_2: Treats hypoxemia and prevents drying/sloughing of mucosal lining of tracheobronchial tree.

Intubation and Mechanical Ventilation: For respiratory distress. Laryngeal edema resolves in 3-5 days; tracheostomy necessary if laryngeal edema prevents intubation.

Fluid Resuscitation: Calculate fluid infusion time from time of injury, not time of hospital admission. Replacement based on body weight and percentage of BSA burned. Colloids avoided during first 24 h because ↑ capillary permeability causes leakage of protein into interstitial tissues, resulting in edema. Crystalloids used in first 24 h, with small amounts of colloids added during second 24 h. Parkland formula, most commonly used, recommends 4 ml fluid/kg body weight/percentage BSA burned. First half infused over first 8 h. Second half infused over following 16 h.

Indwelling Urinary Catheter: Enables accurate measurement of UO.

Gastric Intubation/Suction: Necessary because of potential for paralytic ileus with ≥30% BSA burn or alcohol intoxication.

Pharmacotherapy: All medications, except Td, given IV to avoid sequestration of medication, which then would "flood" vascular system with return of capillary integrity and diuresis of third-spaced fluids.

Td prophylaxis: Given IM to combat *Clostridium tetani,* an anaerobic infection.

Morphine sulfate: For pain management.

Antacids/histamine H_2-receptor antagonists: Maintain gastric pH >5.0 and prevent development of Curling's ulcer.

Bronchodilators and mucolytic agents: Promote ventilation and aid in removal of secretions.

Antibiotics: Prophylactically and as indicated for specific C&S findings.

Diet: High metabolic activity and ↑ protein catabolism r/t burn injury result in significant ↑ in energy requirements and nutritional needs. Positive nitrogen state achieved with high-protein, high-carbohydrate diets. High-fat, low-carbohydrate diets facilitate weaning from ventilator, since high-carbohydrate loads result in ↑ CO_2 production. Method of delivery based on tolerance. Enteral feedings may ↓ GI acidity and ulcer formation. Central PN may be initiated for paralytic ileus or inability to tolerate enteral feedings.

Wound Care: Cleansing, débridement (manual, enzymatic, surgical), and antimicrobial therapy (ie, topical agents: silver sulfadiazine [Silvadene], polymyxin B, povidone-iodine, mafenide, silver nitrate) control bacterial proliferation and provide a wound capable of producing granulation tissue and a capillary network.

Split-Thickness Skin Grafting: Provides closure for full-thickness injuries. Cadaver skin, porcine, cultured epidermal skin, amniotic membranes used for temporary closure before autografting.

Escharotomy (surgical incision through eschar or fascia): Relieves respiratory distress attributable to circumferential burns of neck and trunk, or in extremities to ↓ pressure from underlying edema and restore adequate perfusion. Indications include cyanosis of distal unburned skin, delayed capillary filling, progressive neurovascular changes, pulmonary restriction.

PATIENT-FAMILY TEACHING

- Coughing, deep-breathing exercises, incentive spirometry
- Purpose, expected results, anticipated sensations for all nursing/medical interventions
- Splinting and ROM exercise program for contracture prevention
- Skin care: use of lubricating cream several × day and after bathing; application of padding or dressings to areas that may be traumatized by pressure; avoidance of exposure to sun because healed skin is highly sensitive to UV rays for up to 1 yr
- For darker skinned patient: permanent pigmentation changes likely as a result of destruction of melanocytes; burned areas usually stay pink
- Wound care: dressing change procedure, indicators of infection
- Importance of wearing pressure garment to prevent excessive or hypertrophic scarring
- Medications: drug name, purpose, dosage, schedule, precautions, food-drug and drug-drug interactions, potential side effects
- Addresses and phone numbers of local and other support groups for burn patients, including state's Fire Fighters' Burn Foundation:

  American Burn Association: 800-548-2876

  Shriners Burn Institute: 3229 Burnet Ave, Cincinnati, Ohio, 45229-3095

Nursing Diagnoses/Interventions

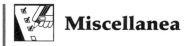 # Miscellanea

Impaired gas exchange r/t smoke inhalation with tracheobronchial swelling, carbonaceous debris, CO retention, pulmonary restriction caused by circumferential burns to neck, thorax
Desired outcome: Within 1 h of intervention, patient exhibits adequate gas exchange: PaO_2 ≥80 mm Hg; O_2 saturation ≥95%; RR 12-20 breaths/min with eupnea; orientation × 3; no adventitious breath sounds.

- Assess, document respiratory status qh, noting rate/depth, breath sounds, LOC. Monitor for upper airway distress (severe hoarseness, stridor, dyspnea, and, less frequently, CNS depression) and lower airway distress (crackles, rhonchi, hacking cough, labored/rapid breathing).
- Monitor ABGs for ↓ PaO_2 and ↑ $PaCO_2$. Check SpO_2 for values <90-94 or progressive decline.
- Administer humidified O_2; titrate to maintain SpO_2 >90%.
- Use high-Fowler's position to promote respiratory excursion.
- Encourage coughing and deep breathing, incentive spirometry, and position changes to mobilize secretions. Note sputum character and amount.
- Perform oropharyngeal or ET suctioning as indicated by adventitious breath sounds and inability to clear airway effectively by coughing.
- As needed, administer bronchodilator treatment (ie, theophylline, sympathomimetics).

Fluid volume deficit r/t active loss through burn wound and leakage of fluid, plasma proteins, and other cellular elements into interstitial space
Desired outcome: Within 24-48 h of this diagnosis, patient becomes normovolemic: BP 110-120/70-80 mm Hg or wnl, peripheral pulses >2+, UO ≥0.5 ml/kg/h.

- Monitor for fluid volume deficit: tachycardia, ↓ BP, ↓ peripheral pulses, UO <0.5 ml/kg/h, thirst, and dry mucous membranes.
- Monitor I&O; administer crystalloids during first 24 h; may use colloid and crystalloid combinations after 24 h. Maintain UO at ≥30-50 ml/h.
- Monitor weight qd. 2-kg acute weight loss may signal 2-L fluid loss.
- Monitor urine specific gravity. ↑ reflects dehydration; ↓ reflects overhydration.
- Monitor serial Hct, Hgb, serum Na^+, and serum K^+ values. As volume is restored, expect ↓ Hct. Hgb values may ↓ secondary to hemolysis within first 1-2 h after burn injury. Transfusions with PRBCs generally required by fifth day postburn. Usually K^+ ↑ during first 24-36 h postburn as a result of hemolysis and lysis of cells. After 72-96 h, hypokalemia may occur as a result of diuresis. Add K^+ to IV solutions as necessary.
- Monitor for fluid volume excess, especially with preexisting respiratory or cardiac disease: crackles, SOB, tachypnea, neck vein distention, S_3 gallop, ↑ CVP/PAWP.
- Use mannitol to promote osmotic diuresis and prevent renal tubular sludging caused by myoglobinuria.
- With onset of diuresis, gradually ↓ infusion rates according to I/O ratio and clinical status.

Pain r/t burn injury
Desired outcomes: Within 1 h of intervention, discomfort improves as documented by pain scale. Nonverbal indicators absent or diminished.

- Assess level of discomfort at frequent intervals, rating discomfort from 0 (no pain) to 10. Patients with partial-thickness burns may experience severe pain because of exposure of sensory nerve endings. Pain tolerance ↓ with prolonged hospitalization and sleep deprivation.
- Monitor for clinical indicators of pain: ↑ BP, tachypnea, dilated pupils, shivering, rigid muscle tone, or guarded position.
- Administer opioid analgesia, tranquilizers, and antidepressants as prescribed. If given PO, administer at ≥30-45 min before painful procedures.
- Provide full explanation of procedures, expected sensations. Use a calm and firm manner.
- Employ nonpharmacologic interventions: relaxation breathing, guided imagery, soft music.
- Ensure periods of uninterrupted sleep (optimally 90 min at a time) by grouping care procedures and limiting visitors.

Impaired tissue integrity/altered peripheral tissue perfusion r/t thermal injury, circumferential burns, edema, and hypovolemia
Desired outcomes: Wound exhibits granulation and healing within acceptable time period.

- Assess, document time and circumstances of burn injury and extent, depth of burn wound.
- In burned extremities, evaluate tissue perfusion qh by monitoring capillary refill, temp, and peripheral pulses. Be alert to ↓ peripheral perfusion: coolness, weak/absent peripheral pulses, and delayed capillary refill. Consult physician immediately for significant findings.
- Cleanse and débride wound. Control ambient temp carefully to prevent hypothermia.
- Apply topical antimicrobial treatments, using aseptic technique.

CONSULT MD FOR

- Severe hoarseness, stridor, restlessness, other indicators of respiratory deterioration
- Fluid volume deficit: ↓ BP, ↓ peripheral pulses, UO <0.5 ml/kg/h, weight loss ≥2 kg in 24 h
- Profound hyperkalemia: usually in first 36 h
- Hypokalemia: usually after 72 h
- Compartment syndrome: ↓ capillary refill, pallor, ↓/absent peripheral pulses, ↑/severe pain, coolness
- Infection: temp ≥38.9° C (102° F), poorly defined burn margins, pockets of purulent material, pale or boggy granulation material, rapid separation of eschar, failure of graft to "take"

RELATED TOPICS

- Antimicrobial therapy
- Compartment syndrome
- Disseminated intravascular coagulation
- Mechanical ventilation
- Metabolic acidosis
- Multiple organ dysfunction syndrome
- Pain
- Renal failure, acute
- Respiratory failure, acute
- Shock, hypovolemic
- Shock, septic

- Elevate burned extremities at heart level to promote venous return and prevent excessive dependent edema formation.
- To prevent pooling of fluid or seroma formation, which contributes to graft loss, express fluid between graft and recipient bed by using a rolling motion with sterile applicators. If prescribed, aspirate hematomas or seromas with tuberculin syringe and 26-gauge needle.
- Monitor type and amount of wound drainage. Bright red bleeding signals graft separation, and purulent exudate indicates infection.
- Maintain immobility of grafted site for ≈ 3 days. Use positioning, splinting, light pressure, and sedation. Restraints, stents, and bulky or occlusive dressings may be required.
- Use bed cradle to prevent bedding from touching open grafted area.
- Provide donor site care as prescribed; be alert to signs of donor site infection.
- Apply compression netting to graft and incision sites.

Altered nutrition: Less than body requirements of protein, vitamins, and calories r/t hypermetabolic state secondary to burn wound healing
Desired outcome: By time of discharge from ICU, patient has adequate nutrition: stable weight, balanced N state per N studies, serum albumin ≥3.5 g/dl, thyroxine-binding prealbumin 20-30 mg/dl, retinol binding protein 4-5 mg/dl, signs of burn wound healing and graft "take."

- Record all intake for qd calorie counts. Measure weight qd.
- Monitor serum albumin, thyroxine-binding prealbumin, retinol binding protein, and urine N measurements. Expect large amounts of N in urine as a result of catabolism. Serum values ↓. ↓ albumin and serum proteins, weight loss, poor graft "take" signal inadequate nutrition.
- Provide high-protein, high-calorie diet. Promote supplemental high-calorie snacks.
- Enteral feedings may be necessary with burns >10% BSA, preinjury illness, other injuries, prolonged ileus.
- Provide/encourage family members to supply desired foods.

Body image disturbance r/t biophysical changes secondary to burn injury
Desired outcomes: Within 72 h of this diagnosis, patient acknowledges body changes and demonstrates movement toward incorporating changes into self-concept. Patient does not exhibit maladaptive responses such as severe depression.

- Assess perceptions and feelings about the burn injury and changes in life-style and relationships, especially those with significant other.
- Involve significant other in as much care as possible.
- Respect patient's need to express anger over body changes.
- Provide information about cosmetic aids and clothing that help conceal burns.
- Praise and encourage attempts to enhance appearance.
- Obtain referral to speech-language pathologist as indicated for speech deficit.

Risk for disuse syndrome r/t immobilization from pain, splints, or scar formation
Desired outcome: Patient displays complete ROM without indicators of discomfort.

- Provide ROM exercises q4h. When possible, combine with hydrotherapy in a Hubbard tank. Premedicate with prescribed analgesic.
- Apply splints as recommended by PT.
- For graft patient, institute ROM exercises and ambulation on fifth postgraft day, or as prescribed. Premedicate with prescribed analgesic.

Risk for infection r/t inadequate primary/secondary defenses secondary to traumatized tissue, bacterial proliferation in burn wounds, invasive lines or urinary catheter, immunocompromise
Desired outcome: Patient infection free: normothermia, WBC count <11,000 μl, negative culture results, defined burn wound margin, and no clinical indicators of burn wound infection.

- Except for eyebrows, clip hair within 2 in wound margin to prevent wound contamination.
- Monitor temp q2h.
- Assess wound qd for state of eschar separation and granulation tissue formation, color, vascularity, sensation, odor. S&S of infection: fever, ↑ WBCs, rapid eschar separation, ↑ exudate, pockets containing purulent material, disappearance of defined burn margin, wound discoloration, color change from pink or mottled red to full-thickness necrosis, superficial ulceration of burned skin at wound margins, pale and boggy granulation tissue, hemorrhagic discoloration of subeschar fat, spongy and poorly demarcated eschar.
- Assess appearance of grafted site: adherence to recipient bed, appearance, color. Failure to adhere, erythema, hyperthermia, ↑ tenderness, purulent drainage, swelling suggest infection.
- Observe for indicators of sepsis: tachypnea, hypotension, disorientation, unexplained metabolic acidosis, and glucose intolerance.
- Obtain wound, blood, sputum, and urine culture specimens for temp >38.9° C (102° F).
- Administer systemic antibiotics and antipyretics as prescribed.
- Place patients 18-60 yrs with burns >30% BSA and patients >60 yrs with burns >20% BSA in protective isolation.

ABBREVIATIONS

ABA: American Burn Association
CO: Carbon monoxide
N: Nitrogen
PRBCs: Packed red blood cells
RBF: Renal blood flow
Td: Combined tetanus diphtheria toxoid
UV: Ultraviolet
VC: Vital capacity

REFERENCES

Burgess MC: Initial management of a patient with extensive burn injury, *Crit Care Nurs Clin North Am* 3(2): 165-179, 1991.

Fakhry SM et al: Regional and institutional variation in burn care, *J Burn Care Rehabil* 16(1): 85-90, 1995.

Garrison JL, Thomas F, Cunningham P: Improved large burn therapy with reduced mortality following an associated septic challenge by early excision and skin allografting using donor-specific tolerance, *Transplant Proc* 27(1): 1416-1418, 1995.

Johnson J: Burns. In Swearingen PL, Keen JH (eds): *Manual of critical care nursing*, ed 3, St Louis, 1995, Mosby.

Williams AI, Baker BM: Advances in burn care management: role of the speech-language pathologist, *J Burn Care Rehabil* 13(6): 642-649, 1992.

Author: **Joyce Young Johnson**

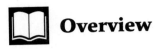 **Overview**

DESCRIPTION
Diagnostic angiographic technique used to assess extent of CAD or structural heart disease; also used to guide therapeutic interventions such as angioplasty. Involves insertion of radiopaque catheter through peripheral vessel into the heart. Dye injected so that heart structures, including coronary arteries, can be visualized with fluoroscopy. Pressure and volume within heart chambers and related vasculature may be measured and cardiac output calculated.

ASSOCIATED PROCEDURES
- Coronary angioplasty, atherectomy, stent placement, valvuloplasty
- Intracoronary thrombolysis
- EP studies to assess conduction system abnormalities
- Transvenous intracardiac pacing wires
- Ablation (laser excision) of diseased conduction pathways

HISTORY/RISK FACTORS
- CAD
- Hypertension
- Valvular heart disease
- Dysrhythmias
- AMI

CLINICAL PRESENTATION
Depends on underlying condition. If catheterization elective, patient may be stable. If AMI evolving, may be unstable. Light sedation, local anesthetic given precatheterization.

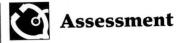 **Assessment**

PHYSICAL ASSESSMENT
Reflects underlying CV disease. With valvular heart disease will have characteristic heart murmur. With CAD may have S_4; with LV failure, crackles and S_3 may be present.

VITAL SIGNS/HEMODYNAMICS
RR: Nl; ↑ with heart failure
HR: Nl; possible dysrhythmias, heart block
BP: Nl or ↑; ↓ if heart failure, cardiogenic shock present
Temp: Wnl
Hemodynamics: If valve is stenotic, valvular pressure gradient measured to determine severity of stenosis (normally, pressure gradient not present). CO measured by thermodilution and other methods; ↓ if there is poor contractility/LV failure. EF (proportion of EDV ejected from LV during systole) may be ↓ because of LV failure; nl is 60%-75%.
> *Right heart catheterization:* ↑ right-sided pressures suggest problems such as pulmonary hypertension, pulmonic regurgitation, severe heart failure.
> *Left heart catheterization:* ↑ left-sided pressures suggest problems such as hypertension, ↓ LV compliance (eg, myocardial ischemia, infarct), cardiomyopathy, aortic or mitral valve disease.

LABORATORY STUDIES
Serum Enzymes: CK-MB level >10% total CK suggests myocardial muscle damage and can occur postcatheterization. ↑ troponin or ↑ myoglobin level is a strong indicator of myocardial damage and assists in diagnosis of AMI.
Mg^{2+}, K^+: Often drop in AMI; low levels associated with ↑ dysrhythmias.
CBC: Establishes baseline levels in case of bleeding or if surgery necessary.
Clotting Studies: Establish baseline if intracoronary thrombolytics used or surgery becomes necessary.

IMAGING
Chest X-ray: To check for cardiomegaly or pulmonary edema.

DIAGNOSTIC PROCEDURES
ECG: Q waves signal MI and meet one of two criteria. They are either wide (>.04 sec) or deep (>25% of total voltage of QRS).

Collaborative Management

PHARMACOTHERAPY
Nitrates and Morphine Sulfate: May be administered and titrated to ↓ or eliminate acute chest pain.
Anticoagulant/Antiplatelet Drugs: Eg, ASA, heparin, Coumadin, dextran, ticlopidine (Ticlid) to prevent additional thrombus formation.
Midazolam (Versed)/Other Benzodiazepines: Used during procedure for light sedation.

CATHETERIZATION PROCEDURES
Right Heart Catheterization: Insertion through femoral or basilic vein and then into right atrium, ventricle, and pulmonary artery. Pressures, volumes, tracings obtained. Left to right shunts detected by measuring O_2 present in blood obtained from sequential locations between IVC and PA. "Step up" in O_2 levels indicates shunt, which can be visualized *via* angiography.
Left Heart Catheterization: Retrograde approach *via* femoral artery to aorta. Pressures, volumes, tracings obtained. Left ventriculography performed to evaluate structure and function of LV, including abnormalities of ventricular wall function seen with prior MI. Coronary arteriography performed to determine presence, extent of lesions within coronary arteries and to assess collateral circulation.
Intraprocedure Complications: Ventricular and other dysrhythmias, myocardial perforation, embolic stroke, MI, allergic reaction to iodinated dye.

PATIENT/FAMILY TEACHING
- Discussion of catheterization and its purpose
- Techniques used intraprocedure: Valsalva's maneuver, coughing, deep breathing
- Importance of bed rest and immobilization of affected extremity postprocedure
- Importance of promptly reporting S&S of hemorrhage, hematoma, embolization

Nursing Diagnoses/Interventions

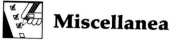

Miscellanea

Altered peripheral tissue perfusion (or risk for same): Involved limb, r/t interruption of arterial blood flow secondary to clot formation in vessel after catheter removal

Desired outcome: Patient has adequate tissue perfusion in involved limb: warm skin, peripheral pulses >2+ on 0-4+ scale, nl skin color, ability to move toes, and complete sensation.

- Monitor circulation to affected limb q30min for 2 h and then q2h thereafter. Assess pulses, temp, color, sensation, and mobility of toes. Be alert to weak or thready pulses, coolness and pallor of extremity, and complaints of numbness and tingling.
- Inspect catheter insertion site for external or subcutaneous bleeding.
- Keep sandbag at insertion site until discontinued.
- Maintain limb immobilization according to hospital protocol.
- Instruct patient to notify staff immediately if numbness, tingling, or pain occurs at affected extremity.

Decreased cardiac output r/t negative inotropic changes secondary to vessel occlusion, infarction, coronary artery spasm, and cardiac tamponade; and r/t electrical factors secondary to catheterization-induced dysrhythmias

Desired outcomes: Within 24 h of this diagnosis, patient has adequate cardiac output: BP wnl, HR 60-100 bpm, NSR on ECG, peripheral pulses >2+ on 0-4+ scale, warm and dry skin, UO ≥0.5 ml/kg/h, CO 4-7 L/min, RAP 4-6 mm Hg, PAP 20-30/8-15 mm Hg, PAWP 6-12 mm Hg, and patient oriented × 3 and free from anginal pain.

- Monitor BP, HR at frequent intervals until stable.
- Monitor ECG for dysrhythmias and ST-segment and T-wave changes. Have atropine, emergency resuscitation equipment immediately available. Run 12/18-lead ECGs as indicated for new-onset dysrhythmias or change in pattern of chest pain.
- Monitor UO qh for first 4 h, and thereafter according to agency protocol.
- Monitor responses to antianginal and coronary vasodilatory medications; report BP < desired range. Hypotension also can occur as a result of acute coronary occlusion or spasm. Treat hypotension immediately. Usually, fluids given and patient placed supine.
- When patient first sits up, ensure that it is done in stages to minimize likelihood of postural hypotension. Monitor VS at frequent intervals during this stage.
- Monitor for bleeding at catheter insertion site. Check Hct level for ↓ from baseline.
- Monitor for cardiac tamponade: hypotension, tachycardia, pulsus paradoxus, JVD, muffled heart sounds, elevation and plateau pressuring of PAWP and RAP and, possibly, enlarged heart silhouette on chest x-ray.
- Monitor mental alertness on an ongoing basis.

CONSULT MD FOR

- UO ≤0.5 ml/kg/h × 2 h
- Delayed hypersensitivity reaction
- Sustained ventricular or other hemodynamically significant dysrhythmias
- Catheter insertion site complications: arterial thrombosis, embolism, pseudoaneurysm, infection

RELATED TOPICS

- Angioplasty/atherectomy, percutaneous transluminal
- Cardiac surgery: CABG
- Coronary artery disease
- Hemodynamic monitoring
- Myocardial infarction, acute

ABBREVIATIONS

EDV: End-diastolic volume
EF: Ejection fraction
EP: Electrophysiologic
IVC: Inferior vena cava

REFERENCES

Keeling A: Reducing time in bed after cardiac catheterization (TIBS II), *Am J Crit Care* 5(4): 277-281, 1996.

Steuble BT: Cardiac catheterication. In Swearingen PL (ed): *Manual of medical-surgical nursing,* ed 3, St Louis, 1994, Mosby.

Vitello-Cicciu J, Eagan J: Data acquisition from the cardiovascular system. In Kinney M, Packa D, Dunbar S (eds): *AACN's clinical reference for critical care nursing,* ed 3, St Louis, 1993, Mosby.

Author: **Janet Hicks Keen**

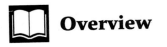 **Overview**

DESCRIPTION
Inadequate blood flow resulting from CAD may cause myocardial ischemia, tissue injury and, ultimately, AMI. CABG is performed when medical treatment for CAD is unsuccessful or disease progression is evident (eg, unstable or persistent angina). Decision for surgery is based on symptoms and angiography results. Surgical technique involves a conduit such as a saphenous vein graft or internal mammary artery as an anastomosis between the aorta and distal coronary artery.

MORTALITY RATE
2%

HISTORY/RISK FACTORS
- CAD and associated risk factors
- COPD, other chronic disorders, which ↑ surgical risk

CLINICAL PRESENTATION
Preop: Patient may be stable and scheduled for elective CABG or may require emergency CABG because of impending MI or ischemic heart failure with cardiogenic shock.
Immediate Postop: Myocardial depression and hypothermia. Expect pallor, coolness, peripheral vasoconstriction, ↓ UO, and nonresponsiveness as a result of anesthesia.
Rewarming: Expect warming of extremities with peripheral vascular dilatation. Diuresis ensues. BP may ↓ because of ↓ SVR.

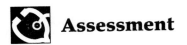 **Assessment**

PHYSICAL ASSESSMENT
IMMEDIATE POSTOP
Neuro: Unresponsiveness or responsive only to vigorous stimulation
Resp: Requires mechanical ventilation
CV: Tachycardia, ventricular dysrhythmias, vasoconstriction with pallor and ↓ capillary refill
GI: Absent bowel sounds
GU: Moderate UO
Other: Chest tube output bloody and ≈ 25-100 ml/h
2-24 H POSTOP
Neuro: Gradual return to baseline LOC
Resp: Resumption of spontaneous ventilation; crackles, wheezes (especially with hx of smoking or heart failure)

CV: Mild tachycardia, hypotension possible with vasodilatation
GI: Return of bowel sounds
GU: Postop diuresis with rewarming
Other: Chest tube output thinner, gradually becoming darker and more serous

VITAL SIGNS/HEMODYNAMICS
RR: ↓ if heavily sedated; ↑ if hypoxic, anemic
HR: ↑; possible ↓ if AV conduction pathways affected by ischemia, surgery
BP: Nl or ↓, depending on vasoconstriction, volume status
Temp: ↓, then nl
PVR: Possible mild to moderate ↑
SVR: Initially ↑, then nl; persistent ↑ with rewarming suggests hypovolemia
CVP: ↓ if hypovolemic; ↑ with advanced heart failure
PAWP: ↓ if hypovolemic; ↑ with LV failure
CO/CI: ↓ until patient rewarms or condition stabilizes
LAP: LA catheter may be inserted during surgery for direct measurement of LAP, which reflects LVEDP. Indicated for significant pulmonary hypertension.
ECG: A-fib common because of swelling and manipulation of atria; ventricular dysrhythmias associated with hypokalemia/diuresis. ST-segment monitoring; 12-lead ECG to rule out ischemia/infarction.

LABORATORY STUDIES
Hgb/Hct: ↓ because of blood loss, cellular hemolysis from bypass.
Electrolytes: Checks for hypokalemia, other abnormalities. K^+ depletion common because of spontaneous diuretic-induced diuresis.
ABGs/Spo$_2$/ET Tube CO$_2$: Assesses oxygenation and for CO_2 retention.
Clotting Studies: PT, PTT, ACT, fibrinogen. Clotting affected as a result of intraoperative anticoagulation, administration of banked blood, induced hypothermia.

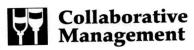 **Collaborative Management**

CABG
Indications: (1) 50% stenosis of left main coronary artery, (2) 3-vessel CAD, (3) unstable angina with 3-vessel disease or severe 2-vessel disease, (4) recent MI, (5) ischemic heart failure with cardiogenic shock, (6) ischemia or impending MI postangiography.

Procedure: Saphenous vein, internal mammary artery, gastroepiploic artery, brachial vein, or Gore-Tex graft used to bypass obstructed portion of coronary artery. Saphenous vein most common, with superior patency rate. Procedure involves general anesthesia, cardiopulmonary bypass, medial sternotomy incision, graft incision(s), placement of catheters for hemodynamic monitoring. Epicardial pacing wires often placed. Chest tubes inserted to drain blood from surgical site and air from pleural cavity.
O$_2$ Therapy: Mechanical ventilation necessary because of intraoperative sedation. Early extubation encouraged to prevent pulmonary infection. High-flow humidified O_2 used after extubation because of anemia, ↑ tissue O_2 demands, ischemic myocardium.
Fluid Management: Crystalloids given immediately postop to maintain PAWP in desired range (usually 6-12 mm Hg). During diuresis phase, PRBCs may be indicated if Hct <30% and patient symptomatic. Fluid status carefully monitored to prevent overhydration and pulmonary edema yet optimize CO.
Rewarming: Postop hypothermia and rapid rewarming may cause shivering and contribute to hypertension or hypotension, ↑ or ↓ SVR, metabolic acidosis, and hypoxia. These problems can ↑ cardiac workload and may potentiate ischemia, dysrhythmias, hemorrhage. Warm blankets, heating blankets, heat lamps, warmed O_2, and warm fluids administered to rewarm at gradual rate of 1° C/h.
IABP: May be used with severe LV failure to ↓ afterload and greatly ↓ cardiac workload.
Afterload Reduction: *Via* arterial vasodilators such as nitroprusside and NTG.
Promotion of Optimal CO: *Via* positive inotropes, such as dobutamine, which is considered superior to dopamine because it promotes mild arterial vasodilatation and ↓ afterload reduction and is less likely to cause tachycardia.
Prevention, Recognition, Treatment of Dysrhythmias: According to ACLS algorithms or other protocol.
Treatment of Pulmonary Hypertension: Caused by progressive cardiopulmonary disease. Pulmonary vasoconstriction is r/t hypoxemia, acidemia, volume overload. Treated by maintaining adequate oxygenation; correcting pH imbalances; giving furosemide, morphine, NTG for venodilatation. Amrinone, isoproterenol, prostaglandin given in severe cases.

Nursing Diagnoses/Interventions

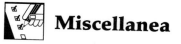 # Miscellanea

Decreased cardiac output (or risk for same) r/t negative inotropic changes secondary to intraoperative subendocardial ischemia and myocardial depressant drugs

Desired outcome: Within 2 h after return to ICU, patient exhibits adequate cardiac output: NSR on ECG, CO 4-7 L/min, CI 2.5-4 L/min/m², peripheral pulses >2+ on 0-4+ scale, warm and dry skin, UO ≥0.5 ml/kg/h, and orientation × 3.

- Monitor ECG continuously for presence of hemodynamically significant dysrhythmias.
- Monitor BP, PAP, RAP, SvO₂ (if available), and heart rate/rhythm on a continuous basis. Monitor PAWP, SVR, and CO qh. Be alert to ↑ PAWP, ↓ CO, ST-segment changes, ↓ SvO₂, or ↑ SVR.
- Monitor for cardiac tamponade: ↑ HR, ↓ BP, paradoxical pulse, plateau pressuring of PAWP or RAP.
- Monitor UO qh, noting output <0.5 ml/kg/h for 2 consecutive h. Monitor BUN and creatinine values prn. Be alert to ↑ BUN (>20 mg/dl) and serum creatinine (>1.5 mg/dl), which can occur with ATN.
- Maintain ventilator settings or provide O₂ therapy as indicated.
- Regulate IV inotropic agents, such as dobutamine, milrinone, amrinone, to maintain CI ≥2.5-4 L/min/m². Monitor for side effects: tachydysrhythmias, ventricular ectopy, headache, angina.
- Administer morphine, other pain medications as needed to ↓ sympathetic response, which will ↑ afterload.
- Regulate afterload-reducing agents such as nitroprusside and NTG to maintain SVR <1200 dynes/sec/cm⁻⁵. Monitor for drug side effects: hypotension, headache, dizziness, nausea, vomiting, cutaneous flushing.
- Monitor Hgb and Hct values prn for ↓, which may signal bleeding and ↓ blood volume, along with ↓ O₂-carrying capacity of the blood.
- Administer diuretic agents as prescribed for ↑ PAWP. Monitor for S&S of hypokalemia (eg, weakness, dysrhythmias).

Risk for fluid volume deficit r/t loss of fluid through nl and abnormal routes secondary to postop diuresis and excessive bleeding

Desired outcome: Patient normovolemic: I = O + insensible losses, RAP ≥4 mm Hg, PAWP ≥6.0 mm Hg, and UO 30-120 ml/h.

- Measure I&O qh. Consult physician for imbalance. Replace excessive chest tube drainage with PRBCs as indicated. Administer IV crystalloids, colloids early postop to equal amount of diuresis and maintain PAWP ≥6 mm Hg and RAP ≥4 mm Hg. Avoid overaggressive fluid resuscitation, which could contribute to bleeding or precipitate pulmonary edema.
- Monitor clotting studies (PT, PTT, ACT, and platelet count), especially if there is unusual bleeding. Be alert to prolongation of PT, PTT, ACT; ↓ platelet count; low fibrinogen value.
- Replace/stabilize clotting factors as indicated with platelets, FFP, cryoprecipitate, protamine, or aminocaproic acid.
- Assess chest x-ray prn for signs of bleeding into pericardial sac and mediastinum, as evidenced by ↑ in cardiac silhouette.

Hypothermia r/t prolonged cooling of body during surgery

Desired outcomes: Body temp returned to nl at a rate ≤1° C/h.

- Continuously measure core temp *via* rectal, tympanic, or thermodilution catheter. If temp <36° C (96.8° F), initiate warming measures, eg, warm blankets, heating lamps, heating blankets, or warmed inspired gases.
- Closely monitor patient during rewarming phase, maintaining rewarming rate of 1° C/h.
- Monitor skin temp, particularly that of extremities, q30min-1h during rewarming. Once extremities are warm, patient should be close to normothermia and warming measures discontinued.
- Monitor BP, pulse, CO, and SVR frequently during rewarming. SVR, BP may fall as peripheral vascular bed dilates.
- If shivering resulting from hypothermia develops, treat immediately with warming measures and drug therapy. Drugs used to treat shivering may include meperidine, morphine, diazepam or other benzodiazepine, or, in extreme instances, NMBA (eg, vecuronium).

CONSULT MD FOR
- CI <2.5 L/min/m²
- UO <0.5 ml/kg/h × 2 h
- Chest tube output >100 ml/h
- Imbalance in I&O ratio
- PAWP <6 or >12 mm Hg or other preestablished range
- SVR >1200 dynes/sec/cm⁻⁵
- Complications: low cardiac output syndrome, hemorrhage, cardiac tamponade, dysrhythmias, atelectasis, hypotension/hypertension, neurologic dysfunction, paralytic ileus, GI bleeding, infection

RELATED TOPICS
- Cardiac tamponade
- Coronary artery disease
- Heart failure, left ventricular
- Hypothermia
- Mechanical ventilation
- Multiple organ dysfunction syndrome
- Pneumonia, hospital-associated

ABBREVIATIONS
ATN: Acute tubular necrosis
CABG: Coronary artery bypass graft
FFP: Fresh frozen plasma
IABP: Intraaortic balloon pump
LVEDP: Left ventricular end-diastolic pressure
NMBA: Neuromuscular blocking agent
PRBCs: Packed red blood cells
SvO₂: Mixed venous oxygen saturation

REFERENCES
Baas LS, Keen JH, Tueller BT: Cardiovascular dysfunctions. In Swearingen PL, Keen JH (eds): *Manual of critical care nursing*, ed 3, St Louis, 1995.

Ley J: Myocardial depression after cardiac surgery: pharmacologic and mechanical support, *AACN Clin Issues in Crit Care Nurs* 4(2): 293-308, 1993.

Osguthorpe S: Hypothermia and rewarming after cardiac surgery, *AACN Clin Issues in Crit Care Nurs* 4(2): 276-292, 1993.

Saint Joseph's Hospital of Atlanta: *Policies and procedures,* 1995-1996.

Shinn J: Management of a patient undergoing myocardial revascularization: coronary artery bypass graft surgery, *Nurs Clin North Am* 27(1): 243-256, 1992.

Author: **Cheryl L. Bittel**

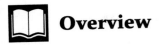 **Overview**

DESCRIPTION
Methods of surgical treatment include valve replacement and commissurotomy.
Valve Replacement: Three types of valves used:
Homograft: Human cadaver valve; seldom used.
Heterograft: From an animal, usually a pig or cow; commonly used.
Artificial: Made of stainless steel, carbon, other durable material.
Clots do not tend to form on natural valves, but duration of use is short—about 5-8 yrs. Clots do tend to form on artificial valves, making lifetime anticoagulant therapy necessary, but they can be used for 10-15 yrs. Valve surgery will ↑ risk for thrombosis and embolism (particularly with mechanical mitral valves), A-fib, and infective endocarditis.
Commissurotomy: Stenotic valve opened by a dilating instrument. When performed early in disease course, chances of success good, although valve regurgitation and recurrent stenosis may result.

HISTORY/RISK FACTORS
- Valvular heart disease
- Acute infective endocarditis
- Traumatic or iatrogenic injury to heart valves (eg, during PBV)

CLINICAL PRESENTATION
Preop: Fatigue, dyspnea on exertion, activity intolerance, all depending on involved valve and severity.
Postop: Myocardial depression, hypothermia. Expect pallor, coolness, peripheral vasoconstriction, ↓ UO, unresponsiveness.

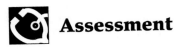 **Assessment**

PHYSICAL ASSESSMENT
IMMEDIATE POSTOP
Neuro: Unresponsiveness or responsive only to vigorous or painful stimulation
Resp: Minimal spontaneous ventilations; requires mechanical ventilation
CV: Tachycardia, ventricular dysrhythmias, vasoconstriction with pallor and ↓ capillary refill
GI: Absent bowel sounds
GU: Moderate UO
Other: Bloody chest tube output
2-24 H POSTOP
Neuro: Gradual return to baseline LOC

Resp: Resumption of spontaneous ventilation; crackles, wheezes (especially with hx of smoking, heart failure)
CV: Mild tachycardia, hypotension possible as SVR returns to nl; ventricular dysrhythmias associated with hypokalemia/diuresis
GI: Bowel sounds probable
GU: Postop diuresis with rewarming
Other: Chest tube output thinner, gradually darkening as fresh bleeding ceases

VITAL SIGNS/HEMODYNAMICS
RR: ↓ if heavily sedated; ↑ if hypoxic, anemic
HR: ↑; possible ↓ if AV conduction pathways affected by ischemia, surgery
BP: Nl or ↓, depending on vasoconstriction, volume status
Temp: ↓, then nl
PVR: Often ↑
SVR: Initially ↑, then nl; persistent ↑ with rewarming suggests hypovolemia
CVP: ↓ if hypovolemic; ↑ with advanced heart failure
PAWP: ↓ if hypovolemic; ↑ with LV failure
CO/CI: ↓ until patient rewarms, condition stabilizes
LAP: Occasionally, LA catheter inserted during surgery and brought through chest wall. LAP directly affects LVEDP and may be indicated if significant pulmonary hypertension present.

LABORATORY STUDIES
Hgb/Hct: ↓ because of blood loss, cellular hemolysis from bypass.
Electrolytes: Monitors for hypokalemia, other abnormalities.
ABGs/Spo₂: Assesses oxygenation. Sample of mixed venous blood from distal PA port may be sent to check O$_2$ saturation. Levels <60% reflect inadequate tissue oxygenation.
Cardiac Enzymes: Generally, CK-MB level >10% of total CK signals myocardial muscle damage. If hx strongly suggestive of MI, and CK total and MB wnl, testing for lactic dehydrogenase (LD) isoenzyme may be helpful. If total LD is elevated and LD$_1$ is the predominant isoenzyme, this is diagnostic of MI.
Clotting Studies: PT, PTT, ACT, fibrinogen. Affected because of intraoperative anticoagulation, administration of banked blood, induced hypothermia.

DIAGNOSTIC PROCEDURES
Cardiac Catheterization: Ventriculogram may assist in visualizing blood flow. Measurement of chamber pressures helps determine type of disorder present and degree of severity.

Echocardiography: To determine ventricular function, chamber size, valve function.
Doppler flow studies: Continuous wave or pulsed wave frequencies to determine blood flow.
Color flow mapping studies: Uses colors to enhance image of blood flowing through heart.
Transesophageal echocardiography: Uses endoscope that produces clear image unimpeded by chest wall.

Collaborative Management

O₂ Therapy: Mechanical ventilation necessary because of intraoperative sedation. Early extubation encouraged to minimize pulmonary infections. High-flow humidified O$_2$ used after extubation because of anemia, ↑ tissue O$_2$ demands, ischemic myocardium.
Fluid Management: Crystalloids given immediate postop to maintain PAWP in desired range. During diuresis, PRBCs may be indicated if Hct ↓. Fluid status carefully monitored to prevent overhydration and pulmonary edema yet optimize CO.
Rewarming: The danger of postop hypothermia in heart surgery is patient warming too quickly and shivering, causing hypertension or hypotension, ↑ or ↓ SVR, metabolic acidosis, and hypoxia. These problems ↑ cardiac workload and may potentiate ischemia, dysrhythmias, or hemorrhage early postop. Warm blankets, heat lamps, warmed O$_2$, warm fluids given to rewarm at rate of 1° C/h.
IABP: May be used during systole to ↓ afterload and greatly ↓ cardiac workload. Not used after aortic valve surgery.
Anticoagulants: Important with mechanical valves or A-fib to prevent thrombosis and embolism. Heparin used initially and then warfarin when patient able to take PO.

PATIENT-FAMILY TEACHING
- Acute infective endocarditis: what it is, how it develops, how it may affect repaired valve
- Antibiotic prophylaxis against endocarditis after valve surgery; taken before dental work or examination by instrument, including teeth cleaning, fillings, extractions, cystoscopy, endoscopy, or sigmoidoscopy; importance of notifying dentists, other physicians about valve surgery before any invasive procedure
- Anticoagulation precautions if artificial valves used
- Phone number for American Heart Association: 800-242-8721

Nursing Diagnoses/Interventions

Decreased cardiac output (or risk for same) r/t negative inotropic changes secondary to intra-operative subendocardial ischemia and administration of myocardial depressant drugs

Note: Long-standing aortic stenosis or ventricular failure caused by mitral valve disease ↑ risk for postop low cardiac output.

Desired outcomes: Within 48-72 h of this diagnosis, patient has adequate cardiac output: NSR on ECG, CO 4-7 L/min, CI ≥2.5 $L/min/m^2$, BP wnl for patient, PAP 20-30/8-15 mm Hg, PAWP 12-18 mm Hg, Svo_2 60%-80%, SVR 900-1200 dynes/sec/cm^{-5}, peripheral pulses >2+ on 0-4+ scale, UO ≥0.5 ml/kg/h, orientation × 3.

- Monitor BP, PAP, RAP, Svo_2 (as available), and ECG continuously. Monitor PAWP, SVR, CO, and UO qh.
- Monitor peripheral pulses and color and temp of extremities q2h.
- Provide O_2 therapy as necessary to maintain Sao_2 >94%.
- Maintain adequate preload (ie, PAWP >6 mm Hg, RAP >4-6 mm Hg) *via* IV fluids. With aortic stenosis and severe LV hypertrophy, a high filling pressure (ie, PAWP >18 mm Hg) may be necessary to ensure adequate cardiac output.
- Maintain nl or ↓ afterload (SVR <1200 dynes/sec/cm^{-5}) by administering IV vasodilating drugs, such as nitroprusside and NTG.
- Maintain NSR by administering antidysrhythmics. A-fib is common and may result in a 20% ↓ in CO. If junctional rhythm or bradycardia occurs, artificial pacing usually becomes necessary.
- Administer inotropic agents (milrinone, dobutamine, dopamine, amrinone) as prescribed to maintain CI ≥2.5 $L/min/m^2$ and SBP >90 mm Hg.

Altered protection r/t risk of bleeding/hemorrhage secondary to anticoagulation

Desired outcome: Throughout hospitalization, patient is free of bleeding or hemorrhage: RAP ≥4 mm Hg, PAWP ≥6 mm Hg, BP wnl for patient, CO ≥4 L/min, CI ≥2.5 $L/min/m^2$, UO ≥0.5 ml/kg/h, urine specific gravity 1.010-1.030, chest tube drainage ≤100 ml/h.

- Patients undergoing aortic valve replacement are at higher risk for postop hemorrhage than those with CABG. Measure chest tube drainage qh. Report drainage >100 ml/h. Maintain chest tube patency.
- Monitor clotting studies. Be alert to and report prolonged PT, PTT, and ACT and ↓ platelet count. For prolonged PTT or ACT, administer IV protamine sulfate as prescribed. Administer platelets, FFP, or cryoprecipitate to replace clotting factors and blood volume.
- Monitor for indicators of hemorrhage or hypovolemia: RAP <4 mm Hg, PAWP <6 mm Hg, ↓ BP, ↓ CO/CI, UO <0.5 ml/kg/h, ↑ urine specific gravity, excessive chest tube drainage (>100 ml/h), ↓ Hct. Administer PRBCs as prescribed to replace blood volume.
- Assess postop chest x-ray for a widened mediastinum, which may signal hemorrhage and possible cardiac tamponade.
- To correct hyperfibrinolytic state (↑ FDPs), administer aminocaproic acid.

Altered cerebral tissue perfusion (or risk for same) r/t impaired blood flow secondary to embolization resulting from cardiac surgery

Note: Particulate embolism from calcified valves and thrombotic emboli from prosthetic valves may lodge in the brain, leading to stroke.

Desired outcome: Throughout hospitalization, patient has adequate brain perfusion: orientation × 3; equal and normoreactive pupils; ability to move all extremities, communicate, and respond to requests.

- Monitor for signs of neurologic impairment: ↓ LOC, pupillary response, ability to move all extremities, response to verbal stimuli.
- Assess orientation and ability to communicate.
- If CNS impairment suspected, administer urea solutions, mannitol, and corticosteroids as prescribed.
- Implement the following for CNS impairment:
  Teach use of unaffected extremities to assist with moving.
  Perform ROM to all extremities qid. Have patient assist as much as possible.
  Progress activity level, as tolerated, with assistance of PT.
- When patient is able to take oral foods and fluids, assess swallowing ability. If hoarseness or coughing present when swallowing, consult physician and speech therapist. NPO status and gastric tube may be necessary until swallowing reflex improves.

Miscellanea

CONSULT MD FOR

- UO <0.5 ml/kg/h × 2 h
- PAWP <6 or >18 mm Hg.
- SVR >1200 dynes/sec/cm^{-5}
- Chest tube output >100 ml/h
- Imbalance in I&O ratio
- Altered LOC or communication deficits
- Complications: hemorrhage, cardiac tamponade, dysrhythmias, atelectasis, hypo/hypertension, neurologic dysfunction, paralytic ileus, GI bleeding, infection, renal failure

RELATED TOPICS

- Aortic regurgitation
- Aortic stenosis
- Cardiac tamponade
- Hemodynamic monitoring
- Mitral regurgitation
- Mitral stenosis
- Shock, cardiogenic
- Stroke: Ischemic

ABBREVIATIONS

FDPs: Fibrin degradation products
FFP: Fresh frozen plasma
IABP: Intraaortic balloon pump
PBV: Percutaneous balloon valvuloplasty
PRBCs: Packed red blood cells
Svo_2: Mixed venous oxygen saturation

REFERENCES

Davis JS, Small BM: Advances in the treatment of aortic stenosis across the life span, *Nurs Clin North Am* 30(2): 317-332, 1995.

Roelandt JRT, Meeter K: Diagnosis and management of valvular heart disease in the elderly, *Cardiol in the Elderly* 1(3): 235-243, 1993.

Treasure T: The pulmonary autograft as an aortic valve replacement, *Lancet:* 343, May 1994.

Valdix S, Puntillo KA: Pain, pain relief, and their recall after cardiac surgery, *Progress in Cardiovasc Nurs* 10(3): 3-11, 1995.

Vitello-Cicciu J, Lapsley D: Valvular heart disease. In Kinney M, Packa D, Dunbar S: *AACN's clinical reference for critical care nursing,* ed 3, 1993, St Louis, Mosby.

Author: **Barbara Tueller Steuble**

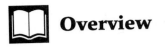 **Overview**

PATHOPHYSIOLOGY

Sudden accumulation of blood or fluid in pericardial space, resulting in heart muscle compression and interference with cardiac filling during diastole and cardiac ejection during systole. ↑ intrapericardial pressure compresses atria, ventricles, and coronary arteries. When these heart chambers no longer can hold their usual volume, the result is ↓ end-diastolic and stroke volume. ↓ cardiac output and poor tissue perfusion also occur.

HISTORY/RISK FACTORS

- Blunt or penetrating cardiac trauma
- Iatrogenic cardiac trauma: cardiac catheterization, PTCA
- Acute MI
- Acute pericarditis
- Anticoagulant therapy
- Cardiac surgery: <24 h postop

CLINICAL PRESENTATION

- Tachycardia, ↓ BP, thready pulse
- Pulsus paradoxus: fall of ≥10 mm Hg in SBP during inspiration
- Shock, pallor, cold and clammy skin
- Confusion, restlessness
- Dyspnea
- Oliguria

Classic Signs: Beck's triad; distended neck veins usually not present in traumatic tamponade because of hypovolemia.

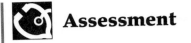 **Assessment**

PHYSICAL ASSESSMENT

Neuro: Confusion, anxiety
Resp: Tachypnea
CV: Muffled heart tones, JVD, paradoxical pulse, ↓ peripheral pulses, delayed capillary refill
GU: ↓ UO

VITAL SIGNS/HEMODYNAMICS

RR: ↑
HR: ↑
BP: ↓; paradox present
Temp: Nl
CVP/PAWP: ↑
CO: ↓
SVR: ↑
Other: Early ↑ in RAP, late ↑ in LVEDP; PASP/PADP/PAWP all ↑ and nearly the same
ECG: ST-segment elevation, nonspecific ST and T-wave changes, electrical alternans (alternation of QRS axis from beat to beat)

IMAGING

Chest X-ray: May show enlarged mediastinum, dilated superior vena cava, nl cardiac silhouette, clear lung fields
Echocardiogram: Echo-free space anterior to RV wall and posterior to LV wall, ↓ in RV chamber size
Transesophageal Echocardiography: May diagnose causes of hemodynamic compromise and differentiate severe RV contusion from acute cardiac tamponade

DIAGNOSTIC PROCEDURES

Pericardiocentesis: Needle aspiration of pericardium to drain pericardial space of excess fluid. Blood removed from pericardium will not clot because of breaking down of clotting factors (defibrination) within pericardial sac by heart action. Surgical exploration recommended after this procedure because of high incidence of recurrent bleeding.

Collaborative Management

Oxygen: 100% O_2 *via* face mask; intubation, mechanical ventilation as needed.
Fluid Resuscitation: Blood products, colloids, or crystalloids used.
Pharmacotherapy: Inotropic agents (eg, dopamine, norepinephrine, phenylephrine, amrinone) to ↑ myocardial contractility and support CO.
Td Immunization: Booster given if hx unknown or booster needed.
Surgical Procedures: Subxiphoid pericardiostomy, a resection of xiphoid process to drain pericardial sac; or pericardiectomy. Immediate thoracotomy for sudden deterioration or cardiac arrest; allows for pericardial sac evacuation, hemorrhage control, internal cardiac massage.

PATIENT-FAMILY TEACHING

- Medications: drug name, purpose, dosage, route, schedule, precautions, drug-drug and food-drug interactions, potential side effects
- Purpose, expected results, anticipated sensations of all nursing/medical interventions
- Follow-up treatment/procedures: type and dates, particularly of ECGs
- Activity limitations after discharge: usually kept at minimum for 2-4 wks

Nursing Diagnoses/Interventions

Decreased cardiac output r/t ↓ preload secondary to ventricle compression by fluid in pericardial sac

Desired outcome: Within 4-6 h after management initiated, patient has adequate cardiac output: CO 4-7 L/min; crisp heart tones; SBP ≥90 mm Hg; HR 60-100 bpm; and no distended neck veins or pulsus paradoxus.

- Assess cardiovascular function by evaluating heart sounds and neck veins qh. Check for muffled heart sounds, irregularities in rate/rhythm, distended neck veins.
- Check for pulsus paradoxus: while slowly deflating BP cuff, listen for first Korotkoff's sound, which occurs during expiration with cardiac tamponade. Note manometer reading when first sound occurs; continue to deflate cuff slowly until Korotkoff's sounds audible throughout inspiration and expiration. Record difference in mm Hg between first and second sounds.
- Measure and record hemodynamic parameters including ↑ RAP with nl BP. Later signs include ↑ PAP with hypotension.
- Evaluate ECG for rate, rhythm, ischemic changes: ST elevation, inverted T-wave.
- Administer blood products, colloids, or crystalloids through large-bore IV lines in the periphery. Be prepared to administer pressor agents if fluid resuscitation does not support BP.
- Have emergency equipment available for immediate PA catheterization, central line insertion, pericardiocentesis, or thoracotomy.

Altered cardiopulmonary, peripheral, cerebral, and renal tissue perfusion r/t interrupted arterial and venous flow secondary to myocardial compression by collection of blood

Desired outcome: Within 4-6 h after fluid management or tamponade evacuation, patient has adequate perfusion: orientation × 3; SBP ≥90 mm Hg; RR 12-20 breaths/min with eupnea; Sao_2 >95%; peripheral pulses >2+; warm, dry skin; brisk capillary refill (<2 sec); UO ≥0.5 ml/kg/h.

- Evaluate the following at least qh: LOC, BP, pulse, pupillary response, skin temp, capillary refill.
- Evaluate UO qh.
- Administer blood products, colloids, or crystalloids.
- Be prepared to administer pressor agents to maintain BP.
- Have equipment available for delivering humidified O_2, intubation, mechanical ventilation.

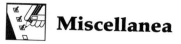 # Miscellanea

CONSULT MD FOR

- Muffled heart tones (new or redevelopment)
- Distended neck veins
- Paradoxical pulse >10 mm Hg
- UO <0.5 ml/kg/h for 2 consecutive h

RELATED TOPICS

- Cardiac surgery: CABG
- Cardiac trauma
- Pericarditis, acute

ABBREVIATIONS

LVEDP: Left ventricular end-diastolic pressure
PA: Pulmonary artery
Td: Combined tetanus diphtheria toxoid

REFERENCES

Chambers J, Sprigings D: Cardiology update: cardiac tamponade, *Nurs Stand* 8(35): 50-51, 1994.

Hancock EW: Cardiac tamponade, *Heart Dis Stroke* 3(3): 155-158, 1994.

Moores DW, Dziuban SW: Pericardial drainage procedures, *Chest Surg Clin North Am* 5(2): 359-373, 1995.

Saadia R et al: Penetrating cardiac injuries: clinical classification and management strategy, *Br J Surg* 81(11): 1572-1575, 1995.

Sommers MS: Acute cardiac tamponade. In Swearingen PL, Keen JH (eds): *Manual of critical care nursing,* ed 3, St Louis, 1995, Mosby.

Author: **Marilyn Sawyer Sommers**

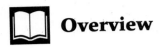
Overview

DESCRIPTION
Surgical procedure for patients who have refractory and intolerable heart failure despite maximal medical treatment (digoxin, diuretics, vasodilators).

Types of Cardiac Transplants
Orthotopic/homotopic/allotransplantation: Recipient's heart, except for posterior atria, replaced with donor heart (most common).
Heterotopic: Donor heart "piggy-backed" to right of recipient's heart. Anastomosis allows for both hearts to function.
Xenotransplantation: Transplant of heart from an animal of one species into a different species.
Donor Procurement: During surgery, the donor heart is exposed and inspected to assess viability. It is cooled with a high-potassium cardioplegia, excised, and protected in plastic bags containing ice-cold NS. It is then transferred *via* ice chest to waiting recipient.

CLINICAL PRESENTATION
Somnolence, disorientation, or unresponsiveness resulting from effects of anesthesia. Tachycardia; two P waves if heterotopic. Pale and cool skin, generalized edema. ET, chest tubes in place.

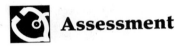
Assessment

PHYSICAL ASSESSMENT
Varies, depending on time of assessment.

Neuro: Initially somnolent. Cerebral perfusion then improves, resulting in ↑ alertness and improved neurologic status relative to baseline.
Resp: Clear breath sounds. If rejection occurring, crackles, rhonchi possible. Ventilator present initially; extubation within 4-6 h postop.
CV: Isoproterenol given initially to ↑ HR and ↓ PVR. All pulses should be palpable. S_1/S_2 present without murmur.
GI: Bowel sounds initially inactive because of anesthesia; may have nausea/vomiting r/t anesthesia and medications.
GU: UO monitored qh *via* indwelling catheter. Should be adequate, depending on CO and volume status.
MS: Although weak at first, will experience more energy as a result of ↑ CO from new heart. Keep HOB flat until extubation.

VITAL SIGNS/HEMODYNAMICS
RR: Nl
Temp: ↓ initially, then nl
CVP/PAWP: ↑ or ↓ initially, then nl
Other: HR maintained at 110 bpm, usually with atrial pacing set at 110 bpm. SBP maintained at >100 mm Hg with MAP >65 mm Hg. CI should be >2.5 L/min/m^2; will improve as heart is warmed and perfused. With rejection, CI will be <2.2 L/min/m^2, BP will ↓, and dysrhythmias may be present.
ECG: Sinus tachycardia; native P wave along with donor P wave if heterotopic. Be alert to atrial dysrhythmias and enlargement of heart.

LABORATORY STUDIES
IMMEDIATE
CBC: ↑ in WBCs suggests infection or rejection. Azathioprine (Imuran) can cause leukopenia.

Hct/Hgb, Platelets: ↓ with postop bleeding.
Chemistries: To assess electrolyte balance, especially K^+ for dysrhythmia management, and blood glucose for blood sugar control.
BUN/Creatinine: To assess renal function, especially with cyclosporine use.
ABGs: Assessed initially; Spo$_2$ later and ET tube CO_2 when weaning from ventilator.
DAILY
Chemistries: Electrolytes, liver enzymes, renal function (BUN/creatinine). Imuran can cause liver dysfunction. Steroids bind with albumin; may need less steroid if albumin low.
PT/PTT: For coagulation status.
Urine/Sputum C&S: To check for bacterial/fungal infections.
CMV/Toxoplasmosis Cultures
Cyclosporine Level: Assessed qd.

IMAGING
Chest X-ray: To determine cardiac enlargement, pulmonary complications.

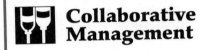
Collaborative Management

GENERAL CONSIDERATIONS
Infection Control: Paramount because of immunosuppression therapy. See "Risk for infection" in Nursing Diagnoses/Interventions.
Rejection: Major concern. Graded based on myocardial biopsies. If untreated, results in complete destruction of heart.
Signs of rejection: Temp >37.5° C (99.5° F), dysrhythmias, ↓ CO, heart failure (syncope, peripheral edema, S_3/S_4, ↓ UO, JVD, hypotension, crackles). Other S&S: malaise, weakness, anorexia, nausea, vomiting, SOB, activity intolerance.

Myocardial biopsies: Tiny pieces of muscle tissue removed from endocardium for assessment. Patient NPO after midnight, except medications. Cannulation site is right internal jugular or femoral vein. Performed at 7 and 14 days postop, then once a wk for 6 wks, every other wk for 3 mos, then once a mo.

Oxygenation: Short ventilator time, with extubation as soon as tolerated. Supplemental O_2 given prn. Encourage frequent coughing/deep breathing.

Fluid Management: I&O checked q1-2h to assess volume status and renal function. Fluid retention common because of steroids and possible renal impairment associated with cyclosporine use. Fluid restricted to 2-3 L/day. Patient weighed qd.

POSTOP CARE

Diet: Initially NG tube to low intermittent suction. Clear liquids after extubation if bowel sounds present. Advanced to low-fat, 4-g sodium diet with fluid restriction of 2-3 L/day as tolerated.

Activity: Turn from side to side q2h if patient stable. After extubation on first postop day, sit in chair. Advance activity as tolerated.

Chest Tube: Initially connected to 20 cm suction. Discontinued first postop day when output <100 ml/8h.

PHARMACOTHERAPY
Immunosuppression

Steroids: Solu-Medrol and prednisone suppress T and B lymphocyte functions, ↓ edema, maintain nl capillary permeability, and prevent vasodilatation. Used to prevent rejection or in higher doses as part of acute rejection protocol.

Cyclosporine: Dose adjusted according to daily blood levels and body weight. *Usual dose:* 0.5 mg/kg/day adjusted to maintain blood levels between 300-500 ng/ml. *Side effects:* renal dysfunction, hypertension, diarrhea, hand tremors, ↑ risk of infection and tumors.

Azathioprine (Imuran): *Maintenance dose:* 2 mg/kg/day; maximum of 150-175 mg/day. Dose adjusted according to WBC level: ↓ or hold if WBCs <5000 µl; hold if WBCs <4000 µl. *Side effects:* ↓ WBCs, toxic hepatitis, mouth sores, muscle wasting.

Orthoclone OKT3: Strong immunosuppressant used in acute rejection; substituted for cyclosporine if perioperative hepatorenal dysfunction present. *Dose:* 5 mg IVP × 10 days. CD3 levels measured qd. *Side effects:* fever, chills, nausea, vomiting, diarrhea, pulmonary edema. Patients comedicated with acetaminophen, famotidine, diphenhydramine.

Antimicrobials: Cefazolin (Kefzol) until chest tubes removed; ganciclovir to prevent/treat CMV. Nystatin (Mycostatin) given after extubation as swish and swallow or lozenge.

Inotropes: NTG to ↓ preload; nitroprusside (Nipride) to ↓ afterload; dobutamine to ↑ contractility/CO; epinephrine to ↑ HR and contractility; norepinephrine to ↑ BP. Amrinone (Inocor) to ↑ contractility/CO and ↓ afterload; dopamine in smaller doses for renal perfusion and in larger doses to ↑ HR and BP; and isoproterenol (Isuprel) to ↑ HR and ↓ PVR. See "Inotropic and Vasoactive Agents" inside front cover.

Calcium Channel Blockers: For hypertension control.

Pain Control: Fentanyl commonly used because it does not cause histamine-mediated drop in BP as does morphine.

Acid-Suppression Therapy: Histamine H_2 blockers (eg, famotidine).

PATIENT-FAMILY TEACHING

- Importance of reporting fever, other signs of infection, including colds or flu-type symptoms, incisional changes or drainage, dental problems (antibiotics necessary for all dental work)
- Necessity of reporting changes in weight >3 lb for 2 consecutive days, ↓ in UO, changes in heart rate/rhythm, SOB, malaise
- Necessity of reporting S&S associated with immunosuppressive therapy: slow healing sores, unusual growths or lumps
- Importance of maintaining daily log including HR, BP, temp, and weight.
- No lifting >10 lb first 2 mos postop; importance of daily exercise, with progression as tolerated
- Use of gloves and mask when gardening or doing yard work to minimize exposure to microorganisms, wearing mask when returning to hospital or in crowded environments
- Diet restrictions, including fluids to 2-3 L/day, low-sodium diet, no concentrated sweets
- Medications: drug name, purpose, dosage, schedule, precautions, drug-drug and food-drug interactions, and potential side effects

Nursing Diagnoses/Interventions

Risk for injury (rejection) r/t immune system response to transplanted heart
Desired outcomes: Levels of immunosuppressant drugs remain in therapeutic range. There are no clinical S&S of rejection: temp >37.5° C (99.5° F), dysrhythmias, ↓ CO, heart failure. Heart muscle biopsies do not reflect rejection.

- Monitor blood levels of cyclosporine, Orthoclone, other immunosuppressants as appropriate.
- Administer medications at precisely scheduled intervals.
- Teach patient to take medication at designated time(s) each day. Never withhold immunosuppressants without consulting physician.
- Instruct patient to attend regularly scheduled appointments as an outpatient with transplant coordinator and to bring along significant other.
- Monitor for S&S of rejection: A-fib or other dysrhythmia, hypotension, temp >37.5° C (99.5° F), ↓ CO; or S&S of heart failure: malaise, nausea, vomiting, SOB, ↓ activity tolerance.

Risk for infection r/t to suppressed immune system secondary to therapy to prevent rejection
Desired outcome: Patient remains infection free.

- Monitor temp q4h. Notify physician/transplant coordinator immediately if temp >37.5° C (99.5° F), WBCs ↑, patient complains of malaise, or there are other obvious signs of infection.
- Implement 5-min Betadine scrub when initially entering patient's room. Maintain good hand washing technique thereafter. Use sterile technique for all dressing and line changes.

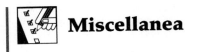

Miscellanea

CONSULT MD FOR
- Svo$_2$ <60%, SBP <90 mm Hg, CI <2.2 L/min/m^2
- S&S of infection: temp >37.5° C (99.5° F), ↑ WBCs, changes in incisional drainage or other body fluids
- S&S of rejection: atrial, ventricular dysrhythmias; temp >37.5° C (99.5° F); ↓ BP; ↓ CO/CI; malaise, anorexia, nausea, vomiting, activity intolerance, SOB
- ↑ chest tube output to >400 ml/h or sudden output cessation

RELATED TOPICS
- Cardiac transplantation: preoperative
- Cardiomyopathy
- Hemodynamic monitoring
- Myocardial infarction, acute
- Organ rejection
- Shock, cardiogenic

ABBREVIATIONS
CMV: Cytomegalovirus
EF: Ejection fraction
Svo$_2$: Mixed venous oxygen saturation

- Ensure that patient wears a mask when outside immediate living area or in public. Caregivers and family members wear masks when entering patient's room during the immediate postop period or according to agency policy.
- Assess incisions, sputum, urine for signs of infection. Check body fluids for alterations in color, odor, consistency. Obtain cultures of any suspicious drainage or other body fluid. Monitor WBCs and culture results on an ongoing basis.
- Avoid contact with transplant patient after being exposed to patients with active infection. Instruct patient to avoid visitors or health care personnel who have active infections. ↓ number of visitors; keep door closed.
- Use leukocyte filter for blood administration to ↓ exposure to potentially antigenic WBCs; discontinue lines and tubes as soon as possible.
- Clean large equipment brought into patient's room with germicide.

Decreased cardiac output r/t rejection, inadequate donor pump, long ischemic time

Desired outcome: Within 2 h postop patient has adequate cardiac output: SBP >90-100 mm Hg, MAP 65-85 mm Hg, CI >2.5 L/min/m^2, RR 12-20 breaths/min, HR >100 bpm with NSR and no ectopy, orientation × 3, UO >0.5 ml/kg/h, I = O, and EF >60%.

- Monitor VS q30min until stable, then qh for 24 h, then q2h and prn.
- Monitor for adequate CO by assessing skin color and temp, pulses, mentation, BP, and HR.
- Monitor I&O qh at first, then q2h. Weigh patient qd.
- With ECG monitoring, watch for atrial and ventricular dysrhythmias. Be aware that dual P waves are expected with heterotopic transplants.
- AV pacing may be necessary prn to keep HR >110 bpm. This is done to maintain CO and prevent bradycardic tendencies resulting from myocardial anoxia during donor heart transport. In addition, mild tachycardia ↓ filling time and keeps the heart from stretching, thus helping prevent RV overload/failure.
- Prepare patient for echocardiogram or myocardial biopsy as indicated. Monitor EF during this procedure.

REFERENCES

Costanzo M et al: Selection and treatment of candidates for heart transplantation: American Heart Association medical/scientific statement, *Circulation* 92(12): 3593-3612, 1995.

Frazier OH, Macris MP: Progress in cardiac transplantation, *Surg Clin North Am* 74(5): 1169-1182, 1994.

Kubo SH et al: Trends in patient selection for heart transplantation, *J Am Coll Cardiol* 21(4): 975-981, 1993.

Logston Boggs R, Wooldridge-King M (eds): *AACN procedure manual for critical care,* ed 3, Philadelphia, 1993, Saunders.

Saint Joseph's Hospital of Atlanta: *Policies, procedures, transplant programs, and transplant classes,* 1995-1996.

Author: **Cheryl L. Bittel**

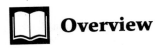 **Overview**

DESCRIPTION
Etiologies for heart failure are numerous but can be categorized in two ways:

Ischemic/Coronary Artery: Results from ischemia or infarction caused by compromised coronary arterial circulation.

Noncoronary Artery: Results from abnormalities of heart muscle or valves; includes cardiomyopathy and valvular disease. Cardiomyopathy can be further defined as follows:

Idiopathic Dilated: Gross heart dilatation caused by damage to myofibrils. Seen in alcohol abuse, pregnancy, viral infection, myocarditis.

Hypertrophic/Obstructive: Abnormal muscle fiber organization. Seen as thickening of interventricular septum with ventricular wall rigidity; probably genetically transmitted.

Restrictive/Constrictive: Endocardial scarring of ventricle with impairment of diastolic function.

CLINICAL PRESENTATION
May be receiving numerous inotropes and on IAPB, ventilator. Will have pronounced weakness, dyspnea with activity; often somnolent.

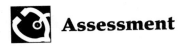 **Assessment**

PHYSICAL ASSESSMENT
Varies, depending on CO and oxygenation

Neuro: Awake, alert; restless and disoriented if fatigued

Resp: Crackles, SOB, exercise intolerance

CV: Tachycardia, hypotension, ↓ CO, S_3/S_4 gallop, ↓ peripheral pulses, JVD, angina

GI: Nl to hypoactive bowel sounds, nausea, vomiting as a result of ↓ perfusion.

GU: Nl or oliguric, depending on CO

VITAL SIGNS/HEMODYNAMICS
RR: ↑
HR: ↑
BP: ↓
Temp: Nl
CVP/PAWP: ↑; may be ↓ if diuresis excessive. Usually requires ↑ PAWP (12-18 mm Hg) to maintain adequate CO.
CO: ↓
ECG: Atrial or ventricular dysrhythmias; axis deviation associated with cardiomegaly.

LABORATORY STUDIES
Chemistries: Electrolytes, liver enzymes, bilirubin

Hematology: CBC with differential, platelet count, PT, and PTT

Antibody Analysis: Blood type, antibody screen, panel of reactive antibodies screen, HLA typing, histoplasmosis and coccidioidomycosis complement fixing antibodies

Serology Testing: For hepatitis B and C, herpes, HIV, CMV, toxoplasmosis, varicella/rubella titers, Epstein-Barr virus

Urine: UA, C&S, viral culture, 12-h creatinine clearance

IMAGING
Right and Left Heart Catheterization: Shows LVEF, usually <30%; helps distinguish heart failure etiology/type

Chest X-ray: Shows enlarged cardiac silhouette, pulmonary congestion

Echocardiogram or MUGA Scan

Sonogram of Gall Bladder

DIAGNOSTIC PROCEDURES
Lung V/Q Testing

Graded Exercises Test with O_2 Consumption

PPD Test: To help r/o active TB

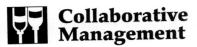 **Collaborative Management**

SELECTION CRITERIA
Patients with These Conditions Considered Viable Candidates
- End-stage heart failure with refractory and intolerable symptoms; failure of maximal medical treatment
- One-year survival expectancy <50%; poor short-term prognosis or functional capacity
- Age <55 yrs (55-65 may be considered)
- LVEF ≤20%-35%
- Chronic unstable angina

Factors That ↑ Urgency
- Intolerance to vasodilators
- ↓ CO; need for inotropic support
- Onset of A-fib
- Cachexia
- Familial dilated cardiomyopathy
- ↑ plasma norepinephrine levels (>600 pg/ml)*
- Peak O_2 consumption ≤14 ml/kg/min*
- Ventricular dysrhythmias refractory to all treatments*

Patients with These Conditions not Considered Viable Candidates: Complicated IDDM with end-organ damage, irreversible liver/kidney dysfunction, comorbid diseases, poor compliance, active infection, severe pulmonary hypertension, active peptic ulcer disease, severe obesity, severe osteoporosis, symptomatic peripheral/cerebral vascular disease

Priority Status
Priority one: Patients that are (1) categorized as New York Heart Association functional

*Associated with higher mortality rate.

class IV in ICU, (2) receiving inotropes or mechanical circulatory support. Exception: patients at home on VAD.

Priority two: All other patients.

DONOR SELECTION
Carefully screened by specially trained team

Acceptable Donor Criteria
- Brain death (diagnosed by 2 MDs)
- Age ≤55 yrs if male; ≤40 yrs if female
- Nl ECG, laboratory and hemodynamic parameters, echocardiogram
- ABO blood group compatibility
- BSA within 10% of recipient's
- Ischemic time (time from donor to recipient) <4 h

Unacceptable Donor Criteria
- Cardiac, liver, autoimmune disease
- Alcohol, drug abuse
- Systemic infection
- Cardiac trauma
- Prolonged hypotension

IMMUNOSUPPRESSIVE THERAPY
Goal: to prevent rejection of transplanted heart while maintaining natural immune response to fight infection.

Cyclosporine: Inhibits T-cell lymphocyte proliferation and activity.

Solu-Medrol: Suppresses T and B lymphocyte functions, reduces/prevents edema, maintains capillary permeability, and prevents vasodilatation. Can be used for maintenance to prevent rejection or as part of acute rejection protocol.

Azathioprine (Imuran): Suppresses cell-mediated hypersensitivity and alters antibody production; suppresses T-cell effect.

MAINTENANCE MEDICATIONS
Inotropes (eg, amrinone, milrinone, dobutamine): Often necessary to support CO until time of surgery.

Diuretics (eg, furosemide, metolazone): Optimize fluid balance. Low-dose dopamine (<5 μg/kg/min) to improve RBF.

Antidysrhythmic Therapy: Common because dysrhythmias often experienced.

CONSULTATIONS
Social services to evaluate psychosocial issues r/t support, finances, compliance; medical nutritionist for complete nutrition assessment

PATIENT-FAMILY TEACHING
- Need for frequent monitoring
- ROM, deep-breathing exercises
- Procedure for cardiac transplantation, including donor selection and wait, immunosuppression therapy, need for careful compliance with medical regimen

Nursing Diagnoses/Interventions

Decreased cardiac output r/t negative inotropic changes in the heart secondary to myocardial cellular destruction and dilatation

Desired outcome: While waiting for transplant, patient has adequate cardiac output: MAP >65 mm Hg; CI >2.5 L/min/m^2; RR 12-20 breaths/min; HR 60-100 bpm; UO ≥0.5 ml/kg/h; I = O + insensible losses; skin warm, dry, and intact; orientation × 3; PAWP ≤18 mm Hg; SVR 900-1200 dynes/sec/cm^{-5}.

- Monitor and assess cardiac output and other hemodynamic parameters q2-4h or after changes in inotropic medication. Consider adjustments in therapy for PAWP >18 mm Hg, CI <2.5 L/min/m^2.
- Assess physical indicators of cardiac output q2-4h: skin color and temp, mentation, UO, BP, HR, lung and heart sounds.
- Monitor I&O q2-4h and weigh patient qd.
- Administer and titrate prescribed medications: nitrates and afterload reducing agents, such as nitroprusside, and preload reducing agents, such as NTG, to maintain SVR within 900-1200 dynes/sec/cm^{-5} and PAWP ≤18 mm Hg; diuretics, such as furosemide and metolazone, to keep PAWP ≤18 mm Hg and UO ≥0.5 ml/kg/h; and inotropic agents, such as dobutamine, milrinone, and amrinone, to keep CI >2.5 L/min/m^2 and SBP >90 mm Hg.
- Minimize cardiac workload by encouraging bed rest or frequent rest periods. Space activities to prevent SOB.
- Encourage active ROM exercises, deep breathing, and position changes q2h.

Powerlessness r/t uncertain future, long stay in ICU, extended wait for transplant, illness-related regimen, and life-style of helplessness

Desired outcome: During hospitalization patient participates in care and decision making, expresses feelings regarding health status, seeks information regarding care, and verbalizes satisfaction with level of control over health status.

- Establish honest communication. Identify patient's perception of situation.
- Assist with identifying strengths, stressors, inappropriate behaviors, and personal needs.
- Explore readiness to participate in care and decision making. Support positive coping behaviors.
- Identify situations in which powerlessness is expected, eg, physician deciding whether patient is a transplant candidate.
- Enable patient to make decisions on important issues r/t medical care, living environment, time schedules. Provide varying environment if possible.
- Allow patient to take responsibility for as much care as possible. Give control and responsibility as appropriate.
- Provide consistent caregivers.
- Include significant others in patient's environment to ↓ social and emotional isolation.
- Encourage sense of partnership with transplant/health care team and support patient's right to ask questions and make health care decisions.

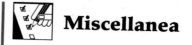

Miscellanea

CONSULT MD FOR
- Inability to maintain SBP >90 mm Hg and CI >2.5 L/min/m^2 or other preestablished range
- UO <0.5 ml/kg/min for 2 consecutive h
- Inability to maintain nutrition: weight loss, cachexia, albumin <3.5 g/dl, transferrin <180 mg/dl, negative nitrogen balance
- Change in mentation
- Signs of infection: eg, ↑ WBCs, fever

RELATED TOPICS
- Cardiomyopathy
- Heart failure, left ventricular
- Myocardial infarction, acute
- Nutritional support, enteral and parenteral
- Organ rejection
- Shock, cardiogenic

ABBREVIATIONS
BSA: Body surface area
CMV: Cytomegalovirus
HLA: Human leukocyte antigen
LVEF: Left ventricular ejection fraction
RBF: Renal blood flow
VAD: Ventricular assist device

REFERENCES
Costanzo M et al: Selection and treatment of candidates for heart transplantation: American Heart Association medical/scientific statement, *Circulation* 92(12): 3593-3612, 1995.
Frazier OH, Macris MP: Progress in cardiac transplantation, *Surg Clin North Am* 74(5): 1169-1182, 1994.
Kubo SH et al: Trends in patient selection for heart transplantation, *J Am Coll Cardiol* 21(4): 975-981, 1993.
Saint Joseph's Hospital of Atlanta: *Policies, procedures, transplant programs, and transplant classes,* 1995-1996.

Author: **Cheryl L. Bittel**

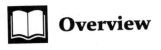 **Overview**

PATHOPHYSIOLOGY
Results from blunt or penetrating injuries.
Blunt: Commonly caused by acceleration-deceleration in which heart muscle injured by (1) compression between sternum and vertebrae, (2) bruising by bony structures, (3) rupture or compression of coronary arteries, or (4) cardiac rupture caused by extreme pressure.
Cardiac concussion: Evidence of cardiac trauma, but no cellular damage. Causes transient myocardial dysfunction, tissue edema, and possibly temporary cardiac dysrhythmias, but there is no ↑ in CK-MB isoenzymes.
Cardiac contusion: Demonstrable cellular damage. Varying degrees of injury and necrosis, with S&S similar to MI. RV wall most often injured because of position directly behind sternum. Cardiac valves also may be injured. Ventricular rupture may occur up to 2 wks after injury if contused area fails to heal but instead softens and weakens.
Penetrating: Gunshot wounds, stab wounds, foreign bodies. Right ventricle, because of its anterior location, most common chamber involved. Most common cause of cardiac tamponade.

HISTORY/RISK FACTORS
- Vehicular collision, sports-related injury
- Acts of violence
- Compression/entrapment injury
- Intoxication, substance abuse
- Thrill-seeking behaviors
- Failure to use safety devices (seat belt, air bag)
- Advanced age, adolescence
- Chronic illness

CLINICAL PRESENTATION
Blunt Injury
- Precordial chest pain
- Bradycardia or tachycardia
- SOB, guarded breathing
Penetrating Injury
- Tachycardia
- SOB
- Weakness
- Diaphoresis
- Acute anxiety
- Cool and clammy skin

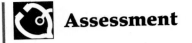 **Assessment**

PHYSICAL ASSESSMENT
Blunt Injury
- Contusion marks on chest
- Flail chest with resulting paradoxical respiratory movement of chest wall
- Murmurs: signal valvular or intraventricular septal injury
- Atrial (S_4) or ventricular (S_3) gallops if injury causes ↓ in ventricular contractility
Penetrating Injury
- Protrusion of penetrating instrument
- External puncture wound
- Signs of cardiac tamponade: pulsus paradoxus, hypotension, muffled heart sounds

VITAL SIGNS/HEMODYNAMICS
RR: ↑
HR: ↑; with contusion may be ↓
BP: usually ↓ because of ↓ CO or hypovolemia
CVP/PAWP: ↓ if hypovolemic; ↑ if impaired contractility caused by contusion or tamponade
ECG: Sinus tachycardia, sinus bradycardia, VT, VF, asystole, ST-segment and T-wave changes, prolonged QT interval. Changes occur in <40% of all myocardial contusions.

LABORATORY STUDIES
Cardiac Enzymes: CK-MB subfraction may ↑ in first 3-4 h after injury to levels >7%-8% total CK. With multiple trauma, however, injury to liver, skeletal muscles, stomach, pancreas, and bowel also ↑ CK-MB.

IMAGING
Chest X-ray: Damage to bony chest structures often an associated finding.
MUGA Scan: With contusion, detects ↓ contractility.
Echocardiography: Detects abnormalities in wall motion and valvular function and presence of intracavity thrombi or pericardial effusion or tamponade.
Transesophageal Echocardiography: May diagnose causes of hemodynamic compromise and differentiate severe RV contusion from acute cardiac tamponade.

Collaborative Management

12-Lead, Continuous ECG Monitoring: To detect dysrhythmias; may show ST-segment elevation with ischemia, Q waves with tissue infarcts.
Activity Restriction: To ↓ myocardial O_2 requirements.
FOR BLUNT INJURIES
Treatment of Dysrhythmias: Antidysrhythmic agents and digitalis for pump failure or tachycardia.
Temporary Pacemaker: For persistent symptomatic bradycardia.
Relief of Acute Pain: Usually with IV morphine sulfate.
Surgical Repair: For ruptured valve, torn papillary muscle, or torn intraventricular septum accompanied by hemodynamic instability.
Treatment of Shock: Crystalloids for fluid resuscitation, PRBCs for ↓ Hct.
Treatment of Myocardial Failure: O_2, diuretics, positive inotropic agents, monitoring with PA catheter for right- and left-sided heart pressures.
FOR PENETRATING INJURIES
Antimicrobial Agents: Control infections caused by contamination from penetrating instrument.
Td Immunization: Booster given if hx unknown or booster needed.
Surgical Intervention: Foreign bodies of reasonable size localized by fluoroscopic examination and removed. Never remove penetrating object until surgeon present.

PATIENT-FAMILY TEACHING
- Purpose, expected results, anticipated sensations of all nursing/medical interventions
- Signs of posttraumatic pericarditis: fever, diaphoresis, precordial chest pain
- Importance of notifying physician promptly if above signs occur
- Medications: drug name, purpose, dosage, schedule, precautions, food-drug and drug-drug interactions, potential side effects

Nursing Diagnoses/Interventions

Altered peripheral, cardiopulmonary, renal, and cerebral tissue perfusion r/t interrupted arterial and venous flow secondary to ↓ cardiac contractility
Desired outcome: Within 12 h after injury, patient has adequate perfusion: SBP ≥90 mm Hg, HR ≤100 bpm, RR 12-20 breaths/min with eupnea, clear lung fields, UO ≥0.5 ml/kg/h, brisk capillary refill (<2 sec), peripheral pulses >2+ on 0-4+ scale, NSR on ECG, orientation × 3.

- Monitor peripheral pulses, heart sounds, capillary refill q4h; monitor heart rate/rhythm and BP qh.
- Administer fluids to maintain SBP at ≥90 mm Hg and UO at ≥0.5 ml/kg/h.
- Maintain continuous cardiac monitoring for first 3-4 days after injury to check for ischemic changes.
- If dysrhythmias occur, prepare to administer antidysrhythmic agent or assist with insertion of transvenous temporary pacemaker.
- If hemodynamic instability occurs, place in supine position if injuries allow; prepare for initiation of PA pressure monitoring.

Pain r/t biophysical injury secondary to myocardial damage and chest wall injury
Desired outcomes: Within 2 h of analgesic therapy, patient discomfort ↓, as documented by pain scale. Nonverbal indicators absent.

- Assess and document location, type, severity, duration of discomfort. Devise pain scale with patient. Administer IV morphine. Pain usually not affected by coronary vasodilators.
- Elevate HOB 30-45 degrees or to position of comfort.
- If pain limits coughing and deep breathing, assist with chest splinting. Intercostal nerve blocks may be necessary for some patients.

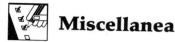 # Miscellanea

CONSULT MD FOR
- Symptomatic dysrhythmias
- New murmurs
- Hemodynamic instability, paradoxical pulse >10 mm Hg
- Neck vein distention
- Muffled heart sounds
- Altered mental status

RELATED TOPICS
- Antidysrhythmic therapy
- Cardiac tamponade
- Multisystem injury
- Shock, cardiogenic
- Vasopressor therapy

ABBREVIATIONS
PRBCs: Packed red blood cells
Td: Combined tetanus diptheria toxoid

REFERENCES
Daleiden A: Clinical manifestations of blunt cardiac injury: a challenge to the critical care practitioner, *Crit Care Nurs Q* 17(2): 13-23, 1994.
End A et al: Elective surgery for blunt cardiac trauma, *J Trauma* 37(5): 798-802, 1994.
Schick EC: Nonpenetrating cardiac trauma, *Cardiol Clin* 13(2): 241-247, 1995.
Thompson EJ: Adenosine thallium imaging: pharmacodynamics and patient monitoring, *Dimens Crit Care Nurs* 13(4): 184-193, 1994.

Author: **Marilyn Sawyer Sommers**

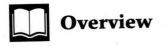 **Overview**

PATHOPHYSIOLOGY

Subacute or chronic disorder affecting cardiac muscle tissue and causing heart failure. Classified according to its effects:

Dilated (congestive): Myocardial fibrils degenerate and heart failure occurs secondary to ↓ systolic EF.

Hypertrophic: Abnormally stiff left ventricle during diastole that restricts ventricular filling. Ventricular septum may be hypertrophic, leading to ventricular outflow tract obstruction (HOCM).

Restrictive or Constrictive: Ventricular walls rigid from fibrosis; inadequate diastolic filling.

Ischemic: Results from CAD. Ventricular wall motion abnormalities and cardiomegaly present. LVEF ↓.

HISTORY/RISK FACTORS

- Infection; virus; toxins (eg, lead, ETOH, arsenic, chemotherapy)
- Uremia
- Neuromuscular disorders, connective tissue disorders
- Nutritional deficiencies
- Family hx of HOCM

CLINICAL PRESENTATION

Fatigue, weakness, palpitations, syncope. Pulmonary congestion can lead to SOB, dyspnea on exertion, orthopnea, peripheral edema, anorexia.

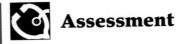 **Assessment**

PHYSICAL ASSESSMENT

Neuro: Somnolence or confusion possible if CO greatly ↓

Resp: Dyspnea, tachypnea, crackles; wet cough, frothy sputum with fluid overload

CV: S_3, S_4, or summation gallop; valvular murmurs of mitral and tricuspid regurgitation; dysrhythmias. Peripheral hypoperfusion may manifest as ↓ pulses, cool skin, and mottling or cyanosis. Cardiomegaly may cause displaced and diffuse PMI.

GI: Hepatosplenomegaly, hepatojugular reflux, nausea, ↓ bowel motility

VITAL SIGNS/HEMODYNAMICS

RR: ↑
HR: ↑
BP: ↓
RAP: ↑
PAP: ↑
PAWP: ↑
CO/CI: ↓
SVR: ↑

ECG: Dysrhythmias, such as sinus tachycardia, A-fib, and ventricular ectopy; possible LV hypertrophy, left bundle branch block, left anterior hemiblock, left axis deviation, nonspecific ST-segment changes, and Q waves

DIAGNOSTIC PROCEDURES

Cardiac Catheterization: To r/o disorders such as ischemic heart disease. Findings may include ↓ CO, ↓ ventricular wall motion, and ↓ EF; ↑ filling pressure; and valvular regurgitation.

Endocardial Biopsy: To identify pathologic agent; can be done during cardiac catheterization.

IMAGING

Chest X-ray: May detect enlarged left ventricle, venous congestion, and Kerley's B lines of interstitial edema.

Echocardiography: To assess LV impairment, dilatation of cardiac chambers, ventricular wall and septal contractility, valvular motion. Two-dimensional echo can detect thrombus formation and estimate EF.

Radionuclide Studies: May show diffuse LV hypokinesis, LVEF <40%, and ↑ end-diastolic and systolic volumes.

Collaborative Management

Pharmacotherapy

Vasodilators: To ↓ preload and afterload and improve CO. Nitrates and nitroprusside used.

Diuretics: To ↓ preload and pulmonary congestion. Lasix (furosemide) used.

Inotropic therapy: To ↑ contractility. Digoxin, dobutamine, amrinone, milrinone used.

Antidysrhythmic agents: To control dysrhythmias; dopamine, isoproterenol (Isuprel) avoided.

Calcium channel blockers (eg, nifedipine): To produce vasodilatation and ↓ cardiac workload.

β Blockers: For hypertrophic cardiomyopathy, to ↓ outflow obstruction and ↓ sympathetic cardiac stimulation.

Anticoagulants: To prevent thrombus formation associated with A-fib.

Potassium supplements: To replace K^+ lost in diuresis.

Antibiotic prophylaxis: Penicillin, other antibiotics taken before dental, surgical, other invasive procedures to prevent endocarditis.

Activity Level: Initially ↓ to ↓ O_2 demand but then ↑ gradually to prevent complications of immobility.

IABP: To ↓ afterload and ↑ coronary artery perfusion.

Cardiac Transplantation: For conditions refractory to medical therapy.

PATIENT-FAMILY TEACHING

- Activity level progression while hospitalized:

  Start with:
  Flexion and extension of extremities qid, 15 × each extremity
  Deep breathing qid, 15 breaths
  Position change from side to side q2h
  Progress to:
  Out of bed to chair as tolerated, tid for 20-30 min
  Then ambulate in room as tolerated, tid for 23-30 min

- Signs of activity intolerance: ↓ in BP >20 mm Hg; ↑ in HR to >120 bpm (or >20 bpm above resting HR in patients receiving β-blocker therapy)

- Importance of avoiding activities that ↑ obstruction (eg, strenuous exercise, Valsalva's maneuvers); stress management techniques

- Phone number for American Heart Association: 1-800-242-8721

Nursing Diagnoses/Interventions

Decreased cardiac output r/t negative inotropic changes in the heart secondary to myocardial cellular destruction and dilatation

Desired outcomes: Within the 24-h period before discharge from CCU, patient has adequate cardiac output: SBP ≥90 mm Hg; CO 4-7 L/min; CI 2.5-4 L/min/m^2; RR 12-20 breaths/min; HR ≤100 bpm; UO ≥0.5 ml/kg/h; I = O + insensible losses; warm, dry skin; orientation × 3; PAWP ≤18 mm Hg; and RAP 4-6 mm Hg.

- Assess for the following factors associated with ↓ CO and LV congestion: JVD, dependent edema, fatigue, weakness, SOB with activity. Additional S&S include:

  Mental status: Restlessness, ↓ responsiveness

  Lung sounds: Crackles, rhonchi, wheezes

  Heart sounds: Gallop, murmur, ↑ HR

  Urinary output: <0.5 ml/kg/h × 2 consecutive h

  Skin: Pallor, mottling, cyanosis, coolness, diaphoresis

  Vital signs: SBP <90 mm Hg, HR >100 bpm, RR >20 breaths/ min, ↑ temp

- Be alert to PAWP >18 mm Hg and RAP >6 mm Hg. Although nl PAWP is 6-12 mm Hg, these patients usually need ↑ filling pressures for adequate preload, with PAWP at 15-18 mm Hg.
- Measure CO/CI q2-4h and prn. Adjust therapy to maintain CO within 4-7 L/min and CI at 2.5-4 L/min/m^2.
- Monitor I&O and weigh patient qd, noting trends. Strict fluid restriction (eg, 1000 ml/day) is often prescribed.
- Minimize cardiac workload by assisting with ADLs when necessary.
- Monitor for compensatory mechanisms, including ↑ HR and BP caused by sodium and water retention.
- Administer medications as prescribed. Observe for the following desired effects:

  Vasodilators: ↓ BP, ↓ SVR, ↑ CO/CI

  Diuretics: ↓ PAWP

  Inotropes: ↑ CO/CI, ↑ BP

- Be alert to the following undesirable effects:

  Vasodilators: Headache, nausea, vomiting, dizziness

  Diuretics: Weakness, hypokalemia

  Inotropes: Dysrhythmias, headache, angina

- Position according to comfort level.

Activity intolerance r/t imbalance between O$_2$ supply and demand secondary to ↓ myocardial contractility

Desired outcome: Within 12-24 h before discharge from CCU, patient exhibits cardiac tolerance to ↑ levels of activity: RR <24 breaths/min, NSR on ECG, BP within 20 mm Hg of nl for patient, HR within 20 bpm of patient's resting HR, peripheral pulses >2+ on 0-4+ scale, and absence of chest pain.

- Plan nursing care to enable extended (at least 90-min) periods of rest.
- Monitor physiologic response to activity, reporting any symptoms of chest pain, new or ↑ SOB, ↑ in HR >20 bpm above resting HR, and ↑ or ↓ in SBP >20 mm Hg.
- To prevent complications of immobility, perform or teach patient and significant others active, passive, and assistive ROM exercises.

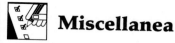 **Miscellanea**

CONSULT MD FOR

- Dysrhythmias: new-onset or associated with hemodynamic instability, especially if occurring after adjustment in therapy (eg, inotropes or antidysrhythmics)
- Inadequate CO: changes in mentation, ↓ BP, oliguria
- Inability to maintain desired hemodynamics: PAWP 15-18 mm Hg, CI >2.5 L/min/m^2, SVR <1200 dynes/sec/cm^{-5}

RELATED TOPICS

- Cardiac transplantation: preoperative
- Heart failure, left ventricular
- Hemodynamic monitoring
- Intraaortic balloon pump
- Vasodilator therapy
- Vasopressor therapy

ABBREVIATIONS

EF: Ejection fraction

HOCM: Hypertrophic obstructive cardiomyopathy

IABP: Intraaortic balloon pump

LVEF: Left ventricular ejection fraction

PMI: Point of maximal impulse

REFERENCES

Dracup K, Dunbar SB, Baker DW: Rethinking heart failure, *Am J Nurs* 95(7): 22-28, 1995.

Keen J, Baird M, Allen J: *Mosby's critical care and emergency drug reference,* ed 2, St Louis, 1996, Mosby.

Nikolic G: Left bundle branch block with right axis deviation, *Heart Lung* 24(4): 345-346, 1995.

Steuble BT: Congestive heart failure/pulmonary edema. In Swearingen PL, Keen JH (eds): *Manual of critical care nursing,* ed 3, St Louis, 1995, Mosby.

Wright JM: Pharmacologic management of congestive heart failure, *Crit Care Nurs Q* 18(1): 32-44, 1995.

Author: **Barbara Tueller Steuble**

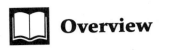 **Overview**

DESCRIPTION
Two types of RRT that manage fluid overload in critically ill patients. Advantage over conventional dialysis is that ultrafiltration occurs gradually, thus avoiding drastic volume changes and rapid fluid shifts. For ultrafiltration to occur there must be a pressure gradient across the membrane that favors filtration. In CAVH or CVVH the major determinants are hydrostatic pressure and oncotic pressure. There is adequate pressure in the blood compartment when SBP 50-70 mm Hg. Negative pressure for ultrafiltration is achieved by lowering the collection container 20-40 cm below the hemofilter. Opposing the hydrostatic pressure is oncotic pressure, which is maintained by plasma proteins. When hydrostatic pressure > oncotic pressure, filtration of water and solutes occurs.

HISTORY/RISK FACTORS (indications for CAVH/CVVH)
- Massive fluid overload: heart failure, ARF, overaggressive fluid resuscitation in multiple trauma
- Fluid overload along with hemodynamic instability
- Cardiogenic shock with pulmonary edema
- Oliguric patient unresponsive to diuretics
- Patient with anuria who requires large volumes of parenteral fluid (eg, TPN): acts as supplement to hemodialysis to maintain fluid balance

CLINICAL PRESENTATION
Fluid volume overload, hemodynamic instability, oliguria

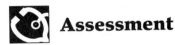 **Assessment**

PHYSICAL ASSESSMENT
Neuro: Altered mental status, lethargy, disorientation
Resp: SOB, Kussmaul's respirations, crackles
CV: S_3 and S_4 gallop, pericardial friction rub, JVD, dysrhythmias, hypertension
GI: Nausea, vomiting, anorexia
GU: Oliguria, anuria
MS: Weakness, muscle tenderness, asterixis

VITAL SIGNS/HEMODYNAMICS
RR: ↑
HR: ↑, irregular
BP: ↑
Temp: Nl; or slight ↑ with infection
Other: Hemodynamics usually reflect fluid volume excess with ↑ CVP/PAWP, ↑ SVR. CO may be ↓ if heart failure present.
ECG: Dysrhythmias common. May show hyperkalemic changes: peaked T waves, prolonged PR interval, ST depression, widened QRS.

LABORATORY STUDIES
Chemistries: BUN, creatinine, uric acid levels ↑ in renal failure, as do K^+, PO_4^{3-}, and possibly Mg^{2+}.
Creatinine Clearance: Most reliable estimation of GFR; usually <50 ml/min.
Urinalysis: Large amounts of protein and many RBC casts common. Sediment wnl when causes are prerenal.
Hematology: Hct may be low because of renal failure; Hct and Hgb fall steadily if bleeding or hemodilution present. PT, PTT may be ↑ because of ↓ platelet adhesiveness.
ABGs: Metabolic acidosis (low $Paco_2$ and plasma pH) if renal failure present.

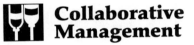 **Collaborative Management**

CAVH/CVVH Therapy: Blood flows from arterial limb of vascular access through the filter and returns through venous limb. Continuous heparin infusion prevents clotting in lines and filter. With CAVH, blood is driven through the system by patient's BP. With CVVH, a pump is used to drive blood flow. As blood flows through filter, water, electrolytes, and many drugs diffuse across the membrane and thus become part of the filtrate. If the objective is removal of large amounts of fluid and solute (urea, potassium, and creatinine), it is necessary to infuse large volumes of FRF to maintain electrolyte balance.

CAVH/CVVH Problems
Hypotension: Correct with positive inotropes/pressors and fluid replacement. Recheck ultrafiltration rate to avoid excessive volume removal.
Poor ultrafiltration: ↓ blood viscosity by predilution fluid replacement. Check for clotted filter; flush if needed. Use pressor support if MAP ↓.

Clotted hemofilter: Adjust heparin infusion to maintain ACT of 150-200. ↑ MAP with fluids or pressors. Check tubing for kinks. May need to change filter and restart therapy.
TPN: To maintain nutritional requirements. Catabolic rate may be 2-3 × nl; this is balanced with TPN.
Predilution Fluid Replacement: If ↑ solute removal required.
FRF: To maintain fluid & electrolyte balance.
Standard fluids infused simultaneously include:
  1 L 0.9 NS with 7.5 ml 10% CaCl
  1 L 0.9 NS with 1.6 ml 50% $MgSO_4$
  1 L 0.9 NS
  1 L D_5W with 150 mEq $NaHCO_3$
Typical final fluid composition:
  Sodium: 150 mEq/L
  Chloride: 114 mEq/L
  Bicarbonate: 37 mEq/L
  Magnesium: 1.6 mEq/L
  Calcium: 2.5 mEq/L
Calculation of FRF
Infusion rate: Equals ultrafiltrate plus other losses/h minus all fluid infused minus net removal rate.
Example: Ultrafiltrate = 600 ml/h + losses (urine, GI) = 100 ml/h; vasopressors 50 ml/h − net fluid removal rate 150 ml/h.

FRF rate: $(600 + 100) − (100 + 50 + 150)$
$$700 − 300$$
$$= 400 \text{ ml/h}$$

Vasopressors: To maintain arterial pressure, which is necessary for driving blood through the hemofilter.

PATIENT-FAMILY TEACHING
- Necessity of vascular access; anticipated sensations during cannula insertion
- Importance of/rationale for limited movement of involved extremity after cannula placement
- Equipment used for procedure (eg, filter, lines, infusion pump)
- Frequency of VS assessment and blood tests for monitoring status during procedure
- Procedure duration: may take ≥24 h until fluid balance attained

Nursing Diagnoses/Interventions

Decreased cardiac output (or risk for same) r/t ↓ preload and electrical changes secondary to fluid and electrolyte shifts occurring with hemofiltration

Desired outcomes: Cardiac output adequate: SBP ≥100 mm Hg, HR 60-100 bpm, RR 12-20 breaths/min, peripheral pulses >2+ on 0-4+ scale, brisk capillary refill (<2 sec), NSR on ECG.

- Assess BP, HR, RR qh first 4 h of hemofiltration, then q2h. Be alert to S&S of fluid volume deficit: SBP ↓ to <100 mm Hg or ↓ >20 mm Hg from baseline, tachycardia, tachypnea.
- Assess peripheral pulses and color, temp, and capillary refill in extremities q2h. Be alert to ↓ amplitude of peripheral pulses and to coolness, pallor, delayed capillary refill in extremities as indicators of ↓ perfusion.
- Measure and record I&O qh. Be alert to loss ≥200 ml/h over desired loss.
- Monitor cardiac rhythm continuously; check for tachycardia, depressed T waves and ST segments; dysrhythmias can occur with hypovolemia and potassium or calcium changes.
- Ensure prescribed rates of ultrafiltration and replacement fluid infusion; adjust if ultrafiltration rate changes. Use infusion pump for replacement fluids to ensure precise rate of infusion. Maintain TPN/IV rates and oral intake within 50 ml of values used to calculate FRF rate. If any parameters change >50 ml, recalculate FRF rate and adjust accordingly.
- Monitor serum electrolyte values, being alert to changes in K^+, Ca^{2+}, PO_4^{3-}, and HCO_3^-.

Risk for fluid volume deficit r/t active loss secondary to excessive ultrafiltration during CAVH or CVVH

Desired outcomes: Patient normovolemic: gradual weight loss (<2.5 kg/day) and UO ≥0.5 ml/kg/h in nonoliguric patients. Ultrafiltration rate remains within 50 ml of desired hourly rate.

- Measure and record I&O q30min first 2 h, then qh. Ensure values within desired limits.
- Weigh patient q8h. Be alert to daily loss ≥2.5 kg.
- Record cumulative ultrafiltrate loss qh. Measure amount in ultrafiltrate container. Difference between this value and total hourly intake is the cumulative loss/h.
- Check FRF rate qh to ensure that it is within prescribed limits, usually 25 ml of calculated rate.
- Monitor for and correct ↑ filtration rate, which may occur because of ↑ BP, or ↑ negative pressure (eg, as a result of lowering of ultrafiltration collection device).
- Monitor VS qh. Changes in BP of ≥10 mm Hg above baseline could ↑ flow through the hemofilter, thereby ↑ rate of ultrafiltration.
- Adjust FRF rate as necessary when ultrafiltration rate ↑.
- Maintain intake (oral, IV, TPN) within 25-50 ml of value used to calculate FRF.

Fluid volume excess (or risk for same) r/t excessive fluid intake associated with ↓ ultrafiltration secondary to hypotension, clogged or clotted filter, or kinked lines

Desired outcome: Patient experiences gradual fluid loss and becomes normovolemic: BP at baseline; ACT 2-3 × baseline; CVP 2-6 mm Hg; HR 60-100 bpm; RR 12-20 breaths/min; and absence of edema, crackles, and other S&S of hypervolemia.

- Monitor BP q30min for first 2 h and then qh. A 10 mm Hg ↓ in BP could ↓ rate of ultrafiltration significantly.
- If ultrafiltration rate is ↓ to 50% of baseline, consult physician and ↓ FRF rate as prescribed.
- Check tubes qh for kinks.
- Monitor clotting time q2h. Maintain constant heparin infusion per infusion pump to maintain ACT at 2-3 × baseline.
- Inspect vascular access filter and lines for patency qh. If clotting or clogging with protein suspected, flush system with 50 ml NS to check patency.
- If clots present, change filter and recheck ACT to ensure necessary adjustment in heparin infusion rate.
- Assess for and document S&S of hypervolemia qh: CVP >6mm Hg, BP ↑ ≥20mm Hg over baseline, tachycardia, JVD, basilar crackles, ↑ edema, tachypnea.

Risk for fluid volume deficit r/t risk of blood loss secondary to line disconnection or membrane rupture

Desired outcome: Patient's membrane and line connections remain intact, and ultrafiltrate test results are negative for blood.

- Tape and secure all connections within system; check connections qh to ensure security; avoid concealing lines, filter, connections with linen.
- Position filter and lines close to the access extremity; secure them with gauze wraps and tape to prevent traction on the connections.
- Inspect ultrafiltrate qh for any signs of blood. If unsure whether it contains blood, check solution with agency-approved test for occult blood.
- If the test is positive for blood, clamp ultrafiltrate port and consult physician.

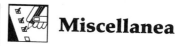

Miscellanea

CONSULT MD FOR

- S&S of fluid volume excess: weight gain >0.5-1 kg/24 h, crackles, tachycardia, significant edema.
- S&S of fluid volume deficit: SBP <100 mm Hg, tachycardia, tachypnea, ↓ peripheral pulses, delayed capillary refill, output ≥200 ml/h over desired fluid loss, daily weight loss ≥2.5 kg.
- Significant electrolyte imbalances: hyperkalemia, hypocalcemia, hypophosphatemia, metabolic acidosis.
- Factors affecting ultrafiltration rate: eg, change in BP ≥10 mm Hg above/below baseline; change in output attributable to vomiting, diarrhea, wound drainage, fever.

RELATED TOPICS

- Hyperkalemia
- Hypocalcemia
- Hypophosphatemia
- Metabolic acidosis, acute
- Renal failure, acute

ABBREVIATIONS

CAVH: Continuous arteriovenous hemofiltration

CVVH: Continuous venovenous hemofiltration

FRF: Filtration replacement fluid

GFR: Glomerular filtration rate

RRT: Renal replacement therapy

REFERENCES

Hagland MR: The management of acute renal failure in the intensive therapy unit, *Intensive and Crit Care Nurs* 9(4): 237-241, 1993.

Kelleher RM: Dialysis in the surgical intensive care patient: a case study, *Crit Care Nurs Q* 14(4): 72-77, 1992.

Strohschein BL et al: Continuous venovenous hemodialysis, *Am J Crit Care* 3(2): 92-99, 1994.

Weiskittel PD: Renal-urinary dysfunctions. In Swearingen PL, Keen JH (eds): *Manual of critical care nursing*, ed 3, St Louis, 1995, Mosby.

Woodrow P: Resource package: haemofiltration, *Intensive and Crit Care Nurs* 9(2): 95-107, 1993.

Author: **Patricia D. Weiskittel**

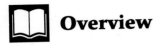

Overview

PATHOPHYSIOLOGY

Localized dilatation of cerebral arterial lumen caused by vessel weakness. Most aneurysms silent until they rupture, although nearly half manifest warning signs caused by expansion and resulting cerebral tissue compression. With rupture, hemorrhage into SAS and basal cisterns results. Patients surviving initial effects of SAH (brain tissue destruction by force of arterial blood, intracerebral hemorrhage, ICP sharply ↑) may also experience rebleeding and cerebral arterial vasospasm, the two common causes of morbidity and mortality.

HISTORY/RISK FACTORS

- Saccular or berry (congenital) aneurysm: 90%
- Septic, miliary, traumatic, fusiform, dissecting aneurysm: 10%

CLINICAL PRESENTATION

In most cases, clinical S&S absent until rupture imminent.

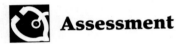

Assessment

PHYSICAL ASSESSMENT

S&S depend on presence/absence of rupture and size, site, and amount of bleeding that occurs.

Warning S&S Before Bleeding: Headache (possibly localized); generalized, transient weakness; fatigue; occasional ptosis and dilated pupils; diplopia, blurred vision, pain above/behind eye

After Initial Bleeding: Meningeal signs, eg, severe headache, nuchal rigidity, fever, photophobia, lethargy, nausea, vomiting; "Sensation of bullet going off in the head"

Hunt-Hess Classification System

Grade 0: Unruptured

Grade I: Asymptomatic or minimal headache, slight nuchal rigidity

Grade Ia: No acute meningeal reactions but fixed neurologic deficit

Grade II: Moderate to severe headache, nuchal rigidity, possible cranial nerve deficit

Grade III: Drowsiness, confusion; mild focal deficit

Grade IV: Stuporous, moderate to severe hemiparesis, possible early decerebrate rigidity and vegetative disturbances

Grade V: Deep coma, decerebrate rigidity, moribund appearance

VITAL SIGNS/HEMODYNAMICS

RR: NI

HR: NI

BP: NI

Temp: NI

Other: VS remain wnl unless aneurysm ruptures with SAH. If that occurs, VS reflect ↑ ICP and catecholamine excess with ↑ or irregular RR and labile HR, BP.

IMAGING

CT Scan: To identify subarachnoid or intracerebral hemorrhage and size, site, and amount of bleeding. If aneurysm is small, it may not appear on the scan.

Cerebral Angiography: Shows size, location, vessels involved and presence of other aneurysms. Also determines accessibility of aneurysm and presence of hematoma, vasospasm, and hydrocephalus. Four-vessel study involving both carotids and vertebrals recommended because of the 15%-20% chance of a second aneurysm.

MRI: To reveal very small aneurysms not visualized with CT or angiography.

Collaborative Management

Pharmacotherapy

Antihypertensives: Hydralazine hydrochloride (Apresoline), reserpine (Serpasil), propranolol (Inderal), nimodipine (Nimotop), labetalol (Normodyne, Trandate), or sodium nitroprusside (Nipride) for persistent hypertension; may be used in combination with a thiazide diuretic.

Loop diuretics: Furosemide (Lasix) may ↓ cerebral edema without causing ↑ in intracranial blood volume that occurs with osmotic diuretics.

Antifibrinolytics: ε-Aminocaproic acid (EACA [Amicar]) or tranexamic acid (TEA) to prevent lysis of aneurysmal clot, which normally occurs 7-14 days postrupture. Delays spontaneous clot breakdown, enabling further stabilization in preparation for surgery. Controversial.

Surgical Interventions: Based on patient status and neurosurgeon preference. Patients with more severe symptoms generally considered poor surgical risks, especially in the period immediately after SAH. Surgery considered for patients with large intracranial clots that cause life-threatening intracranial shift; with cerebral vasospasm, delayed until it subsides.

Cerebral aneurysm repair: Requires a craniotomy with aneurysm clipping, ligation, or coagulation or encasement of the aneurysmal sac in surgical gauze. Method of repair depends on size, site, and number of perforating arteries, as well as patient's status and physician preference.

Interventional Radiology: While surgery remains treatment mainstay, endovascular balloon therapy to occlude the aneurysm or its parent vessel, thus causing thrombosis, may be employed. Patient selection limited to poor surgical candidates or those with surgically difficult aneurysms.

PATIENT-FAMILY TEACHING

- S&S of ruptured aneurysm: severe headache, transient weakness, visual disturbances, pain above/behind eye
- Purpose, expected results, anticipated sensations of all nursing/medical interventions
- Importance of avoiding activities that use isometric muscle contractions (pulling or pushing side rails, pushing against footboard)
- Importance of avoiding straining with bowel movements; measures to prevent constipation
- Rationale for exhaling through mouth when moving in bed or having bowel movement
- Rationale for avoid coughing; importance of opening mouth when sneezing to minimize ↑ in ICP

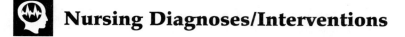

Nursing Diagnoses/Interventions

Decreased adaptive capacity: Intracranial, r/t compromise of fluid dynamic mechanisms secondary to hemorrhage into the SAS

Desired outcome: Patient exhibits adequate cerebral perfusion within 24-72 h of treatment: orientation × 3 (or consistent with baseline); equal and normoreactive pupils; BP wnl for patient; HR 60-100 bpm; RR 12-20 breaths/min with eupnea; bilaterally equal motor function with extremity strength and tone wnl for patient; ICP 0-15 mm Hg; CPP 60-80 mm Hg; and absence of headache, vomiting, and other indicators of ↑ ICP.

- Assess qh for ↑ ICP and herniation (altered mentation, ↑ BP with widening pulse pressure, irregular respirations, ↑ headache, pupillary changes).
- Calculate CPP by means of the formula

$$CPP = MAP - ICP$$
$$\text{where } MAP = \frac{SBP + 2(DBP)}{3}$$

- Assess for ICP >15 mm Hg or CPP <60 mm Hg.
- Assess for and treat conditions that can cause ↑ restlessness with concomitant ↑ in ICP: distended bladder, constipation, hypoxemia, headache, fear, anxiety.
- Implement measures that help prevent ↑ ICP and herniation:
    Maintain complete bed rest.
    Keep HOB elevated 15-45 degrees.
    Avoid neck hyperflexion, hyperextension, or hyperrotation.
    Maintain quiet, relaxing environment.
    Minimize vigorous activity; assist with ADL.
    Maintain adequate ventilation to prevent cerebral hypoxia.
    Monitor ABGs for hypoxemia (Pao_2 <80 mm Hg) or hypercapnia ($Paco_2$ >45 mm Hg), which can lead to ↑ ICP. Administer O_2 to maintain Sao_2 ≥0.94.
    Avoid vigorous, prolonged suctioning.
    Hyperoxygenate with 100% O_2 before/during/after suctioning.
    Limit fluid intake to 1500-1800 ml/24 h as prescribed.
    Monitor and record I&O.
    Teach measures to prevent ↑ ICP.
- Administer antihypertensives to prevent hypertension.
- Administer stool softeners to prevent constipation.
- Administer antitussives to prevent coughing and antiemetics to prevent or treat vomiting.
- If ↑ in ICP occurs suddenly, hyperinflate with a manual resuscitator at ≥50 breaths/min to ↓ $Paco_2$.
- If prescribed for acutely ↑ ICP, administer bolus of mannitol (ie, 1.5-2.0 g/kg as a 15%-25% solution infused over 30-60 min). Monitor carefully to avoid profound fluid & electrolyte disturbances.

Altered protection r/t risk of rebleeding from cerebral aneurysm associated with clotting anomaly secondary to nl fibrinolytic response

Desired outcomes: Patient has no symptoms of rebleeding from ruptured cerebral aneurysm: orientation × 3; equal and normoreactive pupils; BP wnl for patient; HR 60-100 bpm; RR 12-20 breaths/min with eupnea; bilaterally equal motor function; and absence of headache, papilledema, nystagmus, and nausea. ICP 0-15 mm Hg; CPP 60-80 mm Hg.

- Assess for S&S of ↑ ICP with herniation.
- Administer antifibrinolytic agent (ie, EACA) as prescribed to prevent nl hemolytic response and stabilize blood clot around the ruptured aneurysm.
- Use an infusion controller or pump to ensure accurate infusion.
- Follow these nursing implications for administering EACA:
    Rapid administration may induce hypotension, bradycardia, or cardiac dysrhythmias.
    Monitor for side effects: nausea, cramps, diarrhea, dizziness, tinnitus, headache, skin rash, nasal stuffiness, postural hypotension.
    Be alert to clotting or thrombosis, which can be precipitated by this medication. Assess for thrombophlebitis and pulmonary emboli.

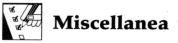

Miscellanea

CONSULT MD FOR
- ICP >15 mm Hg or CPP <60 mm Hg
- Clinical indicators of ↑ ICP: altered mentation, ↑ BP with widening pulse pressure, irregular respirations, pupillary changes
- S&S of fluid overload, hyponatremia

RELATED TOPICS
- Alterations in consciousness
- Hypertensive crisis
- Immobility, prolonged
- Increased intracranial pressure
- Intracranial surgery
- Mechanical ventilation
- Subarachnoid hemorrhage
- Vasodilator therapy

ABBREVIATIONS
CPP: Cerebral perfusion pressure
SAH: Subarachnoid hemorrhage
SAS: Subarachnoid space

REFERENCES
Armstrong SL: Cerebral vasospasm: early detection and intervention, *Crit Care Nurse* 14(4): 33-37, 1994.

Coleman R, Sifri-Steele C: Treatment of posterior circulation aneurysms using platinum coils, *Clin Nurse Spec* 9(2): 123-124, 1995.

Counsell C, Gilbert M, Snively C: Pharmacology update: Nimodipine a drug therapy for treatment of vasospasm, *J Neurosci Nurs* 27(1): 53-56, 1995.

Mitchell PH: Neurological disorders. In Kinney M, Packa D, Dunbar S: *AACN's clinical reference for critical care nursing,* ed 3, St Louis, 1993, Mosby.

Stowe AC: Cerebral aneurysm and subarachnoid hemorrhage. In Swearingen PL, Keen JH (eds): *Manual of critical care nursing,* ed 3, St Louis, 1995, Mosby.

Author: **Ann Coghlan Stowe**

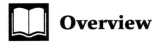 **Overview**

PATHOPHYSIOLOGY

Complex, multidimensional problem; usually categorized by cause

Blunt: Direct, forceful blow to chest; usually "closed" (without communication with outside atmospheric pressure)

Penetrating: Stab or missile wound to chest; considered "open" because of communication between chest cavity and outside atmospheric pressure

Flail Chest: Severe complication of blunt chest trauma occurring when three or more adjacent ribs fracture in two or more places (or sternum fractured, along with ribs adjacent to sternum fracture). Fracture segment moves independently in response to intrathoracic pressure. Hallmark sign is paradoxical chest wall motion.

HISTORY/RISK FACTORS

- Vehicular collision, fall, sports-related injury
- Act of violence
- Intoxication
- Thrill-seeking behaviors
- Failure to use safety devices (seat belt, air bag)
- Chronic illness resulting in debilitation
- Advanced age with osteoporosis

CLINICAL PRESENTATION

Blunt Injury

- Dyspnea, SOB, localized severe chest pain during respirations, asymmetric or paradoxical chest wall motion, inability to clear tracheobronchial secretions
- Agitation, restlessness, anxiety

Penetrating Injury

- Dyspnea, SOB
- Moderate chest pain
- Restlessness, anxiety
- Open wound to chest
- Bloody respiratory secretions/hemorrhage
- Asymmetric or paradoxical chest wall motion, inability to clear tracheobronchial secretions

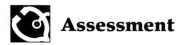 **Assessment**

PHYSICAL ASSESSMENT

Completely undress patient and examine entire body surface for injuries. Use logrolling in event of SCI.

Blunt Injury

Inspection: Use of accessory muscles, ↓ tidal volume, hemoptysis, splinting, cyanosis or pallor, ecchymosis over underlying injury

Palpation: Tracheal deviation, subcutaneous emphysema of neck and upper chest, tenderness at fracture points, step-down at area of flail chest segment, weak pulse, cool and clammy skin, protrusion of bony fragments

Percussion: Dullness over lung fields with hemothorax or atelectasis; hyperresonance over lung fields with pneumothorax

Auscultation: ↓/absent breath sounds, respiratory stridor, bony crepitus over fractures, ↓ BP; bowel sounds in thorax if diaphragm rupture or tear with herniated abdominal contents

Penetrating Injury: Entry sites deceptive, since skin tends to close behind penetrating object, masking injury size and extent. Exit wound usually larger than entrance wound. Do not probe penetrating wound.

Inspection: Use of accessory muscles, ↓ tidal volume, splinting, cyanosis or pallor, ecchymosis over underlying injury. Note presence of penetrating object. Do not remove because object may have caused sealing effect; removal could result in uncontrollable bleeding.

Palpation: Tracheal deviation, subcutaneous emphysema, weak or irregular pulse, cool and clammy skin

Percussion: Dullness over lung fields with hemothorax or atelectasis, hyperresonance over lung fields with pneumothorax

Auscultation: Sucking sound over point of entry during inspiratory phase, ↓ breath sounds, respiratory stridor; bowel sounds in thorax if diaphragm ruptured

VITAL SIGNS/HEMODYNAMICS

RR: ↑

HR: ↑ if hypoxemic or hemorrhaging

BP: ↓ with significant blood loss

Other: Hemodynamics reflect volume status: PAWP and CO ↓ with hemorrhage; CVP/PAWP ↑ with cardiac tamponade

LABORATORY STUDIES

ABGs: Evaluate oxygenation and acid-base status. Typical results: hypoxemia and hypercapnia with respiratory acidosis. Continuous SpO_2 may be used; values <90% reflect impaired ventilation.

Hgb/Hct: Determine need for blood transfusion or fluid volume replacement.

WBC Count: Baseline indicator of infectious process.

IMAGING

Chest X-ray: May confirm air/fluid in pleural space, fractures of bony thorax, and mediastinal shift. With diaphragmatic rupture, loops of bowel may be seen in thoracic cavity.

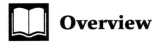 **Collaborative Management**

O_2 Therapy: To maintain SpO_2 ≥92%.

ET Intubation: Maintains patent airway, ↓ respiratory effort, aids in secretion removal, enables mechanical ventilation.

Mechanical Ventilation: For ventilatory failure, severe pulmonary contusion, and stabilization of flail segments.

Thoracentesis: Relieves life-threatening tension pneumothorax. 14-gauge needle inserted into second ICS, MCL to vent pressurized chest cavity.

Chest Tube Insertion: To remove fluid or air from chest cavity. Large-bore (26F-30F) thoracic catheter inserted into chest cavity through second ICS, MCL, or fifth ICS, MAL if hemothorax suspected. Catheter connected to closed chest-drainage system, one-way flutter valve, or, if hemothorax suspected, autotransfusion unit.

Blood Replacement: Usually with crystalloids (eg, NS, LR) rather than colloids (eg, plasma, albumin). PRBCs used as needed to maintain Hct at 28%-30%.

Autotransfusion: Patient's blood, captured from chest tube drainage or operative field, filtered and reinfused immediately.

Analgesia: Manages pain, which interferes with breathing. Opioid analgesics used cautiously because of respiratory depressive effects. Intercostal nerve block may provide local pain relief.

Td Immunization: Booster given if hx unknown or booster needed.

Thoracotomy: Generally avoided unless complications develop after stabilization. *Indications for thoracotomy:* massive air leak in functioning drainage system, continued or ↑ bleeding through chest tube, profound hypovolemic shock, acute deterioration, cardiac tamponade.

PATIENT-FAMILY TEACHING

- Purpose, expected results, anticipated sensations for nursing/medical interventions
- Turning, coughing, deep-breathing exercises
- Use of incentive spirometry
- Medications: drug name, purpose, dosage, schedule, precautions, food-drug and drug-drug interactions, potential side effects

Nursing Diagnoses/Interventions

Impaired gas exchange r/t ↓ alveolar blood flow and ↓ O_2 supply secondary to ↓ pleural pressure

Desired outcome: Within 2-6 h of treatment, patient has adequate gas exchange: Pao_2 ≥60 mm Hg and $Paco_2$ ≤45 mm Hg (or values within 10% baseline), RR ≤20 breaths/min with eupnea, orientation × 3.

- Monitor serial ABGs for hypercapnia or hypoxemia. Monitor O_2 saturation *via* Spo_2.
- Observe for hypoxia: ↑ restlessness, anxiety, changes in mental status.
- Assess for ↑ respiratory distress: ↑ RR, ↑ WOB, ↓/absent chest wall movement on affected side, complaints of ↑ dyspnea, cyanosis.
- Position for full expansion of unaffected lung, usually semi-Fowler's position, or turn with unaffected side down with HOB elevated to ensure better V/Q match.
- Change position q2h to promote drainage/lung reexpansion and facilitate alveolar perfusion.
- Provide analgesia to ↓ discomfort during deep-breathing exercises.
- Ensure delivery of prescribed concentrations of O_2.
- Assess and maintain closed chest-drainage system.
- Keep emergency supplies at bedside: (1) petrolatum gauze pad for insertion site if chest tube becomes dislodged and (2) sterile water in which to submerge chest tube if it becomes disconnected from underwater-seal system. Never clamp chest tube without specific directive from physician; clamping may lead to tension pneumothorax because air cannot escape.

Caution: Follow agency policy for chest tube stripping to maintain patency. It is controversial and associated with high negative pressures in pleural space, which can damage lung tissue. Stripping may be indicated with bloody drainage or visible clots in tubing. Squeezing alternately hand over hand along drainage tube may generate sufficient pressure to move fluid along tube.

Risk for fluid volume deficit r/t active loss secondary to excessive bleeding occurring with chest trauma

Desired outcome: Patient remains normovolemic: BP and HR wnl for patient, UO ≥0.5 ml/kg/h, chest drainage ≤100 ml/h, RR ≤20 breaths/min with eupnea.

- Check sheets underneath patient and dressings at frequent intervals. Report excessive drainage/bleeding. After first 48 h, bleeding should subside, dressing should not require changing more than bid, and drainage should be serosanguineous or serous.
- Monitor drainage in closed chest-drainage system. Amounts >100 ml/h usually considered excessive.
- Estimate need for transfusion/fluids based on amount/rate of bleeding. Record accurate I&O.
- Use autotransfusor to replace blood if bleeding brisk (>100-200 ml/h).
- Be alert to ↓ BP and ↑ HR and RR, which signal impending shock.
- Monitor Hgb as indicator of hemostasis. Be alert to ↓, which can occur with blood loss.

Pain r/t injury resulting from chest tube placement and pleural irritation

Desired outcomes: Within 1 h of analgesia, patient discomfort ↓ as documented by pain scale. Nonverbal indicators absent.

- Inform patient/significant others about chest tube placement and maintenance.
- Assess degree of discomfort, using verbal and nonverbal cues. Evaluate and document analgesia effectiveness based on pain scale.
- Position on unaffected side to minimize discomfort. Give medication 30 min before initiating movement.
- Teach splinting of affected side during coughing, moving, repositioning. Move patient as a unit to promote stability and comfort.
- Schedule activities to provide periods of rest, which may ↑ patient's pain threshold.
- Stabilize chest tube to reduce pull or drag on latex connector tubing. Tape chest tube securely to thorax; loop latex tubing on bed beside patient.
- Teach active ROM on involved side to prevent stiff shoulder from immobility.

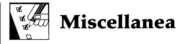

Miscellanea

CONSULT MD FOR
- Respiratory distress
- Tracheal deviation
- Bowel sounds above diaphragm level
- ↑ or bright red chest tube drainage after first 24 h; chest tube drainage >100 ml/h
- Bright red bleeding from operative or other wound after 24-48 h
- Absent or ↓ breath sounds
- New/persistent hypercapnia/hypoxemia
- Hypoxia: restlessness, anxiety, altered mental status

RELATED TOPICS
- Adult respiratory distress syndrome
- Cardiac tamponade
- Cardiac trauma
- Flail chest
- Mechanical ventilation
- Multisystem injury
- Pain
- Pneumonia, hospital-associated
- Pneumothorax
- Respiratory failure, acute
- Shock, hemorrhagic

ABBREVIATIONS
ICS: Intercostal space
MAL: Midaxillary line
MCL: Midclavicular line
PRBCs: Packed red blood cells
Td: Combined tetanus diphtheria toxoid

REFERENCES
Feliciano D, Moore E, Mattox K: *Trauma,* ed 3, Stamford, Conn, 1996, Appleton & Lange.
Hefti D: Chest trauma, *RN* 54(5): 28-33, 1991.
Howard CA: Chest trauma. In Swearingen PL, Keen JH (eds): *Manual of critical care nursing,* ed 3, St Louis, 1995, Mosby.
Hurn PD, Hartsock RL: Blunt thoracic injuries, *Crit Care Nurs Clin North Am* 5(4): 673-686, 1993.
Hurst J: Thoracic trauma, *Respir Care* 37(7): 708-719, 1992.
Mergaert S: S.T.O.P. and assess chest tubes the easy way, *Nursing* 24(2): 52-53, 1994.
Prentice D, Ahrens T: Pulmonary complications of trauma, *Crit Care Nurs Q* 17(2): 24-33, 1994.
Schrader K: Penetrating chest trauma, *Crit Care Nurs Clin North Am* 5(4): 687-696, 1993.
Stanik-Hutt J: Strategies for pain management in traumatic thoracic injuries, *Crit Care Nurs Clin North Am* 5(4): 713-722, 1993.

Author: **Cheri A. Goll**

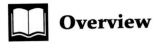 **Overview**

PATHOPHYSIOLOGY

Chronic, irreversible liver disorder characterized by hepatocellular death, scarring, and other structural changes that disrupt blood flow and lead to total liver dysfunction. Complications caused by cellular failure include inability to metabolize bilirubin and presence of jaundice, difficulty producing serum proteins (including albumin and some clotting factors), hyperdynamic circulation and ↓ vasomotor tone, V/Q mismatch and sometimes cyanosis, changes in N metabolism (eg, inability to convert ammonia to urea), and difficulty metabolizing some hormones. Complications r/t blocked blood flow and portal hypertension include ascites, bleeding esophageal and gastric varices, portosystemic collaterals, encephalopathy, and splenomegaly.

HISTORY/RISK FACTORS

- Alcoholic cirrhosis: associated with chronic alcohol abuse
- Postnecrotic cirrhosis: associated with hx of viral hepatitis or hepatic damage from drugs or toxins
- Biliary cirrhosis: associated with posthepatic biliary obstruction

CLINICAL PRESENTATION

- Weakness, fatigability, weight loss, anorexia, nausea, vomiting, abdominal pain, loss of libido, hematemesis
- Dark urine because of presence of bilirubin; light stools because of its absence

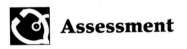 **Assessment**

PHYSICAL ASSESSMENT

- Jaundice, hepatomegaly, ascites, peripheral edema, fetor hepaticus (musty, sweetish odor on breath)
- Changes in personality and behavior; condition can progress to coma: caused by hepatic encephalopathy
- Spider angiomas, testicular atrophy, gynecomastia, pectoral and axillary alopecia: caused by hormonal changes
- Splenomegaly
- Hemorrhoids: caused by portal hypertension complications
- Palmar erythema

VITAL SIGNS/HEMODYNAMICS

RR: Nl or ↑ as a result of V/Q mismatch
HR: Nl or ↑
BP: Nl or ↓
Temp: Nl or ↑ because of predisposition to infection
Hemodynamics: With severe cirrhosis or when stressed by surgery, infection, or bleeding, a hyperdynamic circulatory state similar to SIRS possible with ↓ SVR, ↑ HR, BP slightly ↓, and CO/CI markedly ↑ up to 2-3 × nl.

LABORATORY STUDIES

Hematology: ↓ RBCs attributable to hypersplenism, hemorrhage. WBCs ↓ with hypersplenism and ↑ with infection.
Serum Biochemical Tests
Bilirubin: ↑. If levels very high or persistently ↑, associated with poor prognosis.
Alkalkine phosphatase: Nl to mildly ↑.
ALT, AST: Usually ↑ >300 U with acute failure; nl or mildly ↑ with chronic failure. ALT most specific for hepatocellular damage. AST/ALT ratio >1.0 suggests chronic liver failure or tumor invasion; ratio <1.0 associated with acute or viral hepatitis.
Albumin: ↓, especially with ascites. Persistently low levels suggest poor prognosis.
Na$^+$: Nl to low. Sodium is retained but is associated with water retention, which results in nl serum Na$^+$ levels or even dilutional hyponatremia. Severe hyponatremia often present in terminal stage and associated with tense ascites and hepatorenal syndrome.
K$^+$: Slightly ↓; chronic hypokalemic acidosis common in alcoholic liver disease.
Glucose: ↓ owing to impaired gluconeogenesis and glycogen depletion.
BUN: May be slightly ↓ because of failure of Krebs cycle enzymes in the liver or ↑ because of bleeding or renal insufficiency.
Ammonia: ↑ expected because of inability of failing liver to convert ammonia to urea and shunting of intestinal blood *via* collateral vessels. ↑ intestinal protein from dietary intake or GI hemorrhage ↑ ammonia levels.

Coagulation: PT prolonged and, in severe liver disease, unresponsive to vitamin K therapy.

IMAGING

Barium Swallow: Used in nonemergency situations to verify presence of gastro-esophageal varices.
Radiologic Studies: Ultrasound reveals hepatomegaly and intrahepatic tumors. CT scan of liver/spleen to evaluate size and location of tumors and r/o gallbladder disease.
Angiography: Establishes patency of portal vein and visualizes portosystemic collateral vessels to determine cause and effective treatment for variceal bleeding.

DIAGNOSTIC PROCEDURES

Liver Biopsy: Liver specimen usually obtained percutaneously for microscopic analysis and diagnosis of cirrhosis or other liver disease. Obtained *via* transvenous biopsy if ↑ PT or ↓ platelets present.
Esophagoscopy: Visualizes esophagus and stomach directly *via* fiberoptics. Varices in esophagus and upper portion of stomach identified, and attempts made to identify exact source of bleeding. Variceal bleeding may be treated with sclerotherapy, other procedures, during endoscopic procedure.
EEG: Traces electrical brain impulses to detect/confirm encephalopathy. EEG changes occur very early, usually before behavioral or biochemical alterations.
Psychometric Testing: Evaluates for hepatic encephalopathy.

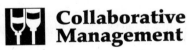 **Collaborative Management**

Correction of Precipitating Factors: Hepatic failure may develop if hepatocellular functioning disrupted. GI hemorrhage or blood loss from other sources requires immediate volume resuscitation. Hypoxia must be corrected immediately. Acute infections treated aggressively with appropriate antibiotics. Electrolyte disturbances resulting from diuretics, diarrhea, or other causes corrected promptly. ETOH and hepatotoxic drugs eliminated.

Fluid, Electrolyte Management: Unless hyponatremia profound, sodium-containing fluids avoided because they contribute to ascites and peripheral edema and may potentiate renal insufficiency. Hypokalemia common and must be corrected with potassium replacements because hypokalemic alkalosis can worsen or precipitate encephalopathy. Albumin and D_5W generally used for fluid resuscitation unless low Hct level signals need for PRBCs. FFP may be used if clotting factors deficient. If unstable, PAP monitoring initiated to ensure adequate tissue perfusion without fluid overload. Hyperdynamic circulatory state supported by fluid administration and sympathomimetic agents (eg, dopamine) as necessary.

Bed Rest: Necessary to ↓ metabolic demands placed on liver during nl daily activity.

Nutritional Therapy: High-calorie, high-protein (80-100 g) diet of high biologic value indicated for patients without evidence of encephalopathy to ensure tissue repair, since the liver is capable of significant regeneration under optimal circumstances. Sodium moderately restricted. If GI function impaired and patient unable to tolerate enteral feedings, PN initiated. For acute hepatic encephalopathy, protein eliminated totally from diet until recovery.

Pharmacotherapy: Drugs with hepatotoxic potential should be discontinued. These include acetaminophen, ETOH, methotrexate, NSAIDs, oral contraceptives, phenytoin, rifampin, many antibiotics, many inhaled anesthetics, chemotherapeutic agents.

Sedatives: Avoided if possible because they can precipitate or contribute to encephalopathy. If necessary, diphenhydramine (Benadryl) or oxazepam (Serax) often selected because they can be eliminated safely in hepatic disease.

Histamine H$_2$-receptor antagonists: To block acid secretion and prevent gastric erosions, which are common with chronic or severe hepatic failure. Ranitidine or famotidine is preferred agent because of cimetidine-related alterations in hepatic metabolism.

Sucralfate (Carafate): Binds to gastric erosions and coats gastric/duodenal mucosa.

Dextrose: In the event of hypoglycemia, a bolus of D_{50} or continual infusion of 10% solution indicated.

Management of Resp Failure: Intubation or mechanical ventilation may be indicated if advanced encephalopathy, aspiration of gastric contents, or ventilatory impairment secondary to ascites is present. Continuous SpO_2 used with respiratory failure or if patient at high risk for same. Need for adequate tissue oxygenation cannot be overemphasized, since hepatic hypoxia is a significant contributor to hepatic failure.

Management of Ascites

Restriction of fluid, sodium intake: If ascites severe, sodium limited to <500 mg/day.

Restriction of physical activity: To ↓ metabolites that must be handled by the liver.

Diuretics: If more conservative measures ineffective in controlling ascites, spironolactone (Aldactone), amiloride, or other potassium-sparing diuretic may be used. If ineffective, more potent diuretics such as furosemide added. For severe ascites, mannitol may be added. Diuresis goal is 1 L/day, as estimated by a 0.5 kg weight loss/day. If diuresis too rapid, may lead to acute hypovolemia, shock, and hepatorenal syndrome.

Albumin: To ↑ intravascular colloidal pressure.

Paracentesis: Removal of ascitic fluid for refractory ascites.

Peritoneal-venous shunt: Shunt system (eg, LeVeen or Denver) may be placed surgically for refractory ascites. Peritoneal cavity drained by a long, perforated catheter that drains into intrathoracic superior vena cava. Device designed so that fluid can flow only in one direction—from peritoneum into bloodstream. Many complications include fluid overload, infection, DIC, peritonitis, shunt occlusion, variceal hemorrhage.

Management of Encephalopathy

Elimination, correction of precipitating factors: Variceal hemorrhage, infection, dehydration, electrolyte imbalance, sedative use, dietary protein intake, constipation.

Elimination of dietary protein: Reintroduced gradually when symptoms improve.

Early, thorough catharsis by magnesium citrate or enemas (usually tap water): To remove intestinal contents.

Administration of neomycin: To ↓ intestinal bacteria that produce ammonia; used only in acute situations.

Administration of lactulose: To create environment unfavorable to ammonia-forming intestinal bacteria and cause osmotic diarrhea. Dose adjusted to produce two or three semiformed stools/day.

Management of Bleeding Complications: FFP and platelets given to correct defects in clotting factors and thrombocytopenia. Vitamin K may be prescribed to help correct bleeding tendencies but may have little effect.

Management of Hepatorenal Syndrome: Often occurs because of overaggressive diuretic therapy, paracentesis, hemorrhage, diarrhea, or dehydration. Prevention, when possible, is essential. Electrolytes corrected and ascites mobilized slowly. Hepatic failure, the causative factor, is treated. Renal dialysis seldom employed because it does not improve survival and can lead to GI hemorrhage and shock.

Hepatic Transplantation: For irreversible, progressive liver disease when supportive therapy has failed. Only therapy available for fulminant hepatic failure; requires highly skilled team of specialists.

PATIENT/FAMILY TEACHING

- Importance of sufficient rest and adherence to prescribed diet
- Availability of alcohol- and drug-treatment programs if alcohol- and drug-related disease has occurred
- Availability of support groups (Alcoholics Anonymous, Al-Anon) for patients and family members when disease is r/t chronic alcohol ingestion
- Importance of avoiding OTC medications without consulting health care provider
- S&S of unusual bleeding, including prolonged mucosal bleeding, very large or painful bruises, dark stools
- Sodium restriction if ascites developed during illness
- Protein restriction if patient has residual or chronic encephalopathy; importance of avoiding constipation
- Necessity of alcohol cessation for > several mos after complete recovery from acute episode; after full recovery, allowance of 1-2 glasses of beer or wine/day if hepatic failure not r/t alcohol ingestion
- Necessity of measuring weight qd and reporting weight loss/gain >5 lbs

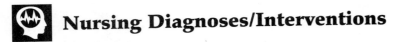

Nursing Diagnoses/Interventions

Fluid volume deficit r/t ↓ intake secondary to medically prescribed restrictions; and r/t ↓ circulating volume secondary to hypoalbuminemia, altered hemodynamics, fluid sequestration, and diuretic therapy

Desired outcome: Within 24 h of this diagnosis, patient normovolemic: MAP ≥70 mm Hg, HR 60-100 bpm, brisk capillary refill (<2 sec), distal pulses >2+ on 0-4+ scale, CVP 2-6 mm Hg, PAP 20-30/8-15 mm Hg, PAWP 6-12 mm Hg, CI ≥3.0 L/min/m^2, SVR 900-1200 dynes/sec/cm^{-5}, UO ≥0.5 ml/kg/h, and orientation × 3.

- Monitor and document HR, BP, ECG, and CV status qh or more frequently for unstable VS. Be alert to MAP ↓ ≥10 mm Hg from previous assessment and to ↑ in HR suggestive of hypovolemia or circulatory decompensation.
- Measure central pressures and thermodilution CO q1-4h. Be alert to low/↓ CVP, PAWP, and CO. Calculate SVR q4-8h or more frequently in unstable patients. ↑ HR, ↓ PAWP, CO less than baseline, or CI <3.0, along with ↓ UO, suggest hypovolemia. Because of altered vascular responsiveness, SVR may not be ↑ with hypovolemic hepatic failure. Be aware that "normal" CO actually may be ↓ for these patients. Monitor Svo$_2$ as available to evaluate adequacy of tissue oxygenation.
- Measure and record UO qh. Be alert to output <0.5 ml/kg/h for 2 consecutive h. If ↓ or other indicators of fluid volume deficit present, consider cautious ↑ in fluid intake (eg, 50-100 ml/h), and then reevaluate volume status. Use extreme caution in giving potent diuretics, since they may precipitate encephalopathy or renal insufficiency by causing rapid diuresis and electrolyte changes.
- Estimate ongoing fluid losses. Measure all drainage from peritoneal or other catheters q2-4h. Weigh patient qd. Compare 24-h intake to output. Weight loss should not exceed 0.5 kg/day because more rapid diuresis can lead to intravascular volume depletion and impair renal function.
- Monitor serum albumin, and administer albumin replacements as indicated.

Fluid volume excess: Interstitial, r/t compromised regulatory mechanisms secondary to acute or chronic hepatic failure

Desired outcomes: Within 48 h of this diagnosis, patient normovolemic: CVP 2-6 mm Hg, PAWP 6-12 mm Hg, HR 60-100 bpm, RR 12-20 breaths/min with eupnea, ↓/stable abdominal girth, and absence of crackles, edema, uncomfortable ascites, and other clinical indicators of fluid volume excess.

- Monitor VS, hemodynamic parameters, and CV status q1-2h. Be alert to CVP >6 mm Hg or PAWP >12 mm Hg.
- Monitor for evidence of pulmonary edema r/t fluid overload. Note presence of dyspnea, orthopnea, basilar crackles that do not clear with coughing, and tachypnea.
- Use minimal amounts of fluids necessary to administer IV medications and maintain IV catheter patency.
- If fluids restricted, offer mouth care and/or ice chips.
- Measure and record abdominal girth qd. Be aware that abdominal girth measurements are subject to error; great care is necessary to ensure accurate measurements. Measure at widest point, and mark this level for subsequent measurement. Measure in the same position each time, preferably supine.
- Monitor serum electrolyte levels, especially sodium and potassium.

Altered nutrition: Less than body requirements, r/t anorexia, nausea, or malabsorption

Desired outcome: By 24 h before hospital discharge, patient verbalizes knowledge of foods permitted/restricted and develops a 3-day menu that includes or excludes these foods appropriately.

- Encourage foods permitted within dietary restrictions. Remember that sodium and fluids are restricted. If ammonia level ↑, protein and foods high in ammonia also will be restricted.
- Monitor I&O; weigh qd.
- Encourage small, frequent meals to ensure adequate nutrition.
- Encourage significant others to bring in desirable foods as permitted.
- Promote bed rest to reduce metabolic demands on the liver.
- Provide a soft diet for esophageal varices. Patients with bleeding esophageal varices are NPO.
- Discuss need for feeding supplements and enteral or parenteral nutrition with physician if appropriate.

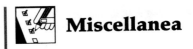

Miscellanea

CONSULT MD FOR

- S&S of fluid volume deficit/excess
- Electrolyte imbalance: hypokalemia, severe hyponatremia (Na$^+$ <120 mEq/L)
- S&S of pulmonary infection, other respiratory complications
- S&S of GI, other hemorrhage: ↓ Hct/Hgb; ↑ BUN; occult blood in stools, gastric contents
- S&S of urinary, bloodstream, other infections

RELATED TOPICS

- Esophageal varices
- Hepatic failure
- Hypervolemia
- Hyponatremia

ABBREVIATIONS

D$_{50}$: 50% dextrose
ETOH: Ethanol
FFP: Fresh frozen plasma
FSPs: Fibrin split products
N: Nitrogen
PRBCs: Packed red blood cells
SIRS: Systemic inflammatory response syndrome

Sensory/Perceptual alterations r/t endogenous chemical alteration (accumulation of ammonia, other CNS toxins with hepatic dysfunction), therapeutically restricted environment, sleep deprivation, and hypoxia

Desired outcomes: By time of hospital discharge, patient exhibits stable personality pattern, age-appropriate behavior, intact intellect appropriate for level of education, distinct speech, and coordinated gross and fine motor movements. Handwriting legible, and psychometric test scores improved from baseline.

- Avoid or minimize precipitating factors:
    Eliminate/↓ dietary protein.
    Avoid/correct constipation.
    Check gastric secretions, vomitus, and stools for occult blood.
    Evaluate Hct and Hgb for evidence of bleeding.
    Monitor for indicators of infection.
    Evaluate serum ammonia levels.
    Be alert for potential sources of electrolyte imbalance (eg, diarrhea, gastric aspiration).
    Avoid use of sedative or tranquilizing agents and hepatotoxic drugs.
    Correct hypoxemia.
- Evaluate for CNS effects such as personality changes, childish behavior, intellectual impairment, slurred speech, ataxia, asterixis.
- Administer daily handwriting or psychometric tests (if appropriate for LOC) to evaluate mild or subclinical encephalopathy.
- Administer enemas to clear colon of intestinal contents that contribute to encephalopathy. Repeat as necessary to ensure thorough colon cleansing.
- Administer neomycin to ↓ intestinal bacteria, which contribute to cerebral intoxicants. Monitor for evidence of ototoxic (ie, ↓ hearing) and nephrotoxic (eg, UO <0.5 ml/kg/h, ↑ creatinine levels) effects caused by neomycin. Avoid giving neomycin in renal insufficiency.
- Administer lactulose to ↓ ammonia formation in intestine. Adjust dose to produce two to three semiformed stools qd.
- Protect confused or unconscious patient from injury.
    Leave side rails up; consider padding them if patient active.
    Have call light within patient's reach at all times.
    Tape all catheters and tubes securely to prevent dislodgement.
- Consider possibility of seizures in severe encephalopathy; have airway management equipment readily available.
- Minimize unnecessary noise, lights, and other environmental stimuli.
- Monitor ICP and CPP. With ↑ ICP, position carefully, and avoid fluid overload, hypercarbia, and hypoxemia. Administer mannitol and furosemide as indicated. Sedation or coma induction may be necessary if cerebral edema does not respond to these measures.

Altered protection r/t clotting anomaly and thrombocytopenia

Desired outcome: Bleeding, if it occurs, is not prolonged.

- Avoid giving IM injections. If necessary, use small-gauge needles and maintain firm pressure over injection sites for several min. Avoid massaging IM injection sites.
- Maintain pressure for several min over venipuncture sites. Inform laboratory personnel of patient's bleeding tendencies.
- Avoid arterial punctures. Consider use of indwelling arterial line.
- Monitor PT levels and platelet counts qd. Consult physician for significant prolongation of PT or of significant ↓ in platelets.
- Assess for signs of bleeding. Note oral and nasal mucosal bleeding and ecchymotic areas, and test stools, vomitus, urine, and gastric drainage for occult blood. Be alert to prolonged bleeding or oozing of blood from venipuncture sites and incisions.
- Use electric rather than straight razor for patient shaving. Provide soft-bristled toothbrush or sponge-tipped applicator and mouthwash for oral hygiene.
- Avoid indwelling gastric drainage tubes; they may irritate gastric mucosa or varices, causing bleeding to occur.
- Administer FFP and platelets as indicated. Monitor carefully for fluid volume overload.
- Administer vitamin K.
- A postshunt coagulopathy may develop in some patients after peritoneal-venous shunt surgery. Monitor these patients closely.
- Be aware that if FSPs are present in the blood and there is significant thrombocytopenia, the patient may have DIC.

REFERENCES

Butler R: Managing the problems of cirrhosis, *Am J Nurs* 94(3): 46-49, 1994.

Covington J: Nursing care of patients with alcoholic liver disease, *Crit Care Nurse* 13(3): 47-57, 1993.

Keen JH: Hepatic failure. In Swearingen PL, Keen JH (eds): *Manual of critical care nursing*, ed 3, St Louis, 1995, Mosby.

Lancaster S, Stockbridge J: PV shunts relieve ascites, *RN* 55(8): 58-60, 1992.

Smith SL, Ciferni M: Liver transplantation for acute hepatic failure: a review of clinical experience and management, *Am J Crit Care* 2(2): 137-144, 1993.

Author: **Janet Hicks Keen**

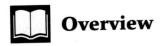

Overview

PATHOPHYSIOLOGY

Surgical emergency that requires rapid intervention to prevent permanent deformity or loss of limb. Occurs when injury or other factor causes ↑ pressure within an anatomic compartment. Pressure ↑ compromises capillary blood flow, resulting in tissue injury. Injured tissues release histamine, resulting in local vasodilatation and ↑ capillary permeability. As pressures eventually exceed capillary pressure, tissue ischemia occurs. Greatly ↑ pressure compresses arterioles and causes spasm. Ischemic tissue begins to necrose, resulting in permanent tissue damage called ischemic myositis.

HISTORY/RISK FACTORS

- Fracture: tibia, fibula, long bone
- Extremity injury: thermal or electrical burns, crush injury, prolonged tourniquet use
- Vascular injury: direct trauma, surgery, IV extravasation
- Constrictive/circumferential dressings, casts, PASG
- Sustained hypotension, shock
- Hypothermia or hyperthermia
- Postischemic swelling
- Venomous bites

CLINICAL PRESENTATION

Early Indicators: Pain out of proportion to injury; ↑ pain with passive motion of involved muscle group. Barriers to communication (intoxication, intubation, coma) may delay diagnosis, since pain is the cardinal symptom.
Late Indicators: If left untreated, necrosed muscle becomes fibrosed and contracted, resulting in a functionally useless compartment (eg, Volkmann's ischemic contracture).

Assessment

PHYSICAL ASSESSMENT

Muscle Involvement: Inability to control pain in patient at risk for compartment syndrome requires closer assessment. Pain on passive extension or digit flexion = early finding of muscle tissue involvement.
Neurovascular Involvement: ↑ extremity circumference, ↓ or loss of two-point discrimination, paresthesias, sluggish capillary refill, and tautness and tenderness over tissue compartments.
Mnemonic 6 Ps: Pain, pallor, polar (coolness), pulselessness, paresthesia, and paralysis

VITAL SIGNS/HEMODYNAMICS

RR: ↑ possible with pain, infection
HR: ↑ possible with pain, infection
BP: slight ↑ possible with pain; ↓ if septic
Temp: ↑ with infection
Other: Hemodynamics may reflect SIRS with ↑ CO and ↓ SVR.

DIAGNOSTIC PROCEDURES

Spo$_2$: Assesses perfusion of distal tissues. Readings compared to those from contralateral, uninvolved extremity.
Intracompartmental Pressure Monitoring: Pressures that indicate need for fasciotomy vary. Delta pressure = MAP − compartmental pressure. If ≤30 mm Hg for 6 h or ≤40 for 8 h, promptly consult physician.
Simple needle manometers: Subject to obstruction from muscle tissue, thus inappropriate for continuous monitoring. Critical value is pressure within 10-30 mm Hg of DBP.
Continuous infusion: Critical value >45 mm Hg.
Wick or slit catheters: Enable continuous pressure monitoring *via* fluid-filled catheters and pressure monitors. Critical value >30-35 mm Hg.

IMAGING

Arteriograms and Venograms: Performed when embolus, thrombus, arteriospasm, or other vascular injury suspected.
Transcutaneous Doppler Venous Flow and/or Duplex Imaging: Detect impaired venous flow.
MRI Spectroscopy: Detects muscle ischemia.

Collaborative Management

Ice and Extremity Elevation: Recommended with fractures to promote vasoconstriction when there is no evidence of impaired microcirculation in extremity. Once microcirculation impaired, however, *ice and extremity elevation contraindicated* because further circulation impairment likely.
Release of External Pressure: Loosening or removing circumferential casts and padding or dressings; escharotomy for circumferential burns or frostbite.
Fasciotomy of Myofascial Compartment: Enables unrestricted swelling. After a few days, fasciotomy is closed primarily; skin grafting may be needed to ensure complete covering of exposed compartments.
Compartment Syndrome Caused by Vascular Injury: Requires exploration of involved vessel to enable application of papaverine (smooth muscle relaxant that causes local vasodilatation), injection of fluid bolus to regain nl internal artery dynamics, and repair of lacerations or resection of involved vessels.
Analgesia: Parenteral opiates (eg, morphine) often with sedative adjuncts.

PATIENT-FAMILY TEACHING

- S&S that necessitate prompt reporting: ↑ pain, paresthesia, paralysis, coolness, ↓ capillary refill, or pulselessness
- Need to report the following indicators of infection: fever, localized warmth, ↑ pain, ↑ wound drainage (especially if purulent), swelling, and redness
- Medications: drug name, purpose, dosage, schedule, precautions, food-drug and drug-drug interactions, potential side effects
- Purpose, expected results, anticipated sensations of all nursing/medical interventions

Nursing Diagnoses/Interventions

Altered peripheral (compartment) tissue perfusion (or risk for same) r/t interruption of capillary blood flow secondary to ↑ pressure within anatomic compartment
Desired outcomes: Throughout duration of hospitalization, patient has adequate perfusion to compartment tissues: brisk (<2 sec) capillary refill; peripheral pulses >2+ on 0-4+ scale; nl tissue pressures (0-10 mm Hg); absence of edema, tautness, and 6 Ps in involved compartment. Within 2 h of admission patient verbalizes understanding of need to report symptoms of impaired neurovascular status.
- Monitor neurovascular status of injured extremity q2h. Assess for ↑ pain on passive digital extension or flexion. Monitor for ↓ capillary refill, loss of two-point discrimination, ↑ limb edema. Use pulse oximetry to assess distal tissue perfusion; report significant differences from uninvolved extremity. Assess for six Ps.
- Loosen circumferential dressings. Apply ice *only* if no S&S of impaired microcirculation.
- Monitor tissue pressures if intracompartmental pressure device present. Be aware of pressures >10 mm Hg or delta pressure ≤30-40 mm Hg for 6-8 h.
- Promote adequate BP, since there is ↑ susceptibility to tissue injury with hypotensive states.

Pain r/t tissue ischemia secondary to compartment syndrome
Desired outcomes: Throughout duration of hospitalization, patient's discomfort ↓ as documented by pain scale. Nonverbal indicators absent or ↓. Within 2 h of admission, patient verbalizes understanding of need to report uncontrolled or increasing pain.
- Assess patient's pain for onset, duration, progression, and intensity. Rate discomfort according to pain scale. Patients with impaired ability to communicate may require visual scale.
- If passive stretching of digits and pressure over limb compartments ↑ pain, compartment syndrome likely.
- Prevent pressure on involved compartment and neurovascular structures.
- After fasciotomy, be aware that if pain does not ↓, it could indicate incomplete fasciotomy. Pain that ↑ several days afterward may signal compartmental infection.
- Continue to monitor neurovascular function with each VS check to assess for recurring compartment syndrome or infection.

Risk for infection r/t inadequate primary defenses secondary to necrotic tissue, wide compartmental fasciotomy, and open wound
Desired outcome: Throughout duration of hospitalization, patient infection free: normothermia, WBC count ≤11,000 μl, no ↑ in pain, and absence of wound erythema and purulent drainage.
- Monitor for fever, ↑ pain, ↑ WBCs, positive cultures.
- Assess exposed wounds and dressings for erythema, ↑ or purulent wound drainage, ↑ wound circumference, edema, and localized tenderness.
- After primary closure or grafting of wound, continue to assess wound for signs of infection.
- Assess for chronic infection and osteomyelitis as potential complications after compartment syndrome.

Body image disturbance r/t physical changes secondary to large, irregular fasciotomy wound and skin grafted scar; loss of function and cosmesis of an extremity; or amputation
Desired outcomes: Within 24-h period before discharge from ICU, patient acknowledges body changes and demonstrates movement toward incorporating changes into self-concept. Patient does not exhibit maladaptive response (eg, severe depression) to wound or functional loss.
- Encourage questions about compartment syndrome, therapeutic interventions, long-term effects, and possible compensatory or cosmetic surgery.
- Provide time for verbalization of feelings. Encourage discussions with patient's significant others.
- Emphasize patient's strengths to promote adaptation to cosmetic and functional loss. Help set realistic goals for recovery.
- Facilitate progression through grieving process.
- Recognize individuality; enable patient to determine when to view or discuss injury.
- If extremity will be amputated, collaborate with physician regarding visit by amputee who has successfully adapted.
- Encourage maximum self-care.

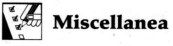 # Miscellanea

CONSULT MD FOR
- Uncontrolled pain
- ↑ pain on passive digital extension/flexion
- Impaired microcirculation: pain, polar, pallor, pulselessness, paresthesia, paralysis
- Delta pressure ≤30-40 mm Hg for 6-8 h
- Intracompartmental pressure >10 mm Hg

RELATED TOPICS
- Angiography
- Burns
- Multisystem injury
- Psychosocial needs, patient
- Shock, hypovolemic
- Systemic inflammatory response syndrome

ABBREVIATION
SIRS: Systemic inflammatory response syndrome

REFERENCES
Mabee JR: Compartment syndrome: a complication of acute extremity trauma, *J Emerg Med* 12: 651-656, 1994.

Moed BR, Thorderson PK: Measurement of intra-compartmental pressure: a comparison of the slit catheter, side-ported needle, and simple needle, *J Bone Joint Surg Am* 75: 231-235, 1993.

Ross DG: Acute compartment syndrome, *Orthop Nurs* (10)2: 33-38, 1991.

Ross DG: Compartment syndrome. In: Swearingen PL, Keen JH (eds): *Manual of critical care nursing,* ed 3, St Louis, 1995, Mosby.

Author: **Dennis G. Ross**

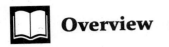 **Overview**

DESCRIPTION
Used during diagnostic procedures and minor surgeries that do not require general or regional anesthesia; inappropriate when large surgical incisions necessary. Process maintains minimally depressed LOC with mood alteration, ↑ pain threshold, and partial amnesia wherein patient is able to respond to physical stimuli and verbal commands and maintain a patent airway. All protective reflexes remain intact. Combinations of medications may be used.

INCIDENCE
Use is ↑ with efforts to ↓ hospital admissions and length of stay.

HISTORY
Likely candidates include patients undergoing:
- Wound dressing changes, abscess drainage
- Bronchoscopy, gastroscopy, colonoscopy, sigmoidoscopy
- Balloon angioplasty, cardioversion
- Closed reduction/immobilization of simple fractures or dislocations
- Podiatric procedures
- Suturing of lacerations

RISK FACTORS
Highly anxious or agitated patients may require large doses of sedatives/analgesics and may be more at risk for respiratory depression.

CLINICAL PRESENTATION (during conscious sedation)
- Somnolent, relaxed, "carefree"
- Speech slow, deliberate, slightly slurred; use of short sentences
- Requires simple questions, since attention span shortened
- Onset of sedation rapid, especially if opioid analgesics given with sedatives

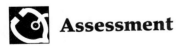 **Assessment**

PHYSICAL ASSESSMENT
Neuro: ↓ LOC, mood alteration, ↑ pain threshold

Resp: Bradypnea, ↓ depth of respirations
CV: Bradycardia, slight hypotension, possible dysrhythmias
GI: Nausea, vomiting possible

VITAL SIGNS/HEMODYNAMICS
RR: Nl or ↓
HR: Nl or ↓
BP: Nl or ↓
Temp: Nl
CVP/PAWP: Nl or slightly ↓
SVR: Nl or ↓
CO: Nl or ↓
12/18-lead ECG: Sinus bradycardia possible. May reveal changes r/t myocardial ischemia if hypotension present. If myocardial perfusion altered, PACs or PVCs may be seen.

LABORATORY STUDIES
ABGs: Checks for hypoxemia and hypercarbia signaling significant respiratory depression.
Drug/Toxicology Screening: If addiction or drug abuse suspected. Tolerance to sedatives or opioid analgesics alters dosage necessary to induce conscious sedation.

IMAGING
Chest X-ray: To validate lungs are nl and without significant disease that may impair ventilation.

DIAGNOSTIC PROCEDURE
ET Intubation: May be necessary in oversedation with loss of protective reflexes that result in loss of patent airway.

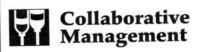 **Collaborative Management**

Goal: to sedate enough for patient to be reasonably comfortable/somnolent yet cooperative throughout procedure.

GENERAL
Supplemental O$_2$: Supports oxygenation to tissues.
Spo$_2$: Monitors O$_2$ saturation.
Continuous ECG Monitoring: Checks for dysrhythmias associated with hypoxemia or medications.
Noninvasive BP Monitoring: Set to measure BP at 1-5 min intervals throughout procedure.

NPO Status: Maintained for minimum of 6 h before elective procedure to ↓ aspiration risk.
Resuscitation Equipment: Includes airway suction equipment and "reversal" medications, which are kept at bedside throughout procedure.

PHARMACOTHERAPY
All agents titrated to patient's response with constant monitoring of VS and hemodynamic parameters if available. When combining agents, dosage of each ↓.
Benzodiazepines
Midazolam (Versed): Onset 3-5 min; maximum effect at 5 min (declines over 30-40 min); dosage 0.5-2.5 mg given slowly in 0.5 mg increments IV to attain sedation. Use 25% of initial dose to maintain sedation.
Diazepam (Valium): Onset 30 sec-2 min; duration 2-4 h with dosage given in 2.5-10 mg increments IV to attain and maintain sedation with or without narcotics.
Opioid Analgesics
Morphine sulfate: Onset 1-3 min; duration 1-3 h; dosage 1-2 mg IV increments given to attain and maintain sedation.
Meperidine (Demerol): Onset 1-3 min; duration 1-3 h; dosage 10 mg IV increments to attain and maintain sedation.
Reversal Agents
Flumazenil (Romazicon): Reverses benzodiazepine effects. Onset 1-2 min; duration 30-60 min; dosage 0.2 mg IV over 15 sec. May repeat if needed, after waiting 45-60 sec.
Naloxone (Narcan): Reverses opioid effects. Onset 2-3 min; duration depends on dosage; dosage 0.1-0.2 mg titrated to patient's response.

PATIENT-FAMILY TEACHING
- Purpose, expected results, anticipated sensations for all medical/nursing interventions throughout sedation procedure
- Loss of memory (common because of sedative effects)
- Postprocedure instructions if patient discharged to home after procedure: no alcohol, operating dangerous machinery, or driving motor vehicle for ≥24 h; written instructions provided, since medication-induced amnesia may impair recall for several h after procedure

Nursing Diagnoses/Interventions

Impaired gas exchange (or risk for same) r/t ↓ O_2 supply secondary to ↓ ventilatory drive associated with use of sedatives/CNS depression

Desired outcome: Throughout conscious sedation, patient has adequate gas exchange: SpO_2 >90%, PaO_2 >80 mm Hg, $PaCO_2$ 35-45 mm Hg, and RR 12-20 breaths/min with eupnea.

- Monitor VS, particularly RR, qmin when initial dosage of sedative given and at least q5min throughout procedure.
- Observe ECG for dysrhythmias, including changes in HR.
- Assess LOC qmin during initial dosage and at least q5min throughout procedure.
- Be sure that emergency airway management equipment is available in room, including manual resuscitator, oral airway ET intubation equipment, suction, and emergency cart with defibrillator.
- Secure at least one additional IV access *stat* if patient exhibits signs of instability.
- Monitor carefully for hypersensitivity reaction, especially during initial dosage.
- Ensure thorough and complete documentation for preprocedure, procedure, and postprocedure periods.
- Continue monitoring for 1-3 h after conscious sedation, paying particular attention to airway patency, RR, and BP.

Miscellanea

CONSULT MD FOR
- ↓ RR, inability to arouse patient, loss of patent airway
- SpO_2 <90%, hypotension, severe bradycardia
- Signs of medication hypersensitivity reaction: difficulty breathing, diaphoresis, tachycardia, itching/rash/wheals on skin.
- Possible complications: hypoventilation, respiratory arrest, lethal dysrhythmias, vomiting with aspiration during/immediately after procedure, severe hypotension, hypoxemia

RELATED TOPICS
- Agitation syndrome
- Anxiety
- Paralytic therapy
- Psychosocial needs, patient

REFERENCES
Association of Operating Room Nurses: Proposed recommended practice: monitoring the patient receiving IV conscious sedation, *AORN J* 56: 316-324, Aug 1992.

Kallar S: Conscious sedation in ambulatory surgery, *Anesthesiology Rev* 18(1): 9-12, 1991.

Keen JH, Baird MS, Allen JH: *Mosby's critical care and emergency drug reference,* ed 2, St Louis, 1996, Mosby.

Murphy EK: Monitoring IV conscious sedation: the legal scope of practice, *AORN J* 57: 512-514, Feb 1993.

Somerson SJ, Husted CW, Sicilia MR: Insights into conscious sedation *Am J Nurs* 95(6): 26-33, 1995.

Authors: **Marianne Saunorus Baird and Robert Aucker**

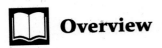 **Overview**

PATHOPHYSIOLOGY

Coronary arteries supply myocardial muscle with O_2 and nutrients necessary for functioning. Atherosclerotic lesions within these arteries are a major cause of obstruction and subsequent ischemia, which ultimately can lead to angina or MI if ischemia is prolonged and causes permanent damage. CAD often diagnosed only after patient is seen for angina or MI. S&S do not appear until there is ≈ 75% artery occlusion.

HISTORY/RISK FACTORS

- Family hx of CAD
- Hyperlipidemia, hypercholesterolemia
- Hypertension, DM, obesity
- Age >65 yrs
- Male; postmenopausal female
- Cigarette smoking
- Anemia, thyrotoxicosis
- ↑ stress
- Sedentary life-style

CLINICAL PRESENTATION

Chronic: Stable or progressively worsening angina that occurs when myocardial demand for O_2 is more than supply, such as during exercise.

Acute/Unstable: Angina occurs more frequently and is unrelieved by NTG and rest, occurs during sleep or rest, or occurs with progressively lower levels of exercise.

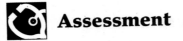 **Assessment**

PHYSICAL ASSESSMENT

Neuro: Anxiety during acute angina attacks; ↓ LOC if severe heart failure present

Resp: Crackles if acute or chronic heart failure present

CV: S_4 heart sound; S_3 heart sound if LV failure present

VITAL SIGNS/HEMODYNAMICS

RR: Nl or ↑ if acute ischemia, heart failure present

HR: Nl or ↑ if acute ischemia, heart failure present

BP: Nl or ↑ during periods of sympathetic stimulation (eg, angina); ↓ if acute or chronic heart failure present

PAWP: ↑ if heart failure present

CO: ↓ if heart failure present

SVR: Nl or ↑ as a result of hypertension or during episodes of ↑ sympathetic stimulation

ECG: If performed during angina, characteristic changes include ST-segment depression in leads over ischemic area. With hx of MI, may show Q waves; with severe or prolonged acute ischemia, ventricular and other dysrhythmias may be present.

LABORATORY STUDIES

Serum Enzymes: Obtained if AMI suspected.

IMAGING

Chest X-ray: To check for evidence of heart failure: pulmonary congestion, enlarged cardiac silhouette.

Radionuclide Studies

SPECT scan: Employs thallium or technetium to identify ischemic or infarcted tissue, which has ↓ uptake (cold spots).

PET scan: Uses radioisotopes to document myocardial perfusion. Can quantify areas of ischemia/infarction and assess collateral circulation.

Infarct imaging: Uses imaging agent, usually technetium, to identify area of infarction.

Coronary Arteriography *via* Cardiac Catheterization: Provides ultimate diagnosis of CAD. Arterial lesions located, and occlusion degree assessed. Feasibility for CABG or angioplasty determined.

DIAGNOSTIC PROCEDURES

Treadmill Exercise Test: Determines amount of exercise that causes angina, as well as degree of ischemia and ECG changes produced. Significant findings include 1 mm or more ST-segment depression or elevation and ventricular ectopic beats.

Ambulatory Monitoring: 24-h ECG that can show activity-induced ST-segment changes or ischemia-induced dysrhythmias.

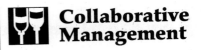 **Collaborative Management**

Management of Risk Factors: Eliminating tobacco, ↓ BP, ↓ serum lipid levels, controlling weight and stress, initiating exercise program.

Oxygen by Nasal Cannula: During angina attacks.

Pharmacotherapy

Sublingual NTG: During angina to ↑ microcirculation, perfusion to myocardium, venodilatation.

β Blockers: To ↓ myocardial O_2 demand.

Angiotensin-converting enzyme such as enalapril: ↓ O_2 demands by ↓ BP and resistance to ventricular contraction (afterload).

Long-acting nitrates or topical NTG: For anginal prophylaxis.

Calcium channel blockers such as nifedipine, diltiazem: To ↓ coronary artery vasospasm and O_2 demand.

Diet: Low in cholesterol, saturated fat, Na, calories, triglycerides, as appropriate.

PTCA: Procedure that improves coronary blood flow by using a balloon inflation catheter to compress plaque material into vessel wall (angioplasty) or removal of atherosclerotic deposits in coronary arteries (atherectomy).

CABG: Surgical procedure for bypass grafting of coronary arteries.

PATIENT/FAMILY TEACHING

- Pathophysiologic processes of cardiac ischemia, angina, infarction
- Precautions and side effects of nitrates and other medications
- Risk factors for CAD and risk factor modification as follows:
  - Diet low in cholesterol and saturated fat
  - Smoking cessation
  - Regular activity/exercise programs
- S&S that necessitate medical attention, such as chest pain unrelieved by NTG
- Medical procedures, such as cardiac catheterization, and surgical procedures, such as PTCA and CABG, if appropriate
- Activity guidelines, including sexual activity, and need to avoid strenuous activity for at least 1 h pc

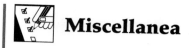

Nursing Diagnoses/Interventions

Pain (angina) r/t ↓ myocardial O_2 supply

Desired outcomes: Within 30 min of onset of pain, subjective perception of angina ↓, as documented by pain scale. Objective indicators, such as grimacing and diaphoresis, are absent.

- Assess location, character, and severity of pain. Record severity on a subjective 0 (no pain) to 10 (worst pain) scale. Also record number of NTG tablets needed to relieve each episode, factor or event that precipitated the pain, and alleviating factors. Document angina relief obtained, using pain scale.
- Keep sublingual NTG within patient's reach, and explain that it is to be administered as soon as angina begins, repeating q5min × 3 if necessary.
- Stay with patient and provide reassurance during periods of angina.
- Monitor HR and BP during episodes of chest pain. Be alert to irregularities in HR and changes in SBP >20 mm Hg from baseline.
- Monitor for headache and hypotension after administering NTG. Keep patient recumbent during angina and NTG administration.
- Administer O_2 to ↑ myocardial O_2 supply.
- Emphasize importance of immediately reporting angina.
- Avoid activities and factors that are known to cause stress and may precipitate angina.
- Administer β blockers and calcium channel blockers to ↓ cardiac work load and O_2 demand.
- Administer long-acting and/or topical nitrates to ↓ O_2 demand and likelihood of angina.

Activity intolerance r/t generalized weakness and imbalance between O_2 supply and demand secondary to tissue ischemia (MI)

Desired outcome: During activity, RPE <3 on 0-10 scale and cardiac tolerance to activity exhibited: RR ≤24 breaths/min, HR ≤120 bpm (or within 20 bpm of resting HR), SBP within 20 mm Hg of resting SBP, and absence of chest pain and new dysrhythmias.

- Assess patient's response to activity. Be alert to chest pain, ↑HR (>20 bpm), change in SBP (20 mm Hg over or under resting BP), excessive fatigue, and SOB. Ask patient to RPE.
- Assist patient with recognizing and limiting activities that ↑ O_2 demands, such as exercise and anxiety.
- Administer humidified O_2 prn or before activity to prevent angina.
- Have patient perform ROM exercises, depending on tolerance and prescribed activity limitations. Because cardiac intolerance to activity can be further aggravated by prolonged bed rest, consult with physician about in-bed exercises and activities that can be performed by patient as condition improves.

Miscellanea

CONSULT MD FOR
- ↑ frequency of angina, angina occurring at rest, angina unrelieved by NTG, or ↓ exercise tolerance without angina
- Hemodynamically significant dysrhythmias
- Sustained hypertension, hypotension
- S&S of complications: unstable angina, AMI, heart failure

RELATED TOPICS
- Angina pectoris
- Angioplasty/atherectomy, percutaneous transluminal coronary
- Cardiac catheterization
- Cardiac surgery: CABG
- Heart failure, left ventricular
- Myocardial infarction, acute

ABBREVIATIONS
CABG: Coronary artery bypass graft
PET: Positron emission tomography
PTCA: Percutaneous transluminal coronary angioplasty/atherectomy
RPE: Rate(d) perceived exertion
SPECT: Single photon emission computed tomography

REFERENCES
Reilly A, Dracup K, Dattolo J: Factors influencing prehospital delay in patients experiencing chest pain, *Am J Crit Care* 3(4): 300-306, 1994.

Steuble BT: Coronary artery disease. In Swearingen PL (ed): *Manual of medical-surgical nursing care,* ed 3, St Louis, 1994, Mosby.

Vitello-Cicciu J, Eagan J: Data acquisition from the cardiovascular system. In Kinney M et al (eds): *AACN's clinical reference for critical care nursing,* ed 3, St Louis, 1993, Mosby.

Author: **Janet Hicks Keen**

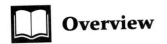 **Overview**

DESCRIPTION

Thrombolytics dissolve or lyse existing clots and thereby reestablish perfusion. With AMI secondary to complete or partial coronary thrombosis, reperfusion salvages myocardial tissue and preserves ventricular function. Indications that lysis has occurred include ↓ chest pain and rapid resolution of ST-segment depression. 80% of cases have reported reperfusion dysrhythmias. Heparin and antiplatelet agents are used as adjuncts to thrombolytic therapy to inhibit action of free thrombin and prevent reocclusion. FDPs are byproducts of thrombolysis. Large amounts result in significant systemic anticoagulation and can trigger bleeding complications.

HISTORY/RISK FACTORS
- Presence of CAD
- Risk factors for CAD

CLINICAL PRESENTATION
- Symptoms of AMI: usually, sudden onset of chest pain/pressure unrelieved by sublingual nitrates lasting >30 min but <6-12 h; possible diaphoresis, nausea, vomiting, anxiety
- Intermittent, severe chest pain for h or days, which may occur with subtotal occlusion secondary to coronary thrombosis

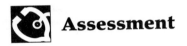 **Assessment**

PHYSICAL ASSESSMENT
- Tachycardia, bradycardia, irregular pulse, hypotension, other findings consistent with AMI.
- Assess for venipuncture attempts, superficial injuries that could become active bleeding sites after thrombolysis.
- Perform baseline neurologic assessment for comparison to subsequent examinations, which are indicated to detect neurologic changes associated with acute stroke.

RELATIVE/ABSOLUTE CONTRAINDICATIONS FOR THROMBOLYTIC THERAPY
Minor Relative
- Recent (within 10 days) minor trauma, including CPR
- Hx of cerebrovascular disease
- Pregnancy
- Likelihood of left-sided heart thrombus
- Acute pericarditis, endocarditis
- Coagulopathy (eg, associated with liver/renal dysfunction)
- Age >75 (controversial)

Major Relative
- Recent (within 10 days) major surgery, serious trauma, obstetric delivery, organ biopsy, puncture of noncompressible vessels
- GI/GU bleeding within 10 days
- Uncontrolled hypertension: SBP >180 or DBP >110 mm Hg

Absolute
- Hypersensitivity to thrombolytic agent
- Active internal bleeding
- Recent (within 2 mos) stroke, intracranial neoplasm, AV malformation/aneurysm
- Recent (within 2 mos) intracranial/intraspinal surgery or trauma
- Bleeding diathesis
- Severe uncontrolled hypertension: DBP >120 mm Hg

VITAL SIGNS/HEMODYNAMICS
Reflect extent of myocardial ischemia/infarction
RR: Mild ↑
HR: Nl, ↑, or ↓
BP: Mild ↑, nl, or ↓
Temp: Wnl
PAWP: ↑ if LV failure present
Other: ↑ sympathetic tone may ↑ HR, BP, SVR
ECG: Ventricular irritability. Reperfusion dysrhythmias associated with clot lysis include accelerated idioventricular rhythm, PVCs, bradycardia, heart block.

LABORATORY STUDIES
Serum Enzymes, Electrolytes, CBC, Clotting Studies: Evaluated before initiating thrombolytic therapy. Heparin-lock device used for specimen collection. Do not delay therapy for confirmation of laboratory values.

DIAGNOSTIC PROCEDURES
ECG: 12/18-lead to determine presence, location, extent of myocardial injury. Localized ST-segment elevation of 1 mm in 2 contiguous leads, significant Q waves, and T-wave inversion are findings associated with AMI. ST-segment elevation that ↓ after sublingual NTG suggests coronary artery spasm (Prinzmetal's angina) and thus thrombolytic therapy is not indicated.

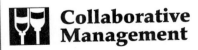 **Collaborative Management**

Thrombolytics: Because time is crucial, therapy may be initiated in prehospital setting or emergency department of a smaller hospital before transfer to definitive care center. In these settings the agent is administered peripherally. In larger centers, it may be started in the catheterization laboratory where it is administered *via* intracoronary route during fluoroscopic examination.
First generation thrombolytics
Streptokinase: Administered IV or *via* intracoronary route. Because it is an antigen, previous exposure to streptococcal organisms may result in antibodies against streptokinase. Steroids or antihistamines administered before therapy to prevent hypersensitivity reaction.
Anistreplase: Induces clot lysis with fewer systemic lytic effects than streptokinase. Allergic and anaphylactic reactions possible.
Urokinase: Enzyme derived from human renal cells. Used for intracoronary infusion and administered in cardiac catheterization laboratory. More expensive than streptokinase but less likely to cause hypersensitivity reactions.
Second generation thrombolytic
Alteplase: Produced by the body; converts plasminogen to plasmin after binding to fibrin clot. Advantageous because it has fewer systemic lytic effects and is nonantigenic.
Adjunctive Therapy: Standard therapy for AMI initiated, including O_2, continuous ECG monitoring, nitrates, IV analgesia, β blockade, and other therapies as indicated. Heparin and antiplatelet agents (eg, aspirin) given concurrently with thrombolytic therapy to prevent reocclusion.
Coronary Angiography: May be performed to assess for patency or reocclusion. Because of systemic lytic effects, it is best to wait 24-48 h after initial thrombolytic therapy.

PATIENT/FAMILY TEACHING
- Atherosclerotic process and expected outcome of thrombolytic therapy; explanation of goal of therapy: to ↓ injury to heart muscle
- Need for monitoring and close postprocedure observation
- Postprocedure patient interventions to prevent reocclusion: take prescribed antiplatelet medications, exercise, comply with dietary modifications, manage or eliminate risk factors such as smoking, hyperlipidemia, hypertension, stress, obesity
- Importance of reporting S&S of MI that occur after hospitalization: unrelenting chest heaviness or pressure; pain that radiates to arm, neck, or jaw; accompanying nausea and diaphoresis; lightheadedness or dizziness

Nursing Diagnoses/Interventions

Altered protection r/t risk of bleeding/hemorrhage secondary to nonspecific thrombolytic effects of therapy

Desired outcome: Symptoms of bleeding complications absent: BP wnl for patient; HR ≤100 bpm; blood-free secretions and excretions; natural skin color; baseline/nl LOC; and absence of back and abdominal pain, hematoma, headache, dizziness, vomiting.

- On admission, obtain thorough hx, assessing for the following:
  - Risk factors for intracranial hemorrhage: uncontrolled hypertension, cerebrovascular pathology, CNS surgery within previous 6 mos
  - Bleeding risks: recent or active GI bleeding, recent trauma, recent surgery, bleeding diathesis, advanced liver/kidney disease
  - Risk of systemic embolization: suspected left-sided heart thrombus
  - Hx of streptococcal infection or previous streptokinase therapy
- Monitor clotting studies per agency protocol. Regulate heparin drip to maintain PTT at 1½-2 × control level or according to protocol.
- Apply pressure dressing over puncture site if cardiac catheterization performed. Inspect site at frequent intervals for evidence of hematoma. Immobilize extremity for 6-8 h after catheterization.
- Avoid unnecessary venipunctures, IM injections, or arterial puncture. Obtain laboratory specimens from heparin-lock device.
- Monitor for indicators of internal bleeding: ↓ Hct/Hgb, back pain, abdominal pain, ↓ BP, pallor, bloody stool or urine.
- Monitor for signs of intracranial bleeding q2h: change in LOC, headache, dizziness, vomiting, confusion.
- Test all stools, urine, vomitus for occult blood.
- Use care with oral hygiene and when shaving patient.

Risk for injury r/t potential for allergic or anaphylactic reaction to streptokinase or anistreplase secondary to antigen/antibody response

Desired outcome: Patient has no symptoms of allergic response: normothermia, RR 12-20 breaths/min with eupnea, HR ≤100 bpm, BP at baseline/wnl, natural skin color, and absence of itching, urticaria, headache, muscular and abdominal pain, nausea.

- Before treatment with streptokinase or anistreplase, question patient about hx of previous streptokinase therapy or streptococcal infection.
- Consult physician for positive findings.
- Administer prophylactic antihistamines/hydrocortisone as indicated.
- Monitor during and for 48-72 h after infusion for indicators of allergy: hypotension (brief or sustained), urticaria, fever, itching, flushing, nausea, headache, muscular pain, bronchospasm, abdominal pain, dyspnea, tachycardia.
- If hypotension develops, ↑ rate of IV infusion/administer volume replacement. Prepare for vasopressor administration if there is no response to volume replacement.
- Treat allergic response with diphenhydramine or other antihistamine, as prescribed.

Decreased cardiac output (or risk for same) r/t alterations in rate, rhythm, and conduction secondary to ↑ irritability of ischemic tissue during reperfusion (usually occurs within 1-2 h after initiation of therapy); or r/t inotropic heart changes secondary to reocclusion and myocardial ischemia

Desired outcomes: Within 12 h of thrombolytic therapy initiation, patient has adequate cardiac output: NSR on ECG, peripheral pulses >2+ on 0-4+ scale, warm and dry skin, and UO ≥0.5 ml/kg/h. Patient awake, alert, and oriented without palpitations, chest pain, or dizziness.

- Monitor ECG continuously during thrombolytic therapy for evidence of dysrhythmias.
- With any dysrhythmia, check VS and note accompanying S&S, such as dizziness, lightheadedness, syncope, palpitations.
- Ensure availability of emergency drugs and equipment: lidocaine, atropine, dopamine, epinephrine, defibrillator/cardioverter, external and transvenous pacemaker.
- Evaluate response to medications and emergency treatment.
- Monitor for signs of reocclusion: chest pain, nausea, diaphoresis, dysrhythmias.
- Obtain 12/18-lead ECG if reocclusion suspected.
- Anticipate and prepare patient for cardiac catheterization, PTCA, or repeated thrombolytic therapy.
- Initiate standard therapies for AMI, including O₂, nitrates, morphine, other therapies as indicated.

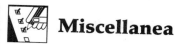

Miscellanea

CONSULT MD FOR
- S&S of intracranial, other internal bleeding
- S&S of reocclusion
- S&S of hypersensitivity reaction
- Sustained or hemodynamically significant dysrhythmias

RELATED TOPICS
- Anaphylaxis
- Cardiac catheterization
- Coronary artery disease
- Myocardial infarction, acute

ABBREVIATIONS
FDPs: Fibrin degradation products

REFERENCES

Daily E: Clinical management of patients receiving thrombolytic therapy, *Heart Lung* 20(5 part 2): 552-565, 1991.

Keen JH, Baird M, Allen J: *Mosby's critical care and emergency drug reference*, ed 2, St Louis, 1996, Mosby.

Keen JH: Caring for patients undergoing coronary artery thrombolysis. In Swearingen PL, Keen JH (eds): *Manual of critical care nursing*, ed 3, St Louis, 1995, Mosby.

Majoros K: Comparisons and controversies in clot buster drugs, *Crit Care Nurs Q* 16(2): 58, 1993.

Rapaport E: Overview: rationale of thrombolysis in treating acute myocardial infarction, *Heart Lung* 29 (5 part 2): 538-541, 1991.

Weiner B: Thrombolytic agents in critical care, *Crit Care Nurs Clin North Am* 5(2): 355-366, 1993.

Author: **Janet Hicks Keen**

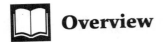 **Overview**

PATHOPHYSIOLOGY
Result of impaired cognitive function occurring primarily in cerebral hemispheres. Has acute onset, is transient, and is caused by either organic or nonorganic factors. Interruption in neurotransmission may be caused by inadequate O_2 or glucose. ↑ brain dopamine also may contribute *via* stimulation of neurons that regulate temp, ANS, hormone release, and emotions. Resulting cognitive deficits reflected in thought processes, learning, and memory.

RISK FACTORS FOR NONORGANIC CAUSES
Sensory Overload
Noise: Especially if high-pitched, unexpected, of long duration
Smell: Unfamiliar and unpleasant odors
Visual: Bright, unending light; constant activity
Taste: NPO, airway suctioning, ET tubes, drugs that affect taste
Sensations: Pain and pressure from catheters, dressings, injury, disease process
Sensory Deprivation: Can occur in midst of multiple stimuli because of lack of meaningful or familiar stimulation.
Sleep Deprivation: Usually occurs 2-7 days after admission. Continual interruption of sleep cycles ↓ amount of REM sleep necessary for emotional and psychologic rest.
Psychologic Stress: Sudden, unexpected, life-threatening illness concurrent with anxiety, loneliness, powerlessness.
Immobilization: Caused by equipment, restraints, therapeutic mobility, restrictions, infrequent position changes.

RISK FACTORS FOR ORGANIC CAUSES
- CNS disorders, hypo/hyperthermia
- Fluid & electrolyte imbalance (especially dehydration)
- ETOH or drug overdose
- Renal, liver disease
- Heart failure, MI, CABG, hypotensive event
- Advanced age
- Pain

CLINICAL PRESENTATION
Hallucinations, illusions, delusions. Initial onset and ↑ intensity usually occur at night.
Cognitive Changes: Short attention span, rambling or inappropriate speech, ↓ LOC.
Disturbance in Sleep-Wake Cycle: Hyperactive/hyperalert state (agitated, combative) or hypoactive/hypoalert state (sleepy, dreamlike state). May alternate between the two.
Impaired Short-Term Memory: Disorientation, self-extubation, removal of IV lines and catheters.

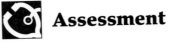 **Assessment**

PHYSICAL ASSESSMENT
Neuro: Glasgow Coma Scale score often remains high despite delirium. Nystagmus/↓ DTRs if sleep deprived; pupils dilated, equal, responsive; ↓ attention span; inappropriate or nonsensical speech; nonpurposeful or inappropriate activity; absent short-term memory
Resp: Shallow, rapid respirations
CV: Tachycardia, possible ↑ BP
GI: ↓ appetite, ↓ bowel sounds
Other: Talking or mumbling to self, fixed gaze or stare, picking at unseen objects

VITAL SIGNS/HEMODYNAMICS
RR: ↑
HR: ↑
BP: ↑; postural changes may occur with haloperidol therapy
MAP/PAP/PAWP/CO/SVR: ↑ as a result of ↑ sympathetic tone
ECG: Tachycardia, prolongation of QT interval can occur with agitation and further prolonged with haloperidol, ↑ risk of torsades de pointes (atypical VT)

LABORATORY STUDIES
ABGs: To determine presence of hypoxia, hypercapnia, acidosis as contributing factors
Electrolytes: To determine imbalance, particularly of Na^+, K^+, and Ca^{2+}
Serum Glucose Levels: To check for hypoglycemia, which is needed for cerebral metabolism
Serum Drug Levels: To detect toxicity, eg, of aminophylline, digitalis, quinidine
Toxicology Screen: To check for presence of benzodiazepines, opiates, other drugs affecting CNS function

Collaborative Management

Identification/Treatment of Delirium Cause: See **RISK FACTORS**
Medications affecting mentation: Corticosteroids, opiates, nifedipine, nitroprusside, NSAIDs, anticholinergics, cardiac drugs, theophylline, antibiotics (eg, amphotericin B, captopril). Discontinuation of one drug rarely resolves delirium. Neurologic, hepatic, or renal function should be evaluated, and contraindicated medications discontinued or doses adjusted.
Treatment of Symptoms
Haloperidol: An antipsychotic; drug of choice for delirium control. ↓ hallucinations, paranoia, and motor activity. Minimal effects on CV system. IV route investigational but widely used in ICU because of fewer side effects than IM route. Not usually used for delirium associated with anticholinergic intoxication or ETOH or drug withdrawal. Droperidol or chlorpromazine also used.
Benzodiazepines: Eg, diazepam, lorazepam, midazolam used for sedation to control agitation; especially useful for ETOH withdrawal. Combination of haloperidol and lorazepam frequently used. Propofol infusion also used for sedative effect.
Opiate analgesics: For pain relief.
Neuromuscular blockers/paralytic therapy: Last resort for extreme agitation and delirium.
Nutritional Therapy: May need ↑ protein or supplemental vitamins because of depletion by hyperactive state. Vitamin B_{12} may be indicated.

PATIENT-FAMILY TEACHING
- Explanation that S&S of delirium (hallucinations, delusions, illusions) are temporary and will resolve.
- Reorientation methods family can use with patient.
- Explanations of all procedures, unfamiliar surroundings and sounds, using clear, simple, short sentences.

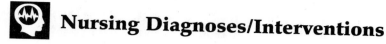

Nursing Diagnoses/Interventions

Sensory/Perceptual alterations r/t impaired perceptions of reality secondary to organic and nonorganic causes

Desired outcome: Within 48 h of treatment, patient displays appropriate perception of reality: orientation $\times$ 3; short-term recall; no evidence of hallucinations, illusions, or delusions.

- Optimize continuity by having same personnel provide care. Staff should employ a consistent, structured manner, using individualized plan of care calmly and unhurriedly.
- Orient to time and place at frequent intervals. Place clocks and calendars in room. Have patient in windowed room if possible.
- Avoid restraints, if possible, which may ↑ paranoid ideas and ↑ autonomic response.
- Speak in a soft, even-toned voice. Repeat explanations often because patient is unable to remember.
- Enable regular and liberal visitations by significant others. Keep personal belongings at bedside to ↑ meaningful stimulation and facilitate reality orientation *via* exposure to familiar persons and objects.
- Use therapeutic touch if it is not culturally offensive to patient or if patient is not experiencing hallucinations, illusions, or delusions. Encourage family to touch patient.
- Assess for hallucinations, illusions, delusions. Avoid arguing with or confronting patient experiencing them. Be aware that delusional thoughts cannot be changed with logic. Remain with patient. Confirm reality and acknowledge patient's feelings.
- Provide comfort measures such as mouth care, repositioning, and adjusting dressings or tubes that pull or itch.
- Provide adequate light as much as possible. Change alarm sensitivity as patient improves; ↓ intercom level.
- Call patient by name on entering room; avoid abruptly turning on lights.
- Monitor for and treat cause(s) of delirium according to protocol (eg, administer analgesics for pain, treat hypoglycemia, administer appropriate O_2 support for hypoxia).

Sleep pattern disturbance r/t sensory overload/deprivation, psychologic stress, delirium

Desired outcome: Within 48 h of treatment initiation, patient's sleep pattern reestablished: 2-3 periods of 2-4 h of uninterrupted sleep at night and ↓ in symptoms of delirium.

- Identify medications that may affect sleep cycle, eg, barbiturates, benzodiazepines, chloral hydrate, morphine sulfate.
- Assess customary day/night sleep cycle routine. Implement individual nighttime rituals.
- Provide comfort measures to facilitate sleep (back rub, repositioning, pain relief).
- Do not restrict naps during daytime; doing so actually may ↑ problem. Morning naps usually include REM sleep.
- Maintain room temp at patient's comfort level. Temp that is too warm ↓ REM and NREM sleep.
- Plan care to provide periods of at least 2 h of uninterrupted sleep during the night if possible.
- Suggest use of music therapy, relaxation techniques, massage.
- ↓ stimuli that prevent or interrupt sleep (ie, ↓ noise, light).
- Simulate day and night with modifications in activity level and lighting (ie, ↓ at night, ↑ during day).
- Critically assess need of waking patient for care or procedures (ie, for baths, lab work, VS).

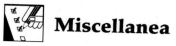

Miscellanea

CONSULT MD FOR
- ↑ symptoms of delirium despite implementation of prescribed therapy
- Psychologic changes that signal ↓ hemodynamic or neurologic status

RELATED TOPICS
- Agitation syndrome
- Alterations in consciousness
- Anxiety
- Paralytic therapy
- Psychosocial needs, patient
- Sleep disturbances

ABBREVIATIONS
ANS: Autonomic nervous system
DTR: Deep tendon reflex
NREM: Non-REM
REM: Rapid eye movement

REFERENCES
Felver L: Patient-environment interactions in critical care, *Crit Care Nurs Clin North Am* 7(2): 327-334, 1995.

Geary SM: Intensive care units psychosis revisited: understanding and managing delirium in the critical care setting, *Crit Care Nurs Q* 17(1): 51-63, 1994.

Halm MA, Alpen MA: The impact of technology on patients and families, *Nurs Clin North Am* 28(2): 443-457, 1993.

Harvey MA: Managing agitation in critically ill patients, *Am J Crit Care* 5(1): 7-16, 1996.

Parker KP: Promoting sleep and rest in critically ill patients, *Crit Care Nurs Clin North Am* 7(2): 337-349, 1995.

Author: **Marguerite J. Murphy**

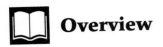 **Overview**

PATHOPHYSIOLOGY

Results from profound ADH deficiency or ↓ renal responsiveness to ADH. May be neurogenic, involving deficiency in ADH synthesis in the hypothalamus, or ↓ release from the posterior pituitary (central), or may be nephrogenic, resulting from ↓ water permeability of collecting tubules as a result of ↓ ADH effect. Although in some cases DI is permanent, it is usually temporary, typically lasting 5-7 days.

COMPLICATIONS

Dehydration, hypotension, hypovolemic shock, ↑ blood viscosity with risk of thromboemboli

HISTORY/RISK FACTORS

Central (Neurogenic) DI
- Head injury
- Meningitis, encephalitis
- Brain tumor
- Neoplasms: eg, lung, breast cancer
- Surgery in area of pituitary gland (eg, transsphenoidal hypophysectomy)
- Intracranial hemorrhage
- ↑ ICP, cerebral hypoxia

Nephrogenic DI
- Congenital disorder
- Hypercalcemia, hypokalemia
- Medications (lithium, demeclocycline HCl [Declomycin])

CLINICAL PRESENTATION

Characteristic feature is excretion of large quantities (as much as 5-12 L/day) of hypotonic urine. Extreme thirst also present.

Assessment

PHYSICAL ASSESSMENT

Unremarkable if patient can satisfy thirst. If not, the following may be present.
Neuro: Altered LOC if serum hyperosmolality and hypernatremia develop; altered LOC, neurologic changes also r/t precipitating event
CV: Orthostatic hypotension, hypotension, tachycardia
GU: UO >200 ml/h for 2 consecutive h or >500 ml/h
Integ: Poor skin turgor, dry mucous membranes

VITAL SIGNS/HEMODYNAMICS

RR: Abnormal pattern if ↑ ICP present
HR: ↑
BP: ↓
Temp: May be ↑ if ↑ ICP present
CVP: ↓
PAWP: ↓

LABORATORY STUDIES

Urine: Osmolality ↓ to <200 mOsm/kg; may be higher if volume depletion present. Specific gravity <1.007.
Serum Osmolality: ↑ to >300 mOsm/kg.
Serum Sodium: ↑ to >147 mEq/L.
Plasma ADH: ↓ in central DI.
Water Deprivation Test: Baseline weight, serum/urine osmolality, urine specific gravity obtained. Fluid intake prohibited. Aforementioned values measured qh. *Negative results:* urine specific gravity >1.020 and urine osmolality >800 mOsm/kg. *Positive results:* ≥5% of body weight lost or urine specific gravity does not ↑ for 3 consecutive h.
Vasopressin Test: Vasopressin (exogenous ADH) administered SC. Urine specimens collected q30min for 2 h and evaluated for quantity and osmolality. Urine osmolality generally ↑ significantly in response to ADH unless DI nephrogenic in origin, in which case response may be minimal.

Collaborative Management

Rehydration: Hypotonic IV solutions often used to replace free water lost in urine. Fluid replacement rapid until patient stabilized, then based on UO.
Exogenous ADH (vasopressin): Several preparations available; dosage adjusted to response. Side effects include hypertension, angina, or MI r/t its vasoconstrictive effects on blood vessels; abdominal cramping and ↑ peristalsis from smooth muscle excitation; water intoxication. Desmopressin popular because it produces fewer side effects.
Thiazide Diuretics/Low-Sodium, Low-Protein Diet: Major therapy for nephrogenic DI to ↓ solute excretion and urine production. Chlorpropamide also may be given to enhance action of ADH.

PATIENT-FAMILY TEACHING

- Appropriate administration of exogenous vasopressin and its side effects.
- Importance of weighing qd at same time of day and in same clothing and reporting weight gains/losses to physician.
- Method for accurate measurement of urine specific gravity and importance of keeping accurate records of test results.
- S&S that necessitate medical attention, including those of dehydration and water intoxication.
- Importance of obtaining Medic-Alert bracelet and ID card.

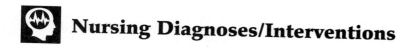

Nursing Diagnoses/Interventions

Fluid volume deficit r/t failure of regulatory mechanisms (resulting in polyuria) secondary to ADH deficiency or altered ADH action

Desired outcome: Within 12 h of therapy initiation, patient becomes normovolemic: BP 110-120/70-80 mm Hg (or wnl for patient), CVP ≥2 mm Hg, PAWP ≥6 mm Hg, HR 60-100 bpm, I = O + insensible losses, and stable weight.

- Keep careful I&O records. Be alert for UO >200 ml/h for 2 consecutive h or ≥500 ml/h. Additional therapy may be necessary.
- Provide adequate fluids. Keep water pitcher full and within easy reach. Administer hyperosmolar tube feedings or solutions with extreme caution. They can induce osmotic diarrhea and worsen fluid losses.
- Administer IV fluids as prescribed. Usually, a hypotonic solution administered as follows: 1 ml IV fluid for each 1 ml UO. In patients with brain injury, moderate diuresis may be permitted to avoid need for osmotic diuretics. Hypernatremia, if present, must be corrected slowly to prevent cerebral edema, seizures, permanent neurologic damage, or death.
- Administer vasopressin; document effects. Be alert to side effects: hypertension, cardiac ischemia, hyponatremia.
- Weigh patient qd, at the same time and using same scale and garments to prevent error.
- Monitor for continuing fluid volume deficit: poor skin turgor; dry mucous membranes; rapid and thready pulse; and SBP, CVP, or PAWP below baseline.
- Monitor serum sodium and serum/urine osmolality. Monitor urine specific gravity qh to evaluate response to therapy. Patients may be allowed to develop hypotonic polyuria between doses of vasopressin to demonstrate persistence of DI when transient DI is suspected.

Risk for injury r/t altered cerebral function secondary to hyperosmolality, dehydration, hypernatremia, or associated conditions such as ↑ ICP

Desired outcome: Patient verbalizes orientation × 3; nl breath sounds auscultated over airways; and oral cavity and musculoskeletal system remain intact and free of injury.

- Monitor orientation, LOC, and respiratory status at frequent intervals. Keep oral airway, manual resuscitator and mask, and supplemental O₂ at bedside.
- Reduce likelihood of injury caused by falls by maintaining bed in lowest position, with side rails up at all times, and using soft restraints as necessary.
- Place gastric tube to intermittent suction in comatose patient to ↓ likelihood of aspiration.
- Elevate HOB to 45 degrees to minimize risk of aspiration.
- Initiate seizure precautions as necessary.

Altered peripheral tissue perfusion r/t interruption of blood flow (thromboembolism) secondary to ↑ blood viscosity, ↑ platelet aggregation and adhesiveness, and immobility

Desired outcome: By time of discharge, patient has adequate peripheral perfusion: peripheral pulses >2+ on 0-4+ scale, brisk capillary refill (<2 sec), warm skin, and absence of swelling, bluish discoloration, erythema, and discomfort in calves and thighs.

- Monitor Hct. With proper fluid replacement, values should return to nl.
- Assess peripheral pulses q2-4h. Be alert for any ↓ in amplitude/absence of pulse.
- Be alert to S&S of DVT: erythema, pain, tenderness, warmth, swelling, bluish discoloration, prominence of superficial veins, especially in lower extremities. Arterial thrombosis may produce cyanosis with delayed capillary refill, mottling, and coolness of the extremity.
- Assist with or perform ROM exercises to all extremities q4h to ↑ blood flow to tissues.
- Apply pneumatic sequential compression stockings or similar device to lower extremities to aid in prevention of thrombosis.

Miscellanea

CONSULT MD FOR
- UO >200 ml/h × 2h or ≥500 ml/h
- Weight loss >1 kg/day
- Electrolyte imbalance: hypernatremia r/t ADH deficiency; hyponatremia or rapid ↓ in Na⁺ r/t vasopressin therapy
- Serious side effects of vasopressin therapy: hypertension, angina, dysrhythmias, ECG changes
- Complications: dehydration, hypovolemic shock, thromboemboli

RELATED TOPICS
- Hypernatremia
- Hyponatremia
- Increased intracranial pressure
- Shock, hypovolemic
- Transsphenoidal hypophysectomy

ABBREVIATION
ADH: Antidiuretic hormone

REFERENCES
Bell TN: Diabetes insipidus, *Crit Care Nurs Clin North Am* 6(4): 675-685, 1994.

Horne MM: Endocrinologic dysfunctions. In Swearingen PL, Keen JH (eds): *Manual of critical care nursing,* ed 3, St Louis, 1995, Mosby.

Loos F: Understanding diabetes insipidus: recognition and management in critical care, *CAACN* 3(3): 18-22, 1992.

Rose BD: *Clinical physiology of acid-base and electrolyte disorders,* ed 4, New York, 1994, McGraw-Hill.

Author: **Mima M. Horne**

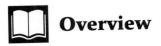

Overview

PATHOPHYSIOLOGY

Chronic disease with metabolic, vascular, and neurologic disorders resulting from dysfunctional glucose transport into body cells. Glucose transport impaired owing to ↓/absent insulin secretion and/or ineffective insulin action. Carbohydrate, fat, and protein metabolism are abnormal, and there is inability to store glucose in the liver and muscle as glycogen, store fatty acids and triglycerides in adipose tissue, and transport amino acids into cells normally.

Types of DM
Non-insulin-dependent diabetes mellitus (NIDDM)/type II: Moderate to severe lack of effective endogenous insulin, causing severe hyperglycemia without ketosis. Up to 25% of patients require periodic to regular insulin administration for blood glucose control. Oral hypoglycemics are used by 50% of these patients, while 25% control blood glucose using only a structured ADA diet for maintenance of ideal body weight. Accounts for 80%-90% of individuals with DM. Untreated hyperglycemia can result in HHNS.

Insulin-dependent diabetes mellitus (IDDM)/type I: Complete lack of effective endogenous insulin, causing hyperglycemia and ketosis. Majority of patients manifest at <30 yrs of age. Dependence on insulin for survival and prevention of DKA.

Gestational diabetes: Intolerance to glucose that develops during pregnancy.

Other: Formerly termed secondary diabetes.
- *Pancreatic diseases that destroy beta islet cells:* Pancreatitis, cystic fibrosis
- *Drug-induced by insulin antagonists:* Eg, phenytoin, steroids (hydrocortisone, dexamethasone), catecholamines (epinephrine, dopamine)
- *Endocrine dysfunction/hormonal diseases:* Eg, acromegaly, Cushing's syndrome, pheochromocytoma
- *Insulin resistance:* Caused by dysfunctional insulin receptors

INCIDENCE
6% of total population (12 million Americans)

HISTORY/RISK FACTORS
NIDDM
- Obesity
- Advanced age

IDDM
- Genetic predisposition
- Altered immune response
- Environmental stressors

Other Types
- Pregnancy
- Pancreatic/hormonal disorders

CLINICAL PRESENTATION (early indicators)
Fatigue, weakness, weight loss, mild dehydration, symptoms of hyperglycemia (polyuria, polydipsia, polyphagia).

LONG-TERM COMPLICATIONS
Macroangiopathy: Vascular disease affecting coronary arteries and larger vessels of brain and lower extremities. May result in MI, stroke, peripheral vascular disease.

Microangiopathy: Thickening of capillary basement membranes resulting in retinopathy, nephropathy, and delayed healing. May result in blindness, renal failure, chronic ulcerations.

Neuropathy: Affects peripheral and autonomic nervous systems, resulting in impaired or slowed nerve transmission, eg, numbness or lack of sensation, particularly in the feet, and orthostatic hypotension, neurogenic bladder, and impaired gastric emptying.

MORNING HYPERGLYCEMIA
Blood glucose elevation on awakening. Causes include:

Insufficient Insulin

Dawn Phenomenon: Glucose remains nl until ≈ 3 AM, when effect of nocturnal growth hormone may ↑ glucose in type I DM.

Somogyi phenomenon: Hypoglycemia occurs during night. Compensatory mechanisms to ↑ glucose levels are activated and result in overcompensation. Corrected by ↓ evening dose of intermediate-acting insulin and/or eating more substantial bedtime snack.

PROBLEMS WITH INSULIN
Insulin Resistance: Experienced by most individuals with DM when daily insulin requirement >200 U to control hyperglycemia and prevent ketosis. Typically results from profound/complete insulin deficiency in type I DM and obesity in type II. May be treated by changing insulin to a purer preparation or changing from animal source (beef or pork) to human insulin.

Lipodystrophy: Local disturbance in fat metabolism resulting in loss of fat (lipoatrophy) or abnormal fatty masses at injection sites (lipohypertrophy). Rarely seen since development of U-100 human source insulins. Rotation of injection sites helps prevent lipohypertrophy. Treatment involves changing to U-100 human source insulin and injecting subsequent scheduled doses into periphery of affected area(s).

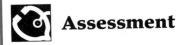

Assessment

PHYSICAL ASSESSMENT
Impending Type I (IDDM) Crisis (DKA): Profound dehydration and hyperglycemia, electrolyte imbalance, metabolic acidosis resulting from ketosis, altered mental status, Kussmaul's respirations, acetone breath, possible hypovolemic shock, abdominal pain, strokelike symptoms

Impending Type II (NIDDM) Crisis (HHNS): Severe dehydration, hypovolemic shock, severe hyperglycemia, shallow respirations, altered mental status, slight lactic acidosis or nl pH, strokelike symptoms

VITAL SIGNS/HEMODYNAMICS
RR: NI; ↑ with DKA, HHNS
HR: NI; ↑ with DKA, HHNS
BP: NI; ↓ with DKA, HHNS
Temp: NI; may be ↑ with DKA, HHNS
Hemodynamics (with crises)
CVP/PAWP: ↓ markedly
PAP: ↓ because of severe hypovolemia
CO/CI: ↓ because of severe hypovolemia
SVR: ↑ early; ↓ later

LABORATORY STUDIES
WHO defines these diagnostic criteria for DM in nonpregnant adults:
Fasting Blood Sugar: Value >140 mg/dl indicative of glucose intolerance if found on at least 2 occasions.

Oral Glucose Tolerance Test: 2-h sample during test >200 mg/dl on at least 2 occasions.

Random Plasma Glucose: >200 mg/dl on at least 2 occasions.

Glycosylated Hgb: Nl range is 4%-7%. Individuals with DM have values >7%. Measured to assess control of blood glucose over preceding 2-3 mo period. The larger the percentage of glycosylated Hgb, the poorer the blood glucose control.

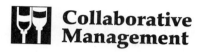
Collaborative Management

Diet: Individually based on ideal body weight and adjusted to metabolic and activity needs. Typical ADA diet composed of 50%-60% carbohydrates, 12%-20% protein, and 20%-30% fat. Focus on weight reduction for type II DM necessitates significant carbohydrate restriction if treated by diet alone. Type I DM necessitates day-to-day consistency in diet and exercise to prevent hypoglycemia. Fat and protein should be present in all meals and snacks to prevent rapid ↑ in postprandial blood glucose. Adding 10-15 g of fiber slows digestion of monosaccharides and disaccharides. For all types of DM, refined and simple sugars should be ↓, and complex carbohydrates (breads, cereals, pasta, beans) encouraged.

Blood Glucose Monitoring: Control of blood glucose facilitated by glycohemoglobin monitoring device. Shown to ↓ incidence and severity of long-term complications.

Oral Hypoglycemics (sulfonylureas): Used in type II DM when diet alone cannot control hyperglycemia. Primary action is to ↑ insulin production by affecting existing beta-cell function. Most serious side effect is hypoglycemia, which can be severe and persistent. Oral hypoglycemics omitted several days before planned surgery. Common factors causing hypoglycemia are fasting for diagnostic purposes, skipping meals, malnour-

ishment r/t illness, other medication therapy.

Insulin: In the critically ill it is sometimes necessary to discontinue intermediate and long-acting insulins and use continuous infusion of regular insulin, which is more easily titrated to frequently obtained blood glucose levels. This measure often necessary because of physiologic instability and frequent use of agents such as steroids and catecholamines, which antagonize hypoglycemic effects of insulin.

Insulin Delivery Systems

Continuous subcutaneous insulin infusion/portable insulin pumps: Deliver constant basal rate of insulin throughout day and night with capability of delivering bolus at mealtime. Patients program pumps based on self-monitoring of blood glucose.

Injection ports: SC access ports inserted into subcutaneous fat. Patients may use port for injection rather than puncturing skin.

Jet injectors: Deliver insulin in fine, pressurized stream through skin without injection needle. Thorough patient training necessary. Typically, onset and peak action occur earlier using these devices.

Insulin pens: Small, prefilled insulin cartridges, inserted into penlike holder. Although patients must use needles for injection, there is no need for insulin to be drawn up from multidose vials.

Exercise: As important as diet and insulin in treating DM. Lowers blood glucose levels, helps maintain nl cholesterol levels, and ↑ circulation. These effects ↑ the body's ability to metabolize glucose and help ↓ therapeutic dose of insulin for most patients.

Transplantation: Complete or partial pancreatic transplants have been performed on a small number of patients, usually in conjunction with kidney transplantation. Transplantation of only beta islet cells currently under investigation as an alternative to other methods.

PATIENT/FAMILY TEACHING
- Use of insulin, including injection tech-

nique, site rotations, storage precautions
- Importance of using appropriate syringe (eg, U-100 syringe with U-100 insulin) and avoiding mixing types/sources of insulin; if prescription is for mixture of insulins, instruction in drawing up of regular insulin into syringe first
- Technique and timing for home monitoring of blood glucose using commercial kit
- Importance of carrying diabetic identification card and wearing Medic-Alert bracelet or necklace
- Recognizing warning signs of hyperglycemia and hypoglycemia, treatment, factors that contribute to both conditions; reminder that stress from illness or infection can ↑ insulin requirements and that ↑ exercise necessitates additional food intake to prevent hypoglycemia
- Importance of daily exercise, maintenance of nl body weight, regular medical evaluation
- Diet low in fat and high in fiber as effective means of controlling blood fats, especially cholesterol and triglycerides; necessity of adequate nutrition and controlled calories to maintain normoglycemia
- Necessity of rotating injection sites and injecting insulin at room temp
- Importance of meticulous skin, wound, foot care
- Importance of annual eye examinations and regular dental checkups
- Drugs that potentiate hyperglycemia: eg, estrogens, corticosteroids, thyroid preparations, diuretics, phenytoin, glucagon, medications that contain sugar (eg, cough syrup)
- Drugs that potentiate hypoglycemia: eg, salicylates, sulfonamides, tetracyclines, methyldopa, anabolic steroids, acetaminophen, MAO inhibitors, ETOH, haloperidol, marijuana; propranolol and other β adrenergic blocking agents mask signs of and inhibit recovery from hypoglycemia
- Local chapter of ADA; American Diabetes Association Membership Center, Box 2055, Harlan, IA 51593-0238

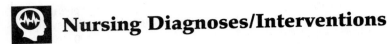

Nursing Diagnoses/Interventions

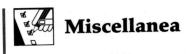

Miscellanea

Altered peripheral, cardiopulmonary, renal, cerebral, and GI tissue perfusion (or risk for same) r/t interrupted blood flow secondary to development and progression of macroangiopathy and microangiopathy

Desired outcome: Optimally, patient has adequate tissue perfusion: warmth, sensation, brisk capillary refill time (<2 sec), and peripheral pulses >2+ on 0-4+ scale in the extremities; BP wnl for patient; UO ≥30 ml/h; baseline vision; good appetite; and absence of nausea and vomiting.

- Compliance with therapeutic regimen is essential for promoting optimal tissue perfusion. Check blood glucose ac and at hs. Encourage performance of regular home blood glucose monitoring.
- Hypertension is a common complication. Careful control of BP is critical in preventing or limiting development of heart disease, retinopathy, or nephropathy. Administer antihypertensive agents.
- Patients may experience ↓ sensation in extremities as a result of peripheral neuropathy. In addition to sensation, assess capillary refill, temp, peripheral pulses, and color. Protect patients with impaired peripheral perfusion from injury with sharp objects or heat. Teach prevention of venous stasis by avoiding pressure at back of knees and constricting garments on extremities and lower body.
- Provide safe environment for patients with ↓ eyesight caused by diabetic retinopathy. Orient to location of water, tissues, glasses, call light.
- Approximately half of all persons with type I DM develop CRF or ESRD. Monitor for changes in renal function (eg, ↑ in BUN/creatinine and altered UO). Proteinuria is an early indicator of developing CRF. Exogenous insulin needs ↓ as renal function ↓.
- Be alert to S&S of hypoglycemia: changes in mentation, apprehension, erratic behavior, trembling, slurred speech, staggering gait, seizure activity. Treat hypoglycemia with rapid-acting sugar (fruit juice, table sugar) or D_{50}.
- Multiple problems may result from autonomic neuropathy, such as the following:
    Orthostatic hypotension: Assist when getting up suddenly or after prolonged recumbency. Check for orthostatic hypotension prn.
    Impaired gastric emptying with nausea, vomiting, and diarrhea: Administer metoclopramide ac. Keep a record of all stools. Nausea, vomiting, and anorexia can signal developing uremia in progressive renal failure.
    Neurogenic bladder: Encourage voiding q3-4h during the day, using manual pressure (Credé's method) if necessary. Intermittent catheterization may be necessary in severe cases. Avoid indwelling urinary catheters because of high risk of infection.

Risk for infection r/t chronic disease process (eg, hyperglycemia, neurogenic bladder, poor circulation)

Desired outcome: Patient infection free: normothermia, negative cultures, and WBC ≤11,000 µl.

- Monitor temp q4h. Be aware that infection is the most common cause of DKA.
- Maintain meticulous sterile technique when changing dressings, performing invasive procedures, or manipulating indwelling catheters.
- Monitor for indicators of URI, UTI, systemic sepsis, and infection at localized (IV) sites.
- Obtain culture specimens for blood, sputum, and urine during temp spikes, or for wounds that produce purulent drainage.

CONSULT MD FOR
- S&S of infection, new ulcerations or injuries
- S&S of complications: hyperglycemia, hypoglycemia, DKA, HHNS, altered mental status
- UO <0.5 ml/kg/h × 2 h or other S&S of deteriorating renal function

RELATED TOPICS
- Diabetic ketoacidosis
- Hyperosmolar hyperglycemic nonketotic syndrome
- Hypoglycemia
- Hypovolemia
- Renal failure, acute

ABBREVIATIONS
ADA: American Diabetes Association
D_{50}: 50% dextrose
ESRD: End-stage renal disease
HHNS: Hyperosmolar hyperglycemic nonketotic syndrome
WHO: World Health Organization

Impaired tissue integrity (or risk of same) r/t altered circulation and sensation secondary to peripheral neuropathy and vascular pathology

Desired outcomes: Patient's lower extremity tissue remains intact. Within 24-h period before hospital discharge, patient verbalizes and demonstrates knowledge of proper foot care.

- Assess skin integrity and evaluate lower extremity reflexes by checking knee and ankle DTRs, proprioceptive sensations, and vibration sensation (using a tuning fork on the medial malleolus). If sensations are impaired, anticipate inability to respond appropriately to harmful stimuli. Monitor peripheral pulses, comparing quality bilaterally. Be alert to pulses $\leq 2+$ on 0-4+ scale.
- Use foot cradle on bed, spaceboots for ulcerated heels, elbow protectors, and pressure-relief mattress to prevent pressure points and promote comfort.
- To alleviate acute discomfort yet prevent hemostasis, minimize activities and incorporate progressive passive and active exercises into daily routine. Discourage extended rest periods in the same position.
- Perform/teach these steps for foot care:
  Wash feet qd with mild soap and warm water; check water temp with water thermometer or elbow.
  Inspect feet qd for erythema or trauma. Prevent infection from moisture or dirt by changing socks qd and using cotton or wool blends.
  Use gentle moisturizers to soften dry skin.

Fluid volume deficit r/t failure of regulatory mechanism secondary to profound hyperglycemia with resultant osmotic diuresis and intravascular depletion

Desired outcomes: Within 12 h of initiating treatment, hypovolemia resolved: BP $\geq$90/60 mm Hg (or within 10% of nl for patient), HR 60-100 bpm, CVP 2-6 mm Hg, PAWP 6-12 mm Hg, UO $\geq$0.5 ml/kg/h, firm skin turgor, NSR on ECG.

- Ensure that measures for rapid rehydration have been initiated as soon as possible. Patient may need 1-3 L of replacement fluid infused during the first h of treatment.
- Monitor VS q15min until condition stable for 1-2 h.
- Consider use of hemodynamic monitoring to assist with rehydration measures. Observe for $\uparrow$ CVP, PAWP, and CO. If PAWP rapidly $\uparrow$ to >15 mm Hg, reduce volume infusion; this may be a sign of early LV failure/pulmonary edema.
- Auscultate breath sounds and heart tones qh. Observe for development of basilar crackles/rales or S_3 gallop, possible signals of circulatory overload.
- Monitor serum electrolyte values closely, especially K^+ and Na^+. Anticipate rapid shifts in K^+, since osmotic diuresis will cause hypokalemia and insulin administration will cause movement of K^+ from plasma into body cells. As pH corrected, K^+ will move from intracellular to intravascular spaces.
- Measure I&O qh and weight qd. $\downarrow$ UO may signal diminishing intravascular fluid volume or impending renal failure.
- Monitor ECG continuously, observing for resolution of tachycardia and possible ventricular dysrhythmias. Cardiac irritability results from hypokalemia, other fluid and electrolyte imbalances.
- Perform neurologic assessments qh. Patients can experience strokelike symptoms as a result of hyperglycemia and actual nonhemorrhagic stroke secondary to profound hypovolemia leading to clotting in the vasculature.

REFERENCES

Baird MS: Diabetes mellitus. In Swearingen PL (ed): *Pocket guide to medical-surgical nursing,* ed 2, St Louis, 1996, Mosby.

Brody GM: Diabetic ketoacidosis and hyperosmolar hyperglycemic nonketotic coma, *Top Emerg Med* 14(1): 12-22, 1992.

Horne MM: Endocrinologic dysfunctions. In Swearingen PL, Keen JH (eds): *Manual of critical care nursing,* ed 3, St Louis, 1995, Mosby.

Sherwin RS: Diabetes mellitus. In Bennett JC, Plum F: *Cecil textbook of medicine,* ed 20, Philadelphia, 1996, Saunders.

Siperstein MD: Diabetic ketoacidosis and hyperosmolar coma, *Endocrinol Metab Clin North Am* 22(2): 303-328, 1993.

Author: **Marianne Saunorus Baird**

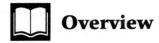 **Overview**

PATHOPHYSIOLOGY

Life-threatening complication of DM. Occurs when insulin deficiency prevents serum glucose use, causing breakdown of fat and protein for energy. Ketones accumulate in blood, resulting in metabolic ketoacidosis, and hyperglycemia causes ↑ serum osmolality. Osmotic diuresis ensues, with losses of Na^+, K^+, PO_4^{3-}, Mg^{2+}, and water, leading to severe dehydration and possible hypovolemic shock. Despite K^+ loss in urine, plasma K^+ may be wnl/↑ because of K^+'s dramatic shift out of the cells as a result of insulin deficiency, acidosis, and tissue catabolism.

COMPLICATIONS

↑ blood viscosity with thromboembolism, impaired tissue perfusion, lactic acidosis, profound CNS depression and, ultimately, death. Cerebral edema can occur with treatment, especially in children.

HISTORY/RISK FACTORS

- IDDM
- Physical stressor: infection (most likely cause), illness (eg, silent MI), trauma, surgery
- Insufficient exogenous insulin replacement
- Nonadherence to diabetes regimen

CLINICAL PRESENTATION

Polyuria, polydipsia, polyphagia, weight loss, weakness, fatigue, nausea, vomiting, abdominal pain, Kussmaul's respirations, fruity or acetone odor to breath

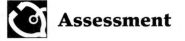 **Assessment**

PHYSICAL ASSESSMENT

Neuro: Irritability, lethargy, coma
Resp: Kussmaul's pattern, ketone breath
CV: Tachycardia, hypotension, dysrhythmias
Integ: Dry and flushed skin, dry mucous membranes, poor skin turgor

VITAL SIGNS/HEMODYNAMICS

RR: ↑
HR: ↑
BP: ↓
Temp: Although infection frequently precipitates DKA, may be nl or ↓ because of acidosis.
CVP/PAPs: ↓ as a result of dehydration
ECG: Initially, dysrhythmias associated with *hyperkalemia:* peaked T waves, widened QRS complex, prolonged PR intervals, flattened-to-absent P wave. After insulin therapy, dysrhythmias associated with *hypokalemia* possible: depressed ST segments, flat or inverted T waves, ↑ ventricular dysrhythmias. 12-lead evaluated to rule out silent MI.

LABORATORY STUDIES

Serum Glucose: 200-800 mg/dl
Serum Ketones: ↑
Urine Glucose/Acetone: Positive, "large"
Serum Osmolality: 300-350 mOsm/L
ABGs: HCO_3^- <15 mEq/L; pH <7.2; $Paco_2$ ↑, reflecting compensatory response
Serum Electrolytes: K^+ nl or ↑ >5.0 mEq/L initially; Na^+ ↑, nl, or ↓; total CO_2, PO_4^{3-}, Mg^{2+}, Cl^- all ↓; anion gap ↑
Hct: ↑ as a result of osmotic diuresis and hemoconcentration
BUN/Creatinine: ↑
WBCs: Initial ↑ may reflect dehydration and ↑ adrenocortical secretion. ↑ also possible as a result of infection.

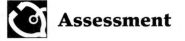 **Collaborative Management**

Rehydration: Usually, isotonic saline (0.9%) administered rapidly (1-2 L during first h) to correct fluid deficit, which is typically 4-6 L. After initial replacement, 0.45% saline administered. To prevent rebound hypoglycemia, dextrose is added to IV line once blood glucose ↓ to 200-300 mg/dl.

Rapid-Acting Insulin: Loading dose of regular insulin, followed by continuous IV insulin infusion, ≈0.1 U/kg/h, or intermittent IM or IV injections. Blood glucose must be reduced gradually to ↓ risk of cerebral edema. Insulin drip discontinued temporarily if serum glucose drops to <100 mg/dl. Flush IV tubing with 100 ml insulin solution to saturate tubing with insulin and improve accuracy of delivery.

Restoration of Electrolyte Balance: K^+ closely monitored and replaced once insulin administered and K^+ returns to intracellular compartment. Replacement essential to prevent severe hypokalemia. PO_4^{3-} replacement (usually as potassium phosphate) indicated if severe depletion resulting from prolonged acidosis has occurred. Monitoring PO_4^{3-} and Ca^{2+} levels essential because supplemental PO_4^{3-} may depress plasma Ca^{2+} levels.

IV Bicarbonate: For severe acidosis (pH <7.0). Not routinely given in DKA because of risk of paradoxical CSF acidosis and hypokalemia.

Insertion of Gastric Tube: Indicated in the comatose or obtunded when risk of vomiting and aspiration high.

Treatment of Underlying Cause: Eg, infection treated with appropriate antibiotics.

PATIENT-FAMILY TEACHING

- Purpose, expected results, anticipated sensations of all nursing/medical interventions.
- Relationship of DKA to illness, infection, trauma, and stress. Emphasize importance of adhering to entire diabetic regimen including meal planning, insulin, exercise, monitoring.
- Sick-day guidelines (eg, need for ↑ fluid and insulin with illness).
- Hospital and community resources (eg, diabetes educator, dietitian, social worker, local American Diabetes Association [ADA], support groups).
- Address for ADA: American Diabetes Association, Inc., 1660 Duke St., Alexandria, VA 22314. Toll-free phone number: 800-232-3472.

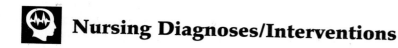

Nursing Diagnoses/Interventions

Fluid volume deficit r/t ↓ circulating volume secondary to hyperglycemia and induced osmotic diuresis

Desired outcomes: Within 12 h of initiating treatment, patient normovolemic: BP ≥90/60 mm Hg (or wnl for patient), MAP ≥70 mm Hg, HR 60-100 bpm, CVP 2-6 mm Hg, PAWP 6-12 mm Hg, balanced I&O, UO ≥0.5 ml/kg/h, firm skin turgor, pink and moist mucous membranes, NSR on ECG.

- Monitor VS q15min until condition stable for 1 h. Be alert to tachycardia, dysrhythmias, hypotension, ↓ CVP/PAWP.
- Monitor for S&S of dehydration: poor skin turgor, dry mucous membranes, sunken and soft eyeballs, tachycardia, orthostatic hypotension.
- Measure I&O. ↓ UO may signal diminishing intravascular fluid volume or impending renal failure. Weigh patient qd.
- Administer prescribed IV fluids to rehydrate. Be alert to S&S of fluid overload, which can occur as a result of rapid infusion of fluids: JVD, dyspnea, crackles, CVP >6 mm Hg.
- Monitor laboratory tests for abnormalities. Be alert for hypokalemia, a common complication of treatment.
- Monitor patient continuously on cardiac monitor. Observe for ECG changes typical of hyperkalemia or hypokalemia.
- Observe for S&S of electrolyte imbalance associated with DKA and its treatment.
  Hypokalemia: ECG changes, muscle weakness, hypotension, anorexia, drowsiness, hypoactive bowel sounds
  Hypophosphatemia: Muscle weakness, respiratory failure, ↓ O_2 delivery, ↓ cardiac function
  Hypomagnesemia: Anorexia, nausea, vomiting, lethargy, weakness, personality changes, tetany, tremor or muscle fasciculations, seizures, confusion progressing to coma

Risk for infection r/t inadequate secondary defenses (suppressed inflammatory response) secondary to protein depletion

Desired outcome: Patient free of infection: normothermia, HR ≤100 bpm, BP wnl for patient, WBCs ≤11,000 μl, and negative culture results.

- Assess for evidence of infection. Monitor for ↑ WBCs.
- Ensure good hand washing technique when caring for patient.
- Because patient is at ↑ risk of bacterial infection, limit use of invasive lines. Rotate peripheral IV sites q72h, depending on agency policy. Central lines should be discontinued as soon as feasible. Schedule dressing changes according to agency policy, and inspect site(s) for signs of local infection, including erythema, swelling, or purulent drainage.
- Use meticulous aseptic technique when caring for or inserting indwelling catheters to minimize risk of bacterial entry. Indwelling urethral catheter is indicated only when continuous accurate assessment of UO is essential.
- Provide good skin care to maintain skin integrity. Assess for areas of ↓ sensation on extremities. Use pressure-relief mattress to help prevent skin breakdown.

Risk for injury r/t altered cerebral function secondary to hyperosmolality, dehydration, cerebral edema associated with DKA, or hypoglycemia

Desired outcome: Patient verbalizes orientation × 3; nl breath sounds auscultated over airways; and oral cavity and musculoskeletal system remain intact and free of injury.

- Monitor orientation, LOC, and respiratory status, especially airway patency, at frequent intervals. Keep oral airway, manual resuscitator and mask, and supplemental O_2 at bedside.
- Reduce likelihood of injury caused by falls by maintaining bed in lowest position, with side rails up at all times, and using soft restraints as necessary.
- Place gastric tube to intermittent suction in comatose patient, as prescribed, to ↓ likelihood of aspiration.
- Elevate HOB to 45 degrees to minimize risk of aspiration.
- Initially, monitor blood glucose qh. Be alert to blood glucose that drops faster than 100 mg/dl/h. Once blood glucose <200-300 mg/dl, dextrose should be added to IV fluids.

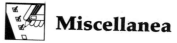

Miscellanea

CONSULT MD FOR

- HR >120 bpm or BP <90/60 mm Hg or ↓ ≥20 mm Hg from baseline, MAP ↓ ≥10 mm Hg from baseline, CVP <2 mm Hg, and PAWP <6 mm Hg.
- UO <0.5 ml/kg/h for 2 consecutive h.
- Blood glucose <200-300 mg/dl or ↓ in blood glucose >100 mg/dl/h
- Serious dysrhythmias: ECG changes found with hyperkalemia and hypokalemia
- S&S of fluid overload resulting from overzealous rehydration: ↑ CVP, crackles, JVD, dyspnea
- Serum electrolyte abnormalities, especially K^+, PO_4^{3-}, and Ca^{2+}, or S&S of electrolyte abnormalities
- Evidence of infection
- Altered LOC or symptoms of cerebral edema

RELATED TOPICS

- Hyperkalemia
- Hyperosmolar hyperglycemic nonketotic syndrome
- Hypokalemia
- Hypophosphatemia
- Metabolic acidosis, acute
- Shock, hypovolemic

REFERENCES

Horne MM: Endocrinologic dysfunctions. In Swearingen PL, Keen JH (eds): *Manual of critical care nursing,* ed 3, St Louis, 1995, Mosby.

Jones TL: From diabetic ketoacidosis to hyperglycemic hyperosmolar nonketotic syndrome, *Crit Care Nurs Clin North Am* 6(4): 703-721, 1994.

Kitabchi AE, Wall BM: Diabetic ketoacidosis, *Med Clin North Am* 79(1): 9-38, 1995.

Sauve DO, Kessler CA: Hyperglycemic emergencies, *AACN Clinical Issues in Crit Care Nurs* 3(2): 350-360, 1992.

Author: **Mima M. Horne**

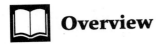 Overview

PATHOPHYSIOLOGY
Commonly acquired coagulopathy with potential to cause profuse bleeding and widespread thrombosis leading to MODS. Characterized by overstimulation of the nl coagulation cascade.

HISTORY/RISK FACTORS
Obstetric: Abruptio placentae, toxemia, septic abortion
GI: Cirrhosis, hepatic necrosis, pancreatitis, necrotizing enterocolitis
Tissue Damage: Surgery, trauma, burns, prolonged extracorporeal circulation, transplant rejection
Vascular: Shock, aneurysm
Miscellaneous: Severe or systemic infection, transfusion reaction or other hemolytic process, fat or pulmonary embolus, snake bite, neoplastic disorder, acute anoxia

CLINICAL PRESENTATION
- Abrupt onset of bleeding or oozing of blood from all invasive sites and mucosal surfaces
- Hematuria, stool or gastric aspirate positive for occult blood; unusual or excessive bruising
- Abnormal thrombosis with extremity pain, ↓ pulses, oliguria/anuria, severe chest pain with SOB, paresis/paralysis, cerebral thrombus, AMI, PE

VITAL SIGNS/HEMODYNAMICS
Usually reflect hemorrhage; may reflect thrombosis (eg, PE, AMI, stroke, peripheral arterial occlusion)
RR: ↑
HR: ↑
BP: ↓
Temp: NI
CVP/PAWP: ↓
CO: ↓
ECG: Dysrhythmias, elevated or depressed ST segment, T-wave inversion

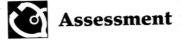 Assessment

PHYSICAL ASSESSMENT
Great variability, depending on predominance of bleeding vs clotting and underlying disorder
Neuro: Confusion, ↓ responsiveness, weakness, paralysis
Resp: Tachypnea, SOB
CV: Tachycardia, dysrhythmias, hypotension, ↓/absent peripheral pulses, pallor, acrocyanosis, delayed capillary refill
GI: ↓/absent bowel sounds, abdominal tenderness, Grey Turner's sign
GU: ↓/absent UO, hematuria
Other: Petechiae, ecchymosis, purpura, mottling of extremities

LABORATORY STUDIES
FDPs/FSPs: ↑ (>10 μg/ml) because of widespread fibrinolysis. *Critical value:* >40 μg/ml.
D-Dimer Assay: Rapid but less sensitive measurement than FDPs. ↑ to >500 caused by ↑ thrombin and plasmin generation.
Fibrinogen Levels: Usually ↓; may remain wnl in early acute phase.
PTT/Activated PTT (APTT): Prolonged as a result of activation of intrinsic pathway causing consumption of coagulation factors. *Critical value:* >70 sec.
PT: Prolonged as a result of activation of extrinsic pathway causing consumption of extrinsic clotting factors. *Critical value:* >40 sec.
Thrombin Time: Prolonged as a result of rapid conversion of fibrinogen into fibrin.
Antithrombin III (AT-III): ↓ because of rapid consumption of this thrombin inhibitor.
Platelets: ↓ (<140,000 μl) because of platelet aggregation during clot formation.
α_2-Antiplasmin: ↓ caused by rapid consumption of same in response to large amounts of plasmin generated. When fully depleted, excessive hyperfibrinolysis (massive, rapid clot lysis) occurs.
Peripheral Blood Smear: For visualization during microscopic examination of schistocytes and burr cells, which indicate deposition of fibrin in small blood vessels.

Collaborative Management

Treatment of Underlying Disease Process: Often corrects secondary DIC. Use of heparin and antifibrinolytic agents controversial, since they have not improved survival and may exacerbate bleeding (heparin) or thrombosis (antifibrinolytic agent).
Continuous IV Heparin Therapy: Three conditions associated with DIC in which heparin often effective:
  Underlying malignancy/carcinoma
  Acute promyelocytic leukemia (APML)
  Purpura fulminans/extreme purpura, often seen with severe sepsis
Low-dose (5-10 U/kg/h) therapy considered. Heparin binds to antithrombin, which then inhibits proteases involved in intrinsic and common coagulation pathways, resulting in a strong anticoagulant effect.
Antifibrinolytic Agents: ε-aminocaproic acid (Amicar), tranexamic acid used to inhibit fibrinolysis for bleeding resulting from a variety of causes. Used with extreme caution in DIC as they may convert a bleeding disorder into a thrombotic problem. In DIC, used with heparin to minimize potential for thrombosis.
Blood Component Replacement: Clotting factors and inhibitors replaced *via* FFP. PT used to guide plasma replacement. Markedly ↓ fibrinogen levels may require cryoprecipitate, which contains 5-10 × more fibrinogen than plasma. Platelet transfusions rarely needed unless there is impaired platelet production and profuse bleeding.
RBC Replacement: PRBCs may be given to ↑ O_2-carrying capacity with Hgb value <9 mg/dl or >20% below baseline with chronic anemia.
Vitamin K_1 (Phytonadione) and Folate: Patients at high risk for deficiency of these substances and are recommended to supplement.
Investigational Agents: Gabexate, nafamostat, transylol, AT-III have been used in limited clinical trials.
Vasoactive Drugs: If patient severely hypotensive, inotropes, vasopressors, vasodilators may be considered. Underlying disease and myocardial ischemia must be considered when initiating vasopressor therapy. See inside front cover for table of inotropic and vasoactive agents.

PATIENT-FAMILY TEACHING
- Importance of avoiding vitamin K–inhibiting and platelet aggregation–inhibiting medications (eg, NSAIDs, certain antimicrobials, sulfonamide derivatives, ethanol), which promote bleeding

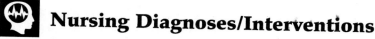 **Nursing Diagnoses/Interventions**

Altered protection r/t bleeding resulting from overstimulation of clotting cascade and rapid consumption of clotting factors
Desired outcome: Within 48-72 h of treatment initiation, patient free of symptoms of bleeding: absence of frank bleeding from invasive sites and mucosal surfaces, secretions and excretions negative for blood, absence of large/↑ ecchymoses, ↓ purpura, and HR, RR, BP within 10% of baseline.

- Assess prior hx of bleeding problems: gingival bleeding, skin bleeding, hematuria, tarry/bloody stools, muscle bleeding, hemoptysis, vomiting of blood, epistaxis, prolonged bleeding from small wounds or following tooth extraction, unusual or "easy" bruising tendency.
- Question patient with no previous hx of bleeding regarding drugs that may promote bleeding, including OTC preparations (eg, NSAIDs, certain antimicrobials, sulfonamide derivatives, ethanol).
- Monitor coagulation/clotting tests qd. Be alert for values that exceed nl by 15%.
- Monitor closely for ↑ bleeding, bruising, petechiae, and purpura. Assess for internal bleeding by testing suspect secretions for blood.
- Monitor neurologic status q2h by assessing LOC, orientation, pupillary reaction, and movement and strength of extremities. Changes in status can indicate intracranial bleeding.
- Use alcohol-free mouthwash and swabs for oral care to minimize risk of bleeding from gum injury. Use NS or solution of NS and sodium bicarbonate (500 ml NS with 15 ml bicarbonate) to irrigate oral cavity. Massage gums gently with a sponge-tipped applicator to help remove debris. Do not attempt to remove large clots from mouth, since profuse bleeding may ensue.
- Use electric rather than straight razor for shaving.
- Avoid giving unnecessary venipunctures and IM injections.
- If patient undergoes an invasive procedure, manually hold pressure over insertion site ≥3-5 min for IV catheters and ≥10-15 min for arterial catheters or until bleeding subsides.

Risk for fluid volume deficit r/t bleeding/hemorrhage
Desired outcomes: Patient normovolemic: HR and RR within baseline, BP within baseline (or SBP >90 mm Hg), warm extremities, distal pulses >2+ on 0-4+ scale, UO ≥0.5 ml/kg/h, capillary refill <2 sec. Within 24 h of initiating treatment, patient exhibits orientation × 3.

- Monitor VS at least q2h, noting ↑ in HR and RR and ↓ in BP and pulse pressure. If patient bleeding actively, measure VS q15-30min. Insertion of an arterial line for continuous monitoring of BP may become necessary.
- Measure UO q2-4h. Be alert to output <0.5 ml/kg/h.
- Monitor CBC qd for significant alterations in Hct, Hgb, and platelets.
- Assess for signs of impending shock: pallor, diaphoresis, cool extremities, delayed capillary refill, ↓ peripheral pulses, restlessness, agitation, disorientation.
- Inspect all invasive sites for frank bleeding; assess all dressings covering wounds.
- Maintain at least one 18-gauge or larger IV catheter for use during shock management, at which time rapid infusion of blood products or IV fluids may be necessary.

Altered peripheral, cardiopulmonary, cerebral, renal tissue perfusion (or risk for same) r/t blood loss or presence of microthrombi
Desired outcomes: Patient has adequate perfusion: peripheral pulses >2+ on scale of 0-4+; brisk capillary refill (<2 sec); BP wnl for patient; CVP ≥5 cm H_2O or ≥2 mm Hg; PAWP 6-12 mm Hg; HR regular and ≤100 bpm; oriented × 3; UO ≥0.5 ml/kg/h; O_2 saturation >90%.

- Monitor BP and assess for early signs of perfusion deficit at least q2h, including dizziness, confusion, and ↓ UO.
- Monitor for ↓ myocardial or pulmonary perfusion as evidenced by chest pain, ST-segment depression or elevation, T-wave inversion. Monitor for S&S of PE: sharp, stabbing chest pain; dyspnea; pallor; cyanosis; pupillary dilatation; rapid, irregular pulse; profuse diaphoresis; anxiety. Administer supplemental O_2.
- Monitor PAWP frequently. ↓ pressures signal hypovolemia/hemorrhage. ↑ PADP may signal PE.
- Monitor CO; calculate SVR, PVR, CI. Anticipate ↑SVR/vasoconstriction with hypovolemia. CO may ↑ or ↓ from nl, depending on cardiac contractility. PVR will ↑ in presence of PE.
- Monitor GI status by observing tolerance to diet or tube feedings, bowel habits, character of stool (tarry, bloody), and presence/absence of bowel sounds. Palpate for abdominal tenderness and monitor abdominal girth q8h.
- Assess for changes in sensorium (confusion, lethargy) and for S&S of stroke, including weakness, paralysis.

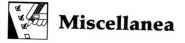 **Miscellanea**

CONSULT MD FOR
- New/↑ bleeding from GI/GU tracts, mucosa, venipunctures
- S&S of stroke, myocardial ischemia/infarction, pulmonary embolus, peripheral arterial thrombosis
- PTT ≥70 sec, PT ≥40 sec, platelet count ≤100 μl
- UO <0.5 ml/kg/h × 2

RELATED TOPICS
- Myocardial infarction, acute
- Pulmonary embolus, thrombotic
- Shock, hemorrhagic
- Stroke: hemorrhagic
- Stroke: ischemic

ABBREVIATIONS
FDP: Fibrin degradation product
FFP: Fresh frozen plasma
FSP: Fibrin split product
MODS: Multiple organ dysfunction syndrome
PE: Pulmonary embolus
PRBCs: Packed red blood cells

REFERENCES
Atkins PJ: Postoperative coagulopathies, *Crit Care Nurs Clin North Am* 5(3): 459-471, 1993.
Baird MS: Hematologic dysfunctions. In Swearingen PL, Keen JH (eds): *Manual of critical care nursing*, ed 3, St Louis, 1995, Mosby.
Bell TN: Disseminated intravascular coagulation, *Crit Care Nurs Clin North Am* 5(3): 389-410, 1993.
Coffland FI, Shelton DM: Blood component replacement therapy, *Crit Care Nurs Clin North Am* 5(3): 543-556, 1993.
Lottman MS, Thompson KS: Assessment of the hematologic system. In Phipps WJ et al (eds): *Medical-surgical nursing: concepts & clinical practice*, ed 5, St Louis, 1995, Mosby.
Lottman MS, Thompson KS: Management of persons with hematologic problems. In Phipps WJ et al (eds): *Medical-surgical nursing: concepts & clinical practice*, ed 5, St Louis, 1995, Mosby.

Author: **Marianne Saunorus Baird**

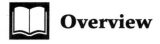 **Overview**

PATHOPHYSIOLOGY
Survival for >24 h after asphyxia caused by submersion. Categorized as follows:

Near Drowning with Aspiration (wet): Aspirant either submersion fluid or gastric contents. Hypoxia results from laryngospasm, bronchospasm, airway obstruction, pulmonary edema.

Freshwater (hypotonic): Causes loss of lung surfactant. Alveoli collapse and lung compliance ↓. Atelectasis and pulmonary edema lead to V/Q mismatch.

Saltwater (hypertonic): Results in rapid shift of water and plasma proteins from circulation into alveoli. Fluid-filled alveoli unventilated, which leads to V/Q mismatch and hypoxia. Aspirated contaminants (eg, algae, chemicals, sand) contribute to obstruction and asphyxiation. Bacterial and aspiration pneumonia often develop.

Near Drowning without Aspiration (dry): Results from asphyxiation secondary to airway obstruction caused by laryngospasm. Laryngospasm often caused by water entering airway but can be triggered by fear or pain.

Hypothermia: Can be significant. Progression causes muscle activity and vital functions to cease and VF to occur. Hypothermia may protect brain from permanent damage, depending on victim's age and its degree. Resuscitation possible, even after 30 min of submersion, and needs to be continued for at least 1 h or until body temp ≥32° C.

HISTORY/RISK FACTORS
- Alcohol or drug ingestion
- Seizure disorder
- Myocardial infarction
- C-spine fracture
- Craniocerebral trauma

CLINICAL PRESENTATION
Severe pulmonary demise may not develop for ≥24 h after event.
- Alterations in mental status, unconsciousness, seizures
- Dyspnea, coughing, pink and frothy sputum
- Vomiting
- Substernal burning or pleuritic chest pain
- Mottled and cold skin, cyanosis

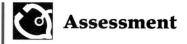 **Assessment**

PHYSICAL ASSESSMENT
Inspection: Tachypnea, pallor, cyanosis, use of accessory muscles, shallow or gasping respirations, fixed and dilated pupils
Percussion: Resonance over lung fields
Auscultation: Crackles, rhonchi, wheezing, stridor

VITAL SIGNS/HEMODYNAMICS
RR: ↑
HR: ↑; irregular
BP: Variable; ↑ with early hypothermia; ↓ in later hypothermia or during rewarming
Temp: ↓ if prolonged submersion; ↑ if pneumonia present
SVR: Variable; ↑ with early hypothermia; ↓ in later hypothermia or during rewarming
ECG: Tachycardia, supraventricular dysrhythmias, bradycardia, VF; Osborne or J waves possible with profound hypothermia

LABORATORY STUDIES
ABGs: Initially hypoxemia and hypercapnia with metabolic and respiratory acidosis. $Paco_2$ may return to nl but hypoxemia persists. Respiratory status can deteriorate quickly, thus serial monitoring essential. Continuous Spo_2 monitoring indicated.
CBCs: To determine baseline hematologic status, presence of infection.
Serum Electrolytes: Disturbances r/t quantity and tonicity of water aspirated. Hypernatremia with saltwater exposure; hyponatremia with freshwater exposure.
BUN/Creatinine: Determine effects of hypoxia on renal tubular function.

IMAGING
Chest X-ray: Serial x-rays check presence of infiltrates, atelectasis, pulmonary edema.
Skull/Spine X-rays: To rule out CNS trauma.

Collaborative Management

O$_2$ Therapy: 100% initiated immediately to treat hypoxia. High concentrations continued, even with good spontaneous ventilation, because of hypoxia risk. Warmed O_2 (40°-43° C) if patient hypothermic.
ET Intubation: May be required for maintaining patent airway.
Mechanical Ventilation: When lung compliance ↓ or patient unable to maintain effective respiratory effort. Freshwater aspiration requires 1½-2 × nl tidal volume at slower rates to optimize alveolar ventilation.
PEEP: Required when pulmonary edema or hypoxia present and unresponsive to ↑ levels O_2 (Fio_2 ≥0.50 to maintain Pao_2 ≥60) and for maintaining clear airways. Used after freshwater aspiration because it keeps alveoli open in absence of adequate surfactant.
Bronchoscopy: To remove aspirated contaminants.
Pharmacotherapy: Profound metabolic acidosis treated with $NaHCO_3$ according to arterial pH. If bronchospasm present, bronchodilators such as epinephrine or isoproterenol HCl may be used. Steroid and prophylactic antibiotic use controversial.
Td Immunization: Booster given if hx unknown or booster needed.
Management of Concurrent Event: Eg, alcohol or drug ingestion, seizure, hypothermia, MI, head injury, C-spine fracture.

PATIENT-FAMILY TEACHING
- Turning, coughing, deep breathing, suctioning
- Use of incentive inspirometry
- Medications: drug name, purpose, dosage, schedule, precautions, food-drug and drug-drug interactions, potential side effects
- Purpose, expected results, anticipated sensations of nursing/medical interventions
- Water safety
- Organ donations
- Existing support systems

Nursing Diagnoses/Interventions

Impaired gas exchange r/t alveolar-capillary membrane changes secondary to fluid accumulation in lung or loss of surfactant

Desired outcome: Within 12 h of treatment, patient has adequate gas exchange: $Pao_2 \geq 60$ mm Hg and $Paco_2$ 35-45 mm Hg. Within 3 days RR ≤ 20 breaths/min with eupnea, breath sounds clear/bilaterally equal, patient oriented $\times$ 3.

- Auscultate lung fields. Note adventitious breath sounds: crackles, rhonchi, friction rubs.
- Monitor ABGs, Spo_2. Progressive hypoxemia may require $\uparrow$ concentrations of O_2 or mechanical ventilation.
- Assess for SOB, tachypnea, use of accessory muscles, nasal flaring, grunting, restlessness, anxiety.
- Place in semi-Fowler's position.
- Assess need for suctioning. Document color, consistency, amount of sputum.
- Use PEEP adapter on manual resuscitator when suctioning patients receiving high levels PEEP. In-line suction device may prevent hypoxia associated with suctioning.
- Provide rest periods between activities to $\downarrow$ O_2 demands.
- Explain all procedures, and provide emotional support to $\downarrow$ anxiety, which can contribute to O_2 consumption.

Hypothermia r/t prolonged exposure to cold water during submersion

Desired outcomes: Within 24 h of therapy, core temp $\uparrow$ to 35°-37° C. BP, RR, and HR wnl for patient.

- Use temp probe or PA catheter to obtain continuous core temp.
- Do not attempt surface or external warming until core temp 35°-37° C. Administer warm fluids and warmed, humidified O_2.
- Be aware of likelihood of $\downarrow$ drug metabolism during hypothermic period.

Risk for infection r/t $\uparrow$ environmental exposure secondary to aspiration of water and contaminants present in water

Desired outcome: Patient infection free: body temp $\leq 37.5°$ C after first 24 h, WBC count wnl for patient, clear sputum, negative culture results.

- Monitor temp q2h. $\uparrow$ temp up to 38° C common during first 24 h. After 24 h, $\uparrow$ temp may signal infection.
- Monitor WBC count for $\uparrow$.
- Inspect sputum for changes in color, consistency, amount.
- Use meticulous aseptic technique when suctioning.
- Collect sputum for C&S if infection suspected.

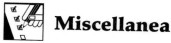 **Miscellanea**

CONSULT MD FOR
- Significant change in breath sounds
- New onset fever >38° C
- Progressive deterioration in Sao_2
- Thick or purulent sputum production
- Changes in mental status: $\downarrow$ LOC, $\uparrow$ agitation

RELATED TOPICS
- Acute tubular necrosis
- Adult respiratory distress syndrome
- Disseminated intravascular coagulation
- Head injury
- Hypervolemia
- Hypothermia
- Mechanical ventilation
- Renal failure, acute
- Spinal cord injury, cervical

ABBREVIATION
Td: Combined tetanus diphtheria toxoid

REFERENCES

Borta M: Psychosocial issues in water related injuries, *Crit Care Nurs Clin North Am* 3(2): 325-329, 1991.

Glanker D: Caring for the victim of near drowning, *Crit Care Nurse* 13(4): 25-32, 1993.

Howard CA: Near drowning. In Swearingen PL, Keen JH (eds): *Manual of critical care nursing*, ed 3, St Louis, 1995, Mosby.

Nemiroff M: Near drowning, *Respir Care* 37(6): 600-608, 1992.

Uustal D: Ethical issues in caring for patients who have suffered water-related injuries, *Crit Care Nurs Clin North Am* 3(2): 361-371, 1991.

Walsh EA, Ioli JG: Childhood near drowning: nursing care and primary prevention, *Pediatr Nurs* 20(3): 265-269, 1994.

Author: **Cheri A. Goll**

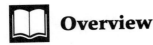 **Overview**

PATHOPHYSIOLOGY

One of the most common drug overdoses. Most patients will admit to having taken this medication. Acute ingestion ≥20 g in adults may cause hepatic necrosis, which can lead to hepatic failure, signaled by hypoglycemia, metabolic acidosis, thrombocytopenia.
Routes: Oral (most common); rectal (suppository)

HISTORY/RISK FACTORS

- Liver disease
- Coingestion of alcohol ↑ risk of toxicity

CLINICAL PRESENTATION

- Onset of S&S usually 1-2 days after ingestion
- Nausea, vomiting, right-sided abdominal pain
- Mild alterations in consciousness with severe lung damage

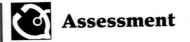 **Assessment**

PHYSICAL ASSESSMENT

Neuro: Confusion, somnolence, asterixis, coma
Resp: Compensatory hyperventilation
CV: Tachycardia, dysrhythmias
GI: Hepatosplenomegaly, jaundice
GU: ↓ UO
Assoc Findings: Include impaired cardiac contractility (as a result of release of myocardial depressants from damaged liver/pancreas), transient renal tubular necrosis, hypophosphatemia, hypothermia, hemorrhagic pancreatitis

VITAL SIGNS/HEMODYNAMICS

RR: ↑
HR: ↑
BP: ↓
Temp: ↓
CVP/PAWP: ↓ as a result of dehydration
Other: Acute fulminant hepatic failure may trigger hyperdynamic circulatory state with ↓ SVR, ↑ CO. CO may ↓ if myocardial depression/injury present.
ECG: Dysrhythmias; T-wave inversion and ST-segment elevation if myocardial injury present.

LABORATORY STUDIES

Serum Levels of Acetaminophen: Initially drawn 4 h postingestion if possible. Subsequently drawn periodically (eg, q4h) until values are below predicted hepatotoxic range.
Chemistries: Serum Na^+, K^+, CO_2, BUN/creatinine, blood glucose, liver enzymes, bilirubin, amylase
Hematology: PT; coagulation studies; CBC
ABGs: To evaluate oxygenation, acid-base values

Collaborative Management

Support of CV, Resp Systems: Oxygen supplementation. If ABGs indicate trend toward respiratory failure, mechanical ventilation is possible. Continuous ECG monitoring for dysrhythmias, which are treated according to ACLS guidelines.
Removal of Acetaminophen from System
Combination activated charcoal/N-acetylcysteine (Mucomyst): Given orally or *via* gastric tube. Greatest effectiveness if given soon after ingestion, but may be effective 8-10 h postingestion or even later. Binds with acetaminophen until passed *via* GI tract. After loading dose of 140 mg/kg, *N*-acetylcysteine given q4h × 17 doses or until acetaminophen levels ↓ well below hepatotoxic range.
Lavage: To remove drug or assess stomach contents for drug ingestion.
Ipecac: Option if ingestion is recent, but vomiting delays use of activated charcoal and *N*-acetylcysteine.
Fluid Replacement: *Via* LR or D_5NS.
Antiemetics: Usually promethazine hydrochloride (Phenergan) for nausea and vomiting.
Rewarming: Heating blanket for hypothermia.
Treatment of Hypoglycemia: D_{50} bolus and continuous infusion of D_5W, based on serum glucose results.
Treatment of Acute Hepatic Failure: To minimize complications and prevent further damage.

PATIENT-FAMILY TEACHING

- Purpose, expected results, anticipated sensations for all nursing/medical interventions
- Importance of avoiding alcohol ingestion with acetaminophen; necessity of abstaining from alcohol consumption if liver damage present

Nursing Diagnoses/Interventions

Ineffective airway clearance r/t presence of tracheobronchial secretions; obstruction; ↓ sensorium

Desired outcome: Within 2-24 h of intervention/treatment, patient has clear airway: clear breath sounds over upper airways and lung fields, RR 12-20 breaths/min with eupnea, Pao_2 ≥80 mm Hg, $Paco_2$ 35-45 mm Hg, pH 7.35-7.45, and Spo_2 ≥92%.

- Assess respiratory function frequently. Be alert to secretions; stridor; gurgling; shallow, irregular, labored respirations; use of accessory muscles; restlessness, confusion; cyanosis.
- Suction oropharynx or *via* ET tube prn.
- Monitor ABG values for hypoxia (Pao_2 <80 mm Hg) and respiratory acidosis ($Paco_2$ >45 mm Hg, pH <7.35).
- Monitor respiratory patterns; provide continuous apnea monitoring if available.
- Monitor for airway obstruction, eg, sounding of high-pressure alarm.
- Monitor Spo_2 continuously for values <92%, depending on baseline, clinical presentation.
- Administer and evaluate effects of antiemetics.
- Place patient in side-lying position during vomiting to ↓ aspiration risk.

Fluid volume deficit r/t ↓ intake secondary to medically prescribed restrictions; and ↓ circulating volume secondary to hypoalbuminemia, altered hemodynamics, and fluid sequestration

Desired outcome: Within 24 h of this diagnosis, patient normovolemic: MAP ≥70 mm Hg; HR 60-100 bpm; distal pulses >2+ on 0-4+ scale; CVP 2-6 mm Hg; PAWP 6-12 mm Hg; CI ≥3.0 L/min/m²; SVR 900-1200 dynes/sec/cm⁻⁵; UO ≥0.5 ml/kg/h; and orientation × 3.

- Monitor and document BP, HR, ECG, and CV status at least qh. Be alert to MAP ↓ ≥10 mm Hg from previous measurement. ↑ HR suggests hypovolemia, circulatory decompensation, or fever caused by infection or cerebral edema.
- Measure central pressures and thermodilution CO q1-4h. Be alert to low or ↓ CVP, PAWP, CO, which, along with ↑ HR and ↓ UO, suggest hypovolemia. Because of altered vascular responsiveness, SVR may not be ↑ with hypovolemic acute hepatic failure. A "normal" CO may be inadequate for these patients. Monitor Svo_2 to evaluate adequacy of tissue oxygenation.
- Measure and record UO qh. Be alert to output <0.5 ml/kg/h for 2 consecutive h. If UO inadequate, consider cautious ↑ in fluid intake (eg, 50-100 ml/h), then reevaluate. Use extreme caution in administering potent diuretics, since they may precipitate encephalopathy or renal disease by causing rapid diuresis and electrolyte changes.
- Estimate ongoing fluid losses. Weigh patient qd, using same scale and method. Compare 24-h intake to output. Weight loss should not exceed 0.5 kg/day because more rapid diuresis can lead to intravascular volume depletion and impair renal function.
- Monitor serum albumin; administer albumin replacements as prescribed.

Sensory/Perceptual alterations r/t CNS depression, hypoglycemia, accumulation of ammonia/other CNS toxins occurring with hepatic dysfunction, therapeutically restricted environment, sleep deprivation, hypoxia

Desired outcomes: By time of hospital discharge, patient exhibits stable personality pattern, age-appropriate behavior, intact intellect appropriate for education level, distinct speech, coordinated gross and fine motor movements. Handwriting legible; psychometric test scores > baseline.

- Avoid or minimize factors that may contribute to encephalopathy: dehydration/electrolyte imbalance, sedatives/hypnotics, infection.
- Evaluate for CNS effects such as personality changes, childish behavior, intellectual impairment, slurred speech, ataxia, and asterixis.
- Eliminate dietary protein in patients with severe encephalopathy. Reintroduce protein gradually after clinical symptoms improve (ie, greater alertness, improved neuromuscular coordination). Limit protein to 40-60 g/day in patients with recent encephalopathy.
- Administer enemas to clear colon of intestinal contents contributing to encephalopathy.
- Administer neomycin to reduce intestinal bacteria, which contribute to production of cerebral intoxicants. Monitor for ototoxic and nephrotoxic effects of neomycin.
- Administer lactulose to produce two to three semiformed stools qd. Avoid lactulose-related diarrhea because it may cause dangerous dehydration and electrolyte imbalance.
- Protect confused or unconscious patient from injury: leave side rails up; consider padding them if patient active. Have call light available; tape all catheters and tubes securely.
- Consider possibility of seizures with severe encephalopathy; have airway management equipment readily available.
- Monitor serum glucose frequently until stable. Administer D_{50} and D_5W as necessary.
- Minimize unnecessary noise, lights, and other environmental stimuli.

Miscellanea

CONSULT MD FOR
- S&S of worsening hepatic function: ↓ LOC, ↑ bilirubin, jaundice
- UO <0.5 ml/kg × 2 h
- Complications: ↓ CO, ↓ BP, hypoglycemia, electrolyte imbalance

RELATED TOPICS
- Delirium: ICU psychosis, acute confusional state
- Hepatic failure
- Metabolic acidosis, acute
- Renal failure, acute

REFERENCES
Keen JH, Baird MS, Allen JH: *Mosby's critical care and emergency drug reference,* ed 2, St Louis, 1996, Mosby.

Malseed R, Goldstein F, Balkon N: *Pharmacology: drug therapy and nursing considerations,* Philadelphia, 1995, Lippincott.

Stiesmeyer JK: Drug overdose. In Swearingen PL, Keen JH (eds): *Manual of critical care nursing,* ed 3, St Louis, 1995, Mosby.

Author: **Johanna K. Stiesmeyer**

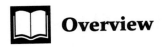 Overview

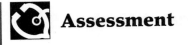 Assessment

Collaborative Management

PATHOPHYSIOLOGY

Amphetamines are potent CNS stimulants. Although precise mechanism is unknown, these chemicals obstruct reuptake of epinephrine and dopamine, leading to significant CNS and CV stimulation. The myocardium may be injured as a result of ↑ O_2 demands by the body and myocardial workload, which may result in myocardial ischemia and infarction.

Street Names: Methamphetamine, speed, crystal, meth, white crosses, ice

Routes: Oral, IV, IM, smoked

CLINICAL PRESENTATION

Confusion, irritability, aggressive behavior, hyperactivity, hallucinations; may progress to seizures, coma

PHYSICAL ASSESSMENT

Neuro: Convulsions, delusions, tremens, memory loss, stupor, stroke, coma

Resp: Hyperventilation

CV: Tachycardia, hypertension, myocardial ischemia/infarction, CV collapse

GU: Renal failure r/t dehydration and rhabdomyolysis

Assoc Findings: Mydriasis, fasciculations, hyperthermia, thrombocytopenic purpura

VITAL SIGNS/HEMODYNAMICS

RR: ↑

HR: ↑

BP: ↑

Temp: ↑

SVR: ↑

CO: ↑; ↓ if myocardial ischemia/infarction occurs

ECG: Atrial or ventricular dysrhythmias, especially tachycardic rhythms, evidence of ischemia or infarction

LABORATORY STUDIES

Toxicology Screen: To detect presence/level of amphetamine, other substances of abuse.

Chemistries: Dehydration, hypokalemia, or hypoglycemia may be present; rhabdomyolysis may precipitate ARF, leading to ↑ BUN/creatinine and electrolyte disturbances.

Cardiac Enzymes: With isoenzyme fractionations, monitored to evaluate presence/degree of myocardial injury.

Support of CV, Resp Systems: Antidysrhythmic agents (verapamil, adenosine, digitalis) given for tachydysrhythmias. Ischemia treated with nitrates; MI treated with thrombolytic therapy, PTCA, CABG.

Removal of Substance from System: For oral ingestion, activated charcoal administered orally or *via* gastric tube to bind with ingested substance in the stomach, often followed by gastric lavage. Ipecac not recommended.

Treatment of Hypertension: Usually with antihypertensives, eg, nitroprusside (Nipride) (or NTG for myocardial ischemia); titrated to ↓ BP.

Prevention/Treatment of Seizures: IV diazepam 0.1-0.2 mg/kg given slowly and repeated q5min until sedation achieved. Haldol can be used IM at a dosage of 0.1-0.2 mg/kg.

Treatment of Hyperthermia: Cooling blanket, antipyretics.

Treatment of Dehydration: Fluid replacement, such as LR solution and D_5NS.

Anticipation/Treatment of Rhabdomyolysis: Usually treated with sodium bicarbonate, mannitol, or furosemide (Lasix). Patient kept well hydrated to prevent ATN.

PATIENT-FAMILY TEACHING

Addresses, phone numbers of local substance abuse programs and support groups

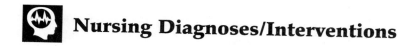 ## Nursing Diagnoses/Interventions

Risk for fluid volume deficit r/t altered intake or excessive losses secondary to vomiting or diaphoresis

Desired outcome: Patient normovolemic: UO ≥0.5 ml/kg/h, moist mucous membranes, balanced I&O, BP wnl for patient, HR ≤100 bpm, stable weight, urine specific gravity 1.010-1.020, CVP 2-6 mm Hg, PAWP 6-12 mm Hg.

- Monitor hydration status on an ongoing basis. Be alert to continuing dehydration as evidenced by poor skin turgor, dry mucous membranes, thirst, weak pulse with tachycardia, and postural hypotension.
- Assess for electrolyte imbalance, in particular hypokalemia: irregular pulse, cardiac dysrhythmias, and serum K^+ <3.5 mEq/L.
- Monitor I&O qh; assess for output ↑ out of proportion to intake, bearing in mind insensible losses, especially if hyperthermia present.
- Monitor laboratory values, including serum electrolytes and serum and urine osmolality. Be alert to BUN ↑ out of proportion to creatinine (indicator of dehydration rather than renal disease), high urine specific gravity, low urine Na^+, and ↑ Hct and serum protein concentration.
- Maintain fluid intake as prescribed; administer prescribed electrolyte supplements.

Hyperthermia r/t toxic effects of amphetamines

Desired outcome: Optimally, within 24-72 h of intervention, patient becomes normothermic.

Note: With massive overdose, temp regulation may never be achieved.

- Monitor for hyperthermia: temp >38.3° C (>101° F), pallor, no perspiration, and torso warm to the touch. If available, provide continuous monitoring of temp. Otherwise, measure rectal, core, or tympanic temp qh and prn.
- Provide and monitor effects of cooling blanket, cooling baths, and ice packs to the axillae and groin.
- Maintain fluid replacement as prescribed. Monitor hydration status and trend of I&O and urine specific gravity (optimal range: 1.010-1.020).
- Monitor neurologic status qh and prn until stabilized.
- Monitor VS continuously or qh and prn until stabilized. Be alert to ↑ BP, HR, and RR.
- Administer and evaluate effects of antipyretic medications.

Risk for violence (self-directed) r/t mind-altering drug or depressed state

Desired outcome: Patient remains free of self-inflicted injury.

- If condition stable, provide auxiliary staff member, such as orderly or nursing assistant, to watch patient when awake.
- Speak in a quiet, calm voice, using short sentences. Limit interventions.
- Administer and evaluate effectiveness of sedation to calm patient.
- Keep all sharp instruments out of patient's room. Follow agency protocol accordingly.
- If necessary, restrain patient. Start with soft restraints but progress to leather restraints if patient is threatening to self or staff.

Miscellanea

CONSULT MD FOR

- ECG evidence of ischemia, infarction, or hemodynamically significant dysrhythmias
- Uncontrolled hypertension
- Complications: seizures, rhabdomyolysis (S&S: reddish-brown urine, ↓UO)

RELATED TOPICS

- Drug overdose: general
- Hypovolemia
- Myocardial infarction, acute
- Status epilepticus
- Supraventricular tachycardia

ABBREVIATION

ATN: Acute tubular necrosis

REFERENCES

Braitberg G, Kunkel D: Amphetamines and amphetamine-like drugs. In Tintinalli JE, Ruiz E, Krome RL (eds): *Emergency medicine: a comprehensive study guide,* ed 4, New York, 1996, McGraw-Hill.

Keen JH, Baird MS, Allen JH: *Mosby's critical care and emergency drug reference,* ed 2, St Louis, 1996, Mosby.

Malseed R, Goldstein F, Balkon N: *Pharmacology: drug therapy and nursing considerations,* Philadelphia, 1995, Lippincott.

Stiesmeyer JK: Drug overdose. In Swearingen PL, Keen JH (eds): *Manual of critical care nursing,* ed 3, St Louis, 1995, Mosby.

Author: **Johanna K. Stiesmeyer**

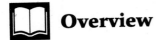 **Overview**

PATHOPHYSIOLOGY
Barbiturates depress the sensory cortex, ↓ motor activity, and alter cerebellar function. Overdosage results in profound CNS and respiratory depression, hypotension, hypothermia, coma, and death. Often have a long half-life, some as great as 4-5 days.
Examples: Secobarbital [Seconal], pentobarbital [Nembutal], secobarbital/amobarbital [Tuinal]
Routes: Oral, IV, IM
Street Names: Yellow jackets, reds, barbs

HISTORY/RISK FACTORS
Legitimate prescription for seizure prophylaxis, sedation

CLASSIFICATION OF BARBITURATE INTOXICATION (McCarron et al, 1982)
Alert: No signs of CNS depression
Drowsy: CNS depression from alert to stuporous
Stuporous: Markedly sedated; responsive to verbal and tactile stimuli
Coma 1: Responsive to painful but not to verbal and tactile stimuli; no change in respirations or BP
Coma 2: Unconscious, unresponsive to pain, no change in respirations or BP
Coma 3: Unresponsive to pain; slow, shallow, or rapid spontaneous respirations; low but adequate BP
Coma 4: Unresponsive to pain; apnea or inadequate BP or both

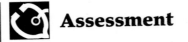 **Assessment**

PHYSICAL ASSESSMENT
Neuro: Headache, vertigo, dizziness, lethargy, ataxia, stupor, flaccidity, seizures, absent doll's eye reflex, coma, loss of DTRs, nystagmus
Resp: Depression, hypoventilation, apnea, respiratory arrest
CV: Hypotension, bradycardia, cardiac arrest
GU: Oliguria, ARF
Assoc Findings: Hypothermia, nausea, vomiting, opposite reactions of euphoria and excitability before nl sedative effects occur; withdrawal symptoms of tremens and convulsions possible

VITAL SIGNS/HEMODYNAMICS
RR: ↓
HR: ↓
BP: ↓
Temp: ↓
Hemodynamics: Reflect vascular relaxation, bradycardia: ↓ CVP/PAWP, SVR, CO
ECG: Sinus or other bradycardias

LABORATORY STUDIES
Toxicology Screen: To check drug levels.
Chemistries: Serum K^+, Na^+, CO_2, BUN/creatinine, glucose, liver and renal function studies evaluated.
CBC: To establish baseline; check for anemia, infection.
ABGs: To evaluate adequacy of ventilation.

Collaborative Management

Support of CV, Resp Systems: Electrical rhythm monitored; bradydysrhythmias treated according to ACLS guidelines. After fluid replacement, vasopressor therapy (eg, dopamine) may be initiated for hypotension. Mechanical ventilation may be required, depending on degree of hypoxia and CO_2 retention.
Removal of Substance from System: Ipecac to promote vomiting; activated charcoal given orally or *via* gastric tube to bind with substance in the stomach; gastric lavage; hemodialysis, which may be used for Coma 4 stage.
Prevention/Treatment of Seizures: Phenytoin or diazepam may be given.
Sedation for Withdrawal Symptoms: Typically the ingested barbiturate is tapered gradually to zero.
Prevention of Aspiration: Gastric tube to low suction.
Treatment of Nausea, Vomiting: Antiemetics, usually IV promethazine hydrochloride.
Treatment of Hypothermia: Warming blanket.

PATIENT-FAMILY TEACHING
- S&S of toxicity; S&S of withdrawal
- Purpose, expected results, anticipated sensations for all nursing/medical interventions
- Drug rehabilitation programs, as appropriate

Nursing Diagnoses/Interventions

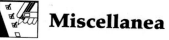 **Miscellanea**

Ineffective airway clearance r/t presence of tracheobronchial secretions or obstruction or ↓ sensorium

Desired outcome: Within 2-24 h of intervention/treatment, patient has clear airway: clear breath sounds over upper airways and lung fields, RR 12-20 breaths/min with eupnea, PaO_2 ≥80 mm Hg, $PaCO_2$ 35-45 mm Hg, pH 7.35-7.45, and SpO_2 ≥92%.

- Assess respiratory function frequently. Be alert to any respiratory distress, restlessness and confusion, or cyanosis.
- Monitor respiratory patterns; provide continuous apnea monitoring if available.
- Suction oropharynx or *via* ET tube prn.
- Monitor ABG values for hypoxia (PaO_2 <80 mm Hg) and respiratory acidosis ($PaCO_2$ >45 mm Hg, pH <7.35).
- Monitor O_2 saturation continuously. Be alert to values <92%, depending on baseline and clinical presentation.
- Administer and evaluate effects of antiemetics.
- Place patient in side-lying position during vomiting to ↓ aspiration risk.

Decreased cardiac output r/t bradycardia and ↓ preload and afterload secondary to vasodilatation

Desired outcome: Within 4 h of treatment initiation, patient has adequate cardiac output: BP ≥90/60 mm Hg, peripheral pulses >2+ on scale of 0-4+, CO ≥4.0 L/min, CI ≥2.5 $L/min/m^2$, SVR ≥900 $dynes/sec/cm^{-5}$; UO ≥0.5 ml/kg/h; and NSR on ECG.

- Assess for physical and hemodynamic indicators of ↓ CO: ↓ BP, MAP, CO/CI, and amplitude of peripheral pulses. Calculate SVR. Vasodilatation may ↓ afterload and CO.
- Assess electrical rhythm *via* ECG for bradycardia. As necessary, administer atropine, dopamine, epinephrine, or isoproterenol. Consider transcutaneous or transvenous pacing if bradycardia persistent.
- As prescribed, administer epinephrine to stimulate vasoconstriction, ↑ SVR, and ↑ myocardial contractility. Observe for therapeutic effects: ↑ SVR, CO/CI, BP, MAP, and UO; stronger peripheral pulses; warming of extremities; and ↑ UO (indicator of ↑ renal perfusion).
- Administer fluid replacement therapy. Up to 2-3 L may be required to attain adequate vascular volume. During fluid resuscitation, assess for S&S of fluid volume excess: crackles, JVD, and ↑ PAP, PAWP, RAP.

Sensory/Perceptual alterations r/t chemical alterations secondary to ingestion of barbiturates

Desired outcome: Within 48 h of intervention, patient verbalizes orientation to time, place, and person.

- Establish and maintain calm, quiet environment to minimize sensory overload. Dim lights when possible.
- At frequent intervals, assess orientation to time, place, and person. Reorient as necessary.
- Orient to the unit and explain all procedures before performing them. Include significant others in orientation process.
- Do not leave patient alone if he or she is agitated or confused.

    As appropriate, try to involve family/significant others because patient may have more trust in them.

    Tell patient you will check on him or her at frequent intervals (eg, q5-10min) or that you will stay at patient's side.

CONSULT MD FOR
- SpO_2 <90%, hypoventilation, other indicators of ↓ ventilation/inadequate oxygenation
- Persistent or unresponsive bradycardia, hypotension
- Deteriorating LOC
- UO <0.5 ml/kg/h × 2 h

RELATED TOPICS
- Bradycardia
- Mechanical ventilation
- Shock, hypovolemic
- Status epilepticus

ABBREVIATION
DTR: Deep tendon reflex

REFERENCES
Keen JH, Baird MS, Allen JH: *Mosby's critical care and emergency drug reference,* ed 2, St Louis, 1996, Mosby.

McCarron MM et al: Short-acting barbiturate overdose, *JAMA* 248(1): 55-61, 1982.

Malseed R, Goldstein F, Balkon N: *Pharmacology: drug therapy and nursing considerations,* Philadelphia, 1995, Lippincott.

Ryan P. Barbiturates. In Tintinalli J, Ruiz E, Krome RL (eds): *Emergency medicine: a comprehensive study guide,* ed 4, New York, 1996, McGraw-Hill.

Stiesmeyer JK: Drug overdose. In Swearingen PL, Keen JH (eds): *Manual of critical care nursing,* ed 3, St Louis, 1995, Mosby.

Author: **Johanna K. Stiesmeyer**

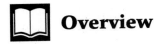 # Overview

PATHOPHYSIOLOGY
Benzodiazepines act on the CNS to facilitate action of GABA, a major inhibitory neurotransmitter. Usual doses ↓ anxiety and cause sedation. Overdosage leads to deep sedation, coma, hypotension, seizures. Also may cause respiratory depression, especially if IV or combined with ETOH.

Common Benzodiazepines
- Chlordiazepoxide (Librium)
- Diazepam (Valium)
- Lorazepam (Ativan)
- Furazepam (Dalmane)
- Temazepam (Restoril)
- Alprazolam (Xanax)

Routes: Oral, IM, IV

HISTORY/RISK FACTORS
Legitimate prescription for seizure prophylaxis, sedation, anxiety relief

CLINICAL PRESENTATION
Slurred speech, CNS sedation, depression; possibility of withdrawal manifested by seizures

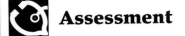 # Assessment

PHYSICAL ASSESSMENT
Neuro: Drowsiness, ataxia, coma
Resp: Respiratory depression, arrest
CV: Hypotension, tachycardia
GU: Renal failure caused by rhabdomyolysis
Assoc Findings: Hypothermia

VITAL SIGNS/HEMODYNAMICS
RR: NI or ↓
HR: ↑
BP: ↓
Temp: ↓
Hemodynamics: Reflect vascular relaxation, bradycardia: ↓ CVP/PAWP, SVR, CO
ECG: SVT or other tachycardias

LABORATORY STUDIES
Toxicology Screen: To check drug levels.
Chemistries: Serum K^+, Na^+, CO_2, BUN/creatinine, glucose, liver and renal function studies evaluated.
CBC: To establish baseline values.
ABGs: To evaluate adequacy of ventilation.

Collaborative Management

Support of CV System: Electrical rhythm monitored; tachydysrhythmias treated with verapamil. Hypotension treated with fluid replacement and dopamine or norepinephrine (Levophed) as necessary.

Support of Resp System: Apnea monitoring and mechanical ventilation may be indicated.

Removal of Substance from System: Ipecac to induce vomiting; activated charcoal to bind with substance in the stomach; gastric lavage.

Prevention of Seizures: Administration of phenytoin and diazepam, but seizures unlikely because benzodiazepines ↑ the seizure threshold.

Prevention of Aspiration: Insertion of gastric tube, placed at low intermittent suction.

Identification of Rhabdomyolysis: Seizure activity and breakdown of muscle causes protein to precipitate in the kidneys, leading to renal failure. Detected by ↑ BUN, creatinine, and protein values in urine.

Treatment of Hypothermia: Warming blanket if indicated.

Specific Antidote: Effects may be reversed by flumazenil (Romazicon). Repeat doses may be necessary. Use cautiously if at all with established benzodiazepine use, since rapid ↓ in benzodiazepine levels may trigger seizures. Be aware that in mixed drug overdose, presence of benzodiazepines may aid in seizure prophylaxis.

PATIENT-FAMILY TEACHING
- S&S of toxicity; S&S of withdrawal
- Purpose, expected results, anticipated sensations of all nursing/medical interventions
- Drug rehabilitation programs, as appropriate

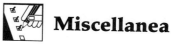

Nursing Diagnoses/Interventions

Ineffective airway clearance r/t presence of tracheobronchial secretions; obstruction; ↓ sensorium

Desired outcome: Within 2-24 h of intervention/treatment, patient has clear airway: clear breath sounds over upper airways and lung fields, RR 12-20 breaths/min with eupnea, PaO_2 ≥80 mm Hg, $PaCO_2$ 35-45 mm Hg, pH 7.35-7.45, and SpO_2 ≥92%.

- Assess respiratory function frequently. Be alert to respiratory distress, restlessness and confusion, or cyanosis.
- Suction oropharynx or *via* ET tube prn.
- Monitor ABG values for hypoxia (PaO_2 <80 mm Hg) and respiratory acidosis ($PaCO_2$ >45 mm Hg, pH <7.35).
- Monitor respiratory patterns; provide continuous apnea monitoring if available.
- Monitor O_2 saturation continuously. Be alert to values <92%, depending on baseline and clinical presentation.
- Administer and evaluate effects of antiemetics.
- Place patient in side-lying position during vomiting to ↓ aspiration risk.

Decreased cardiac output r/t ↓ preload and afterload secondary to vasodilatation

Desired outcome: Within 4 h of treatment initiation, patient has adequate cardiac output: BP ≥90/60 mm Hg, peripheral pulses >2+ on 0-4+ scale, CO ≥4.0 L/min, CI ≥2.5 L/min/m², SVR ≥900 dynes/sec/cm^{-5}, UO ≥0.5 ml/kg/h, and NSR on ECG.

- Assess for physical and hemodynamic indicators of ↓ CO: ↓ BP, MAP, CO/CI, and amplitude of peripheral pulses. Calculate SVR. Vasodilatation may ↓ afterload and CO.
- Assess electrical rhythm *via* ECG for tachydysrhythmias. Be sure to distinguish supraventricular from ventricular dysrhythmias and treat according to ACLS guidelines.
- As prescribed, administer epinephrine to stimulate vasoconstriction, ↑ SVR, and ↑ myocardial contractility. Observe for therapeutic effects: ↑ SVR, CO/CI, BP, MAP, and UO; stronger peripheral pulses; warming of extremities; and ↑ UO (indicator of ↑ renal perfusion).
- Administer fluid replacement therapy. Up to 2-3 L may be required to attain adequate vascular volume. During fluid resuscitation, assess for S&S of fluid volume excess: crackles, JVD, and ↑ PAP, PAWP, RAP.

Sensory/Perceptual alterations r/t chemical alterations secondary to ingestion of benzodiazepines

Desired outcome: Within 48 h of intervention, patient verbalizes orientation to time, place, and person.

- Establish and maintain calm, quiet environment to minimize sensory overload. Dim lights when possible.
- At frequent intervals, assess orientation to time, place, and person. Reorient as necessary.
- Orient to the unit, and explain all procedures before performing them. Include significant others in orientation process.
- Do not leave patient alone if he or she is agitated or confused.
  - As appropriate, try to involve family/significant others because patient may have more trust in them.
  - Explain that you will check on patient at frequent intervals (eg, q5-10min) or that you will stay at patient's side.

Miscellanea

CONSULT MD FOR
- SpO_2 <90%, hypoventilation, other indicators of ↓ ventilation/inadequate oxygenation
- Persistent or unresponsive hypotension, hemodynamically significant tachycardia
- Deteriorating LOC
- UO <0.5 ml/kg/h × 2 h

RELATED TOPICS
- Mechanical ventilation
- Shock, hypovolemic
- Status epilepticus
- Supraventricular tachycardia

REFERENCES

Bosse G: Benzodiazepines. In Tintinalli JE, Ruiz E, Krome RL (eds): *Emergency medicine: a comprehensive study guide,* ed 4, New York, 1996, McGraw-Hill.

Keen JH, Baird MS, Allen JH: *Mosby's critical care and emergency drug reference,* ed 2, St Louis, 1996, Mosby.

Malseed R, Goldstein F, Balkon N: *Pharmacology: drug therapy and nursing considerations,* Philadelphia, 1995, Lippincott.

Stiesmeyer JK: Drug overdose. In Swearingen PL, Keen JH (eds): *Manual of critical care nursing,* ed 3, St Louis, 1995, Mosby.

Author: **Johanna K. Stiesmeyer**

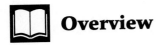 **Overview**

PATHOPHYSIOLOGY
Cocaine causes CNS excitation and excessive SNS activity. Effects are highly variable and depend on amount of drug taken.
Cutting Agents: Substances may be used to ↑ bulk in pure cocaine and include procaine, phencyclidine (angel dust), amphetamine, quinine, talc, and strychnine. Can become emboli that shower into cerebral and pulmonary circulation with subsequent deleterious effects.
Street Names: Crack, rock, freebase, snow
Routes: Nasal or IV (cocaine, snow); smoked (crack, rock, freebase)

HISTORY/RISK FACTORS
Massive overdose can result when cocaine-filled condoms rupture in GI tract during illicit transport.

CLINICAL PRESENTATION
Hyperexcitable, aggressive state; headache, seizures common. Initially may seem well coordinated but may deteriorate to tremens and fasciculations. Stupor, coma possible with large overdose.
Withdrawal: Poor concentration, absence of sweating, bradykinesia, sleep disturbance, ↓ libido, intense cocaine craving, depression, suicidal tendencies

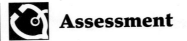 **Assessment**

PHYSICAL ASSESSMENT
Neuro: Paranoia, delirium, tactile/visual hallucinations, tremens, aggression, tonic-clonic seizures
Resp: Sharp pleuritic pain, hemoptysis, pneumothorax, bronchospasm, pulmonary edema, respiratory failure
CV: Hypertension, sinus tachycardia, sinus bradycardia, ventricular dysrhythmias, MI, heart failure, cardiomyopathy, acute endocarditis, aortic dissection; profound hypotension and shock also possible
GU: Renal failure r/t profound hypotension and rhabdomyolysis
Assoc Findings: Hyperthermia, perforated nasal septum, track marks r/t IV use, and mydriasis

VITAL SIGNS/HEMODYNAMICS
RR: ↑
HR: ↑
BP: ↑
Temp: Profound ↑ as high as 43° C (109° F) rectally
SVR: ↑
CO: ↑ unless heart failure, myocardial ischemia present
ECG: Dysrhythmias, especially PVCs, VT, VF; may show ischemic changes: T-wave inversion or ST-segment elevation or depression

LABORATORY STUDIES
Toxicology Screen: Will show presence of cocaine; actual levels usually of little diagnostic value.
Chemistries: Serum K^+, Na^+, CO_2, BUN/creatinine, glucose, and renal function studies analyzed.
ABGs: To check for metabolic acidosis.

Collaborative Management

Support of CV System: SVTs may be treated with propranolol (Inderal) or verapamil; ventricular dysrhythmias treated with antidysrhythmics such as lidocaine, procainamide (Pronestyl), and bretylium. Antihypertensives or vasopressors as indicated to maintain/control BP.
Support of Resp System: O_2 therapy to meet ↑ tissue demands. If comatose, may require mechanical ventilation.
X-rays: Abdominal films may identify cocaine-filled condom. If present, surgery may be performed to remove it. Oral/NG activated charcoal may be given to bind with the cocaine; laxative or suppository used to facilitate rectal expulsion.
IV Fluids: LR solution or D_5NS to correct fluid volume deficit.
Seizure Control: Phenytoin for active seizures; phenobarbital for maintenance.
Treatment of Hyperthermia: Cooling blanket, ice, acetaminophen; core temp monitored for most accurate measurements.
Prevention of Aspiration: Gastric tube inserted and placed to continuous low suction.

PATIENT-FAMILY TEACHING
- S&S of toxicity; S&S of withdrawal
- Purpose, expected results, anticipated sensations for all nursing/medical interventions
- Drug rehabilitation programs as appropriate, eg, Narcotics Anonymous (consult local phone book)

Nursing Diagnoses/Interventions

Hyperthermia r/t toxic effects of cocaine

Desired outcome: Optimally, within 24-72 h of intervention, patient becomes normothermic. **Note:** With massive overdose, temp regulation may never be achieved.

- Monitor for hyperthermia: temp >38.3° C (>101° F), pallor, no perspiration, and torso warm to the touch. If available, provide continuous monitoring of temp. Otherwise, measure rectal, core, or tympanic temp qh and prn.
- Provide and monitor effects of cooling blanket, cooling baths, and ice packs to the axillae and groin.
- Maintain fluid replacement as prescribed. Monitor hydration status and trend of I&O and urine specific gravity (optimal range: 1.010-1.020).
- Monitor neurologic status qh and prn until stabilized.
- Monitor VS continuously or qh and prn until stabilized. Be alert to ↑ BP, HR, and RR.
- Administer and evaluate effects of antipyretic medications.

Risk for fluid volume deficit r/t altered intake or excessive losses secondary to vomiting or diaphoresis

Desired outcome: Patient normovolemic: UO ≥0.5 ml/kg/h, moist mucous membranes, balanced I&O, BP wnl for patient, HR ≤100 bpm, stable weight, urine specific gravity 1.010-1.020, CVP 2-6 mm Hg, PAWP 6-12 mm Hg.

- Monitor hydration status on an ongoing basis. Be alert to continuing dehydration as evidenced by poor skin turgor, dry mucous membranes, thirst, weak pulse, tachycardia, postural hypotension.
- Assess for electrolyte imbalance, in particular hypokalemia: irregular pulse, ventricular dysrhythmias, and serum K$^+$ <3.5 mEq/L. Replace electrolytes as necessary.
- Monitor I&O qh; assess for output elevated out of proportion to intake, bearing in mind insensible losses, especially if hyperthermia present.
- Monitor laboratory values, including serum electrolytes and serum and urine osmolality. Be alert to BUN ↑ out of proportion to creatinine (indicator of dehydration rather than renal disease), high urine specific gravity, low urine Na$^+$, and ↑ Hct and serum protein concentration.
- Maintain fluid intake so that positive fluid state is maintained (eg, 50-100 ml > hourly losses).

Sensory/Perceptual alterations r/t chemical alterations secondary to ingestion of mind-altering drugs

Desired outcome: Within 48 h of intervention, patient verbalizes orientation to time, place, and person.

- Establish and maintain calm, quiet environment to minimize sensory overload. Dim lights when possible.
- At frequent intervals, assess orientation to time, place, and person. Reorient as necessary.
- Orient to the unit and explain all procedures before performing them. Include significant others in orientation process.
- Do not leave patient alone if he or she is agitated or confused.
- Administer antianxiety agents as prescribed.
- If patient hallucinating, intervene in the following ways:

    Be reassuring. Explain that hallucinations may be very real to patient but that they are not real; they are caused by the substance patient consumed, and they will go away eventually.

    As appropriate, try to involve family/significant others because patient may have more trust in them.

    Explain that restraints are necessary to prevent harm to patient and others. Reassure patient that restraints will be used only as long as they are needed.

    Explain that you will check on patient at frequent intervals (eg, q5-10min) or that you will stay at patient's side.

Miscellanea

CONSULT MD FOR

- Seizure activity
- Hemodynamically significant dysrhythmias
- Crackles, S$_3$, other S&S of heart failure, pulmonary edema
- UO <0.5 ml/kg/h × 2 h

RELATED TOPICS

- Hypovolemia
- Myocardial infarction, acute
- Pulmonary edema
- Status epilepticus
- Ventricular tachycardia

REFERENCES

Keen JH, Baird MS, Allen JH: *Mosby's critical care and emergency drug reference,* ed 2, St Louis, 1996, Mosby.

Malseed R, Goldstein F, Balkon N: *Pharmacology: drug therapy and nursing considerations,* Philadelphia, 1995, Lippincott.

Perrone J, Hoffman R: Cocaine. In Tintinalli JE, Ruiz E, Krome RL (eds): *Emergency medicine: a comprehensive study guide,* ed 4, New York, 1996, McGraw-Hill.

Renzl F: Cocaine poisoning. In Rippe J et al (eds): *Intensive care medicine,* ed 3, Boston, 1996, Little, Brown.

Stiesmeyer JK: Drug overdose. In Swearingen PL, Keen JH (eds): *Manual of critical care nursing,* ed 3, St Louis, 1995, Mosby.

Author: **Johanna K. Stiesmeyer**

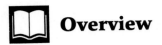 Overview

PATHOPHYSIOLOGY

Toxicity results in ↓ LOC, profound CV instability, and conduction disturbances and other ECG changes. Progressive widening of QRS signals worsening toxicity. Pulmonary edema and ARDS may occur, as well as ATN caused by rhabdomyolysis. In some cases, acute pancreatitis, AMI, and cardiac arrest possible.
Examples: Amitriptyline hydrochloride (Elavil), doxepin hydrochloride (Sinequan), imipramine hydrochloride (Tofranil), trimipramine maleate (Surmontil)
Route: Oral

CLINICAL PRESENTATION

Somnolence, lethargy, stupor, seizures; may progress to coma

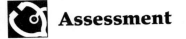 Assessment

PHYSICAL ASSESSMENT

Neuro: Coma, seizures, delirium, hallucinations
Resp: Hyperventilation, crackles, ↓ breath sounds, respiratory arrest
CV: Hypotension, sinus tachycardia, SVT, ventricular dysrhythmias, hypertension
GU: Oliguria, anuria
Assoc Findings: Hyperthermia or hypothermia

VITAL SIGNS/HEMODYNAMICS

RR: ↓ or ↑
HR: ↑
BP: ↓ or ↑
Temp: ↑ or ↓
Hemodynamics: Unstable; CO usually ↓ because of rhythm disturbances
ECG: Widened QRS complex, tachydysrhythmias, ventricular irritability, ischemia/infarction patterns, possible fatal dysrhythmias (eg, VF, asystole)

LABORATORY STUDIES

Drug Screening: Blood, plasma, urine, gastric contents analyzed for presence, amount of drug.
Chemistries: Serum K^+, Na^+, CO_2, BUN/creatinine, glucose, and liver and renal studies evaluated.
Cardiac Enzymes and Isoenzyme Fractionations: To determine presence and degree of myocardial damage.

Collaborative Management

If patient is symptom free, monitor for minimum of 6-8 h, noting VS and width of QRS complex.
Support of CV System: Electrical rhythm monitored for ≥6 h to assess for widening QRS complex (signal of worsening toxicity). Widened QRS with QT prolongation may lead to torsades de pointes, in which case $MgSO_4$ may be prescribed. SVTs treated with verapamil; ventricular dysrhythmias treated with lidocaine. Atropine and pacing may be indicated for symptomatic bradycardia.
Removal of Substance from System: Activated charcoal given *via* gastric tube to bind with ingested substance in the stomach, facilitating its removal *via* gastric lavage. Ipecac to promote vomiting not recommended, since vagal stimulation may induce dysrhythmias.
Reversal of Drug Effects: Alkalosis *via* sodium bicarbonate to promote excretion. An alternative approach is to promote a state of respiratory alkalosis by ↑ RR *via* mechanical ventilation.
Prevention/Treatment of Seizures: Phenytoin and diazepam.
Resp Support: Mechanical ventilation. Pulmonary edema treated with nitrates, morphine, diuretics, potassium replacement, and IPPB treatments.
Treatment of Hypotension: Fluid replacement, followed by dopamine and norepinephrine bitartrate (Levophed) as indicated.
Treatment of Hyperthermia or Hypothermia: Cooling or warming blanket as indicated.
Prevention of Aspiration: Insertion of gastric tube, which is connected to low suction.

PATIENT-FAMILY TEACHING

As indicated, community resources for psychiatric follow-up

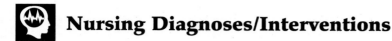 # Nursing Diagnoses/Interventions

Decreased cardiac output (or risk for same) r/t changes in rate, rhythm, and conduction secondary to cyclic antidepressant effects or myocardial ischemia

Desired outcomes: Within 24 h of this diagnosis, patient has adequate cardiac output: BP within acceptable range, NSR on ECG, QRS complex ≤0.10 sec, HR 60-100 bpm, warm and dry skin, UO ≥0.5 ml/kg/h, measured CO 4-7 L/min, PAWP ≤12 mm Hg, orientation × 3.

- Monitor heart rate and rhythm continuously. Monitor BP/CO frequently. Be alert to widening QRS, ↓ CO, ST-segment changes, and symptomatic dysrhythmias. Treat dysrhythmias according to ACLS guidelines. Have pacemaker immediately available.
- Administer $NaHCO_3$; use mechanical ventilation to induce alkalosis and promote drug excretion.
- Provide O_2 therapy or maintain ventilator settings.
- Monitor UO qh, noting output <0.5 ml/kg/h for 2 consecutive h. Monitor BUN/creatinine values closely. ↑ BUN (>20 mg/dl) and serum creatinine (>1.5 mg/dl) can occur with low UO and ATN.
- If patient hypotensive, administer fluids. If response inadequate, start dopamine. Use norepinephrine for severe hypotension. Monitor for side effects: tachydysrhythmias, ventricular ectopy, angina.
- Provide a quiet environment conducive to stress reduction.

Ineffective airway clearance r/t presence of tracheobronchial secretions or obstruction or ↓ sensorium

Desired outcome: Within 2-24 h of intervention/treatment, patient has clear airway: clear breath sounds over upper airways and lung fields, RR 12-20 breaths/min with eupnea, Pao_2 ≥80 mm Hg, $Paco_2$ 35-45 mm Hg, pH 7.35-7.45, and Spo_2 ≥92%.

- Assess respiratory function frequently. Be alert to stridor; gurgling; shallow, irregular, or labored respirations; restlessness; confusion; and cyanosis. Provide continuous apnea monitoring if available.
- Suction oropharynx or *via* ET tube prn.
- Monitor ABG values for hypoxia (Pao_2 <80 mm Hg) and hypercarbia. As indicated, maintain mild respiratory alkalosis to promote urinary excretion of cyclic antidepressant.
- If patient has been placed on mechanical ventilation, monitor for airway obstruction.
- Monitor O_2 saturation continuously. Be alert to values <92%, depending on baseline and clinical presentation.
- Administer and evaluate effects of antiemetics.
- Place in side-lying position during vomiting to ↓ aspiration risk.

Risk for violence (self-directed) r/t mind-altering drugs or depressed state

Desired outcome: Patient remains free of self-inflicted injury.

- If condition stable, provide auxiliary staff member, such as orderly or nursing assistant, to watch patient when awake.
- Speak in a quiet, calm voice, using short sentences. Limit interventions.
- Administer and evaluate effectiveness of sedation to calm patient.
- Keep all sharp instruments out of patient's room. Follow agency protocol accordingly.
- If necessary, restrain patient. Start with soft restraints but progress to leather restraints if patient is threat to self or staff.
- As indicated, consult psychiatric clinical nurse specialist or clinical psychologist.

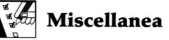 # Miscellanea

CONSULT MD FOR
- Progressive widening of QRS complex, prolongation of QT, which ↑ risk of torsades de pointes
- Hemodynamically significant dysrhythmias
- Deteriorating LOC, seizures

RELATED TOPICS
- Hypovolemia
- Mechanical ventilation
- Respiratory alkalosis, acute
- Status epilepticus
- Supraventricular tachycardia
- Ventricular tachycardia

ABBREVIATION
ATN: Acute tubular necrosis

REFERENCES
Aaron C: Cyclic antidepressant poisoning. In Rippe J, Irwin R, Fink M (eds): *Intensive care medicine,* ed 3, Boston, 1996, Little, Brown.

Keen JH, Baird MS, Allen JH: *Mosby's critical care and emergency drug reference,* ed 2, St Louis, 1996, Mosby.

Malseed R, Goldstein F, Balkon N: *Pharmacology: drug therapy and nursing considerations,* Philadelphia, 1995, Lippincott.

Mills K: Tricyclic antidepressants. In Tintinalli JE, Ruiz E, Krome RL (eds): *Emergency medicine: a comprehensive study guide,* ed 4, New York, 1996, McGraw-Hill.

Stiesmeyer JK: Drug overdose. In Swearingen PL, Keen JH (eds): *Manual of critical care nursing,* ed 3, St Louis, 1995, Mosby.

Author: **Johanna K. Stiesmeyer**

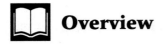

Overview

DESCRIPTION
Affects all ages, races, socioeconomic levels. Can be categorized in several ways: deleterious reaction to street drugs during first-time use, chronic abuse of street drugs, chronic abuse of medically prescribed drugs, unintentional overdose experienced by elders r/t untoward effects of prescribed medications. Drug type, amount, and route affect outcome, prognosis, and clinical presentation. Alcohol and other mixed substance ingestion common.

HISTORY/RISK FACTORS
- Illicit drug use
- Multiple drug use (illicit or prescribed)
- Hepatic, renal, cardiopulmonary impairment
- Sensory impairment (eg, visual disturbances)
- Neurologic impairment (eg, memory disorders)
- Depression
- Female gender (suicide attempts by drug ingestion more common than in males)
- Extremes of age (toddlers, preschoolers, elders)

CLINICAL PRESENTATION
Variable; usually an extension of drug effects. Often altered LOC, nausea, vomiting. Cardiopulmonary instability if severe.

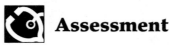

Assessment

PHYSICAL ASSESSMENT
Acetaminophen: S&S of acute hepatic necrosis develop 24-48 h after ingestion
Alcohol: Confusion, aggression, stupor, coma, ↓ DTR, hypoglycemia, hypokalemia
Amphetamines: CNS and CV stimulation; seizures, stroke possible
Barbiturates: CNS and cardiopulmonary depression; cardiac and respiratory arrest possible
Benzodiazepines: CNS depression, muscle relaxation; profound hypotension, respiratory arrest possible
Cocaine: CNS, CV stimulation; seizures, AMI possible
Cyclic Antidepressants: Hypotension, dysrhythmias, pulmonary edema, ATN possible
Opiates: CNS, respiratory depression, stupor, coma, respiratory or cardiac arrest possible

VITAL SIGNS/HEMODYNAMICS
Depend on drug ingested. Mild to severe hemodynamic instability common. Dehydration, hypovolemia often present, resulting in ↓ CVP/PAWP, CO.

LABORATORY STUDIES
Toxicology Screen: Baseline blood levels drawn to check for suspected causative agent. Treatment should not be delayed while awaiting results. In some instances (eg, with acetaminophen) levels will guide antidote administration.
Additional Tests: Serum Na^+, K^+, CO_2, BUN/creatinine, blood glucose, liver enzyme, and bilirubin values; PT, coagulation studies, CBC, protein, amylase, ABGs, and renal function assays. Cardiac enzymes with isoenzyme fractions may be prescribed to check for presence of myocardial injury.

Collaborative Management

Note: Treatment depends on type of drug ingested, amount, rate of absorption, route of administration, and time span between ingestion and delivery of care.

Drug Removal

Ipecac: Depends on length of time from ingestion to treatment and patient's mental status.

- May be inappropriate if drug ingested >1 h before seeking treatment, especially if drug ingested in liquid form, which is rapidly absorbed.
- Contraindicated with altered mental status; aspiration of gastric contents a possibility.
- May cause bradycardia. In combination with vomiting, may cause hemodynamic compromise, particularly if cardiotoxic drugs such as digoxin or cyclic antidepressant involved.
- Other considerations:

  Has patient already vomited?

  Has patient ingested a hydrocarbon or caustic substance?

  Is there an oral antidote?

- When ipecac administered, vomiting expected within 20 min. If it does not occur, repeat dose. If ineffective, proceed to gastric lavage.

Activated charcoal: Effectiveness enhanced when mixed with sorbitol, but diminished when food present in GI tract. If multidose administration necessary, provide subsequent doses within 2-6 h. Does not bind with lithium, potassium, potassium chloride, ETOH, or iron.

Gastric lavage: Important adjunct in treatment of ingested overdose; results in prompt emptying of gastric contents. Essential to protect airway when using this therapy. Lavage should continue until fluid is clear of fragments, which may take 10-30 min. Use Ewald or other large-diameter tube to ensure effective removal of particles. Standard NG tube usually ineffective in removing recently ingested tablets or capsules.

Support of CV, Resp Systems: O_2 supplementation. If ABGs indicate trend toward respiratory failure or breathing effort weak or absent, mechanical ventilation provided.

Fluid Replacement: LR or NS. Dextrose-containing solutions used if hypoglycemic. IV K^+ replacement at rates ≤10-20 mEq/L.

Specific Antidotes: Given if available: eg, naloxone (Narcan) for opiates, *N*-acetylcysteine (Mucomyst) for acetaminophen, flumazenil (Romazicon) for benzodiazepines, digoxin-immune Fab (Digibind) for digoxin.

Identification of Rhabdomyolysis: Possible with drug overdose, especially if extreme hyperthermia or seizures present. Accumulation of protein in kidneys, detected by ↑ BUN/creatinine and protein in urine. Seizure activity and breakdown of muscle cause protein to precipitate in the kidneys, leading to renal failure. Prevention of seizures is the best treatment for preventing rhabdomyolysis.

PATIENT-FAMILY TEACHING

- Referrals to psychiatric facility, mental health, or other community resources as appropriate
- Drug rehabilitation programs, eg, Narcotics Anonymous

Nursing Diagnoses/Interventions

Ineffective airway clearance r/t presence of tracheobronchial secretions; obstruction; ↓ sensorium

Desired outcome: Within 2-24 h of intervention/treatment, patient has clear airway: clear breath sounds over upper airways and lung fields, RR 12-20 breaths/min with eupnea, PaO_2 ≥80 mm Hg, $PaCO_2$ 35-45 mm Hg, pH 7.35-7.45, SpO_2 ≥92%.

- Assess respiratory function frequently. Be alert to secretions; stridor; gurgling; shallow, irregular, or labored respirations; use of accessory muscles; restlessness and confusion; cyanosis.
- Suction oropharynx or *via* ET tube prn.
- Monitor ABG values for hypoxia (PaO_2 <80 mm Hg) and respiratory acidosis ($PaCO_2$ >45 mm Hg and pH <7.35).
- Monitor respiratory patterns; provide continuous apnea monitoring if available.
- Monitor O_2 saturation continuously. Be alert to values <92%, depending on baseline and clinical presentation.
- Administer and evaluate effects of antiemetics.
- Place patient in side-lying position during vomiting to ↓ aspiration risk.

Hyperthermia r/t toxic effects of cocaine, hallucinogens, phencyclidine, salicylates, or cyclic antidepressants

Desired outcome: Optimally, within 24-72 h of intervention, patient becomes normothermic. **Note:** With massive overdose, temp regulation may never be achieved.

- Monitor for hyperthermia: temp >38.3° C (>101° F), pallor, absence of perspiration, and torso that is warm to the touch. If available, provide continuous monitoring of temp. Otherwise, measure rectal, core, or tympanic temp qh and prn.
- Provide and monitor effects of cooling blanket, cooling baths, and ice packs to the axillae and groin.
- Maintain fluid replacement as prescribed. Monitor hydration status and trend of I&O and urine specific gravity (optimal range: 1.010-1.020).
- Monitor VS and neurologic status frequently according to patient's condition. Be alert to ↑ BP, HR, and RR.
- Administer and evaluate effects of antipyretic medications.

Risk for fluid volume deficit r/t altered intake or excessive losses secondary to vomiting or diaphoresis

Desired outcome: Patient normovolemic: UO ≥0.5 ml/kg/h, moist mucous membranes, balanced I&O, BP wnl for patient, HR ≤100 bpm, stable weight, urine specific gravity 1.010-1.020, CVP 2-6 mm Hg, and PAWP 6-12 mm Hg.

- Monitor hydration status on an ongoing basis. Be alert to continuing dehydration as evidenced by poor skin turgor, dry mucous membranes, complaints of thirst, weak pulse with tachycardia, and postural hypotension.

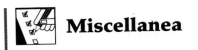

Miscellanea

CONSULT MD FOR

- Respiratory decompensation/pulmonary edema: crackles, use of accessory muscles, restlessness, confusion, cyanosis, SpO_2 <92%
- Hemodynamically significant dysrhythmias
- Infection: temp >38.33° C (101° F); ↑/new onset rhonchi, other adventitious sounds; ↑/change in sputum production

ABBREVIATIONS
ATN: Acute tubular necrosis
DTR: Deep tendon reflex

RELATED TOPICS

- Alterations in consciousness
- Drug overdose: specific drug(s) involved
- Hypovolemia
- Mechanical ventilation
- Renal failure, acute

- Assess for electrolyte imbalance, in particular hypokalemia: irregular pulse, cardiac dysrhythmias, and serum K^+ <3.5 mEq/L.
- Monitor I&O qh; assess for output elevated out of proportion to intake, bearing in mind insensible losses, especially if hyperthermia present.
- Monitor laboratory values, including serum electrolytes and serum and urine osmolality. Be alert to BUN elevated out of proportion to creatinine (indicator of dehydration rather than renal disease), high urine specific gravity, low urine Na^+, and ↑ Hct and serum protein concentration.
- Maintain fluid intake as prescribed; administer prescribed electrolyte supplements.

Sensory/Perceptual alterations r/t chemical alterations secondary to ingestion of mind-altering drugs

Desired outcome: Within 48 h of intervention, patient verbalizes orientation to time, place, and person.

- Establish and maintain calm, quiet environment to minimize sensory overload. Dim lights when possible.
- At frequent intervals, assess orientation to time, place, and person. Reorient as necessary.
- Orient to the unit and explain all procedures before performing them. Include significant others in orientation process.
- Do not leave patient alone if he or she is agitated or confused.
- Administer antianxiety agents as prescribed.
- If patient hallucinating, intervene in the following ways:

   Be reassuring. Explain that hallucinations may be very real to the patient but that they are not real; they are caused by the substance patient consumed, and they will go away eventually.

   As appropriate, try to involve family/significant others because patient may have more trust in them.

   Explain that restraints are necessary to prevent harm to patient and others. Reassure patient that restraints will be used only as long as they are needed.

   Tell patient you will check on him or her at frequent intervals (eg, q5-10min) or that you will stay at patient's side.

Risk for violence (self-directed) r/t mind-altering drugs or depressed state

Desired outcome: Patient remains free of self-inflicted injury.

- If condition stable, provide auxiliary staff member, such as orderly or nursing assistant, to watch patient when awake.
- Speak in a quiet, calm voice, using short sentences. Limit interventions.
- Administer and evaluate effectiveness of sedation to calm patient.
- Keep all sharp instruments out of patient's room. Follow agency protocol accordingly.
- If necessary, restrain patient. Start with soft restraints but progress to leather restraints if patient is threat to self or staff.

REFERENCES

Keen JH, Baird MS, Allen JH: *Mosby's critical care and emergency drug reference,* ed 2, St Louis, 1996, Mosby.

Malseed R, Goldstein F, Balkon N: *Pharmacology: drug therapy and nursing considerations,* Philadelphia, 1995, Lippincott.

Stiesmeyer JK: Drug overdose. In Swearingen PL, Keen JH (eds): *Manual of critical care nursing,* ed 3, St Louis, 1995, Mosby.

Author: **Johanna K. Stiesmeyer**

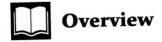 **Overview**

PATHOPHYSIOLOGY
Variety of substances that act to stimulate the CNS, producing visual, auditory, and other hallucinations.
Common Agents: Lysergic acid diethylamide (LSD), mescaline, morning glory seeds, nutmeg, ecstasy
Routes: Oral, IV, nasal, smoked

CLINICAL PRESENTATION
LSD: Description of tasting or hearing colors, mental dissociation
Mescaline: Sense of being followed by moving geometric shapes
Ecstasy: Heightened sexual libido

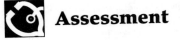 **Assessment**

PHYSICAL ASSESSMENT
Neuro: Hallucinations, paranoid behavior patterns, tremors, seizures, coma
Resp: Apnea, respiratory arrest
Assoc Findings: Hyperthermia, diaphoresis

VITAL SIGNS/HEMODYNAMICS
RR: Usually ↑; may be ↓ if in coma
HR: ↑
BP: ↑
Temp: ↑
Hemodynamics: Monitoring usually not indicated

LABORATORY STUDIES
Toxicology Screen: Serum plasma analyzed for presence of the drug.
Chemistries: Serum K^+, Na^+, CO_2, BUN/creatinine, glucose, and liver and renal studies evaluated.

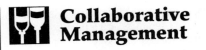 **Collaborative Management**

Support of Cardiopulmonary System: O_2 therapy; IV fluids if dehydrated.
Removal of Substance from System: If orally ingested, ipecac to induce vomiting; activated charcoal given orally or *via* gastric tube to bind with substance in stomach; gastric lavage.
Prevention of Seizures: Anticonvulsants such as phenytoin, diazepam.
Sedation: Chlorpromazine 0.5 mg/kg IM may be prescribed.

PATIENT-FAMILY TEACHING
• Purpose, expected results, anticipated sensations for all nursing/medical interventions given in simple, clear language for patients who are actively hallucinating
• Drug rehabilitation program, as indicated

⊕ Nursing Diagnoses/Interventions

Hyperthermia r/t toxic effects of hallucinogens

Desired outcome: Optimally, within 24-72 h of intervention, patient becomes normothermic.

Note: With massive overdose, temp regulation may never be achieved.

- Monitor for hyperthermia: temp >38.3° C (>101° F), pallor, absence of perspiration, and torso that is warm to the touch. If available, provide continuous monitoring of temp. Otherwise, measure rectal, core, or tympanic temp qh and prn.
- Provide and monitor effects of antipyretics, cooling blanket, cooling baths, and ice packs to the axillae and groin.
- Maintain fluid replacement as prescribed. Monitor hydration status and trend of I&O and urine specific gravity (optimal range: 1.010-1.020).
- Monitor neurologic status qh and prn until stabilized.
- Monitor VS continuously or qh and prn until stabilized. Be alert to ↑ BP, HR, and RR.

Risk for fluid volume deficit r/t altered intake or excessive losses secondary to vomiting or diaphoresis

Desired outcome: Patient normovolemic: UO ≥0.5 ml/kg/h, moist mucous membranes, balanced I&O, BP wnl for patient, HR ≤100 bpm, stable weight, urine specific gravity 1.010-1.020, CVP 2-6 mm Hg, PAWP 6-12 mm Hg.

- Monitor hydration status on an ongoing basis. Be alert to continuing dehydration as evidenced by poor skin turgor, dry mucous membranes, complaints of thirst, weak pulse with tachycardia, and postural hypotension.
- Assess for electrolyte imbalance, in particular hypokalemia: irregular pulse, cardiac dysrhythmias, and serum K^+ <3.5 mEq/L.
- Monitor I&O qh; assess for output elevated out of proportion to intake, bearing in mind insensible losses, especially if hyperthermia present.
- Monitor laboratory values, including serum electrolytes and serum and urine osmolality. Be alert to BUN elevated out of proportion to creatinine (indicator of dehydration rather than renal disease), high urine specific gravity, low urine Na^+, and ↑ Hct and serum protein concentration.
- Maintain fluid intake as prescribed; administer prescribed electrolyte supplements.

Sensory/Perceptual alterations r/t chemical alterations secondary to ingestion of mind-altering drugs

Desired outcome: Within 48 h of intervention, patient verbalizes orientation to time, place, and person.

- Establish and maintain calm, quiet environment to minimize sensory overload. Dim lights when possible.
- At frequent intervals, assess orientation to time, place, and person. Reorient as necessary.
- Orient to the unit and explain all procedures before performing them. Include significant others in orientation process.
- Do not leave patient alone if he or she is agitated or confused.
- Administer antianxiety agents as prescribed.
- If patient hallucinating, intervene in the following ways:

  Be reassuring. Explain that hallucinations may be very real to patient but that they are not real; they are caused by the substance patient consumed, and they will go away eventually.

  As appropriate, try to involve family/significant others because patient may have more trust in them.

  Explain that restraints are necessary to prevent harm to patient and others. Reassure patient that restraints will be used only as long as they are needed.

  Tell patient you will check on him or her at frequent intervals (eg, q5-10min) or that you will stay at patient's side.

▦ Miscellanea

CONSULT MD FOR

- Seizure activity
- Hemodynamically significant dysrhythmias
- UO <0.5 ml/kg/h × 2 h

RELATED TOPICS

- Delirium
- Drug overdose: general
- Hypovolemia
- Status epilepticus

REFERENCES

Cisek J: Hallucinogens. In Tintinalli JE, Ruiz E, Krome RL (eds): *Emergency medicine: a comprehensive study guide,* ed 4, New York, 1996, McGraw-Hill.

Keen JH, Baird MS, Allen JH: *Mosby's critical care and emergency drug reference,* ed 2, St Louis, 1996, Mosby.

McCarron M: Phencyclidine and hallucinogens. In Rippe J, Irwin R, Fink M (eds): *Intensive care medicine,* ed 3, Boston, 1996, Little, Brown.

Malseed R, Goldstein F, Balkon N: *Pharmacology: drug therapy and nursing considerations,* Philadelphia, 1995, Lippincott.

Stiesmeyer JK: Drug overdose. In Swearingen PL, Keen JH (eds): *Manual of critical care nursing,* ed 3, St Louis, 1995, Mosby.

Author: **Johanna K. Stiesmeyer**

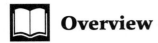 # Overview

PATHOPHYSIOLOGY

Produce analgesia and cause sedation, CNS depression, including depression of respiratory centers in the brainstem. Also cause peripheral vasodilatation/↓ SVR and may lead to profound hypotension. Chronic drug injectors at risk for infections, including bloodstream infection.

Examples: Codeine, fentanyl, heroin, hydrocodone, hydromorphone hydrochloride (Dilaudid), meperidine hydrochloride (Demerol), methadone (Dolophine Hydrochloride), morphine, opium, oxycodone hydrochloride (Percocet, Tylox)

Cutting Agents: Heroin may be mixed (cut) with other substances to ↑ volume (eg, mannitol, starch) or potentiate pharmacologic effects (eg, dextromethorphan, lidocaine, scopolamine). Presence of cutting agents results in mixed overdosage and complicates therapeutic management.

Routes: Oral, IV, IM, smoked, inhaled

CLINICAL PRESENTATION (hallmark indicators)

Stupor or coma, pinpoint pupils, respiratory depression, acute pulmonary edema

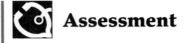 # Assessment

PHYSICAL ASSESSMENT

Neuro: Range from ↓ mental alertness to profound coma, seizures, miosis.

Resp: Respiratory depression, including hypoventilation, periods of apnea; bronchospasm; wheezing, rhonchi. Crackles and frothy sputum if acute pulmonary edema present.

CV: Profound hypotension, bradycardia, CV collapse, sudden death.

GU: Oliguria, anuria, ATN associated with profound hypotension and rhabdomyolysis.

Assoc Findings: Track marks, scarring on arms and in hidden body locations.

Cut with Scopolamine: Anticholinergic activity, including tachycardia, hypertension, dilated pupils, dry skin/mucous membranes, ↓ bowel sounds, urinary retention, agitation, combativeness. These effects may not be apparent until opioid effects reversed with naloxone.

VITAL SIGNS/HEMODYNAMICS

RR: ↓
HR: ↓
BP: ↓
Temp: Nl
PAP: ↑ if pulmonary edema present
CVP: ↓ if dehydration, CV collapse
CO: ↓
ECG: Sinus bradycardia, other bradydysrhythmias

LABORATORY STUDIES

Toxicology Scan: Urine sampling is the best way to identify the drug.

CBC: To establish baseline and check WBCs to detect infection (ie, bloodstream, respiratory tract).

ABGs: To detect hypoxemia, hypercapnia.

Chemistries: To check for ↓ K^+, ↑ Na^+, which may be present as a result of dehydration. Glucose and renal, hepatic function also evaluated.

IMAGING

Chest X-ray: May demonstrate atelectasis, pulmonary edema, infiltrates r/t aspiration.

Collaborative Management

Support of CV System To Prevent Collapse: Electrical rhythm monitored; bradydysrhythmias treated with atropine and pacemaker. Vasopressor therapy for hypotension after fluids have been replaced.

Removal of Drug from System: If oral ingestion suspected, ipecac to induce vomiting, activated charcoal orally or *via* gastric tube to bind with opiates.

Reversal of Opioid Effects: Administration of naloxone hydrochloride (Narcan). After initial dose, patient must be monitored closely, since additional doses may be required. Effects last between 2-3 h. If narcotic effects last longer than effects of naloxone, patient may slip into coma once naloxone wears off. In this case, continuous naloxone infusion considered. Excessive doses of naloxone may precipitate acute withdrawal in chronic opiate users.

Support of Resp System: Pulmonary edema treated with diuretics, restriction of IV fluid intake. Mechanical ventilation may be required.

Prevention of Aspiration: Gastric tube inserted and placed to continuous, low suction.

Prevention/Treatment of Seizure Activity: Anticonvulsant therapy, such as phenytoin.

Treatment of Drug Withdrawal Symptoms: Hallucinations treated with haloperidol (Haldol).

Identification/Treatment of Rhabdomyolysis: Seizure activity and breakdown of muscle cause protein to precipitate in the kidneys, leading to renal failure. Detected by ↓ UO and ↑ BUN, creatinine, and protein in urine.

Management of Associated Toxicities: With concurrent scopolamine overdose, benzodiazepines such as lorazepam (Ativan) or physostigmine (Antilirium) may be used for sedation or to reverse anticholinergic effects. Consult Poison Control Center for management of mixed agent overdosage.

PATIENT-FAMILY TEACHING

- Purpose, expected results, anticipated sensations of all nursing/medical interventions
- Drug rehabilitation programs, eg, Narcotics Anonymous (consult local phone book)

Nursing Diagnoses/Interventions

Ineffective airway clearance r/t presence of tracheobronchial secretions; obstruction; ↓ sensorium

Desired outcome: Within 2-24 h of intervention/treatment, patient has clear airway: clear breath sounds over upper airways and lung fields, RR 12-20 breaths/min with eupnea, Pao_2 ≥80 mm Hg, $Paco_2$ 35-45 mm Hg, pH 7.35-7.45, Spo_2 ≥92%.

- Assess respiratory function frequently. Be alert to secretions; stridor; gurgling; shallow, irregular, or labored respirations; use of accessory muscles; restlessness and confusion; and cyanosis.
- Suction oropharynx or *via* ET tube prn.
- Monitor ABGs for hypoxemia (Pao_2 <80 mm Hg) and respiratory acidosis ($Paco_2$ >45 mm Hg and pH <7.35).
- Monitor respiratory patterns; provide continuous apnea monitoring if available.
- If patient is on mechanical ventilation, monitor for airway obstruction.
- Monitor O_2 saturation continuously. Be alert to values <92%, depending on baseline and clinical presentation.
- Place in side-lying position during vomiting to ↓ aspiration risk.
- Use NG tube to remove stomach contents, thereby ↓ risk of aspiration.

Risk for fluid volume deficit r/t altered intake or excessive losses secondary to vomiting or diaphoresis

Desired outcome: Patient normovolemic: UO ≥0.5 ml/kg/h, moist mucous membranes, balanced I&O, BP wnl for patient, HR ≤100 bpm, stable weight, urine specific gravity 1.010-1.020, CVP 2-6 mm Hg, and PAWP 6-12 mm Hg.

- Monitor hydration status on an ongoing basis. Be alert to continuing dehydration as evidenced by poor skin turgor, dry mucous membranes, complaints of thirst, weak pulse with tachycardia, and postural hypotension.
- Assess for electrolyte imbalance, in particular hypokalemia: irregular pulse, cardiac dysrhythmias, and serum K^+ <3.5 mEq/L.
- Monitor I&O qh; assess for output elevated out of proportion to intake, bearing in mind insensible losses, especially if hyperthermia present.
- Monitor laboratory values, including serum electrolytes and serum and urine osmolality. Be alert to BUN elevated out of proportion to creatinine (indicator of dehydration rather than renal disease), high urine specific gravity, low urine Na^+, and ↑ Hct and serum protein concentration.
- Maintain fluid intake as prescribed; administer prescribed electrolyte supplements.

Miscellanea

CONSULT MD FOR

- Respiratory failure/pulmonary edema: crackles, use of accessory muscles, restlessness, confusion, cyanosis, Spo_2 <92%
- Hemodynamically significant dysrhythmias
- Infection: temp >38.33° C (101° F); ↑/new onset rhonchi, other adventitious sounds; ↑/change in sputum production
- Complications: aspiration, septic shock, ATN

RELATED TOPICS

- Acute tubular necrosis
- Drug overdose: general
- Mechanical ventilation
- Pneumonia, aspiration
- Pulmonary edema

ABBREVIATION

ATN: Acute tubular necrosis

REFERENCES

Centers for Disease Control and Prevention: Scopolamine poisoning among heroin users New York City, Newark, Philadelphia, and Baltimore, 1995 and 1996, *MMWR* 45(2): 457-460, 1996.

Keen JH, Baird MS, Allen JH: *Mosby's critical care and emergency drug reference*, ed 2, St Louis, 1996, Mosby.

Malseed R, Goldstein F, Balkon N: *Pharmacology: drug therapy and nursing considerations*, Philadelphia, 1995, Lippincott.

Schauber J: Opiate overdose. In Rippe J, Irwin R, Fink M (eds): *Intensive care medicine*, ed 3, Boston, 1996, Little, Brown.

Stiesmeyer JK: Drug overdose. In Swearingen PL, Keen JH (eds): *Manual of critical care nursing*, ed 3, St Louis, 1995, Mosby.

Author: **Johanna K. Stiesmeyer**

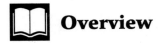 **Overview**

PATHOPHYSIOLOGY

CNS stimulant/illicit drug with no recognized therapeutic effects. Hypoglycemia is common. Rhabdomyolysis and myoglobinuria may occur and precipitate renal failure. Chemically r/t ketamine HCl (Ketalar).
Street Names: PCP, angel dust, mist
Routes: Oral, nasal, smoked

CLINICAL PRESENTATION

Effects are dose dependent and variable, ranging from hyperexcitability and psychotic behavior to stupor and coma.

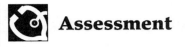 **Assessment**

PHYSICAL ASSESSMENT

Neuro: Hyperreflexia, muscle rigidity, paranoia, stupor, seizures, coma; eyes open in a blank stare, nystagmus, and pinpoint pupils also possible
Resp: Respiratory depression, respiratory arrest, bronchospasm, laryngeal stridor
CV: Profound hypertension, tachycardia
RU: Myoglobinuria, oliguria
Assoc Findings: Hypothermia or hyperthermia

VITAL SIGNS/HEMODYNAMICS

RR: ↑
HR: ↑
BP: ↑
Temp: ↑ or ↓
Hemodynamic Monitoring: Not usually necessary
ECG: Sinus, supraventricular, other tachydysrhythmias

LABORATORY STUDIES

Toxicology Screen: Urine assay to determine presence of PCP.
Chemistries: K^+, Na^+, CO_2, BUN/creatinine, glucose, liver and renal studies may be evaluated.
ABGs: To check for metabolic acidosis.

Collaborative Management

Support of CV System: Electrical rhythm monitored and tachydysrhythmias treated with verapamil or according to ACLS guidelines. IV nitroprusside or labetalol used for hypertensive emergencies. Other β-blockers or calcium channel blockers *not* recommended for hypertension or dysrhythmias. NTG may be given to dilate myocardial vasculature.
Removal of Drug from System: No specific antidote available, although standard practice is multiple administrations of charcoal to bind with ingested substance in the stomach. First dose of charcoal accompanied with sorbitol to prevent constipation.
Prevention/Treatment of Seizure Activity: Diazepam, phenytoin given. Haldol may be given to control psychosis. Effects usually occur within 5-10 min of administration.
Resp Support: Pulmonary edema treated with diuretics and restriction of IV fluid intake. Persons with hypoxia and deteriorating respiratory integrity placed on apnea monitor and potentially on mechanical ventilation.
Prevention of Aspiration: Gastric tube inserted and connected to low suction.
Identification of Rhabdomyolysis: Seizure activity and breakdown of muscle causes protein to precipitate in the kidneys, leading to renal failure. Detected by ↑ urine BUN, creatinine, and protein values.
Treatment of Hypothermia or Hyperthermia: Warming or cooling blanket as appropriate. Acetaminophen may be given rectally for hyperthermia.

PATIENT-FAMILY TEACHING

- Purpose, expected results, anticipated sensations for all nursing/medical interventions given in simple, clear language with patients who are actively hallucinating
- Drug rehabilitation program, as indicated

Nursing Diagnoses/Interventions

Sensory/Perceptual alterations r/t chemical alterations secondary to ingestion of mind-altering drugs

Desired outcome: Within 48 h of intervention, patient verbalizes orientation to time, place, and person.

- Establish and maintain calm, quiet environment to minimize sensory overload. Dim lights when possible.
- At frequent intervals, assess orientation to time, place, and person. Reorient as necessary.
- Orient to the unit and explain all procedures before performing them. Include significant others in orientation process.
- Do not leave patient alone if he or she is agitated or confused.
- Administer antianxiety agents as prescribed.
- If patient hallucinating, intervene in the following ways:

    Be reassuring. Explain that hallucinations may be very real to patient but that they are not real; they are caused by the substance patient consumed, and they will go away eventually.

    As appropriate, try to involve family/significant others because patient may have more trust in them.

    Explain that restraints are necessary to prevent harm to patient and others. Reassure patient that restraints will be used only as long as they are needed.

    Tell patient you will check on him or her at frequent intervals (eg, q5-10min) or that you will stay at patient's side.

Risk for violence (self-directed) r/t mind-altering drugs or depressed state

Desired outcome: Patient remains free of self-inflicted injury.

- If condition stable, provide auxiliary staff member, such as orderly or nursing assistant, to watch patient when awake.
- Speak in a quiet, calm voice, using short sentences. Limit interventions.
- Administer and evaluate effectiveness of sedation to calm patient.
- Keep all sharp instruments out of patient's room. Follow agency protocol accordingly.
- If necessary, restrain patient. Start with soft restraints but progress to leather restraints if patient is threatening to self or staff.

Hyperthermia r/t toxic effects of phencyclidine

Desired outcome: Optimally, within 24-72 h of intervention, patient becomes normothermic.

Note: With massive overdose, temp regulation may never be achieved.

- Monitor for hyperthermia: temp >38.3° C (>101° F), pallor, absence of perspiration, and torso that is warm to the touch. If available, provide continuous monitoring of temp. Otherwise, measure rectal, core, or tympanic temp qh and prn.
- Provide and monitor effects of cooling blanket, cooling baths, and ice packs to the axillae and groin.
- Maintain fluid replacement as prescribed. Monitor hydration status and trend of I&O and urine specific gravity (optimal range: 1.010-1.020).
- Monitor neurologic status qh and prn until stabilized.
- Monitor VS continuously or qh and prn until stabilized. Be alert to ↑ BP, HR, and RR.
- Administer and evaluate effects of antipyretic medications.

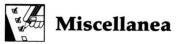 # Miscellanea

CONSULT MD FOR
- S&S of rhabdomyolysis: ↓ UO, reddish-brown discoloration of urine
- Persistent or severe hypertension
- Complications, including pulmonary edema, hemodynamically significant tachydysrhythmias, hypoglycemia, seizures

RELATED TOPICS
- Agitation syndrome
- Hypertensive crisis
- Renal failure, acute
- Status epilepticus
- Supraventricular tachycardia

REFERENCES

Cisek J: Hallucinogens. In Tintinalli JE, Ruiz E, Krone RL (eds): *Emergency medicine: a comprehensive study guide,* ed 4, New York, 1996, McGraw-Hill.

Keen JH, Baird MS, Allen JH: *Mosby's critical care and emergency drug reference,* ed 2, St Louis, 1996, Mosby.

McCarron M: Phencyclidine and hallucinogens. In Rippe J, Irwin R, Fink M (eds): *Intensive care medicine,* ed 3, Boston, 1996, Little, Brown.

Malseed R, Goldstein F, Balkon N: *Pharmacology: drug therapy and nursing considerations,* Philadelphia, 1995, Lippincott.

Stiesmeyer JK: Drug overdose. In Swearingen PL, Keen JH (eds): *Manual of critical care nursing,* ed 3, St Louis, 1995, Mosby.

Author: **Johanna K. Stiesmeyer**

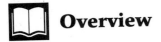 # Overview

PATHOPHYSIOLOGY

Mild intoxication may cause salicylism: tinnitus, headache, confusion, palpitations, hyperventilation. More severe intoxication leads to CNS stimulation and possible cerebral edema, respiratory alkalosis followed by metabolic acidosis, profound hypokalemia. Other possible findings include dehydration, renal failure (caused by ↓ GFR, rhabdomyolysis), pulmonary edema, hepatitis/hepatic failure.

Examples: Aspirin, bismuth subsalicylate
Routes: Oral, rectal (suppository)

HISTORY/RISK FACTORS

Prolonged use of high doses: eg, for RA, osteoarthritis

CLINICAL PRESENTATION

Altered mental status, impaired hearing or vision, sweating, dizziness, GI bleeding, S&S of dehydration

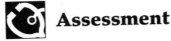 # Assessment

PHYSICAL ASSESSMENT

Neuro: Initially confusion, headache, tinnitus; later delirium, convulsions, coma
Resp: Hyperventilation, hyperpnea, pulmonary edema
GU: Oliguria, anuria
Hep: ↑ liver enzymes, jaundice
Assoc Findings: Hyperthermia, thrombocytopenia, bleeding, anemia

LABORATORY STUDIES

Salicylate Levels: Blood plasma analyzed for presence and amount of salicylate and repeated q4-6h, especially if salicylates ingested in sustained release form.
Chemistries: To check for hypokalemia, other electrolyte imbalances, hypoglycemia, hyperglycemia.
CBC: To check for ↓ platelets, ↓ RBC as a result of bleeding.
Clotting Studies: To check for excessive anticoagulation; prolonged bleeding time.

Collaborative Management

Removal of Substance from System: Ipecac to induce vomiting; activated charcoal given orally or *via* gastric tube to bind with substance in the stomach; gastric lavage; and hemodialysis, which may be necessary if substance has been absorbed into the system. Several doses of activated charcoal may be necessary to achieve 10:1 ratio of charcoal to salicylate.
Fluid Replacement: 1-3 L D_5.45NS or D_5NS (with or without $NaHCO_3$ [1 mEq/kg/h] and potassium [10-20 mEq/L]) over first 1-2 h.
Treatment of Prolonged Bleeding Time: Phytonadione (vitamin K_1), FFP, platelets, PRBCs.
Treatment of Hyperthermia: Cooling blanket or ice applications.
Treatment of Cerebral Edema: Hyperventilation (*via* mechanical ventilation), mannitol.
Resp Support: Mechanical ventilation as indicated.
Treatment of Pulmonary Edema: Nitrates, morphine, diuretics, potassium replacement, IPPB.
Prevention of Aspiration: Insertion of gastric tube, which is then connected to low suction.
Replacement of Blood Loss: Delivery of blood and blood products.

PATIENT-FAMILY TEACHING

- S&S of salicylism: headache, tinnitus, hearing loss, palpitations, sweating, vomiting
- S&S of actual or impending GI hemorrhage: pain, nausea, vomiting of blood, dark stools, lightheadedness, passage of frank blood in stools; importance of seeking medical attention promptly if signs of bleeding occur

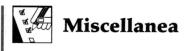

Nursing Diagnoses/Interventions

Fluid volume deficit r/t dehydration or active loss secondary to hemorrhage from GI tract or other sources

Desired outcome: Within 8 h of this diagnosis, patient normovolemic: MAP $\geq$70 mm Hg, HR 60-100 bpm, CVP 2-6 mm Hg, PAWP 6-12 mm Hg, CI $\geq$2.5 L/min/m^2, and UO $\geq$0.5 ml/kg/h.

- Monitor postural VS q4-8h or more frequently if recurrence of active bleeding suspected. $\downarrow$ SBP >10 mm Hg or $\uparrow$ in HR of 10 bpm in sitting position suggests significant intravascular volume deficit, with $\approx$ 15%-20% loss of volume.
- Measure central pressures and thermodilution CO q1-4h. Be alert to low or $\downarrow$ CVP, PAWP, and CO. Calculate SVR q4-8h or more frequently if unstable. $\uparrow$ HR, $\downarrow$ PAWP, $\downarrow$ CO (CI <2.5 L/min/m^2), and $\uparrow$ SVR suggest hypovolemia and the need for volume restoration.
- Monitor BP q15min during episodes of rapid active blood loss or unstable VS. Be alert to MAP $\downarrow$ of >10 mm Hg from previous reading.
- Use D$_5$.45NS or D$_5$NS to replace fluids; promote forced alkaline diuresis by administering sodium bicarbonate 1 mEq/kg/h *via* continual infusion. Replace K$^+$ as necessary.
- If there is evidence of acute blood loss, replace volume with a combination of crystalloid and blood products as indicated *via* large-bore IV ($\geq$18 gauge) catheter.
- Measure UO qh. Be alert to output <0.5 ml/kg/h for 2 consecutive h.
- Check all stools and gastric contents for occult blood.
- Measure and record all GI blood losses from hematemesis, hematochezia, melena.

Ineffective airway clearance r/t presence of tracheobronchial secretions; obstruction; $\downarrow$ sensorium

Desired outcome: Within 2-24 h of intervention/treatment, patient has clear airway: clear breath sounds over upper airways and lung fields, RR 12-20 breaths/min with eupnea, Pao$_2$ $\geq$80 mm Hg, Paco$_2$ 35-45 mm Hg, pH 7.35-7.45, and Spo$_2$ $\geq$92%.

- Assess respiratory function frequently. Be alert to secretions; stridor; gurgling; shallow, irregular, or labored respirations; use of accessory muscles; restlessness and confusion; and cyanosis.
- Suction oropharynx or *via* ET tube prn.
- Monitor ABGs for hypoxia (Pao$_2$ <80 mm Hg) and respiratory acidosis (Paco$_2$ >45 mm Hg and pH <7.35).
- Monitor respiratory patterns; provide continuous apnea monitoring if available.
- If patient is on mechanical ventilation, monitor for airway obstruction.
- Monitor O$_2$ saturation continuously. Be alert to values <92%, depending on baseline and clinical presentation.
- Administer and evaluate effects of antiemetics.
- Place in side-lying position during vomiting to $\downarrow$ aspiration risk.

Hyperthermia r/t toxic effects of salicylates

Desired outcome: Optimally, within 24-72 h of intervention, patient becomes normothermic.

Note: With massive overdose, temp regulation may never be achieved.

- Monitor for hyperthermia: temp >38.3° C (>101° F), pallor, absence of perspiration, and torso that is warm to the touch. If available, provide continuous monitoring of temp. Otherwise, measure rectal, core, or tympanic temp qh and prn.
- Provide and monitor effects of cooling blanket, cooling baths, and ice packs to the axillae and groin.
- Maintain fluid replacement as prescribed. Monitor hydration status and trend of I&O and urine specific gravity (optimal range: 1.010-1.020).
- Monitor neurologic status qh and prn until stabilized.
- Monitor VS continuously or qh and prn until stabilized. Be alert to $\uparrow$ BP, HR, and RR.
- Administer and evaluate effects of antipyretic medications.

Miscellanea

CONSULT MD FOR

- Hemodynamically significant dysrhythmias; ECG evidence of hypokalemia
- $\downarrow$ UO or UO <0.5 ml/kg/h × 2 h
- Occult or frank blood in stool, vomitus, or other evidence of bleeding
- S&S of $\uparrow$ ICP: $\downarrow$ LOC, pupillary changes, widened pulse pressure, irregular respiratory pattern, bradycardia, seizures

RELATED TOPICS

- Gastrointestinal bleeding: upper
- Hypokalemia
- Hypovolemia
- Increased intracranial pressure
- Mechanical ventilation
- Metabolic acidosis, acute
- Psychosocial support, patient

ABBREVIATIONS

FFP: Fresh frozen plasma
GFR: Glomerular filtration rate
PRBCs: Packed red blood cells
RA: Rheumatoid arthritis

REFERENCES

Curry S: Salicylates. In Tintinalli JE, Ruiz E, Krome RL (eds): *Emergency medicine: a comprehensive study guide,* ed 4, New York, 1996, McGraw-Hill.

Keen JH, Baird MS, Allen JH: *Mosby's critical care and emergency drug reference,* ed 2, St Louis, 1996, Mosby.

Linden C: Salicylate and other nonsteroidal antiinflammatory drug poisonings. In Rippe J, Irwin R, Fink M (eds): *Intensive care medicine,* ed 3, Boston, 1996, Little, Brown.

Malseed R, Goldstein F, Balkon N: *Pharmacology: drug therapy and nursing considerations,* Philadelphia, 1995, Lippincott.

Stiesmeyer JK: Drug overdose. In Swearingen PL, Keen JH (eds): *Manual of critical care nursing,* ed 3, St Louis, 1995, Mosby.

Author: **Johanna K. Stiesmeyer**

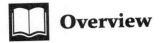

Overview

DESCRIPTION

No two people age in the same way. There is interdependence among social, physiologic, and psychologic aspects of life as well as in physiologic reserve and variability in disease presentation and functional parameters (ie, ability to perform ADLs). For elders (>65 yrs), success in aging depends on genetics, environmental factors, life-style, presence/effect of chronic disease.

HISTORY/RISK FACTORS (for impaired physiologic/functional parameters)

- Medications
- Immobility
- Incontinence
- Sleep disorders
- Chronic disease

CLINICAL PRESENTATION

May include one or more of the following: change in function (ADLs), acute confusion, fatigue, pain, falls, gait disturbance, incontinence, anorexia, weight loss, syncope, dyspnea

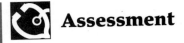

Assessment

PHYSICAL ASSESSMENT

Variable, depending on life-style, environment, chronic disease

Neuro: Scattered loss of neurons, slowed nerve impulse conduction, ↓ peripheral nerve function leading to ↓ ability to maintain homeostasis, slowed response/recovery to stressors, ↑ permeability of blood-brain barrier leading to ↑ sensitivity to medications and ↓ O_2 and glucose levels, ↓ ability to deal with multiple stimuli

Resp: ↓ lung compliance, ↓ diffusing capacity, ↑ physiologic dead space, V/Q imbalance, loss of elastic recoil (can lead to nonsignificant crackles), ↓ chemoreceptor responsiveness to hypoxemia or hypercapnia, ↓ mucociliary clearance (defense mechanism), ↓ IgA production (↑ susceptibility to viruses and bacteria), impaired cough mechanism

CV: NSR wnl, end-diastolic volume not ↓ in healthy elders, compensatory S_4 possible as a result of vigorous atrial contraction, ↓ baroreceptor sensitivity, ↓ β-adrenergic receptors, ↓ cardiac reserve

GI: ↓ hepatic blood flow resulting in ↓ metabolism of some medications and ↓ first-pass extraction of some drugs (ie, propranolol, verapamil)

GU: ↓ sense of thirst, ↓ RBF and GFR, ↓ ability to concentrate urine, ↓ ability to conserve Na^+, ↓ response to ADH, constance of urine production over 24 h (loss of diurnal rhythm), ↓ renin activity, ↓ bladder capacity; *incontinence is not normal*

MS: ↓ muscle mass, ↓ total body water, ↑ body fat, presence of osteoarthritis

Integ: Thin epidermis, ↓ vascularity, ↓ sweat glands, ↓ number of nerve cells, ↓ elasticity (↓ turgor), ↓ thermoregulation

Endo: ↓ sensitivity of peripheral receptors to insulin

VITAL SIGNS/HEMODYNAMICS

Vary with presence/absence of chronic disease

RR: Nl without disease 20-22 breaths/min
HR: 80-100 bpm
BP: Nl; ↑ SBP possible if CV disease present

Temp: 35.56-36.11° C (96-97° F)
ECG: NSR nl; occasional to rare asymptomatic PVCs

LABORATORY STUDIES

Serum Creatinine: Does not reflect renal status of elders well; overestimates renal function

Creatinine Clearance: Slight ↓

T_3: ↓

TSH: ↑

Fasting Blood Glucose: Nl to slight ↑

Glucose Tolerance Test: ↑

Albumin: Possible ↓ resulting from poor diet

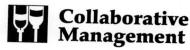 **Collaborative Management**

Fluid Management: Carefully monitor I&O in all elders. Hypo/hypertonic IV solutions that can lead to cardiac overload or dehydration given cautiously. Correct deficits slowly to prevent heart failure.

Temp: Do not take axillary temp in elders because of ↓ peripheral circulation. Skin temp may be cooler than core temp. Tympanic = oral equivalent.

Activity: Immobility leads to deconditioning, depression, ↑ dependence. Can ↑ risk of orthostatic hypotension, ↑ HR. Thrombophlebitis, negative protein and nitrogen states possible. Encourage involvement in ADL, ROM exercises. Provide PT evaluation.

Medical Immobilization Devices: Used cautiously if at all. Vest restraints ↓ respiratory excursion, compromise oxygenation. Wrist restraints lead to helplessness, hopelessness and promote wrist/arm ulceration if too tight. Can be psychologically damaging, particularly with past traumatic events, such as concentration camps, hx of physical abuse.

Nutrition: Monitor nutritional status. Check albumin, total protein. Provide nutritional consult. Parenteral, enteral nutrition if unable to eat. Assess swallowing ability, ability to handle secretions, coughing after eating, pocketing of food in oral cavity. Provide OT/speech consult as indicated.

Skin Care: Monitor for impaired skin integrity; turn q2h if unable to turn self.

Urinary Care: Avoid indwelling catheter. If one must be used, remove it as soon as possible.

Pharmacologic Considerations: ↓ hepatic blood flow, ↓ albumin, and other physiologic changes ↑ risk of adverse reactions. Note use of nonprescribed/OTC medications, nutritional supplements, homeopathic remedies, folk remedies, street/recreational drugs. Consult with pharmacist regarding age-appropriate dosage of medications.

PATIENT/FAMILY TEACHING

- Information about recovery from acute illness/surgery: prolonged in elders and based on preillness/surgical functional level
- Importance of open communication between staff and patient/family regarding care, environment, ethical issues
- Importance of family bringing in familiar items, pictures to ↓ risk of acute confusion caused by new environment

Nursing Diagnoses/Interventions

Risk for fluid volume deficit r/t ↓ fluid intake or ↑ losses secondary to vomiting, diarrhea, draining tubes, excessive diaphoresis, exacerbation of chronic disease, third spacing of fluids caused by disease, hypotonic IV fluids, osmotic agents, tube feedings

Desired outcomes: Patient normovolemic: mental status; VS; urine specific gravity, color, consistency, and concentration remain wnl for patient. Skin turgor nl; tongue and mucous membranes remain moist. I = O + insensible losses. CVP, MAP, PAWP, Na^+, K^+, and creatinine remain wnl.

- Assess and document skin turgor. Check hydration status by pinching skin over sternum or forehead; assess tongue and mucous membranes for moistness.
- Measure UO qh until ≥0.5 ml/kg/h.
- Monitor HR, ECG, CV status q15min until stable.
- Monitor values for Na^+, BUN, blood osmolality to ensure they are wnl.
- Expect to correct fluid deficit slowly over 2-3 days.
- Monitor for S&S of third spacing, including peripheral edema, especially sacral.
- Monitor cardiac and respiratory systems for signs of fluid volume overload, pulmonary edema as a result of therapy.

Hypothermia r/t age-related changes in thermoregulation and/or environmental exposure

Desired outcome: Temp and mental status wnl for patient or returning to nl at a rate of 1°/h after intervention.

- Monitor temp using low-range thermometer if possible. Nl temp may be as low as 35.56° C (96° F).
- Assess and document mental status. ↑ disorientation or atypical behavior may signal hypothermia.
- Be alert to risk factors for development of environmental hypothermia: sedatives, hypnotics, anesthesia, muscle relaxants (these agents ↓ shivering).
- Elders are at risk for environmental hypothermia at ambient temps of 22.22°-23.89° C (72°-75° F). Ensure that patient is kept warm with blankets, especially when sent to other departments.
- Initiate slow external rewarming: raise room temp to ≥ 23.89° C (75° F) and use warm blankets, head covers, warm circulating air blankets.
- If temp fails to ↑ 1° F qh using above techniques, suspect a cause other than environmental. In this event, anticipate laboratory tests for sepsis, hypothyroidism, and hypoglycemia. Temp will not return to nl until underlying conditions have been corrected.

Risk for infection r/t age-related changes in immune and integumentary system; r/t suppressed inflammatory response secondary to chronic medication use (eg, antiinflammatory agents, steroids, analgesics); r/t slowed ciliary response; or r/t poor nutrition

Desired outcome: Patient infection free: orientation × 3; behavior wnl for patient; respiratory rate/pattern, lung sounds, core temp, HR wnl for patient; skin intact with color and temp nl for patient.

- Assess baseline VS, including LOC and orientation. A change in mentation is a leading sign of infection in elders. Also be alert to HR >100 bpm and RR >24 breaths/min. Auscultate lung fields for adventitious sounds. Be aware, however, that crackles may be a nl finding when heard in lung bases, especially in elders >75 yrs.
- Monitor temp using low-range thermometer if possible. Be aware that temp of 35.56° C (96° F) may be nl. In that case, temp of 36.67°-37.22° C (98° F) may be considered febrile.
- To ensure the core temp is accurately determined, obtain readings *via* central line or rectum.
- Assess skin for tears, breaks, redness, or ulcers. Document condition on admission for ongoing comparison.
- Assess urine quality and color. UTI, manifested by cloudy, foul-smelling urine without painful urination, is the most common infection in elders. Urinary incontinence also may signal UTI.
- Because of ↑ risk of infection, avoid use of indwelling urinary catheters unless mandatory. Remove as soon as possible.
- Obtain drug hx in reference to antiinflammatory or immunosuppressive drugs or chronic use of analgesics or steroids. These drugs can mask fever.
- If infection suspected, anticipate antibiotics, blood and urine cultures, and urinalysis to isolate bacteria type and WBCs to determine immune response. Expect chest x-ray in order to rule out

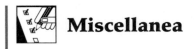 # Miscellanea

CONSULT MD FOR
- S&S of dehydration, hypovolemia
- Acute changes in mental status
- Tachydysrhythmias, A-fib, bradydysrhythmias
- ↓ UO with adequate hydration
- ↓ O_2 level
- ↑ RR

RELATED TOPICS
- Alterations in consciousness
- Heart failure, left ventricular
- Hypovolemia
- Pneumonia, aspiration
- Pulmonary edema
- Renal failure, acute
- Shock, septic

ABBREVIATIONS
A-fib: Atrial fibrillation
GFR: Glomerular filtration rate
PT: Physical therapist
RBF: Renal blood flow
T_3: Triiodothyronine
TSH: Thyroid-stimulating hormone
UTI: Urinary tract infection

pneumonia. WBCs ≥11,000 µl can be a late sign of infection in elders because their immune system is slow to respond to insult.

Altered thought processes r/t ↓ cerebral perfusion secondary to age-related ↓ physiologic reserve or cardiac dysfunction; r/t electrolyte imbalance secondary to age-related ↓ renal function; r/t altered sensory-perceptual reception secondary to poor vision or hearing; or r/t ↓ brain oxygenation secondary to illness state and ↓ functional lung tissue

Desired outcome: Mental status returns to wnl for patient within 3 days of treatment. Patient sustains no evidence of injury or harm as a result of altered mental status.

- Assess and document baseline LOC and mental status. Have patient perform a 3-step task (eg, "Raise your right hand, place it on your left shoulder, and then place the right hand by your right side.") Test short-term memory by showing patient how to use call light, having patient return demonstration, and then waiting at least 5 min before having patient demonstrate use of call light again. Inability to remember beyond 5 min indicates poor short-term memory.
- Document actions in behavioral terms. Describe the "confused" behavior.
- Obtain preconfusion functional and mental status abilities from significant others.
- Identify cause of acute confusion (eg, assess oxygenation levels, serum glucose, WBCs). Assess hydration status; monitor I&O q8h.
- Review cardiac status. Watch for hemodynamically significant or new dysrhythmias.
- Monitor ABGs or Spo₂ for impaired oxygenation.
- Review current medications, including OTC drugs. Consult with pharmacist as indicated. Toxic levels of certain medications such as digoxin or theophylline cause acute confusion.
- Monitor results of creatinine clearance test. In aging, lower muscle mass produces lower creatinine; "normal" serum creatinine levels in a well-hydrated elder can therefore signal renal insufficiency.
- Have patient wear glasses and hearing aid, or keep them within easy reach for use.
- Keep urinal and other routinely used items nearby. Toilet or offer urinal or bedpan q2h while patient awake and q4h during the night. Do not expect patient with short-term memory problems to use the call light.
- Place patient close to nurses' station if possible. Arrange for a nonstimulating and safe environment. Provide music but not TV (confused individuals often think TV action is happening in their room).
- Encourage significant others to bring in familiar items, including blankets, bedspread, pictures of family and pets.
- Reorient to surroundings as needed. Keep clock or calendar at bedside. Verbally remind patient of date and day as needed. Tell patient in simple terms what is occurring (eg, "It's time to eat breakfast").
- If patient becomes angry or argumentative during reorientation, stop this approach. Do not argue with patient's interpretation of the environment. State, "I can understand why you may (hear, think, see) that."
- If patient displays hostile behavior or misperceives your role (nurse becomes thief, jailor, etc.), leave the room. Return in 15 min. Introduce yourself as though you had never met. Begin dialogue anew. Patients who are acutely confused have poor short-term memory and may not remember previous encounter.
- Have significant others talk by phone or come in and sit with patient if patient requires frequent checking.
- If patient is attempting to pull out tubes, hide them (eg, under blankets). Put stockinette mesh dressing over IV lines. Tape feeding tubes to side of face using paper tape and drape tube behind ear. Remember: out of sight; out of mind. Tell patient to leave the tube alone and explain, "Don't pull that; it helps you breathe."
- Evaluate continued need for therapy that may have become an irritating stimulus (eg, if patient is now drinking, discontinue IV).
- Use medical immobilization devices with caution, if at all. Restraints can ↑ agitation.
- Use medications cautiously for controlling behavior. Neuroleptics such as haloperidol can be used successfully in calming patients with dementia or psychiatric illness (contraindicated with parkinsonism). However, if patient experiencing acute confusion or delirium, short-acting benzodiazepines (eg, lorazepam) may ↓ anxiety and fear.

REFERENCES

Abrahms W, Beers M, Berkow R (eds): *The Merck manual of geriatrics*, ed 2, Whitehouse Station, New Jersey, 1995, Merck Research Laboratories.

Jansen P: Caring for older adults. In Swearingen PL (ed): *Pocket guide to medical-surgical nursing*, ed 2, St Louis, 1996, Mosby.

Kane R, Ouslander J, Abrass I (eds): *Essentials of clinical geriatrics*, ed 3, New York, 1994, McGraw-Hill.

Mattson M, McConnell E, Linton A (eds): *Gerontological nursing: concepts and practice*, ed 2, Philadelphia, 1996, Saunders.

Author: **Patricia R. Jansen**

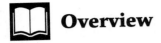 **Overview**

PATHOPHYSIOLOGY
Degenerative process characterized by enlargement of air spaces distal to terminal bronchioles, accompanied by alveolar wall destruction. As a result, air trapped and distal airways hyperinflated, with risk of rupture or collapse. Total disability possible because all available energy used for breathing. In later stages, pulmonary hypertension develops, leading to RV failure (cor pulmonale).

HISTORY/RISK FACTORS
- Cigarette smoking
- Air pollution
- Occupational exposure to dust/gases
- α_1-antitrypsin genetic abnormality

CLINICAL PRESENTATION
Chronic: Nonproductive cough (unless bronchitis also present), dyspnea on exertion
Acute (exacerbation): ↑ dyspnea, productive cough, fever, peripheral edema, fatigue

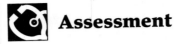 **Assessment**

PHYSICAL ASSESSMENT
Emaciation, ↑ A-P chest diameter, pursed-lip breathing, hypertrophy of accessory muscles of respiration, ↓ thoracic excursion, ↓ fremitus over affected lung fields, hyperresonance over affected lung fields, ↓ breath sounds, prolonged expiratory phase. Digital clubbing occurs late in the disease.

VITAL SIGNS/HEMODYNAMICS
RR: ↑
HR: ↑
BP: ↓ if heart failure present
Temp: ↑ if infection present
PAP: ↑ as a result of pulmonary hypertension
CVP: May be ↑ because of RV heart failure
PAWP: Necessary to reflect accurate hydration status with advanced disease
ECG: May reveal atrial and ventricular dysrhythmias. Most patients will have atrial dysrhythmia because of atrial dilatation and RV hypertrophy caused by pulmonary hypertension.

LABORATORY STUDIES
ABGs: May reveal slight ↓ in Pao_2. As disease progresses, Pao_2 continues to ↓; $Paco_2$ may ↑ as a result of hypoventilation and CO_2 retention. Early in the disease, however, $Paco_2$ may be nl if a good V/Q match is present. The pH will be low to nl once CO_2 retention begins.
CBC: May reveal chronically ↑ RBCs (polycythemia) later in the disease as a compensatory response to chronic hypoxemia.
Sputum Culture: To determine presence of pulmonary infection.

IMAGING
Chest X-ray: Shows lung hyperinflation, ↑ A-P diameter, lowered and flattened diaphragm, and small cardiac silhouette.

DIAGNOSTIC PROCEDURES
Pulmonary Function Tests: Show ↑ total lung capacity, ↑ residual volume, and ↓ forced expiratory reserve volume. VC wnl or slightly ↓.

Collaborative Management

O₂ Therapy: To treat hypoxemia. Used cautiously at a low flow rate (1-2 L/min) with chronic CO_2 retention in which hypoxemia stimulates respiratory drive.
Intubation/Mechanical Ventilation: Intubation may be necessary if unable to maintain patent airway as a result of tenacious or copious secretions, ineffective cough, or fatigue. Mechanical ventilation required if unable to maintain adequate ABGs (Pao_2 >60 mm Hg) with supplemental O_2; decision for use made carefully, since weaning may be difficult.
Hydration: IV fluids may be necessary to replace fluids lost from insensible sources (eg, tachypnea, diaphoresis with fever).
Pharmacotherapy
Bronchodilators: To open airways by relaxing smooth muscles.
Steroids (eg, prednisone): To ↓ inflammation, thereby ↑ air flow. Acute adrenal insufficiency can develop if drugs discontinued abruptly.
Antibiotics: Based on sensitivity studies from sputum cultures.
Chest Physiotherapy: To help loosen and mobilize pulmonary secretions.
Diuretics/Na Restriction: To reduce fluid overload in heart failure.

PATIENT-FAMILY TEACHING
- Use of home O_2, including instructions for when to use it, importance of not ↑ prescribed flow rate, precautions, community resources for replacement.
- S&S of RV heart failure that necessitate medical attention: ↑ dyspnea, fatigue; ↑ coughing; changes in amount, color, consistency of sputum; swelling of ankles, legs; fever; sudden weight gain.
- Avoiding infectious individuals, especially those with URIs. Importance of receiving flu and pneumococcal vaccines.
- Review of Na-restricted diet; importance of good nutrition in treating this disorder.
- Importance of pacing activity level to conserve energy.
- Pursed-lip breathing technique:
  Sit upright with hands on thighs or lean forward with elbows propped on over-the-bed table.
  Inhale slowly through nose with mouth closed.
  Form lips in "O" shape as though whistling.
  Exhale slowly through pursed lips. Exhalation should take twice as long as inhalation (eg, count to 5 on inhalation; count to 10 on exhalation).

Nursing Diagnoses/Interventions

Ineffective breathing pattern r/t ↓ lung expansion secondary to chronic air flow limitations
Desired outcome: Following treatment/intervention, patient's breathing pattern improves as evidenced by ↓/absence of dyspnea and movement toward state of eupnea (or baseline).
- Assess respiratory status q2h, being alert for indicators of respiratory distress. Auscultate breath sounds; report ↓ breath sounds or ↑ adventitious breath sounds.
- Teach pursed-lip breathing, which may prevent airway collapse during expiration.
- Administer bronchodilator therapy as prescribed. Monitor for side effects, including tachycardia and dysrhythmias.
- Monitor response to prescribed O_2 therapy. Be aware that high concentrations can depress respiratory drive in chronic CO_2 retention.
- Monitor serial ABGs. Patients with chronic CO_2 retention may have chronically compensated respiratory acidosis with low to nl pH (7.35-7.38) and $Paco_2$ >45 mm Hg.

Activity intolerance r/t imbalance between O_2 supply and demand secondary to inefficient WOB
Desired outcome: Patient reports ↓ dyspnea during activity or exercise and rates perceived exertion at ≤3 on 0-10 scale.
- Maintain prescribed activity levels and explain rationale to patient.
- Monitor respiratory response to activity. Activity intolerance indicated by excessively ↑ respiratory rate (eg, >10 breaths/min above baseline) and depth, dyspnea, and use of accessory muscles. Ask patient to rate perceived exertion. If activity intolerance noted, instruct patient to stop activity and rest.
- Organize care so that periods of activity are interspersed with periods of at least 90 min of undisturbed rest.
- Assist with ROM exercises to prevent deconditioning and other complications of immobility.

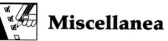 ## Miscellanea

CONSULT MD FOR
- Respiratory decompensation: agitation, restlessness, ↓ LOC, use of accessory muscles, Spo_2 <90%
- URI: change in amount, color of sputum; respiratory distress; ↑ adventitious breath sounds
- Heart failure: ↑ PAWP associated with pulmonary crackles, JVD, S_3 gallop

RELATED TOPICS
- Bronchitis, chronic
- Heart failure, right ventricular
- Immobility, prolonged
- Mechanical ventilation
- Pneumonia, community-acquired

ABBREVIATIONS
URI: Upper respiratory infection
VC: Vital capacity

REFERENCES
Braun SR et al: Comparison of six oxygen delivery systems for COPD patients at rest and during exercise, *Chest* 102(3): 694-698, 1992.
Harrigan MR: A large thin-walled cavity with air-fluid level in chest radiograph, *Respir Care* 39(10): 994-998, 1994.
Howard C: Chronic bronchitis. In Swearingen PL (ed): *Manual of medical-surgical nursing care,* ed 3, St Louis, 1994, Mosby.
Johannsen JM: Chronic obstructive pulmonary disease: current comprehensive care for emphysema and bronchitis, *Nurse Pract* 19(1): 59-67, 1994.
Schulman LL et al: Pulmonary vascular resistance in emphysema, *Chest* 105(3): 798-805, 1994.
Weaver TE, Narsavage GL: Physiological and psychosocial variables related to functional status in chronic obstructive pulmonary disease, *Nurs Res* 41(5): 286-287, 1992.

Author: **Cheri A. Goll**

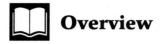 **Overview**

PATHOPHYSIOLOGY
Infection of endocardium caused by bacteria, viruses, fungi, or rickettsiae. Aortic and mitral valves commonly affected. Once infection begins, valvular dysfunction manifested by insufficiency with regurgitant blood flow can occur, ultimately resulting in ↓ CO. Vegetations may become so large that valve obstruction occurs, mimicking valvular stenosis and further ↓ CO. Vegetation pieces may break off and embolize to vital organs. Cerebral vasculature a common site and can result in ischemic stroke.

MORTALITY
20%-50%

RECURRENCE
10%-20%

HISTORY/RISK FACTORS
- Invasive procedures: PA catheter insertion, TUR, endoscopy, surgery, dental work
- Preexisting valvular disorder
- IV drug abuse
- Immunosuppression

CLINICAL PRESENTATION
Fever, diaphoresis, fatigue, anorexia, joint pain, weight loss, abdominal pain

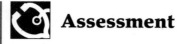 **Assessment**

PHYSICAL ASSESSMENT
General Findings: New or changed murmur. *If LV heart failure present:* fine crackles, S_3/S_4 heart sound. *If RV heart failure present:* edema, JVD, positive hepatojugular reflex, jaundice, and ascites. *Late findings:* anemia, petechiae, finger clubbing.
Classic Findings: Splinter hemorrhages, Janeway lesions, Osler's nodes.
Note: If vegetative emboli occur, S&S of cerebral, peripheral vascular, myocardial, renal, or mesenteric infarct will be seen.

VITAL SIGNS/HEMODYNAMICS
RR: ↑
HR: ↑; ↓ if conduction system block occurs
BP (with aortic stenosis): ↓, narrow pulse pressure
BP (with aortic insufficiency): ↑ SBP, widened pulse pressure
BP (with mitral stenosis or insufficiency): Possible ↓
CO: ↓
Other: With aortic valve problems, LVEDP ↑. With mitral valve problems, pulmonary congestion present.
ECG: AV node or bundle of His may be affected as infection spreads. RA, LA, or ventricular enlargement may be seen. Atrial dysrhythmias frequently seen.

LABORATORY STUDIES
Blood Cultures: Definitive diagnosis of infecting organism. If results negative, may be past acute infective phase.
Hematology Studies: Will show ↑ WBCs, ↑ eosinophils, and anemia.
Cardiac Enzyme Levels: ↑ if MI occurred as a result of emboli of vegetations in coronary arteries.
ABGs: Pulmonary dysfunction caused by cardiac disorder may result in ↓ Pao₂.

IMAGING
Echocardiogram: Reveals valvular involvement and vegetation size and defines severity of valvular dysfunction. Transoesphageal echocardiograms may be more useful in detecting vegetations.
Additional Studies: To assess for embolization to other organs (eg, renal, mesenteric, or peripheral arteriograms or CT scan).

Collaborative Management

Fluid and Sodium Limitations: Based on severity of symptoms to prevent fluid volume overload.
Bed Rest: Recommended initially, with activity limitations throughout remainder of treatment.
Diet: High in protein and calories to prevent cardiac cachexia.
Pharmacotherapy
Antibiotics: Usually 4-6 wks of IV antibiotics, with selection based on results of blood C&S studies.
Diuretics and vasodilators: To ↓ preload.
Positive inotropic agents (eg, digoxin, dobutamine, amrinone): To ↑ contractility and cardiac output.
Nitroprusside: To ↓ afterload.
Sedation: To allay anxiety during long period of hospitalization.
O₂: To maintain Pao₂ >60 mm Hg and O₂ saturation at >95%. Pulse oximetry used to verify satisfactory O₂ saturation.
Prophylaxis Regimen: Antibiotics given to individuals at risk who undergo dental, oral, upper respiratory tract, GU, or GI procedures.
Valve Replacement: Required when hemodynamic function deteriorates or if infection does not respond to antibiotic therapy.

PATIENT-FAMILY TEACHING
- To prevent IE recurrence, prophylactic antibiotics according to most recent AHA guidelines
- Stress-reduction techniques
- Importance of reporting S&S of *recurring infections:* fever, malaise, flushing, anorexia; *heart failure:* dyspnea, tachypnea, tachycardia, digital clubbing, edema, ascites, weight gain, jaundice

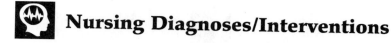

Nursing Diagnoses/Interventions

Decreased cardiac output r/t altered preload, afterload, or contractility secondary to valvular dysfunction

Desired outcomes: Within 72 h after therapy initiation, patient has adequate hemodynamic function: NSR or controlled A-fib on ECG, HR ≤100 bpm, BP ≥90/60 mm Hg, stable weight, I = O + insensible losses, RR ≤20 breaths/min with eupnea, and absence of clinical signs of heart failure.

- Assess heart sounds q2-4h. Change in the characteristics of heart murmur may signal progression of valvular dysfunction.
- Monitor heart rhythm continuously. Dysrhythmias or conduction defects may signal spread of infection or atrial volume overload.
- Monitor for LV heart failure: crackles, S_3/S_4 sounds, dyspnea, tachypnea, digital clubbing, ↑ pulse pressure and LVEDP, and ↓ BP and CO.
- Monitor for RV heart failure: ↑ CVP, JVD, positive hepatojugular reflex, edema, jaundice, ascites.
- Monitor I&O qh, and measure weight qd.
- If PAP or RAP high, ↓ preload by limiting fluid and sodium intake and administering diuretics and venous dilators as prescribed.
- If MAP high, ↓ afterload with prescribed arterial dilators.
- If afterload low, ↑ afterload with vasopressors. To prevent further ↓ caused by vasodilatation, avoid morphine sulfate or rapid rewarming.
- ↑ contractility with positive inotropes.
- Limit patient care activities; schedule activities to tolerance.
- Provide sedation as needed to ↓ O_2 consumption caused by anxiety/agitation.
- Prevent orthostatic hypotension by changing patient's position slowly.

Risk for infection r/t presence of invasive catheters and lines and inadequate secondary defenses r/t prolonged antibiotic use

Desired outcomes: Patient free of secondary infection: clear urine, wound healing within acceptable time frame, and absence of erythema, warmth, and purulent drainage at insertion sites for IV lines. On resolution of acute stage of IE, patient remains normothermic with WBC count ≤11,000 μl and negative culture results.

- Ensure strict aseptic technique for insertion site care for all invasive devices and IV lines.
- Provide mouth care q4h to ↓ oropharyngeal bacteria.
- For patients with indwelling urinary catheters, cleanse urinary meatus with soap and water during daily bath. Inspect urine for evidence of infection.
- Monitor temp, WBCs, and HR for ↑.
- Calculate SVR whenever CO measurements are obtained. Septic shock is demonstrated by ↑ CO, ↓ SVR, and ↑ Svo_2 during early stages.

Altered renal, gastrointestinal, peripheral, cardiopulmonary, and cerebral tissue perfusion (or risk for same) r/t interrupted arterial blood flow secondary to vegetative emboli

Desired outcome: Patient has adequate perfusion: UO ≥0.5 ml/kg/h, active bowel sounds, peripheral pulses >2+ on 0-4+ scale, BP ≥90/60 mm Hg, RR 12-20 breaths/min with eupnea, NSR on ECG, and orientation × 3.

- Monitor I&O for oliguria, which may be a sign of renal infarct.
- Monitor bowel sounds. Hypoactive or absent bowel sounds may be the result of mesenteric infarct.
- Assess peripheral pulses, color, and temp of extremities. ↓ pulses ≤2+ and pale and cool extremities may denote embolization.
- Monitor for confusion and changes in sensorimotor capabilities or cognition. Alterations can occur with cerebral emboli.
- Assess for chest pain, ↓ BP, SOB, ischemic or injury pattern on ECG, or ↑ cardiac enzymes. These may be signs of MI caused by migration of vegetative emboli to coronary arteries.
- Assess for splinter hemorrhages, Osler's nodes, Janeway lesions.

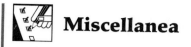

Miscellanea

CONSULT MD FOR
- Dysrhythmias; A-fib with rapid ventricular response
- LV heart failure: crackles, S_3 and S_4, dyspnea, ↓ BP, ↑ LVEDP, ↓ CO
- RV heart failure: ↑ CVP, JVD, positive hepatojugular reflex, edema, ascites
- Weight gain >1 kg/24 h
- Evidence of infection: eg, CV site, GU, bloodstream
- New-onset splinter hemorrhages, Osler's nodes, Janeway lesions
- Evidence of major organ/tissue infarction:
  Cerebral: Altered mental status, motor weakness
  Coronary: ST-segment elevation/depression, T-wave inversion, Q waves, chest pain, ↑ cardiac enzymes
  Extremites: ↓ pulses, coolness, pallor
  GI: ↓/absent bowel sounds, distention
  GU: UO <0.5 ml/kg/h × 2 h

RELATED TOPICS
- Antimicrobial therapy
- Aortic regurgitation
- Aortic stenosis
- Cardiac surgery: valvular disorders
- Heart failure, left ventricular
- Heart failure, right ventricular
- Hemodynamic monitoring
- Mitral regurgitation
- Mitral stenosis
- Shock, cardiogenic

ABBREVIATIONS
LVEDP: Left ventricular end-diastolic pressure
TUR: Transurethral resection

REFERENCES
Armstrong J: Antibiotic prophylaxis in patients undergoing endoscopic procedures, *Gastroenterol Nurs* 18(1): 36-37, 1995.

Baas LS, Steuble BT: Cardiovascular dysfunctions. In Swearingen PL, Keen JH (eds): *Manual of critical care nursing,* ed 3, 1995, St Louis, Mosby.

Blake GJ: Managing antibiotic prophylaxis for dental and upper respiratory tract procedures: how to protect susceptible patients from bacterial endocarditis, *Nursing* 25(1): 18-21, 1995.

Dajani AS et al: Prevention of bacterial endocarditis: recommendations of the American Heart Association, *JAMA* 264: 2919-2922, 1990.

Author: **Linda S. Baas**

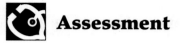 Overview

PATHOPHYSIOLOGY
Formed when there is a GI-cutaneous communication. High-output proximal small bowel fistulas, which have output >500 ml/24 h, are the most difficult to manage. Drainage is hypertonic; rich in enzymes, electrolytes, proteins; thin in consistency; often copious. Extensive skin and tissue breakdown often occurs because of activated pancreatic enzymes in fistula drainage. Fluid, electrolyte, and protein loss great. Drainage from distal sites, eg, ileum and colon, thick and has less volume. Sepsis, hypercatabolism, and malnutrition frequently associated with bowel fistulization.

HISTORY/RISK FACTORS
- Direct trauma to GI system, especially bowel
- Infection of surgical wound, drainage tract, peritoneum
- Prolonged catabolic state in association with bowel injury, GI neoplasm, GI abscess, or severe inflammatory bowel disease
- Complex GI surgical procedures

CLINICAL PRESENTATION
- Discharge of obvious bile, enteric contents, gas through surgical incision
- Sudden ↑ in drainage from surgical incision or drainage catheter
- Change in nature of drainage from serous or serosanguineous to yellow, green, brown, or foul-smelling
- S&S of dehydration, SIRS, sepsis
- With persistent fistulization: loss of weight, muscle mass resulting from protein loss and hypercatabolism

Assessment

PHYSICAL ASSESSMENT
- Sunken eyes, poor skin turgor, dry oral mucosa
- Peripheral edema, muscle wasting as a result of protein loss
- ↓/absent bowel sounds if peritonitis or ileus present
- Discomfort, guarding over abdominal mass (abscess) or near drain site or surgical incision
- Tenderness, erythema, pain at incision/fistula site because of irritation from fistula output or infection
- Muscle weakness, irregular HR if hypokalemia present

VITAL SIGNS/HEMODYNAMICS
RR: ↑
HR: ↑
BP: NI or ↓
Temp: ↑ if infection present
PAP: ↓ because of dehydration
CO: ↓
Other: SVR ↓ and CO ↑ if SIRS, sepsis present
ECG: Sinus tachycardia; hypokalemic changes, including PVCs, S-T segment depression, flattened T wave

LABORATORY STUDIES
Culture: Fistula effluent from stomach, duodenum, biliary tree, and pancreas may be cultured for evidence of infection. Small and large bowel fistulas generally not cultured because of expected presence of bacteria.

IMAGING
Radiography: Water-soluble contrast medium injected into suspected fistula (fistulography) to identify tract. CT scan may be used to identify and direct drainage of abscesses associated with fistulization.

DIAGNOSTIC PROCEDURES
Biopsy: May be obtained with neoplastic disease to identify malignancy.

Collaborative Management

Nutritional Support: With distal small bowel and colonic fistulas, enteral elemental diets may be infused into proximal small bowel if patient capable of proximal absorption. With proximal fistulas, feedings may be infused distal to fistula into the jejunum. Small bowel fistulas, prolonged adynamic ileus, or extensive intraabdominal sepsis usually requires TPN. Providing sufficient calories, protein, electrolytes, and fluids for high-output fistulas a challenge, but malnutrition associated with high mortality rates, and need for nutritional support imperative.

Fluid, Electrolyte Replacement: Balanced salt solutions, usually containing potassium, administered to maintain fluid and electrolyte balance. Often, amount to be delivered prescribed in direct relation to fistula output. Effluent from each fistula measured separately for accurate estimation of specific electrolyte and fluid losses.

Local Fistula Management: Drainage from each fistula collected separately to assess individual activity and healing. Systems of gravity or gentle suction drainage and barrier skin protection devised.

Antibiotics: As indicated for infection.

Surgery: Indicated in these instances: (1) to close fistulas that continue to drain significant amounts despite absence of infection and appropriate nutritional support, (2) to explore and drain fistula tracts not identified or drained by less invasive techniques, (3) if overwhelming sepsis fails to respond to antibiotics and supportive therapy. Usual operation to close persistently draining fistulas is resection with end-to-end anastomosis.

Postop: PN and antibiotic coverage continued. Gastrostomy usually created to enable prolonged intestinal decompression and drainage. Patient expected to remain NPO for 1-2 wks after surgery.

Nursing Diagnoses/Interventions

Impaired tissue integrity r/t chemical trauma, infection, or malnutrition
Desired outcome: Within 72 h of this diagnosis, tissue adjacent to fistula free of erythema, excoriation, and edema.
- Assess extent of problem: size, shape, location of fistula; potential leakage tracts created by skinfolds; condition of adjacent skin, tissue; consistency, character of fistula output. Be alert for damage to adjacent tissue (ie, severe local erythema, excoriation, edema, maceration).
- Establish drainage and collection system for each fistula. Use continuous wound suction device(s) as indicated.
  Clean intact skin with nonirritating antibacterial cleanser.
  Remove pooled drainage from wound and surrounding area.
  Apply barrier powder (eg, karaya, Orahesive) to excoriated skin.
  Protect intact skin with flexible transparent dressing (eg, OpSite).
  Attach collecting bag to barrier sheet base.
  For high-output fistulas, urostomy bag and collecting system may be necessary.
- Reposition frequently or use rotating bed to optimize gravity drainage of fistula output.
- If ↑ fistula output results from oral or enteral feedings, eliminate or modify these feedings.
- Consult ostomy nurse for recommendations in pouching complex or multiple fistulas.

Altered nutrition: Less than body requirements, r/t protein loss *via* fistula output, disruption of GI tract continuity, or absorptive disorder
Desired outcome: By time of hospital discharge, patient has adequate nutrition: food intake ↑ to RDA; body weight returns to baseline or within 10% of patient's ideal weight.
- Collaborate with physician, dietitian, and pharmacist to estimate metabolic needs based on activity level, estimated metabolic rate, baseline nutritional status.
- Monitor for bowel sounds q8h. If absent, withhold oral or enteral feedings.
- If fistula output ↑ in response to enteral feedings, ↓ rate of infusion or reduce feeding strength. If patient tolerates oral feedings but fistula output ↑, ↑ feeding frequency and ↓ amount consumed at each feeding.
- Be aware that when entire intestine is not available for nl absorption, elemental feeding formulas may be more readily absorbed.
- Prepare patient for parenteral feedings as necessary.

Risk for infection r/t inadequate primary defenses, hypercatabolic state, presence of invasive lines, and protein loss/malnutrition
Desired outcome: Patient free of infection: core or rectal temp <37.8° C (100° F), negative culture results, HR 60-100 bpm, RR 12-20 breaths/min, BP wnl for patient, and orientation × 3.
- Check for ↑ rectal or core temp q4h.
- If there is a sudden ↑ in temp, assess likely sites for infection.
- Evaluate orientation and LOC q4h. Document and report significant deviations from baseline.
- Monitor BP, HR, RR, CO, and SVR q4h. Be alert to ↑ HR and RR associated with temp elevations. ↑ CO and ↓ SVR suggest sepsis or SIRS.
- Give parenteral antibiotics in a timely fashion. Reschedule antibiotics if dose delayed >1 h. Failure to administer antibiotics on schedule can result in inadequate blood levels and treatment failure. Aminoglycosides used frequently; monitor for nephrotoxicity, ototoxicity.
- Optimize gravity drainage of fistula by prone or upright positioning as tolerated.
- Wear gloves when contact with drainage possible. Wash hands thoroughly before/after caring for patient and dispose of dressings and drainage carefully.

Fluid volume deficit r/t active loss secondary to fistula drainage
Desired outcome: Within 8 h of this diagnosis, patient normovolemic: balanced daily I&O, UO ≥0.5 ml/kg/h, urine specific gravity 1.010-1.020, moist mucous membranes, good skin turgor, HR ≤100 bpm, CVP/RAP 2-6 mm Hg, and PAWP 6-12 mm Hg.
- Evaluate fluid balance by calculating and comparing daily I&O. With high-output fistulas, evaluate total I&O q8h. Record all sources of output, including fistula drainage. Replace fistula output with prescribed fluid (usually a balanced salt solution containing potassium).
- Measure UO q1-4h. Be alert for UO <0.5 ml/kg/h or ↑ specific gravity with ↓ urine volume.
- Assess and document condition of mucous membranes and skin turgor. Dry membranes and inelastic skin indicate inadequate fluid volume and need for ↑ fluid intake.
- Measure and evaluate VS, CVP, and PAP (when available) q1-4h, depending on hemodynamic stability. Be alert to ↑ HR, ↓ CVP, and ↓ PAP, which indicate inadequate intravascular volume. Encourage ↑ oral fluid intake as appropriate.
- Control sources of insensible fluid loss by humidifying O_2, maintaining comfortable environment, and controlling fever with antipyretics such as acetaminophen.

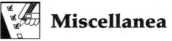

Miscellanea

CONSULT MD FOR
- Unanticipated ↑ in fistula output
- Hypokalemic ECG changes, hemodynamically significant dysrhythmias
- S&S of surgical site, bloodstream, or other infection
- Fluid, electrolyte imbalance including S&S of hypovolemia, hypokalemia, hyponatremia, hypoalbuminemia

RELATED TOPICS
- Fecal ostomies/diversions
- Hypovolemia
- Nutritional support, parenteral
- Shock, septic
- Systemic inflammatory response syndrome
- Vancomycin-resistant entercocci

ABBREVIATION
SIRS: Systemic inflammatory response syndrome

REFERENCES
Keen JH: Enterocutaneous fistulas. In Swearingen PL, Keen JH (eds): *Manual of critical care nursing,* ed 3, St Louis, 1995, Mosby.
Krumberger J: Gastrointestinal disorders. In Kinney M, Packa D, Dunbar S (eds): *AACN's clinical reference for critical care nursing,* ed 3, St Louis, 1993, Mosby.
Lange MP et al: Management of multiple enterocutaneous fistulas, *Heart Lung* 18(4): 386-390, 1989.

Author: **Janet Hicks Keen**

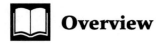 **Overview**

PATHOPHYSIOLOGY
When blood flow is obstructed through the liver, collateral vessels develop to divert blood from portal circulation into systemic circulation. These high-pressure collateral vessels are known as varices. Their rupture leads to dramatic hematemesis and hemorrhage, which is difficult to control and is exacerbated by thrombocytopenia and clotting disorders often found with hepatic disease. Problems associated with portosystemic shunting of blood include impaired liver function, encephalopathy, septicemia, and metabolic abnormalities. Acute variceal bleeding results in hypoxic damage to liver cells and complications such as jaundice, ascites, and encephalopathy. Mortality rate related directly to degree of hepatocellular failure.

HISTORY/RISK FACTORS
- Cirrhosis, hepatitis, biliary disease
- Traumatic portal vein injury, tumor invasion
- Events that may precipitate bleeding in gastroesophageal varices: insertion of gastric tube, coagulopathy and/or heparin therapy, mechanical irritants (eg, rough or unchewed food), Valsalva's maneuver, vigorous coughing

CLINICAL PRESENTATION
Sudden, massive hematemesis. Average amount of blood lost during single bleeding episode is 10 U. Melena, with or without hematemesis, another frequent occurrence. Rapid blood loss initially causes thirst, then dizziness, and ultimately hypovolemic shock as hemorrhage continues.

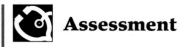 **Assessment**

PHYSICAL ASSESSMENT
Cool and pale skin, altered mental status, pale and dry oral mucosa, cracked lips. Yellowing of skin and sclera associated with jaundice. Mild to marked peripheral edema and ascites. Splenomegaly commonly associated with portal hypertension. Cirrhotic liver usually small and firm. Enlarged, tender liver associated with hepatic inflammation. If aspiration of gastric contents has occurred, coarse crackles and rhonchi may be auscultated.

VITAL SIGNS/HEMODYNAMICS
RR: ↑
HR: ↑
BP: ↓
Temp: NI
CVP/PAP: ↓
CO: ↓
SVR: ↑
Other: In hepatic failure, hyperdynamic CV state may be present. Associated findings include ↑ CO, ↓ PVR, bounding pulses, and warm, flushed extremities. Hyperdynamic state more apparent with volume resuscitation and portal decompression surgery.
ECG: Sinus tachycardia. Ischemic changes possible if profound acute anemia present, especially with preexisting CV disorders.

LABORATORY STUDIES
Hematology: ↓ Hct, Hgb. Platelets and WBCs may be ↓ because of splenic enlargement. PT prolonged because of clotting factor deficiency with hepatocellular disease.
Biochemistry: Severity of liver damage estimated by ↑ serum total bilirubin, ↓ serum albumin, prolonged PT. Serum ammonia ↑ as blood is shunted from liver by collateral vessels and failing liver is unable to convert ammonia to urea. Large protein load from GI bleeding may result in greatly ↑ ammonia levels. BUN ↑ because of hypovolemia and ↑ protein load. ↑ BUN/creatinine suggests onset of ARF.
Blood Alcohol: May be tested on admission to help distinguish acute intoxication from encephalopathy.
Occult Blood: Tests for blood in stool, gastric secretions.

IMAGING
Portal Venography: Establishes portal vein patency and visualizes portosystemic collateral vessels to determine cause and effective treatment. HVWP measured by introducing balloon catheter into femoral vein and threading it into a hepatic vein branch. NI HVWP 5-6 mm Hg; values of ≈ 20 mm Hg typical with cirrhosis.
Transhepatic Portography: Obliteration of varices *via* injection of thrombin or Gelfoam into veins that supply the varices.
Barium Swallow: Used in nonemergency situations to verify presence of gastroesophageal varices.

DIAGNOSTIC PROCEDURES
Esophagoscopy: Varices in esophagus and upper portion of stomach identified, and attempts made to identify exact source of bleeding. Variceal bleeding may be treated by injection sclerotherapy during this procedure. Serious complications: aspiration, cardiac dysrhythmias. ET intubation may be performed before procedure to protect airway.
Liver Biopsy: Liver specimen obtained by direct puncture or other methods.

Collaborative Management

Fluid Resuscitation: Combinations of isotonic IV solutions, albumin, PRBCs, FFP used. Until blood products available, emergency resuscitation with D_5W and albumin, sodium chloride, or LR initiated. Excessive saline infusions usually avoided to prevent ascites. LR not recommended with significant liver dysfunction because the damaged liver may be unable to convert lactate to bicarbonate, thereby contributing to metabolic acidosis. FFP helpful in restoring deficient clotting factors. Platelets given only if platelet count markedly ↓ or if spontaneous bleeding occurs from nonvariceal sites. Hemodynamic monitoring essential to prevent hypovolemic shock while avoiding overtransfusion, which can ↑ variceal pressure and trigger rebleeding.

Vasopressin (Pitressin): Potent vasoconstrictor that controls variceal hemorrhage by constricting mesenteric, splenic, and hepatic arteriolar beds, causing ↓ blood flow to portal vein and ↓ portal venous pressure. Typically, 20 U in 100 ml D_5W given IV over a 20-min period, followed by continuous IV infusion of 0.1-0.4 U/min. IV nitroglycerin may be given concurrently to counter vasopressin-induced cardiac side effects such as vasoconstriction and to ↓ portal venous constriction.

Gastric Intubation: Insertion of gastric tube may trigger additional bleeding; usually avoided if bleeding source known to be variceal.

Endoscopic Sclerotherapy: During endoscopy, varices injected with sclerosing solution such as sodium tetradecyl sulfate or morrhuate to contract varix and stop bleeding. Sclerosing solution causes variceal inflammation, venous thrombosis, and eventual scar tissue. Repeated injections strengthen scar tissue in esophageal wall and ↓ risk of recurrent hemorrhage. Esophageal ulceration a serious complication of sclerotherapy. Ulcer prophylaxis with antacids, H_2-receptor blockers, sucralfate may be initiated.

Esophageal Balloon Tamponade: Achieves temporary control of variceal hemorrhage *via* inflation of esophageal and gastric balloons until balloon pressure > variceal pressure, thereby tamponading bleeding vessels. Multilumen (S-B, Minnesota) tube passed through mouth into stomach. Gastric and esophageal balloons inflated. Firm traction exerted by taping tube to mouth guard of a football helmet, which maintains correct positioning. Complications numerous, including pharyngeal obstruction with possible asphyxia and mucosal erosion with variceal rupture. Useful for controlling acute bleeding until definitive therapy available (eg, sclerotherapy, surgery), but balloon should not be inflated for >24 h.

TIPS: Invasive radiologic intervention in which expandable metal stent is inserted through the liver parenchyma *via* angiographically directed balloon catheter. Stent expansion provides a vascular shunt between portal and hepatic veins. Portal pressure ↓; varices decompressed. *Potential complications:* puncture of vascular structures or viscera resulting in hemorrhage or septicemia.

Surgical Management: Emergency surgery for variceal bleeding is associated with significant mortality rate. It is desirable to control acute bleeding medically and schedule elective surgery when condition has stabilized.

Portosystemic shunts: Lower portal pressure by joining portal vein with vena cava. *Disadvantage:* total diversion of portal blood flow and consequent disabling encephalopathy in many patients.

Distal splenorenal shunt: Diverts blood from troublesome varices *via* short gastric and splenic veins to the renal vein. Portal blood flow to liver preserved, and incidence of encephalopathy greatly reduced.

Other surgical methods: Include stapling transection of lower esophagus and devascularization procedures.

PATIENT/FAMILY TEACHING

- S&S of actual/impending hemorrhage: nausea, dark stools, lightheadedness, vomiting of blood, passing of frank blood in stools; importance of seeking medical attention promptly if these S&S appear
- Importance of medical follow-up for management of variceal bleeding
- Medications: drug name, purpose, dosage, schedule, precautions, food-drug and drug-drug interactions, potential side effects
- Necessity of avoiding heavy lifting, straining, other activities associated with Valsalva's maneuver
- Importance of avoiding mechanically irritating foods, such as nuts, corn chips, unchewed food, and ingestion of NSAIDs and alcohol, which irritate esophageal and gastric mucosa

Nursing Diagnoses/Interventions

Fluid volume deficit r/t active loss of circulating blood volume secondary to variceal bleeding, invasive interventions, or surgery

Desired outcome: Within 12 h of this diagnosis, patient normovolemic: MAP >70 mm Hg, HR 60-100 bpm, brisk capillary refill (<2 sec), CVP 2-6 mm Hg, PAWP 6-12 mm Hg, CI ≥3.0 L/min/m^2, UO ≥0.5 ml/kg/h, orientation × 3.

- Administer prescribed fluids at rapid rate (wide open for active, massive bleeding). Minimize IV infusion of sodium-containing solutions, which can contribute to ascites and precipitate hepatorenal syndrome in susceptible patients.
- Monitor HR, BP, ECG, and CV status q15min, or more frequently with active bleeding or if using vasopressin or similar agents. Be alert to ↑ HR, ↓ MAP of ≥10 mm Hg less than baseline, and delayed capillary refill. Anticipate vasopressin-induced reflex bradycardia; consult physician if bradycardia severe (HR <60 bpm) or compromises tissue perfusion.
- Measure central pressures and thermodilution CO/CI q1-2h or more frequently if unstable. Be alert to low/↓ CVP and PAWP. Assess for signs of overaggressive fluid resuscitation: ↑ CVP, PAP, PAWP, and aggravation of variceal bleeding in some patients. Anticipate compensatory ↑ in CO/CI, with CI usually ≥3.0. Monitor Svo$_2$ as available to evaluate adequacy of tissue oxygenation. Evaluate volume status by noting ↑ or ↓ in PAWP and UO.
- Measure UO qh. Be alert to output <0.5 ml/kg/h for 2 consecutive h. Anticipate ↓ UO after initial dose of vasopressin. Expect diuresis after vasopressin discontinued.
- Monitor for physical indicators of hypovolemia, including cool extremities, capillary refill ≥2 sec, absent/↓ amplitude of distal pulses, change in LOC.
- Measure and record all GI blood losses from hematemesis, hematochezia (red blood through rectum), melena. Test all stools and gastric contents for occult blood.
- Administer vasopressin. Ensure patency of IV catheter qh to avoid severe necrosis associated with extravasation. Monitor for serious side effects such as bradycardia, ventricular irritability, chest pain, abdominal cramping, hyponatremia, water intoxication, oliguria. Administer concurrently with IV nitroglycerin to ↓ adverse CV effects and improve efficacy.
- Avoid use of indwelling gastric tubes for routine gastric drainage because they can irritate varices and prolong or renew bleeding.
- Be alert to adverse side effects of esophageal sclerotherapy: infection, pulmonary complications (ie, Pao$_2$ <80 mm Hg, basilar crackles, ↓ breath sounds), and esophageal ulceration (ie, difficulty in swallowing, pain, continued bleeding). Anticipate mild retrosternal pain and transient fever postprocedure.
- Monitor for complications r/t TIPS: hepatic or vascular bleeding (↓ BP, ↓ Hct/Hgb, ↓ CO, ↑ abdominal girth; inadvertent puncture of gallbladder, other viscera with subsequent gram-negative sepsis (↓ BP, ↑ HR, ↓ UO, fever).

Decreased cardiac output r/t altered rate or rhythm secondary to myocardial ischemia from prolonged, massive bleeding or vasopressin-induced coronary vasoconstriction; r/t ↓ preload secondary to acute blood loss; or r/t ↑ afterload secondary to vasoconstrictive effects of shock or vasopressin therapy

Desired outcome: Within 24 h of this diagnosis, patient's cardiac output adequate: NSR on ECG, CI wnl or ↑ (≥3.0 L/min/m^2), MAP >70 mm Hg, Svo$_2$ 60%-80%.

- Monitor BP, HR, ECG, PAP (see first three bulleted entries in preceding nursing diagnosis/intervention).
- Administer O$_2$ and adjust as necessary to maintain Spo$_2$ ≥92% or Sao$_2$ ≥80. Place patient in semi-Fowler's position to optimize oxygenation.
- Monitor Hct; administer PRBCs as necessary for values <28/100 ml.
- Monitor for evidence of myocardial ischemia if Hgb greatly ↓ or if patient receiving vasopressin. Observe for ventricular dysrhythmias and ST-segment changes. Instruct patient to report chest discomfort promptly. Administer nitrates as indicated.

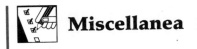 # Miscellanea

CONSULT MD FOR
- Serious side effects of vasopressin therapy: hemodynamically significant bradycardia, ventricular dysrhythmias, chest pain, ischemic ECG changes, severe bowel cramping, water intoxication, oliguria
- Displacement of multilumen tube
- S&S of complications: hemorrhagic shock, hepatic encephalopathy, hepatorenal failure

RELATED TOPICS
- Cirrhosis
- Pneumonia, aspiration
- Shock, hemorrhagic
- Systemic inflammatory response syndrome
- Transfusion therapies

ABBREVIATIONS
FFP: Fresh frozen plasma
HVWP: Hepatic vein wedge pressure
PRBCs: Packed red blood cells
S-B: Sengstaken-Blakemore
Svo$_2$: Mixed venous oxygen saturation
TIPS: Transjugular intrahepatic portosystemic shunt

- Minimize patient's activity during acute bleeding episode to ↓ myocardial O_2 demands. Explain and encourage adherence to total bed rest regimen. As available monitor Svo_2 to evaluate adequacy of tissue oxygenation.
- Measure thermodilution CO q1-2h. Be aware that a "normal" CO may be a low value in a hyperdynamic circulatory state associated with cirrhosis. Compare to baseline or watch for trend of ↓ values. Maintain CI $\geq$3.0 L/min/m^2.

Ineffective airway clearance r/t tracheobronchial obstruction by esophageal balloon device; tracheobronchial obstruction by pharyngeal secretions above the inflated esophageal balloon device; or perceptual/cognitive impairment secondary to encephalopathy

Desired outcome: Within 4 h of this diagnosis, patient's airway clear: nl breath sounds, absence of adventitious sounds, and RR 12-20 breaths/min with eupnea.

- Place in side-lying position during vomiting episodes unless patient *fully* alert and more comfortable in upright position.
- As necessary, suction oropharynx with Yankauer or similar suction device to remove blood and secretions.
- Auscultate lung fields during/after vomiting episodes for rhonchi, which can signal aspiration of gastric contents.
- Provide oral care at frequent intervals to assist in mobilizing oropharyngeal secretions. A dilute solution of hydrogen peroxide and NS may be helpful in removing tenacious secretions or dried blood from teeth and oral mucosa.
- Monitor for early signs of respiratory failure: ↑ RR, WOB, and $Paco_2$; ↓ Spo_2 and Pao_2.
- Implement these interventions for patients with S-B or similar tube:
    Verify proper tube placement by immediate chest x-ray.
    Be certain that oral secretions are suctioned from above the inflated esophageal balloon *via* proximal tube or additional lumen in the tube for this purpose. Label proximal tube or lumen with the warning, "Do not irrigate."
    Ensure patency of gastric and esophageal drainage lumens. Irrigate *gastric* lumen q1-2h and prn to ensure patency.
    Be aware that proximal migration of the esophageal balloon or rupture of the gastric balloon may result in total airway obstruction. Keep scissors in an obvious place near patient in order to immediately deflate all lumens of the S-B tube should respiratory distress occur.
    Check security of tape, tube connections, and traction initially and q2h. Firm traction established by taping the tube to a helmet or a firm, padded retainer.
    Document quantity, characteristics of gastric drainage q4h.

Altered esophageal tissue perfusion (or risk of same) r/t interruption of venous and arterial blood flow secondary to pressure on esophageal tissue from balloon tamponade

Desired outcomes: Esophageal balloon pressure maintained within prescribed range (usually 20-45 mm Hg). Patient has no symptoms of esophageal perforation: BP wnl for patient, HR 60-100 bpm, and absence of sudden substernal or back pain.

- Check esophageal balloon pressure q2-4h. Maintain pressure within prescribed range (usually 20-45 mm Hg). Release pressure at prescribed intervals.
- Carefully document date and time of balloon inflation and deflation. Tissue necrosis likely to occur if balloons left inflated for >24 h.
- After 24 h, assist physician in relieving traction and deflating esophageal balloon. Tube remains in place with gastric balloon inflated for next 24 h, and patient closely monitored for rebleeding. If there is no further rebleeding, the gastric balloon is deflated and the tube removed.
- Be alert for signs of esophageal perforation: sudden epigastric or substernal pain, back pain, shock state.

REFERENCES

Bouley G et al: Transjugular intrahepatic portosystemic shunt: an alternative, *Crit Care Nurse* 16(1): 23-29, 1996.

Butler R: Managing the complications of cirrhosis, *Am J Nurs* 94(3): 46-49, 1994.

Covington J: Nursing care of patients with alcoholic liver disease, *Crit Care Nurse* 13(3): 47-57, 1993.

Keen JH: Bleeding esophageal varices. In Swearingen PL, Keen JH (eds): *Manual of critical care nursing,* ed 3, St Louis, 1995, Mosby.

Kerber K: The adult with bleeding esophageal varices, *Crit Care Nurs Clin North Am* 5(1): 153-162, 1993.

Author: **Janet Hicks Keen**

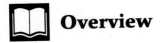 **Overview**

PATHOPHYSIOLOGY

It is sometimes necessary to interrupt continuity of the bowel because of trauma, intestinal disease, or associated complications. The resulting fecal diversion can be located anywhere along the bowel, depending on site of diseased or injured portion; it can be permanent or temporary. Most common sites are the colon and ileum.

HISTORY/RISK FACTORS

- Diverticulitis
- Colorectal cancer
- Polyps/familial adenomatous polyposis
- Ulcerative colitis, Crohn's disease
- Abdominal trauma
- Mesenteric ischemia/bowel infarction
- Atonic colon, Hirschprung's disease

CLINICAL PRESENTATION

Depends on underlying disease process

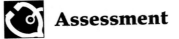 **Assessment**

PHYSICAL ASSESSMENT (immediate postop)

Ostomy Appearance: Bright-to-beefy red and moist stoma.

Bowel Sounds: Hypoactive for 24-48 h.

Abdominal Distention: May be present first 24-72 h postop until peristalsis returns and passage of flatus occurs.

Ostomy Output

Colostomy: Initial (24-72 h) usually serosanguineous drainage. Initial stool output (3-5 days) usually thick brown liquid. Later, will be mushy to semiformed to formed.

Ileostomy (conventional [Brooke] or temporary): Initial (24-48 h) usually serosanguineous drainage. Initial effluent (48-72 h) usually viscous, shiny, dark green liquid. Later, pastelike and light to medium brown.

Continent ileostomy (Kock pouch): Initial (24-48 h) usually serosanguineous with/without blood clots draining through stoma catheter and into pouch. Later, pastelike and light to medium brown.

VITAL SIGNS/HEMODYNAMICS

Reflect clinical status rather than actual procedure.

Evidence of Hemorrhagic Shock: ↑ RR, HR; ↓ BP, CVP/PAP, CO

Evidence of Infection: ↑ RR, ↑ HR, ↓ BP, ↑ temp

Early Sepsis: ↓ SVR with ↑ CO

Late Sepsis: ↑ SVR with ↓ CO

LABORATORY STUDIES

CBC: To check for presence of infection caused by bowel perforation (preop) or surgical site infection (postop). Hct, Hgb checked to monitor for acute blood loss.

Chemistries: To check for electrolyte imbalance, especially hypokalemia caused by fluid shifts/dehydration.

IMAGING

Abdominal X-rays: Flat plate and upright to check for obstructions, ↑ air/fluid levels in bowel, or free air under diaphragm, which suggests bowel perforation/disruption.

Upper GI Series with Small Bowel Followthrough, Hypaque or Gastrografin Enema, CT Scan with Oral Contrast: To assess for perforation, abscess, or fistula.

Collaborative Management

Colostomy: Created when a portion of the colon is brought to the abdominal skin surface. An opening in the exteriorized colon permits elimination of flatus and stool through the stoma.

Transverse: Temporary means of diverting the fecal stream. Performed before definitive surgery when bowel obstruction or colon perforation present. Stool is soft, unformed, and eliminated unpredictably. May be double-barreled, with a proximal stoma through which stool is eliminated and a distal stoma adjacent to proximal stoma called a mucus fistula.

Descending or sigmoid: Usually a permanent fecal diversion; often performed for rectal cancer. Stool is usually formed and predictable.

Ileostomy

Conventional (Brooke): Distal portion of ileum is brought up and out onto skin surface of abdominal wall. Some indications include ulcerative colitis, Crohn's disease, and familial adenomatous polyposis.

Temporary: Usually a loop stoma with or without a supporting rod in place beneath ileal loop until exteriorized loop of ileum becomes affixed to skin. Diverts fecal stream away from a more distal anastomosis or fistula repair site until healing occurs. Output is usually liquid or pastelike, contains digestive enzymes, and eliminated continually. Pouch necessary to collect gas and fecal discharge.

Continent (Kock pouch): Intraabdominal pouch constructed from ≈ 30 cm of distal ileum. A portion of ileum is intussuscepted to form an outlet valve from the pouch to the abdominal skin, where a stoma is constructed. The intraabdominal pouch is continent for gas and fecal discharge and emptied ≈ qid by inserting a catheter through the stoma. A small dressing is worn over the stoma to collect mucus.

Ileoanal reservoir: To preserve fecal continence and prevent need for permanent ileostomy. During first stage after total colectomy, an ileal reservoir is constructed just above ileal junction and anal canal; the ileal outlet from the reservoir is brought down through the rectal muscle cuff and anastomosed to the anal canal. Anal sphincter is preserved, and resulting ileal reservoir provides a storage place for feces. A temporary diverting ileostomy required for 2-3 mos to allow healing of anastomosis. Second stage occurs when the diverting ileostomy is taken down and fecal continuity is restored.

PATIENT-FAMILY TEACHING

- Importance of dietary management to promote nutritional and fluid maintenance
- Care of incision, dressing changes, permission to take baths or showers once sutures/drains are removed
- Care of stoma, peristomal, perianal skin; use of ostomy equipment; method for obtaining supplies
- Gradual resumption of ADL, excluding heavy lifting, pushing, or pulling for 6-8 wks
- Referral to community resources including home health care agency, ET nurse, and local chapter of United Ostomy Association (toll-free number: 800-826-0826)
- Importance of follow-up care with physician and ET nurse; confirm date and time of next appointment
- Importance of reporting S&S that necessitate medical attention, such as change in stoma color from nl bright and shiny red; peristomal or perianal skin irritation; any significant changes in appearance, frequency, and consistency of stools; fever, chills, abdominal pain, or distention; and incisional pain, drainage, swelling, or redness

Nursing Diagnoses/Interventions

Risk for impaired peristomal skin integrity r/t exposure to effluent or sensitivity to appliance material

Impaired stomal tissue integrity (or risk of same) r/t improperly fitted appliance resulting in impaired circulation

Desired outcome: Patient's stomal and peristomal skin and tissue remain intact.

AFTER COLOSTOMY OR CONVENTIONAL ILEOSTOMY

- Apply a pectin, methylcellulose-based, solid-form skin barrier around stoma to protect peristomal skin from contact with stool, which causes irritation.

    Cut an opening in the skin barrier about 1/16 to 1/8 in larger than the stoma, remove release paper, and apply sticky surface directly to peristomal skin.

    Remove skin barrier and inspect skin q3-4days. Peristomal skin should look like other abdominal skin. Changes such as erythema, erosion, serous drainage, bleeding, or induration signal infection, irritation, or sensitivity to materials placed on the skin.

    Because stomas become less edematous for some wks after surgery, the skin barrier opening must be remeasured each time it is changed.

- Apply a two-piece pouch system, pouch with access cap, or transparent pouch so that the stoma can be inspected for viability q8h. A matured stoma will be red in color with overlying mucus. A nonmatured stoma will be red and moist where mucous membrane is exposed, but can be a darker, mottled, grayish-red with a transparent or translucent film of serosa elsewhere.

- When removing skin barrier and pouch for routine care, cleanse skin with warm tap water, using soap only if skin is covered with sticky stool. Rinse off any residual and pat dry gently.

- To maintain a secure pouch seal, empty the pouch when it is ⅓-½ full of stool or gas.

AFTER CONTINENT ILEOSTOMY (KOCK POUCH)

- A 28F or 30F catheter is inserted through the stoma and into the pouch and sutured to peristomal skin. Avoid stress on the suture, and monitor for erythema, induration, drainage, or erosion. As prescribed, maintain catheter on low, continuous suction or gravity drainage to prevent stress on the nipple valve, and maintain pouch decompression.

- Check catheter q2h for patency, and irrigate with sterile saline (30 ml) to prevent obstruction. Confer with physician if unable to instill solution, if there is no return, or if leakage of irrigating solution or pouch contents appears around the catheter.

- Change 4×4 dressing around stoma q2h or as often as it becomes wet. Drainage will be serosanguineous at first and mixed with mucus.

- Assess stoma for viability with each dressing change. A stoma that is pale or dark purple to black or dull in appearance can indicate circulatory impairment and should be reported immediately.

AFTER ILEOANAL RESERVOIR

- Perform routine care for diverting ileostomy (see earlier).

- After the operation's first stage, there may be incontinence of mucus. Maintain perineal/perianal skin integrity by gently cleansing the area with water and cotton balls, soft tissues, or commercial perianal cleanser. Avoid soap, which can cause itching or irritation. Use absorbent pad at night to absorb incontinence of mucus. Irrigate pouch qd as prescribed.

- After the operation's second stage (when the ileostomy is taken down), expect patient to experience frequency and urgency of defecation.

- Wash perineal/perianal area with warm water or commercial perianal/perineal cleansing solution, using squeeze bottle, cotton balls, or soft tissues. Do not use toilet paper because it can cause irritation.

- Provide sitz baths to promote comfort and help clean perineal/perianal area.

- Apply protective skin sealants or ointments. Avoid skin sealants on irritated or eroded skin.

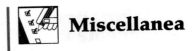 **Miscellanea**

CONSULT MD FOR

- Changes in peristomal skin: erythema, erosion, serous drainage, bleeding, induration, separation of stoma from peristomal skin/abdominal surface
- Impaired stomal viability: stoma that is pale, dark purple, black, or dull in appearance
- Frank bleeding from stoma, Kock pouch, ileoanal reservoir, or surgical site
- S&S of complications: hemorrhagic shock, septicemia, paralytic ileus, peritonitis, anastomotic leak, obstruction, stomal ischemia/necrosis

RELATED TOPICS

- Abdominal trauma
- Hypovolemia
- Peritonitis
- Shock, hemorrhagic
- Shock, septic

Bowel incontinence r/t disruption of nl function with fecal diversion

Desired outcomes: Within 2-4 days after surgery, patient has bowel sounds and eliminates gas and stool *via* fecal diversion. Within 3 days after teaching has been initiated, patient verbalizes understanding of measures that will maintain nl elimination pattern and demonstrates care techniques specific to the fecal diversion.

AFTER COLOSTOMY AND CONVENTIONAL ILEOSTOMY

- Empty stool from the pouch's bottom opening, and assess stool quality/quantity to document return of bowel function.
- If the colostomy is not eliminating stool after 3-4 days and bowel sounds have returned, gently insert a gloved, lubricated finger into the stoma to determine presence of stricture at the skin or fascial levels and note presence of any stool. Colostomy irrigation may be prescribed to stimulate elimination of gas and stool.

AFTER CONTINENT ILEOSTOMY (KOCK POUCH)

- Monitor I&O, and record color and consistency of output.
- Expect aspiration of bright red blood or serosanguineous liquid drainage from the Kock pouch during the early postop period.
- As GI function returns after 2-4 days, expect drainage to change in color from blood-tinged to greenish-brown liquid. When ileal output appears, suction (if present) is discontinued and the pouch catheter is placed to gravity drainage.
- As the diet progresses from clear liquids to solid food, ileal output thickens. Check and irrigate catheter q2h and prn to maintain patency. If patient reports abdominal fullness in pouch area along with ↓ fecal output, check catheter placement and patency.

AFTER ILEOANAL RESERVOIR

- Monitor I&O, observing quantity, quality, and consistency of output from diverting ileostomy and reservoir. Monitor for temp ↑ accompanied by perianal pain and discharge of purulent, bloody mucus from drains and anal orifice.
- If drains are present, irrigate as prescribed to maintain patency, ↓ stress on suture lines, and ↓ incidence of infection.
- After the operation's first stage, patient may experience mucus incontinence. Patient can wear small pad to avoid soiling of garments.
- After the operation's second stage (when the ileostomy is taken down), expect incontinence and 15-20 bowel movements/day with urgency when patient is on a clear-liquid diet. Assist patient with perianal care, and apply protective skin care products. To ↓ incontinence at night, catheter can be placed in reservoir and connected to gravity drainage bag.
- When patient is on solid foods the number of bowel movements will ↓ to 6-12/day and consistency will thicken.
- Administer hydrophilic colloids and antidiarrheals as indicated to ↓ frequency and fluidity of stools.

Body image disturbance r/t presence of fecal diversion

Desired outcome: Within 5-7 days after surgery, patient demonstrates acceptance of the fecal diversion and incorporates changes into self-concept as evidenced by acknowledging body changes, viewing the stoma, and participating in care of the fecal diversion.

- Expect the following fears, which may be expressed by patients experiencing a fecal diversion: physical, social, and work activities will be curtailed significantly; rejection, isolation, and feelings of uncleanliness will occur; odor will be present and loss of voluntary control may occur.
- Encourage discussion of feelings and fears; clarify any misconceptions. Involve family members in discussions because they, too, may have anxieties and misconceptions.
- Provide calm and quiet environment for patient and significant others to discuss the surgery. Initiate open and honest discussion.
- Encourage acceptance of fecal diversion by having patient participate in care. Assure patient that education offers a means of control.
- Consult with surgeon about a visit by another ostomate.

REFERENCES

Adrien L: Fecal diversions. In Swearingen PL (ed): *Manual of medical-surgical nursing care,* ed 3, St Louis, 1994, Mosby.

Hampton BG, Bryant PA: *Ostomies and continent diversions: nursing management,* St Louis, 1992, Mosby.

Hull TL, Erwin-Toth P: The pelvic pouch procedure and continent ostomies: overview and controversies, *J Wound, Ostomy, Continence Nurs* 23(3): 156-165, 1996.

Paulford-Lecher N: Teaching your patient stoma care, *Nursing* 23(9): 47-49, 1993.

Author: **Lolita Adrien**

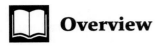 **Overview**

PATHOPHYSIOLOGY
Severe and potentially fatal complication of blunt chest trauma. Occurs when three or more adjacent ribs fracture in two or more places (or sternum fractures, along with ribs adjacent to fracture). Fracture segment moves independently in response to intrathoracic pressure: retracting on inspiration and bulging on expiration. Forces required to fracture multiple ribs or sternum usually great; underlying lung tissue may be seriously damaged. Pulmonary contusion likely, and pneumothorax a common complication.

HISTORY/RISK FACTORS
- Vehicular collision, sports-related injury, fall
- Auto/pedestrian trauma
- Act of violence
- Intoxication
- Thrill-seeking behaviors
- Failure to use safety devices (air bag, seat belt)
- Chronic illness resulting in debilitation
- Advanced age, eg, resulting in osteoporosis

CLINICAL PRESENTATION
- Paradoxic chest wall motion: hallmark symptom
- Dyspnea, SOB, tachypnea
- Agitation, restlessness, anxiety
- Localized severe chest pain during respirations

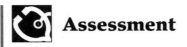 **Assessment**

PHYSICAL ASSESSMENT
Inspection: RR >20 breaths/min, use of accessory muscles, ↓ tidal volume, hemoptysis, asymmetric/paradoxic chest wall motion, inability to clear tracheobronchial secretions, splinting, cyanosis or pallor, ecchymosis over underlying injury
Palpation: Subcutaneous emphysema of neck and upper chest, tenderness at fracture points, stepdown at area of flail chest segment, protrusion of bony fragments
Percussion: Dullness over lung fields, which can signal hemothorax or atelectasis; hyperresonance over lung fields, which can signal pneumothorax
Auscultation: ↓ breath sounds, respiratory stridor, bony crepitus over fracture sites

VITAL SIGNS/HEMODYNAMICS
RR: ↑
HR: ↑ if hypoxemic or hemorrhaging
BP: ↓ according to degree of blood loss
Other: Hemodynamics reflect volume status; PAWP and CO ↓ if hemorrhaging

LABORATORY STUDIES
ABGs: Evaluate oxygenation and acid-base status. Typical results reflect Pao_2 <80 and $Paco_2$ >45 with respiratory acidosis (pH <7.35). Continuous Spo_2 monitoring may be used. Values <90%-92% reflect impaired ventilation.
Hgb/Hct: Reflect need for blood transfusion or fluid volume replacement.
WBCs: Baseline indicator of infectious process.

IMAGING
Chest X-ray: Confirms presence of air/fluid in pleural space, fractures of the bony thorax, and mediastinal shift.

Collaborative Management

Humidified O_2: Given by mask or cannula to maintain Spo_2 ≥92%.
Analgesia: Manages pain, which interferes with WOB. Opioid analgesics used cautiously because of respiratory depressive effects. Intercostal nerve block possible for local pain relief. Epidural/intrapleural analgesics considered most effective.
Stabilization/Fixation Flail Chest: Most stabilize within 10-14 days without surgery. Internal fixation uses volume-cycled ventilator with PEEP or CPAP to stabilize fracture(s). External fixation involves wiring or otherwise attaching segment to intact bony structures.
Chest Tube Insertion: Removes fluid or air from chest cavity. Large-bore (26F-30F) thoracic catheter inserted into chest cavity through second ICS, MCL, or fifth ICS, MAL if hemothorax suspected. Catheter connected to closed chest-drainage system or one-way flutter valve or to combined chest-drainage, autotransfusion unit. Latter used if hemothorax suspected.
Fluid Replacement: Depending on presence/extent of shock. Generally, LR or NS given to restore fluid volume.
ET Intubation: Maintains patent airway, ↓ airway resistance and respiratory effort, provides easy removal of airway secretions, enables manual or mechanical ventilation, as necessary.
Mechanical Ventilation: For extreme respiratory distress, decompensation, or ventilatory collapse.
Thoracentesis: Relieves life-threatening tension pneumothorax. 14-gauge needle inserted into second ICS, MCL to vent pressurized chest cavity.
Thoracotomy: Generally avoided unless complications develop after stabilization. Indications for thoracotomy: massive air leak in functioning drainage system, continued or ↑ bleeding through chest tube, refractory hypotension, acute deterioration, cardiac tamponade.
Tetanus Immunization: Booster given if needed or hx unknown.

PATIENT-FAMILY TEACHING
- Turning, coughing, deep-breathing exercises
- Use of incentive spirometry
- Purpose, expected results, anticipated sensations of nursing/medical interventions
- Medications: drug name, purpose, dosage, schedule, precautions, food-drug and drug-drug interactions, potential side effects

Nursing Diagnoses/Interventions

Impaired gas exchange r/t ↓ alveolar blood flow and ↓ O_2 supply secondary to ↓ pleural pressure

Desired outcome: Within 2-6 h of treatment, gas exchange adequate: Pao_2 ≥60 mm Hg and $Paco_2$ ≤45 mm Hg (or values within 10% of baseline), RR ≤20 breaths/min with eupnea, orientation × 3.

- Check serial ABGs for continued hypercapnia or hypoxemia. Continuously monitor Spo_2. Deliver prescribed concentrations O_2.
- Observe for hypoxia: ↑ restlessness, anxiety, changes in mental status.
- Assess for ↑ respiratory distress: ↑ RR, ↑ WOB, ↓/absent movement of chest wall on affected side, complaints of ↑ dyspnea, cyanosis.
- Position for full expansion of unaffected lung (semi-Fowler's position usually provides comfort and enables adequate chest wall expansion), or turn with unaffected side down with HOB elevated to promote V/Q match.
- Change position q2h to promote drainage/lung reexpansion and facilitate alveolar perfusion.
- Encourage deep breaths. Provide analgesia to ↓ discomfort during deep breathing.
- Assess and maintain closed chest-drainage system.
- Keep emergency supplies at bedside: (a) petrolatum gauze pad to cover insertion site if chest tube becomes dislodged and (b) sterile water in which to submerge chest tube if it disconnects from underwater-seal system. Avoid chest tube clamping, since air cannot escape and it may lead to tension pneumothorax.
- Follow agency policy regarding chest tube stripping. It has been associated with high negative pressures in the pleural space, which can damage lung tissue. Gentle "milking" may be indicated with bloody drainage or visible clots in tubing. Squeezing alternately hand-over-hand along drainage tube may generate sufficient pressure to move fluid along tube.

Pain r/t injury caused by chest tube placement and pleural irritation

Desired outcomes: Within 1 h of giving analgesia, discomfort ↓ as documented by pain scale. Nonverbal indicators absent.

- Inform patient/significant others about chest tube placement and maintenance.
- Assess degree of discomfort, using verbal and nonverbal cues. Devise pain scale with patient. Evaluate and document analgesia effectiveness based on pain scale.
- Position on unaffected side to minimize discomfort. Medicate 30 min before initiating movement or therapies.
- Teach splinting of affected side during coughing, moving, repositioning. Move patient as a unit to promote stability and comfort.
- Schedule periods of rest throughout activities to help ↑ pain threshold.
- Stabilize chest tube to reduce pull or drag on latex connector tubing. Tape chest tube securely to thorax; loop latex tubing on bed beside patient.
- Encourage active ROM on involved side to prevent stiff shoulder from immobility.

Risk for infection (hospital-associated pneumonia) r/t inadequate primary defenses (eg, ↓ ciliary action) and invasive procedures (eg, intubation)

Desired outcome: Patient infection free: normothermia, WBCs wnl for patient, sputum clear to whitish in color.

- Perform hand washing before/after contact with respiratory secretions or equipment
- Identify candidates at ↑ risk for pneumonia: >70 yrs old, obese, hx COPD or smoking, intubation, antimicrobial therapy, colonization of oropharynx or trachea by aerobic gram-negative bacteria.

  Give written instructions and demonstrations of turning, coughing, deep-breathing exercises.

  Most patients need encouragement to expand their lungs effectively. Use incentive spirometer to promote periodic, voluntary lung expansion > tidal volume.

  If secretions cannot be removed effectively by coughing, perform gentle chest physiotherapy, including breathing exercises, postural drainage, and percussion (may be contraindicated with severe, extensive injury).

  For patient with ET or tracheostomy tube, provide a fast, deep breath with manual resuscitator to stimulate cough receptors.

- Suction "as needed" rather than routinely; frequent suctioning can ↑ risk of trauma and cross-contamination; consider "in-line" suction device to ↓ risk of infection or contamination.

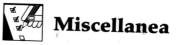 # Miscellanea

CONSULT MD FOR
- Respiratory distress
- Hypoxemia: restlessness, anxiety, altered mental status
- Green, yellow, purulent, or bloody respiratory secretions
- ↓ lung compliance: eg, ↑ inspiratory flow pressures required to deliver prescribed tidal volume, frequent sounding of high pressure alarm
- New/persistent hypercapnia/hypoxemia

RELATED TOPICS
- Adult respiratory distress syndrome
- Cardiac tamponade
- Cardiac trauma
- Chest trauma
- Mechanical ventilation
- Multisystem injury
- Pain
- Pneumonia, hospital-associated
- Pneumothorax
- Respiratory failure, acute

ABBREVIATIONS
ICS: Intercostal space
MAL: Midaxillary line
MCL: Midclavicular line

REFERENCES
Feliciano D, Moore E, Mattox K: *Trauma,* ed 3, Stamford, Conn, 1996, Appleton & Lange.
Howard CA: Chest trauma. In Swearingen PL, Keen JH (eds): *Manual of critical care nursing,* ed 3, St Louis, 1995, Mosby.
Hurn PD, Hartsock RL: Blunt thoracic injuries, *Crit Care Nurs Clin North Am* 5(4): 673-686, 1993.
Stanik-Hutt J: Strategies for pain management in traumatic thoracic injuries, *Crit Care Nurs Clin North Am* 5(4): 713-722, 1993.
Turney SZ, Rodriguez A, Cowley RA: *Management of cardio-thoracic trauma,* Baltimore, 1990, Williams & Wilkins.

Author: **Cheri A. Goll**

Overview

PATHOPHYSIOLOGY
LGIB less likely to cause hemorrhage than UGIB. Sudden loss of blood from GI tract will ↓ circulating volume, resulting in ↓ venous return and ↓ CO. Release of epinephrine and norepinephrine triggers vasoconstriction, causing ↓ splanchnic flow and possibly mesenteric ischemia. Causes of LGIB include:

Ischemic Disorders: Mesenteric ischemia, ischemic colitis. Associated with acute thrombosis or low flow states and hypoxemia. In addition to blood loss, protein, electrolyte, and fluid losses contribute to hypovolemia. Bowel infarction possible.

Inflammatory Disorders: Involve inflammation of bowel mucosa or submucosa causing friable tissue. May result in massive hemorrhage.

Injury: Blunt or penetrating trauma may involve colon and associated vasculature. Disruption of colon integrity may cause infection.

Neoplasms: Benign or malignant; can cause serious bleeding.

HISTORY/RISK FACTORS
- Ischemic disorders: rheumatic or atherosclerotic heart disease, advanced age, oral contraceptives, severe hypoxemia, LV failure, ↓ CO, chronic heart failure, shock
- Inflammatory Disorders: ulcerative colitis, Crohn's disease, diverticulitis
- Contributing Factors: blood dyscrasias including DIC, thrombocytopenia

CLINICAL PRESENTATION
- Blood loss of 1000 ml in 15 min usually produces S&S of shock. Massive hemorrhage defined as loss of >30% of total blood volume or bleeding episode necessitating 6 U transfusion in 24-h period.
- Syncope and mild to severe colicky pain possible.
- Mild or slow LGIB may cause melena. Massive LGIB associated with dark red "currant jelly" stools or passing of fresh blood with clots (hematochezia).

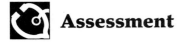

Assessment

PHYSICAL ASSESSMENT
- Shock state present with profuse, active bleeding: Tachycardia, hypotension, cool and diaphoretic extremities, ↓ peripheral pulses, delayed capillary refill (>2 sec), pallor or cyanosis, restlessness, confusion,

↓ UO, obvious bleeding.
- Abdomen may appear large or distended. Auscultation may reveal hyperactive bowel sounds caused by mucosal irritation by blood, or a silent abdomen, which suggests serious complications (ileus, perforation, vascular occlusion). Palpation may reveal tenderness or firmness resulting from distention.

VITAL SIGNS/HEMODYNAMICS
RR: ↑
HR: ↑
BP: ↓
Temp: NI
CVP/PAP: ↓
CO: ↓
SVR: ↑
Other: Postural VS measured. ↓ SBP >10 mm Hg or HR ↑ 10 bpm indicates recent intravascular loss of ≥1000 ml in adults.
ECG: May reflect severe cardiac ischemia resulting from hypoperfusion, including T-wave depression or inversion.

LABORATORY STUDIES
Hematology: Serial Hgb and Hct values reflect amount of blood lost. First Hct value may be near nl, but subsequently expected to ↓ dramatically as volume is restored and extravascular fluid mobilizes into vascular space. Platelet count ↑ within 1 h of hemorrhage; leukocytosis follows.

Chemistries: Excessive vomiting, gastric suction may cause hypochloremic, hypokalemic state accompanied by ↑ serum HCO_3^- level. ↑ BUN without corresponding ↑ creatinine occurs because of excess intestinal protein from digestion of RBCs. Plasma protein may ↑ in response to ↑ hepatic production. Mild hyperglycemia is a compensatory response to stressful stimuli. Hyperbilirubinemia is caused by breakdown of reabsorbed blood and its pigments.

IMAGING
Radiology: Flat-plate abdominal x-ray may reveal free air under diaphragm, suggesting perforation.

Angiography: If bleeding rapid and suspected of being arterial or from a large vein, angiography of various GI arterial systems may locate bleeding site(s). If bleeding site clearly identified, therapeutic embolization may be attempted during angiography.

DIAGNOSTIC PROCEDURES
Proctosigmoidoscopy: Rectum and sigmoid colon visualized directly *via* endoscopy. Mucosal bleeding, polyps, hemorrhoids, other lesions may be seen. Biopsy specimens may be obtained.

Collaborative Management

Fluid, Electrolytes: Volume replacement performed as quickly as possible. Two large-bore IV lines (14-16 gauge) inserted for rapid fluid resuscitation. Crystalloid replacement initiated until dramatic blood loss or differential diagnosis warrants use of colloids or blood products. If bleeding massive, LR is the preferred crystalloid volume expander because electrolyte disturbances are minimized.

Blood Products: PRBCs and FFP balanced to provide replacement of cells and clotting components. Generally FFP required after infusion of 6 U PRBCs. Large transfusions cause calcium to bind with citrate from stored blood and deplete free calcium levels.

Resp Support: Because of ↓ O_2-carrying capacity of RBCs in massive blood loss, O_2 therapy initiated and adjusted as needed to ensure adequate oxygenation.

Nutritional Support: TPN started when status likely to remain NPO for days to wks. Enteral or oral feedings started if there is no further evidence of GI hemorrhage and bowel function has returned.

Gastric Intubation: Often necessary because of partial or complete ileus. Gastric lavage may be performed to quickly distinguish UGIB from LGIB.

Pharmacotherapy
Corticosteroids: To ↓ inflammation associated with inflammatory bowel disorders.

Analgesics: Codeine, diphenoxylate HCl with atropine (Lomotil) may be used. Opiates not used for diarrhea associated with ulcerative colitis because they may precipitate toxic megacolon.

Vasopressin (Pitressin): May be used for uncontrolled massive bleeding.

Other: α-Stimulating sympathomimetics (eg, norepinephrine, dopamine at doses >10 μg/kg/min) avoided if possible, since they contribute to mesenteric ischemia.

Surgical Management: Many techniques used, depending on lesion location and severity. Massive LGIB difficult to control and may require surgical procedures such as colectomy, with creation of permanent ileostomy or internal ileal pouch.

PATIENT/FAMILY TEACHING
- S&S of LGIB: pain, nausea, dark or "currant jelly" stools, lightheadedness; importance of seeking medical attention promptly if signs of bleeding occur
- Importance of avoiding medications/agents with potential for GI tract irritation: aspirin, NSAIDs, ETOH

Nursing Diagnoses/Interventions

Fluid volume deficit r/t active loss secondary to GI tract hemorrhage; or r/t sequestration of fluid in peritoneum

Desired outcome: Within 8 h of this diagnosis, patient becomes normovolemic: MAP ≥70 mm Hg, HR 60-100 bpm, CVP 2-6 mm Hg, PAWP 6-12 mm Hg, CI ≥2.5 L/min/m^2, and UO ≥0.5 ml/kg/h.

- Monitor postural VS on admission, q4-8h, and more frequently if recurrence of active bleeding suspected: ↓ SBP >10 mm Hg or ↑ HR of 10 bpm in a sitting position suggests significant intravascular volume deficit, with ≈ 15%-20% volume loss.
- Monitor BP, HR, ECG, and CV status qh or more frequently with active bleeding or unstable VS. Be alert to sudden ↑ in HR and ↓ MAP of >10 mm Hg from previous reading.
- Measure central pressures and thermodilution CO. ↑ HR, ↓ PAWP, ↓ CO (CI <2.5 L/min/m^2), and ↑ SVR suggest hypovolemia and need for volume restoration.
- Replace volume with combination of crystalloid and blood products as indicated *via* large-bore IV (≥18-gauge) catheter.
- Measure UO qh. Be alert to output <0.5 ml/kg/h for 2 consecutive h. ↑ fluid intake if ↓ output caused by hypovolemia and hypoperfusion.
- Monitor Hct; be alert to values <28%-30%.
- Measure and record all GI blood losses from hematochezia, melena.
- Check all stools for occult blood.
- Ensure proper function and patency of gastric tubes. Do not occlude air vent of double-lumen tubes because this may cause vacuum occlusion.
- Administer O$_2$ as prescribed to facilitate maximal delivery to the tissues.
- Monitor for hypoxemia. Maintain O$_2$ saturation ≥92%.
- Monitor ECG for evidence of myocardial ischemia: T-wave depression, QT prolongation, ventricular dysrhythmias.
- Monitor for ↓ cardiac output: pallor, cool extremities, capillary refill delayed for >2 sec, and ↓/absent amplitude of distal pulses.

Pain r/t chemical or physical injury of GI mucosal surfaces caused by digestive juices and enzymes or tissue trauma

Desired outcomes: Within 2 h of this diagnosis, subjective evaluation of discomfort improves, as documented by pain scale. Nonverbal indicators of discomfort, such as grimacing, are absent.

- Monitor for and document GI pain or discomfort. Devise pain scale with patient, rating discomfort from 0 (no pain) to 10 (severe). Be aware that pain may disappear concomitant with a bleeding episode, since blood covers and protects eroded tissue.
- Administer opiate analgesics with caution, since vasodilatation and ↓ preload can result in dramatic hypotension with GI bleeding.
- Monitor respiratory rate/depth to avoid opiate-induced respiratory depression.
- Because anxiety reduction contributes to pain relief, ensure consistency and promptness in delivering analgesia.
- Supplement analgesics with nonpharmacologic maneuvers to aid in pain reduction. Modify body position to optimize comfort.

Diarrhea r/t irritation and ↑ motility secondary to blood in GI tract

Desired outcome: By time of hospital discharge, stools are nl in consistency and frequency and negative for occult blood.

- Monitor and record stool amount, frequency, and character.
- Provide or have bedpan or bedside commode readily available.
- Minimize embarrassing odor by removing stool promptly and using room deodorizers.
- Use matter-of-fact approach when assisting with frequent bowel elimination. Reassure that frequent elimination is a common problem for most patients with GI bleeding.
- Evaluate bowel sounds q4-8h. Anticipate nl to hyperdynamic bowel sounds. Absence of bowel sounds (especially if associated with severe pain or abdominal distention) may signal serious complications such as ileus or perforation.
- Monitor serum sodium, potassium, and calcium levels for abnormalities.
- Keep patient NPO until diarrhea episodes have subsided.

Miscellanea

CONSULT MD FOR
- S&S of brisk or renewed bleeding, hypovolemic shock
- UO <0.5 ml/kg/h × 2 h
- S&S of complications: ruptured viscus, bowel infarction, renal insufficiency, peritonitis
- Abnormal serum sodium, potassium, calcium levels

RELATED TOPICS
- Abdominal trauma
- Blood and blood products (see Appendix)
- Gastrointestinal bleeding: upper
- Shock, hemorrhagic
- Transfusion therapies

ABBREVIATIONS
FFP: Fresh frozen plasma
LGIB: Lower gastrointestinal bleeding
PRBCs: Packed red blood cells
UGIB: Upper gastrointestinal bleeding

REFERENCES
Keen JH: Gastrointestinal bleeding. In Swearingen PL, Keen JH (eds): *Manual of critical care nursing,* ed 3, St Louis, 1995, Mosby.

Rush C: Gastrointestinal bleeding: preventing hypovolemic shock, *Nursing* 25(8):33, 1995.

Savides TJ and Jensen DM: Severe gastrointestinal hemorrhage. In Ayres SM (ed): *Textbook of critical care,* ed 3, Philadelphia, 1995, WB Saunders.

Author: **Janet Hicks Keen**

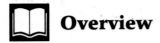 **Overview**

PATHOPHYSIOLOGY

Esophagus: Esophageal varices the most common cause of massive esophageal hemorrhage. Esophagitis and esophageal ulcers/tumors less frequent causes. Maneuvers that ↑ intraabdominal pressure (eg, vomiting, straining, coughing) can lead to Mallory-Weiss tear, a laceration at the esophagogastric junction, which results in massive bleeding.

Stomach and Duodenum: Commonly caused by peptic ulcer disease.

Stress ulcers: Common in the critically ill; tend to be multiple shallow lesions in proximal stomach.

Cushing's ulcers: Occur in esophagus, stomach, duodenum; associated with deeper mucosal invasion than stress ulcers.

Curling's ulcers: Seen with major burn injury. Located in duodenum; tend to be single, deep ulcers.

Gastritis: Usually occurs as slow, diffuse oozing; difficult to control.

Benign/malignant gastric tumors: May cause severe bleeding episodes.

HISTORY/RISK FACTORS

- Critical illness: especially if caused by major injury, surgery, CNS disorder, burns
- Prolonged shock or hypoperfusion; organ failure
- Excessive alcohol, NSAIDs, steroid ingestion
- Hiatal hernia
- Hepatic, pancreatic, biliary tract disease
- Blood dyscrasias
- Familial cancer
- Recent abdominal surgery
- Presence of *Heliobacter pylori*: found in >90% duodenal ulcers and 70% gastric ulcers

CLINICAL PRESENTATION

- Syncope, hematemesis, melena, ↑ GI transit time, diarrhea
- Mild to severe pain: often associated with ulcerative or erosive disease
- If blood loss severe: alterations in LOC, ↓ UO

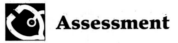 **Assessment**

PHYSICAL ASSESSMENT

Auscultation: Hyperactive bowel sounds caused by mucosal irritation by blood or a silent abdomen, suggesting serious complications such as ileus, perforation, vascular occlusion.

Inspection/Palpation: Epigastric tenderness if peptic ulcer present. Cool and diaphoretic extremities, ↓ peripheral pulses, delayed capillary refill (>2 sec), pallor or cyanosis, restlessness, confusion. Jaundice, vascular spiders, ascites, and hepatosplenomegaly suggest liver disease. Vomitus or gastric aspirate may contain obvious whole blood or coffee ground–appearing old blood.

VITAL SIGNS/HEMODYNAMICS

RR: ↑
HR: ↑
BP: ↓; orthostasis
Temp: Wnl
CVP/PAP: ↓
SVR: ↑
CO: ↓

ECG: May reflect diffuse cardiac ischemia caused by hypoperfusion, including T-wave depression or inversion.

LABORATORY STUDIES

Hematology: Serial Hgb and Hct values reflect amount of blood lost. First Hct value may be near nl, but subsequent values expected to ↓ dramatically as volume restored and extravascular fluid mobilizes into vascular space. Platelet count ↑ within 1 h of hemorrhage; leukocytosis follows.

Chemistries: Excessive vomiting, gastric suction may cause hypochloremic, hypokalemic state accompanied by ↑ serum HCO_3^- level. ↑ BUN without corresponding ↑ creatinine occurs because of excess intestinal protein from digestion of RBCs. Plasma protein may ↑ in response to ↑ hepatic production. Mild hyperglycemia a compensatory response to stressful stimuli. Hyperbilirubinemia caused by breakdown of reabsorbed blood and its pigments.

Coagulation Studies: Depending on preexisting disease, hypocoagulability may be present.

IMAGING

Radiology: Flat-plate abdominal x-ray may reveal free air under diaphragm, which suggests perforation.

Angiography: If bleeding rapid and suspected of being arterial or from a large vein, angiography of various GI arterial systems may locate bleeding site(s). If bleeding site clearly identified, therapeutic embolization may be attempted during angiography.

DIAGNOSTIC PROCEDURES

Esophagogastroduodenoscopy (panendoscopy): Most accurate means of determining source of UGIB. Esophagus, stomach, duodenum visualized directly with fiberoptic endoscope passed through mouth. Usually performed within first 12 h of admission. May be necessary to clear stomach of blood and clots by lavage before procedure. Antacids and sucralfate withheld until after procedure because they alter lesion appearance. Electrocautery, laser, other therapeutic techniques often employed during procedure.

Collaborative Management

Fluid, Electrolytes: Volume replacement performed as quickly as possible. Two large-bore IV lines (14- or 16-gauge) inserted for rapid fluid resuscitation. Crystalloid replacement initiated until dramatic blood loss or differential diagnosis warrants use of colloids or blood products. If bleeding massive, LR is the preferred crystalloid volume expander because electrolyte disturbances are minimized.

Blood Products: PRBCs and FFP balanced to provide replacement of cells and clotting components. Generally FFP required after infusion of 6 U PRBCs. Large transfusions cause Ca^{2+} to bind with citrate from stored blood and deplete free Ca^{2+} levels.

Vasopressors and Inotropics: Used *only* if tissue perfusion remains compromised despite adequate intravascular volume replacement. Hemodynamic monitoring essential for continuous evaluation of volume status, especially if patient >50 yrs of age or with chronic illness such as CV, pulmonary, renal, hepatic disease.

Resp Support: Because of ↓ O_2-carrying capacity of RBCs in massive blood loss, O_2 therapy initiated and adjusted as needed to ensure adequate oxygenation.

Nutritional Support: TPN started when status

likely to remain NPO for days to wks. Enteral or oral feedings started if no further evidence of GI hemorrhage and bowel function returned.

Gastric Intubation: Often necessary. Lavage sometimes performed to clear blood and clots from stomach. Gastric intubation avoided if esophageal varices are suspected bleeding source, since variceal tearing may occur.

Endoscopic Electrocoagulation or Laser Photocoagulation: To treat bleeding ulcers.

Pharmacotherapy: Gastric alkalinization effective in preventing and controlling ulceration. Recent evidence suggests acid-suppression therapy in critically ill associated with ↑ incidence of nosocomial pneumonia. When stomach's acidic environment is neutralized, bacteria ↑ and infection occurs if bacterial count of aspirated gastric juice is ↑.

Antacids: ↑ gastric pH and ↓ corrosiveness of gastric acid. May require continuous gastric infusion or administration qh.

Histamine H_2-receptor antagonists (eg, famotidine, ranitidine): Block gastric acid and pepsin secretion; employed to treat erosive and ulcerative disease. Cimetidine usually avoided in critically ill because it may result in drug interactions.

Sucralfate (Carafate): Combines with gastric acid and forms adhesive protective coating over damaged mucosa; not absorbed from GI tract and frequently leads to constipation.

Misoprostol (Cytotec): Synthetic prostaglandin E_1 that enhances body's nl mucosal protective mechanisms and ↓ acid secretion. Aspirin, other NSAIDs inhibit natural prostaglandin synthesis; therefore misoprostol especially effective for ulceration associated with these drugs.

Omeprazole (Prilosec): Deactivates enzyme system that pumps H^+ from parietal cells,

thus inhibiting gastric acid secretion; may completely inhibit gastric acid secretion.

Vasopressin (Pitressin): Sometimes used for uncontrolled massive bleeding, especially from esophageal varices.

Gastric pH Monitoring: To assess pH of gastric contents (intraluminal pH) or gastric mucosal tissue (intramural pH). Goal of therapy: to maintain gastric pH within 4.0-5.0. Intraluminal pH measured by aspirating gastric secretions and testing with pH indicator paper or by using specially designed gastric tube. GI tonometer and sump tube may be used to measure intramural pH. Because the gut is especially vulnerable to ischemia, intramural pH a valuable early predictor of intestinal ischemia, sepsis, MODS.

Surgical Management: Many surgical techniques used, depending on lesion location and severity. Ulcerative disease requires surgery if lesions continue to bleed despite aggressive medical therapy or if complications such as perforation or obstruction develop. Oversewing of bleeding vessel usually followed by acid-reducing procedure. In unstable patients, vagotomy and pyloroplasty performed. Antrectomy or parietal cell vagotomy may be performed in more stable patients. Common procedure for duodenal ulcers is gastrojejunostomy (Billroth II procedure).

PATIENT/FAMILY TEACHING

- S&S of actual/impending upper GI hemorrhage: pain, nausea, vomiting of blood, dark stools, lightheadedness; importance of seeking medical attention promptly if signs of bleeding occur
- Importance of avoiding medications/agents with potential for gastric irritation: aspirin, NSAIDs, ETOH

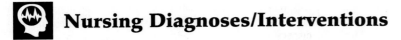 **Nursing Diagnoses/Interventions**

Fluid volume deficit r/t active loss secondary to GI tract hemorrhage; or r/t sequestration of fluid into peritoneum

Desired outcome: Within 8 h of this diagnosis, patient normovolemic: MAP ≥70 mm Hg, HR 60-100 bpm, CVP 2-6 mm Hg, PAWP 6-12 mm Hg, CI ≥2.5 L/min/m^2, and UO ≥0.5 ml/kg/h.

- Monitor postural VS on admission, q4-8h, and more frequently if recurrence of active bleeding suspected: ↓ SBP >10 mm Hg or ↑ HR of 10 bpm in a sitting position suggests significant intravascular volume deficit, with ≈ 15%-20% volume loss.
- Monitor BP, HR, ECG, and CV status qh or more frequently with active bleeding or unstable VS. Be alert to sudden ↑ in HR and ↓ MAP >10 mm Hg from previous reading.
- Measure central pressures and thermodilution CO. ↑ HR, ↓ PAWP, ↓ CO (CI <2.5 L/min/m^2), and ↑ SVR suggest hypovolemia and need for volume restoration.
- Replace volume with combination of crystalloid and blood products as indicated *via* large-bore IV (≥18-gauge) catheter.
- Measure UO qh. Be alert to output <0.5 ml/kg/h for 2 consecutive h. ↑ fluid intake if ↓ output caused by hypovolemia and hypoperfusion.
- Monitor Hct; be alert to values <28%-30%.
- Measure and record all GI blood losses from hematemesis, melena.
- Check all stools and gastric contents for occult blood.
- Ensure proper function and patency of gastric tubes. Do not occlude air vent of double-lumen tubes because this may cause vacuum occlusion.
- Administer O$_2$ as prescribed to facilitate maximal delivery to the tissues.
- Monitor for hypoxemia. Maintain O$_2$ saturation ≥92%.
- Monitor ECG for evidence of myocardial ischemia: T-wave depression, QT prolongation, ventricular dysrhythmias.
- Monitor for ↓ cardiac output: pallor, cool extremities, capillary refill delayed for >2 sec, and ↓/absent amplitude of distal pulses.

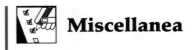 **Miscellanea**

CONSULT MD FOR
- S&S of brisk or renewed bleeding, hypovolemic shock
- UO <0.5 ml/kg/h × 2 h
- S&S of complications: ruptured viscus, bowel infarction, renal insufficiency, peritonitis
- Abnormal serum sodium, potassium, calcium levels

RELATED TOPICS
- Blood and blood products (see Appendix)
- Esophageal varices
- Nutritional support, parenteral
- Peritonitis
- Shock, hemorrhagic
- Transfusion therapies
- Vasopressor therapy

ABBREVIATIONS
FFP: Fresh frozen plasma
MODS: Multiple organ dysfunction syndrome
PRBCs: Packed red blood cells
UGIB: Upper gastrointestinal bleeding

Pain r/t chemical or physical injury of GI mucosal surfaces caused by digestive juices and enzymes or tissue trauma

Desired outcomes: Within 2 h of this diagnosis, patient's subjective evaluation of discomfort improves, as documented by pain scale. Nonverbal indicators of discomfort, such as grimacing, absent.

- Monitor for and document abdominal pain or discomfort. Devise pain scale with patient, rating discomfort from 0 (no pain) to 10 (severe). Be aware that pain may disappear concomitant with a bleeding episode, since blood covers and protects eroded tissue.
- Administer gastric alkalizing agents, sucralfate as indicated to relieve pain.
- Measure gastric pH q2-4h or continuously. If measuring pH *via* gastric aspirate, be sure to use clean syringe and discard first aspirate to ensure accurate results. Adjust gastric alkalizing therapy to maintain pH of 4.0-5.0 or other prescribed range. Avoid excessive alkalization, which has been associated with ↑ risk of nosocomial pneumonia. As available, use GI tonometer to measure gastric mucosal pH.
- Administer opiate analgesics with caution, since vasodilatation and ↓ preload can result in dramatic hypotension with UGIB.
- Monitor respiratory rate and depth to avoid opiate-induced respiratory depression.
- Because anxiety reduction contributes to pain relief, ensure consistency and promptness in delivering analgesia.
- Supplement analgesics with nonpharmacologic maneuvers to aid in pain reduction. Modify body position to optimize comfort. Patients with pain associated with gastric reflux may be more comfortable with HOB elevated if this position does not compromise hemodynamic status.

Diarrhea r/t irritation and ↑ motility secondary to blood in GI tract

Desired outcome: By time of hospital discharge, stools nl in consistency and frequency and negative for occult blood.

- Monitor and record stool amount, frequency, and character.
- Provide or have bedpan or bedside commode readily available.
- Minimize embarrassing odor by removing stool promptly and using room deodorizers.
- Use matter-of-fact approach when assisting with frequent bowel elimination. Reassure that frequent elimination is a common problem for most patients with GI bleeding.
- Evaluate bowel sounds q4-8h. Anticipate nl to hyperdynamic bowel sounds. Absence of bowel sounds (especially in association with severe pain or abdominal distention) may signal serious complications such as ileus or perforation.
- Monitor serum sodium, potassium, and calcium levels for abnormalities.
- Keep patient NPO until diarrhea episodes have subsided.

REFERENCES

Bezzarro ER: Changing perspectives of H_2-antagonists for stress ulcer prophylaxis, *Crit Care Nurs Clin North Am* 5(2): 325-331, 1993.

Generali J: *Heliobacter pylori* update, *Drug Newsletter* 13(5): 39-40, 1994.

Keen JH: Gastrointestinal bleeding. In Swearingen PL, Keen JH (eds): *Manual of critical care nursing,* ed 3, St Louis, 1995, Mosby.

Prevost SS, Overle A: Stress ulceration in the critically ill patient, *Crit Care Nurs Clin North Am* 5(1): 163-169, 1993.

Author: **Janet Hicks Keen**

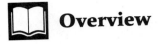 **Overview**

PATHOPHYSIOLOGY

Causes include actual, perceived, or anticipated loss of aspects of self, body part, or function; terminal or life-threatening illness; profound changes in self concept or role function; separation from home, pet, or loved one. Stages of grief:

Protest
- Denial: "No, not me."
- Disbelief: "But I just saw her this morning."
- Anger, hostility, resentment
- Bargaining to postpone loss
- Appeal for help to recover loss
- Loud complaints
- Altered sleep and appetite

Disorganization
- Depression
- Withdrawal, social isolation
- Psychomotor retardation
- Silence

Reorganization
- Acceptance of loss
- Development of new interests and attachments
- Restructuring of life-style
- Return to preloss level of functioning

HISTORY/RISK FACTORS
- Traumatic injury, burn injury, severe disease
- Terminal illness
- Serious dysfunction of any organ or body system
- Sudden critical illness
- Loss of body part
- Organ transplantation

CLINICAL PRESENTATION

Typically, the protest stage occurs first, although the disorganization stage may be present, depending on duration and stage of critical/serious illness. May fluctuate among three stages until reorganization complete.

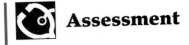 **Assessment**

PHYSICAL ASSESSMENT

Stage of Grieving: Assess behavioral response, then determine grieving stage. Expect disbelief, denial, guilt, anger, and depression. Compare to baseline status.

Related Factors: Assess spiritual, religious, sociocultural expectations related to loss. "Is religion an important part of your life? How do you and your significant others deal with serious health problems?" Also consider previous coping strategies.

VITAL SIGNS/HEMODYNAMICS

RR: Nl or slight ↑ with anxiety
HR: Nl or slight ↑ with anxiety
BP: Nl or slight ↑ with anxiety
Temp: Nl
Other: Release of endogenous catecholamines causes cardiopulmonary stimulation if patient anxious.

Collaborative Management

Developmental Factors: Consider patient's age and developmental stage when planning interventions. Assess impact of disease process on meeting developmental goals.
Family Systems: Assess family constellation, relationships, roles, interactional dynamics, and support systems. Plan strategies to mobilize support if needed. Refer problems to appropriate psychiatric personnel.
Spiritual Needs: Consider impact of beliefs/attitudes about death. Refer to individuals who can assist in meeting religious or spiritual needs.
Pharmacotherapy: Temporary use of anxiolytics (eg, lorazepam [Ativan]), antidepressants, or hypnotics helpful in relieving some extreme symptoms during grieving process. However, overuse retards progression toward reorganization.
Consultations: Case manager, psychiatric clinical nurse specialist, psychiatrist, or other mental health practitioner may be necessary to facilitate grieving process.

PATIENT-FAMILY TEACHING
- Stages of grieving and usual behavioral responses during each stage
- Encouragement for significant others to permit anger within limits
- Referrals to clergy or community support groups as appropriate

Nursing Diagnoses/Interventions

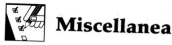

Miscellanea

Anticipatory grieving r/t perceived potential loss of physiologic well-being (eg, expected loss of body function or body part, changes in self-concept or body image, or terminal illness)

Desired outcomes: Patient and family/significant others express grief, participate in decisions about the future, and communicate concerns to health care team members and to one another.

- Assess factors contributing to anticipated loss.
- Assess and accept behavioral response, eg, disbelief, denial, guilt, anger, depression.
- Assess spiritual, religious, and sociocultural expectations related to loss.
- Encourage patient and family/significant others to share concerns; respect their desire not to speak.
- Demonstrate empathy. Touch when appropriate.
- Assess grief reactions of patient and significant others and identify potential for dysfunctional grieving (eg, absence of emotion, hostility, avoidance). Refer to mental health professional as needed.
- When appropriate, assess patient's wishes about tissue donation.

Dysfunctional grieving r/t loss of physiologic well-being or fatal illness

Desired outcomes: Within 24 h of this diagnosis, patient expresses grief, explains meaning of the loss, and communicates concerns with significant others. Patient completes necessary self-care activities.

- Assess grief stage and previous coping abilities. Discuss feelings, meaning of the loss, and goals.
- Acknowledge and permit anger; set limits on expression of anger to discourage destructive behavior.
- Identify suicidal behavior (eg, severe depression, statements of intent, suicide plan, previous hx of suicide attempt). Ensure safety and refer to mental health professional as necessary.
- Encourage participation in ADL and diversional activities. Identify physiologic problems related to loss (eg, eating or sleeping disorders); intervene accordingly.

Spiritual distress r/t separation from spiritual/cultural supports or challenged belief and value system

Desired outcome: Within 24 h of diagnosis, patient verbalizes spiritual or religious beliefs and expresses hope for the future, attainment of spiritual or religious support, and availability of requisites for resolving conflicts.

- Assess spiritual or religious beliefs, values, and practices.
- Explain availability of spiritual aids, such as a chapel or religious services.
- Present a nonjudgmental attitude toward religious or spiritual beliefs and values. Attempt to create an environment conducive to free expression.
- Be alert to comments related to spiritual concerns or conflicts. ("I'm being punished for my sins.")
- Use active listening and open-ended questioning to assist in resolving conflicts related to spiritual issues. ("I understand that you want to be baptized. We can arrange to do that.")
- Provide privacy and opportunities for religious practices, such as prayer and meditation.
- If spiritual beliefs and therapeutic regimens are in conflict, provide honest, concrete information to encourage informed decision making. ("I understand that your religion discourages receiving transfusions. Do you understand that by refusing blood your condition is more difficult to treat?")

CONSULT MD FOR
- Evidence of suicidal behavior (eg, severe depression, statements of intent)
- Failure to show progression toward reorganization

RELATED TOPICS
- Anxiety
- Psychosocial needs, family/significant others
- Psychosocial needs, patient
- Sleep disturbances

REFERENCES
Demi AS, Miles MS: Bereavement, *Annu Rev Nurs Res* 4: 105-123, 1986.
Kozier B et al: *Fundamentals of nursing: concepts, process, and practice*, ed 5, Redwood City, Calif, 1995, Addison-Wesley.
Kübler-Ross E: *On death and dying*, New York, 1969, Macmillan.

Author: **Patricia Hall**

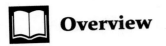 **Overview**

PATHOPHYSIOLOGY

Acute or subacute postinfectious polyneuritis. Frequency of GBS after infection and its occurrence with lymphoid tissue diseases (eg, Hodgkin's disease) suggest an autoimmune disorder. Mainly affects Schwann's cells, which synthesize and maintain the peripheral nerve myelin sheath. Ventral (motor) root axons of anterior horn cells, which innervate voluntary skeletal muscles, primarily involved. Dorsal (sensory) root axons also affected, but to lesser degree. Recovery of neurologic function depends on proliferation of Schwann's cells and axonal remyelination.

RECOVERY

Expected in 85%-95% of cases, with minor residual deficits occurring in <50% of affected patients.

INCIDENCE

Affects 1.5-2.0 individuals per 100,000 population.

HISTORY/RISK FACTORS

- Respiratory or GI illness: 10-14 days before onset of neurologic symptoms, in which viral agent is present (50% of cases)
- Recent vaccination (15% of cases): eg, for influenza
- Recent surgical procedure (5% of cases)

CLINICAL PRESENTATION

Sensory complaints, muscle weakness developing rapidly over 24-72 h
- Weakness: symmetric; generally begins in distal muscle groups and ascends to more proximal muscles
- Ascending flaccid motor paralysis: most common presenting sign, associated with early loss of DTRs
- Muscles of respiration (intercostals and diaphragm) frequently involved; ≈50% of all patients require mechanical ventilation

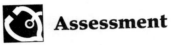 **Assessment**

PHYSICAL ASSESSMENT

General: Symmetric motor weakness, ↓/absent DTRs, hypotonia or flaccidity of affected muscles, respiratory abnormalities (eg, nasal flaring, hypoventilation), facial paralysis, paresthesias, loss of pain/temp sensations, proprioceptive/vibratory dysfunction

ANS Involvement (type of AD): Sinus tachycardia, bradycardia, orthostatic hypotension, hypertension, excessive diaphoresis, bowel and bladder retention, loss of sphincter control, ↑ pulmonary secretions, SIADH, cardiac dysrhythmias (a common cause of death). Sustained ↑ in BP may result in seizures, stroke, intracranial hemorrhage.

Cranial Nerve Involvement: All cranial nerves except I and II may be involved (see Appendix).

VITAL SIGNS/HEMODYNAMICS

RR: ↑ weakness of muscles of respiration
HR: NI; ↑ or ↓ if AD present
BP: Often ↓ because of ↓ vascular tone; may suddenly ↑ if AD present
Temp: NI
Hemodynamics: Usually not indicated unless complications such as prolonged CV instability or septicemia occur. A ↓ in CO may result from autonomic dysfunction and enlarged vascular bed.
ECG: Dysrhythmias possible if hypoxemia or AD present.

LABORATORY STUDIES

LP/CSF Analysis: CSF will show ↑ protein without any ↑ in WBCs. CSF protein, normally between 15-45 mg/100 ml, may peak to levels of several hundred mg/ml 4-6 wks after onset. CSF pressure, normally between 0-15 mm Hg (90-180 mm H_2O), may ↑ in severe cases.

CBC: Moderate leukocytosis may occur early, possibly as a result of inflammatory process associated with demyelination, but CBC level normalizes as disease runs its course.

ABGs: Performed if VC drops to <1 L or if dyspnea, confusion, restlessness, nasal flaring, use of accessory muscles, or breathlessness present. A ↓ in PaO_2 >10-15 mm Hg or ↑ in $PaCO_2$ 10-15 mm Hg > baseline/nl value signals need for urgent intubation.

DIAGNOSTIC PROCEDURES

Pulmonary Function Studies: VC <1 L may signal need for assisted ventilation.

Electrodiagnostic Studies: EMG and NCV demonstrate profound slowing of motor conduction velocities and conduction blocks because of peripheral nerve demyelination. May not appear initially, but becomes apparent several wks into illness. Evoked potentials (auditory, visual, brainstem) used to distinguish GBS from other neuropathologies.

Collaborative Management

Resp Support: Supplemental O_2, ET intubation, tracheostomy with assisted mechanical ventilation, as necessary.

Corticosteroids: May slow or halt demyelinating process and ↓ inflammation along peripheral nerves.

Plasmapheresis: Involves complete exchange of plasma with removal of abnormal circulating antibodies that affect peripheral nerve myelin sheath. Removal of these autoantibodies may ↓ duration and severity of GBS. *Complications:* hypovolemia, abnormal clotting, hypokalemia, hypocalcemia.

Maintenance of CV Function: As necessary, cardiac monitoring initiated for dysrhythmias, arterial pressure monitored to evaluate hypertension or hypotension, and antihypertensives or vasopressors used as indicated.

Management of Bowel, Bladder Dysfunction: Paralytic ileus or hypoperistalsis may occur. NG suction and parenteral infusion may be necessary. Indwelling urinary catheter used for urinary retention.

Nutritional Management: PN given until return of peristalsis. Tube or gastrostomy feedings given for severe dysphagia. With recovery of gag reflex and swallowing ability, diet progresses to semisolid and solid foods.

Management of Motor Dysfunction: Frequent active/passive ROM exercises necessary during all phases of GBS. As condition stabilizes, PT and OT personnel involved in planning rehabilitation process. Strenuous ROM avoided during acute phase, as it may exacerbate weakness and accelerate demyelinating process.

PATIENT-FAMILY TEACHING

- AD: factors likely to precipitate; S&S
- Possibility of respiratory failure and need for mechanical ventilation (Emphasize that this is temporary.)
- Purpose, expected results, anticipated sensations during plasmapheresis
- Purpose, expected results for ROM

Nursing Diagnoses/Interventions

Impaired gas exchange r/t altered O_2 supply associated with ↓ lung expansion secondary to weakness/paralysis of intercostal and diaphragmatic muscles

Desired outcomes: Within 12-24 h of this diagnosis, patient has adequate gas exchange: orientation × 3, RR 12-20 breaths/min with eupnea, HR ≤100 bpm, BP wnl for patient, Pao_2 ≥80 mm Hg, $Paco_2$ ≤45 mm Hg, and O_2 saturation ≥94%.

- Assess neurologic function qh or more often as needed. Ascending motor and sensory dysfunctions usually occur rapidly (over 24-72 h) and can lead to life-threatening respiratory arrest.
- Monitor for respiratory distress: adventitious (crackles, rhonchi), ↓, or absent breath sounds; temp ≥37.8° C (100° F); ↑ HR and BP; tidal volume or VC ↓ from baseline; ↓ in Pao_2 or ↑ in $Paco_2$ ≥10-15 mm Hg from baseline or nl values; abnormal respiratory rate or rhythm; ↑ restlessness or anxiety; confusion. If these S&S present, be prepared to assist with intubation or tracheotomy.
- Suction airway as determined by auscultation findings. As paresis or paralysis subsides (after 2-4 wks, usual time of dysfunction peak), cranial nerve function will begin to return (ie, gag, swallowing, coughing). Evaluate ability to cough.
- Deliver O_2 and humidification as prescribed.
- Unless contraindicated, maintain adequate hydration (up to 2-3 L/day) to minimize thickening of pulmonary secretions.
- Turn and reposition patient at least q2h to prevent stasis of secretions.

Risk for disuse syndrome r/t ascending flaccid paralysis and paresthesias

Desired outcomes: Patient maintains baseline/optimal ROM of all joints and baseline muscle size and strength of all muscles.

- Assess neurologic function qh. Ascending motor and sensory dysfunction usually occurs rapidly, over 24-72 h. Start with lower extremities and work upward to determine level of deficit:

  Assess muscle symmetry by using side-to-side comparison.

  Assess muscle strength by having patient pull against resistance with each extremity.

  Assess DTRs of the Achilles, patellae, biceps, triceps, and brachioradialis. Report ↓ (+1) or absent (0) response.

  Assess for paresthesias, presence/absence of position sense, presence/absence of vibratory sense, and presence/absence of response to light touch or pinprick to determine level of dysfunction and whether or not ascending.

- Turn patient in correct anatomic alignment q2h or more often.
- Ensure that active or passive ROM exercises performed q2h during all phases of GBS. Involve significant others if appropriate.
- As indicated, apply splints to hands/arms and feet/legs to help prevent contracture; alternate splints so they are on for 2 h and off for 2 h.
- Use pneumatic compression device or other prescribed therapy to minimize risk of thrombophlebitis.
- Low air loss or fluidized beds may be used to manage respiratory, autonomic, and musculoskeletal problems that occur with GBS.

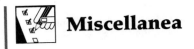 **Miscellanea**

CONSULT MD FOR
- Respiratory compromise: dyspnea, tachypnea, ↓ in Pao_2 >15 mm Hg or ↑ in $Paco_2$ >15 mm Hg over baseline or nl values
- Complications of plasmapheresis: hypovolemia, abnormal clotting, hypokalemia, hypocalcemia
- Sustained AD (>15-30 min)
- Cardiac dysrhythmias, sustained hypotension
- Progressive motor weakness, ↓/absent DTRs, cranial nerve dysfunction

RELATED TOPICS
- Autonomic dysreflexia
- Immobility, prolonged
- Mechanical ventilation
- Nutritional support, enteral and parenteral
- Pneumonia, aspiration
- Psychosocial needs, patient
- Syndrome of inappropriate antidiuretic hormone

ABBREVIATIONS
AD: Autonomic dysreflexia
DTR: Deep tendon reflex
NCV: Nerve conduction velocity
SIADH: Syndrome of inappropriate antidiuretic hormone
VC: Vital capacity

Dysreflexia (or risk for same) r/t noxious stimulus

Desired outcome: Patient has no symptoms of AD as evidenced by nl ECG, HR 60-100 bpm, BP wnl for patient, cool and dry skin, nl strength, and absence of headache and chest/abdominal tightness.

- Assess for signs of AD: cardiac dysrhythmias, HR <60 bpm or >100 bpm, ↑ and sustained BP (eg, ≥250-300/150 mm Hg), facial flushing, ↑ sweating, extreme generalized warmth, profound weakness, and complaints of severe headache or tightening in chest/abdomen.
- Place patient on cardiac monitor during first 10-14 days of hospitalization or if there are S&S of AD.
- Monitor carefully during activities known to precipitate AD: position changes, vigorous coughing, straining with bowel movements, suctioning.
- If indicators of AD present, correct any stimulating factors.
- Consult physician if symptoms do not abate within 15-30 min.
- If there is a sustained ↑ in BP, administer antihypertensive agent.

Sensory/Perceptual alterations (or risk for same) r/t altered sensory transmission secondary to cranial nerve involvement

Desired outcome: Patient relates presence of nl vision and exhibits nl pupillary/gag reflexes, ability to masticate, intact corneas, and full ROM of head and shoulders.

- Evaluate cranial nerves III, IV, and V by checking for extraocular eye movements, pupillary light reflex, degree of ptosis, and diplopia.

  If patient exhibits a deficit, place objects where they can be seen. Assist with ADL as indicated.

  For diplopia, cover one eye with patch or frosted lens; alternate patch or lens q2-3h during waking hours.

  Use eyelid crutches for ptosis.
- Evaluate cranial nerves V and VII by checking facial sensation and movement, ability to masticate, and corneal reflex.

  If a deficit present, assess for corneal irritation or abrasion. Apply artificial tear drops or ointments as prescribed. Secure eyelid in closed position if corneal reflex diminished or absent.
- Evaluate cranial nerves IX, X, and XII by checking for pharyngeal sensation and movement (swallowing), presence/absence of gag reflex, and tongue control.

  If a deficit found, suction during oral hygiene. Do not feed patient an oral diet until gag reflex returns.
- Assess cranial nerve XI by checking ability to shrug shoulders and turn head from side to side.

  If a deficit found, place head in a position of comfort and proper anatomic alignment.

REFERENCES

Barall-Inman RA: Question and answer: Guillain-Barré syndrome, *J Am Acad Nurse Prac* 7(4): 165-169, 1995.

Gregory RJ: Understanding and coping with neurological impairment, *Rehabil Nurs* 20(2): 74-78, 83, 130, 1995.

Stowe AC: Guillain-Barré syndrome. In Swearingen PL, Keen JH: *Manual of critical care nursing*, ed 3, St Louis, 1995, Mosby.

Villaire M: ICU from the patient's point of view, *Crit Care Nurse* 15(1): 80-87, 1995.

Waldock E: The pathophysiology of Guillain-Barré syndrome, *Br J Nurs* 4(14): 818-821, 1995.

Author: **Ann Coghlan Stowe**

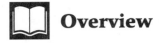

Overview

PATHOPHYSIOLOGY

Results from blunt or penetrating forces. *Blunt injuries* caused by deceleration, acceleration, rotational forces (eg, vehicular collisions, falls). *Penetrating injuries* pierce cranium, damaging underlying brain tissue and support structures. Outcome variable based on injury type and mechanism, coma duration, preinjury medical status, and brainstem integrity.

Direct Injuries

Linear skull fracture: Nondisplaced; associated with low-velocity impact.

Basilar skull fracture: Involves base of cranium's anterior, middle, or posterior fossae.

Depressed skull fracture: Depression over point of impact; may be closed, compressed, or open.

Concussion: Diffuse, axonal brain injuries; mild to severe.

Contusion: Bruising of brain tissue; described as *coup* if injury directly beneath site of impact, *contrecoup* if opposite site of impact.

Secondary Injuries

Epidural hematoma: Occurs after laceration of middle meningeal artery; develops rapidly in space between skull and dura.

Subdural hematoma: Bleeding primarily from veins between dura and arachnoid spaces; classified as acute, subacute, chronic.

SAH: Seen over convexities of brain and in basal cisterns; indicates bleeding into ventricles.

Intracranial hematoma: Results from injury to small arteries and veins; associated with petechiae, contusions, edema.

Herniation: Portion of brain displaced, causing ischemia, necrosis, and, ultimately, death.

Ischemia: Occurs secondary to hypotensive or hypoxic event following initial injury.

INTRACRANIAL PRESSURE DYNAMICS

Pressure created within cranium by brain, blood, and CSF. Nl pressure <15 mm Hg. Any volume ↑ causes pressure ↑. Compensatory mechanisms, eg, shunting of CSF or vasoconstriction, activate to ↓ volume. With brain injury, compensatory mechanisms overwhelmed and extrinsic measures become necessary to maintain nl pressure/volume relationship.

HISTORY/RISK FACTORS

- Vehicular collision, fall, sports-related injury
- Acts of violence
- Intoxication
- Failure to use safety device (helmet, seat belt, air bag)
- Chronic illness
- Advanced age

CLINICAL PRESENTATION

Variable; focal or generalized neurologic deficits, changes in LOC, headache, behavior changes

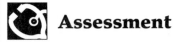

Assessment

PHYSICAL ASSESSMENT

Baseline data include assessment of mental status, cranial nerves, motor status, sensory status, reflexes. Thereafter, neurologic assessment based on clinical status. (See Appendix for Glasgow Coma Scale and Rancho Los Amigos Levels of Cognitive Functioning Scale.) Following are assessment findings related to specific injuries:

Epidural Hematoma/Linear Skull Fracture: Loss of consciousness followed by lucid interval and rapid deterioration; ipsilateral pupil dilatation and contralateral weakness; evidence of brainstem compression: fixed pupils, extension or flexion posturing, irregular respirations

Basilar Skull Fracture: Rhinorrhea and otorrhea; *anterior fossa injuries:* periorbital ecchymosis, epistaxis, damage to cranial nerves I and II, meningitis; *middle and posterior fossa injuries:* tinnitus, hemotympanum, Battle's sign

Compound Depressed Skull Fracture: Changes in LOC, pupillary changes, headache, CSF leaks if dura torn, tympanum rupture, contused brain tissue

Concussion: Brief loss of consciousness, headache, dizziness, vomiting, mild changes in mentation, memory loss, ↓ attention span, ↓ concentration skills

Contusion: Prolonged loss of consciousness; focal or generalized neurologic deficits

Subdural Hematoma/SAH: *Acute:* changing LOC within 24 h, ipsilateral dilated pupil, contralateral extremity weakness. *Subacute:* occurs within 48 h to wks after injury; LOC deteriorates and focal neurologic deficits ensue. *Chronic:* personality changes, headache, and other neurologic signs occur wks or mos after injury. High-risk groups: elders and chronic alcohol users.

SAH: Headache, changes in LOC, nuchal rigidity, ↑ temp, positive Kernig's sign

Other Data: Baseline CV, Resp, GI, GU, and Integ data obtained with ongoing reassessment. Cushing's triad is a late sign indicating mechanical compression or severe metabolic brainstem dysfunction.

VITAL SIGNS/HEMODYNAMICS

RR: ↑, ↓; irregularly irregular

HR: Possible ↓ with brainstem compression

BP: Possible ↑ SBP and ↓ DBP (widened pulse pressure); ↓ with neurogenic shock

Temp: ↓ or ↑ with thermoregulatory failure

Resp Patterns: Apneustic, cluster, ataxic (see Appendix)

Other: ↓ SVR, PAWP, CO if neurogenic shock present

DIAGNOSTIC PROCEDURES

EEG: Detects areas of irritability associated with seizures and generalized brain activity. Anticonvulsants alter brain activity; document their use.

Evoked Responses: Evaluate brain's electrical potentials (responses) to external stimulus—auditory, visual, somatosensory. Determine extent of injury in uncooperative, confused, comatose patients.

LABORATORY STUDIES

CSF Analysis: To determine infection; not done if ↑ ICP present.

IMAGING

Skull X-ray: Detects structural deficits such as skull fractures and facial bone destruction as well as air-fluid level in sinuses, abnormal intracranial calcification, radiopaque foreign bodies.

C-spine X-ray: Shows structural spinal deficits and rules out associated C-spine injuries. C-spine mobilization required until C-1 through T-1 visualized completely and fractures ruled out.

CT Scan: Gray and white matter, blood, CSF detectable; capable of diagnosing cerebral hemorrhage, infarction, hydrocephalus, cerebral edema, structural shifts.

MRI: Provides detailed spatial resolution, can follow trace metabolic processes, detects structural changes.

Cerebral Angiography: Adjunct in diagnosing brain injury; used if CT scan unavailable.

🍷 Collaborative Management

Treatment based on relationship between ICP and CPP where:

$$CPP = MAP - ICP$$

Goal of treatment: to maintain CPP >60 mm Hg and ↓ ICP to <15 mm Hg.

ICP Monitoring: Variety of techniques (intraventricular cannula, subarachnoid screw, epidural or intraparenchymal fiberoptic sensor) used. Monitoring systems provide digital display of ICP, but CPP must be calculated.

CSF Drainage: Intraventricular or ventriculostomy systems used to drain CSF and ↓ ICP. Keep drainage collection bags at level of ear tragus or higher to prevent excessive CSF flow.

Hyperventilation: Controls ICP by ↓ $Paco_2$, thereby vasoconstricting cerebral vessels and causing ↓ cerebral blood volume. Accomplished *via* mechanical ventilation. $Paco_2$ maintained between 30-35 mm Hg and Pao_2 at >80 mm Hg.

Diuresis Therapy: ↓ cerebral brain volume by extracting fluid from brain's intracellular compartment. Dehydration a major complication; strict attention to serum electrolytes and osmolality necessary.

$AVDo_2$ and Jugular Bulb O_2 Saturation: Monitor to help determine if blood flow to brain matches metabolic requirements. Differentiates between ischemia and hyperemia.

Sedating Agents: Use of continuous drips of midazolam HCl (Versed), propofol (Diprivan), and narcotic analgesics, such as fentanyl citrate (Sublimaze) or morphine sulfate, common. Nondepolarizing agents, eg, vecuronium bromide (Norcuron), also used.

Seizure Control: Seizures greatly ↑ brain's metabolic demand; prophylaxis used as necessary. Phenytoin (Dilantin), diazepam (Valium), and phenobarbital commonly used.

Barbiturate Coma: Pentobarbital sodium (Nembutal) is drug of choice. Continuous ICP and hemodynamic monitoring and controlled ventilation necessary because barbiturates induce profound cardiac and cerebral depression.

Maintaining Body Temp: For every 1° C ↑, a 10%-13% ↑ in metabolic rate occurs. Fever etiology important; it influences treatment choice.

Central fever: Directly attributed to brain injury; reflects derangement in hypothalamic function. Characterized by lack of sweating and diurnal variation, plateaulike elevation up to 41° C (105.8° F), absence of tachycardia, persistence for days/wks. Control with external cooling rather than with antipyretics. Hypothermia therapy may ↑ metabolic demand *via* shivering. Wrap distal extremities in bath towels or give chlorpromazine (Thorazine) to control shivering.

Peripheral fever: Associated with wound or CNS infections, other bacterial invasion. Characterized by sweating, diurnal variation, response to antipyretic agents, tachycardia.

Cytokine release: Associated with brain injury; responds to ASA instead of to acetaminophen.

BP Control: Hypotension ↓ cerebral perfusion. Dopamine HCl used at doses between 3-5 μg/kg/min to maintain CPP. Hypertension ↑ capillary permeability and petechial hemorrhage. Manage with labetalol HCl (Normodyne) or nitroprusside sodium (Nipride).

Modifying Nursing Care Activities That ↑ ICP: Sustained ↑ in ICP (>5 min) must be avoided. Space activities such as bathing, turning, and suctioning to prevent stair-step ↑ in ICP.

Suctioning: Only as needed; preoxygenate with 100% O_2; limit 2 passes of ≤10 sec each; follow each pass with 60 sec hyperventilation using 100% O_2; use suction catheter with outer-to-inner diameter ratio of 2:1.

Flexion, extension, lateral movements: Maintain neck in neutral position to prevent flexion and lateral movements that can greatly ↑ ICP. For patients with poor neck control, stabilize with towel rolls or sandbags.

HOB positioning: Adjust based on clinical response. Desired effect is improvement in perfusion and ↓ in ICP.

Rehabilitation: Brain injury highly associated with physical and cognitive impairments. Initiate early consultations, and prepare patient for active rehabilitation program.

Surgical Intervention: To evacuate mass lesions (epidural, subdural, intracranial hematomas), place ICP monitoring system, elevate depressed skull fractures, débride open wounds and brain tissue, repair dural tears or scalp lacerations. Temporal lobectomy may be necessary to control severe ↑ in ICP.

PATIENT-FAMILY TEACHING

- Signs of ↑ ICP: headache (new, worsening), vomiting, confusion, sleepiness, visual disturbances, dizziness
- Importance of avoiding Valsalva maneuver, agitation, continuous coughing
- Support available through National Head Injury Foundation (18A Vernon Street, Framingham, MA 01701) or state chapter of the Head Injury Foundation

Nursing Diagnoses/Interventions

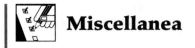 ## Miscellanea

Impaired gas exchange r/t ↓ O_2 supply and ↑ CO_2 production secondary to brainstem injury, aspiration, imposed inactivity, possible neurologic pulmonary edema

Desired outcomes: $Paco_2$ 25-30 mm Hg during hyperventilation, 35-40 as ICP stabilizes, and 35-45 by time of transfer from ICU. By time of transfer, patient has adequate gas exchange: orientation × 3, Pao_2 ≥80 mm Hg, RR 12-20 breaths/min with eupnea, no adventitious breath sounds.

- Assess respiratory rate, depth, rhythm. Auscultate lung fields for breath sounds q1-2h. Monitor for changes in respiratory patterns.
- Deliver O_2 within prescribed limits. Assess for hypoxia: confusion, agitation, restlessness, irritability. Cyanosis is a late indicator.
- Ensure patent airway *via* proper neck positioning and suctioning as necessary. Hyperoxygenate before and after each suction pass.
- Monitor ABGs. Be alert for hypoxemia (Pao_2 <80). Monitor for $Paco_2$ ≥25-30. ↑ levels may ↑ cerebral blood flow and thus ↑ ICP.
- Turn q2h, within limits of injury, to promote lung drainage/expansion and alveolar perfusion.
- Evaluate need for artificial airway in patients unable to maintain airway patency or adequate ventilatory effort.
- Encourage deep breathing at frequent intervals, if patient able, to promote oxygenation.

Risk for infection (CNS) r/t inadequate primary defenses secondary to skull fracture, penetrating wounds, craniotomy, ICP monitoring, or bacterial invasion resulting from pneumonia or iatrogenic causes

Desired outcome: Patient infection free: normothermia, WBCs ≤11,000 μl, negative culture results, HR ≤100 bpm, BP wnl for patient, with no agitation, purulent drainage, or other clinical indicators of infection.

- Assess VS for indicators of CNS infection: ↑ temp, ↑ RR, possible ↓ BP.
- Monitor for systemic infection: discomfort, malaise, agitation, restlessness. Monitor WBCs for ↑ or shift to left.
- Inspect cranial wounds for erythema, tenderness, swelling, purulent drainage. Obtain culture as indicated.
- Apply loose sterile dressing (sling) to collect CSF drainage. Do not pack. Record drainage amount, color, character.
- Caution against coughing, sneezing, nose blowing, or other Valsalva-type maneuvers because these activities can further damage the dura.
- Use orogastric (not NG) tubes with basilar skull fracture or severe frontal sinus fracture.
- Apply restraints *only* if necessary to keep patient from harm. Restraints can ↑ ICP by causing straining.

Decreased adaptive capacity: Intracranial, r/t compromise of pressure/volume dynamics

Desired outcome: Patient exhibits adequate intracranial adaptive capacity within 72 h of treatment: orientation × 3 (or consistent with baseline); equal and normoreactive pupils; BP wnl; HR 60-100 bpm; RR 12-20 breaths/min with eupnea (or controlled ventilation); ICP 0-15 mm Hg; CPP 60-80 mm Hg.

- Assess qh for ↑ ICP and herniation (altered mentation, ↑ BP with widening pulse pressure, irregular respirations, ↑ headache, pupillary changes).
- Calculate CPP by means of the formula

$$CPP = MAP - ICP$$
$$\text{where } MAP = \frac{SBP + 2(DBP)}{3}$$

- Assess for ↑ ICP (ICP ≥15 mm Hg) or CPP <60 mm Hg.
- Assess for and treat conditions that can cause ↑ restlessness with concomitant ↑ ICP: hypoxemia, pain, fear, anxiety.
- Implement measures that help prevent ↑ ICP and herniation:
   Maintain complete bed rest.
   Maintain HOB in position that keeps ICP <15 mm Hg and CPP >60 mm Hg.
   Avoid neck hyperflexion, hyperextension, or hyperrotation.
   Maintain quiet, relaxing environment.
   Minimize vigorous activity; assist with ADL.
   Maintain adequate ventilation to prevent cerebral hypoxia.

CONSULT MD FOR
- Hypercapnia: $Paco_2$ >30 mm Hg during hyperventilation or >40-45 mm Hg as condition stabilizes
- Hypoxemia: Pao_2 <80 mm Hg
- CPP <60-80 mm Hg
- ICP >15 mm Hg
- Sudden changes in LOC
- Widening pulse pressure
- Bradycardia
- Pupillary changes
- UO > 200 ml/h × 2

RELATED TOPICS
- Agitation syndrome
- Cerebral aneurysm
- Diabetes insipidus
- Herniation syndromes
- Immobility, prolonged
- Increased intracranial pressure
- Intracranial surgery
- Syndrome of inappropriate antidiuretic hormone
- Vasodilator therapy

ABBREVIATIONS
$AVDo_2$: Arterial venous difference in oxygen
CPP: Cerebral perfusion pressure
SAH: Subarachnoid hemorrhage

Avoid vigorous, prolonged suctioning.

Hyperoxygenate with 100% O_2 before/during/after suctioning.

Maintain normovolemia.

Monitor and record I&O.

- Administer antihypertensives to prevent hypertension.
- If ↑ ICP occurs suddenly, perform hyperinflation with manual resuscitator at 100% O_2 at ≥50 breaths/min to ↓ $Paco_2$.
- If prescribed for acute ↑ in ICP, administer bolus of mannitol (ie, 1.5-2.0 g/kg as a 15%-25% solution infused over 30-60 min). Monitor carefully to avoid profound fluid and electrolyte disturbances.
- Prevent fluid volume excess, which could ↑ cerebral edema, by precise delivery of IV fluids at consistent rates. Administer mannitol and furosemide at prescribed intervals to promote diuresis and ↓ intracranial brain volume.
- Treat ↑ in ICP immediately by implementing the following:

  Elevate HOB to position that minimizes ICP and maximizes CPP.

  Loosen constrictive objects around neck.

  If recently repositioned, return to original position.

  Assess for contributors to ↑ ICP: hypoxia, fear, anxiety, pain, agitation.

Ineffective thermoregulation r/t trauma associated with injury to or pressure on hypothalamus

Desired outcome: Patient normothermic within 24 h of this diagnosis.

- Monitor for signs of hyperthermia: temp >38.33° C (101° F), pallor, absence of perspiration, torso warm to touch.
- As indicated, obtain specimens for blood, urine, sputum cultures to r/o underlying infection.
- Be alert to signs of meningitis: fever, chills, nuchal rigidity, Kernig's sign, Brudzinski's sign.
- Assess wounds for S&S of infection: erythema, tenderness, purulent drainage.
- If hyperthermic, remove excess clothing and administer tepid baths, hypothermic blanket, or ice bags to axilla or groin.
- Administer antipyretics such as acetaminophen or ASA.

Risk for disuse syndrome r/t immobilization and prolonged inactivity secondary to brain injury, spasticity, or altered LOC

Desired outcome: Patient exhibits baseline/optimal ROM with no verbal or nonverbal indicators of pain.

- Begin passive ROM exercises q4h on all extremities immediately on admission. Monitor ICP during ROM; alter care plan for sustained ↑.
- Teach passive ROM exercises to significant others. Encourage their participation as often as they are able.
- Reposition patient q2h within restrictions of head and other injuries, using logrolling technique as indicated.
- Ensure proper anatomic position and alignment. Support alignment with pillows, trochanter rolls, wrapped sandbags.
- For patients with spasticity or flaccidity, consult OT for use of splints and other supportive devices to prevent contractures and optimize later function.

Fluid volume deficit r/t failure of regulatory mechanisms resulting in polyuria

Desired outcome: Patient remains normovolemic: BP 110-120/70-80 mm Hg (or wnl for patient), CVP ≥2 mm Hg, PAWP ≥6 mm Hg, HR 60-100 bpm, I = O + insensible losses, stable weight.

- Keep careful I&O records. Report UO >200 ml/h for 2 consecutive h.
- Provide adequate fluids. Keep water pitcher full and within reach. Administer hyperosmolar tube feedings/solutions with extreme caution. They can worsen fluid losses by inducing diarrhea osmotically.
- For patients who cannot maintain adequate PO fluid intake, administer IV fluids as prescribed, usually hypotonic solution, as follows: 1 ml IV fluid for each 1 ml of UO. With brain injury, moderate diuresis may be permitted to avoid need for osmotic diuretics. Hypernatremia, if present, must be corrected slowly to prevent cerebral edema, seizures, permanent neurologic damage, or death.
- Administer vasopressin as indicated; observe for and document desired effects as well as these side effects: hypertension, cardiac ischemia, hyponatremia.
- Weigh qd at same time and using same scale and garments to prevent error. Check for weight loss >1 kg/day.
- Monitor for continuing fluid volume deficit: ↓ skin turgor, dry mucosa, rapid/thready pulse, and SBP, CVP/PAWP < baseline.
- Monitor serum sodium, serum and urine osmolality, and urine specific gravity. Monitor urine specific gravity qh to evaluate response to therapy.

REFERENCES

Davis A et al: Neurologic dysfunctions. In Swearingen PL, Keen JH (eds): *Manual of critical care nursing*, ed 3, St Louis, 1995, Mosby.

Eisenhart K: New perspectives in the management of adults with severe head injury, *Crit Care Nurs Q* 17(2): 1-12, 1994.

German K: Intracranial pressure monitoring in the 1990s, *Crit Care Nurs Q* 17(1): 21-32, 1994.

Kerr ME, Lovasik D, Darby J: Evaluating cerebral oxygenation using jugular venous oximetry in head injuries, *AACN Clin Issues in Crit Care Nurs* 6(1): 11-20, 1995.

Prendergast V: Current trends in research and treatment of intracranial hypertension, *Crit Care Nurs Q* 17(1): 1-8, 1994.

Author: **Alice Davis**

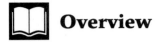 **Overview**

PATHOPHYSIOLOGY

Includes four distinct patterns of impulse conduction disturbance through the AV node.
First-Degree: Impulse conduction delayed from SA node through AV node.
Second-Degree, Type I (Mobitz I, Wenkebach): Impulse conduction originates at SA node; partially blocked at AV node. May manifest as 2:1 conduction or high-grade (advanced) block (>2:1 conduction). Usually results in gradually ↑ PR intervals until one impulse blocked; then cycle begins again.
Second-Degree, Type II (Mobitz II): Intermittent block at AV node. May manifest as 2:1 conduction or high-grade (advanced) block (>2:1 conduction).
Third-Degree (complete heart block): Complete block at AV node. To compensate, AV junction or ventricle develops another pacemaker. Atria and ventricles contract independently of the other because of separate pacing mechanisms.

HISTORY/RISK FACTORS

- CAD, MI, myocardial ischemia, myocarditis, conduction system disease, aortic valve disease, mitral valve prolapse, ASD
- Antidysrhythmic drugs, including digoxin
- β Adrenergic blocking agents
- Calcium channel blocking agents
- Cardioplegia during open heart surgery

CLINICAL PRESENTATION

May be without symptoms or may experience chest discomfort, lightheadedness, dizziness, weakness, unusual fatigue, SOB. May appear pale or cyanotic with cold hands and feet and slightly moist skin and speak with effort.

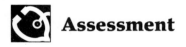 **Assessment**

PHYSICAL ASSESSMENT

Neuro: Altered LOC, syncope, weakness, fainting, vertigo, anxiety, restlessness
Resp: Dyspnea, SOB, crackles in lung bases
CV: Chest discomfort, activity intolerance, sense of "skipped beats"
GI: Nausea, vomiting, heartburn-like pain
GU: ↓ UO
Integ: Diaphoresis, pallor, cyanosis

VITAL SIGNS/HEMODYNAMICS

RR: ↑ or nl
HR: ↓
BP: ↓ or nl
Temp: Nl
CVP/PAWP: Nl, ↑, or ↓
CO: ↓

SVR: ↑

12/18-lead ECG

First-degree: Regular rhythm, atrial and ventricular rates 60-100 bpm, P waves present preceding each QRS, QRS nl, PR interval prolonged (>0.20 sec), P:QRS = 1:1.
Second-degree, type I: Irregular rhythm, atrial rate > ventricular rate, P waves precede each QRS, some P waves nonconducted, QRS usually appears nl, PR interval variable and lengthens progressively with each cycle until one P wave is nonconducted.
Second-degree, type II: Irregular rhythm; atrial rate (60-150 bpm) > ventricular rate; ventricular rate dependent on frequency of blocked sinus impulses at AV node; P waves ≥2 for each QRS, sometimes in set pattern of 2:1, 3:1, 4:1; QRS usually of nl duration; PR interval consistently nl or prolonged on each conducted complex; P>QRS.
Third-degree: Usually regular rhythm; atrial rate of 60-100 bpm > ventricular rate; ventricular rate <50 bpm; P waves occur at regular intervals; QRS <0.12 sec if pacing occurs at AV junction and >0.12 sec if variable ventricular PR interval, exhibiting no relationship between P and QRS.

LABORATORY STUDIES

Electrolytes: ↑ K^+, Mg^{2+} levels may cause ↓ HR and significant changes in rhythm, especially with antidysrhythmics.
Therapeutic Antidysrhythmic Levels: Data necessary for rhythm control and drug toxicity prevention. Digoxin, β blockers, calcium blockers can lead to heart block.
Drug/Toxicology Screening: Identifies cardiotoxic drug overdose (tricyclic antidepressants, sedatives, barbiturates, opiates).
ABGs: May reveal hypoxemia or pH abnormality that can interfere with electrolyte balance and precipitate dysrhythmias.

IMAGING

Chest X-ray: May reflect enlarged cardiac silhouette indicative of heart disease.
Echocardiography: Use of ultrasound to evaluate ventricular pumping action, including estimation of ventricular EF.
Cardiac Catheterization: Assesses for CAD.

DIAGNOSTIC PROCEDURES

24-h Holter Monitoring/Cardiac Event Monitoring/"Full Disclosure": Identifies subtle dysrhythmias during ambulation and throughout day. Abnormal rhythms correlated with symptoms; patient records symptoms as they occur.
Exercise Stress Testing: Used alone or with 24-h Holter monitoring to detect subtle dysrhythmias. May not yield data regarding bradycardia or heart block as readily as tachycardia or cardiac irritability/ischemia.

Collaborative Management

Supplemental O_2: ↑ O_2 delivery to tissue.
Spo₂: Detects ↓ O_2 saturation resulting from dysrhythmias or other causes.
Continuous ECG Monitoring: Detects all dysrhythmias, onset and duration, and termination for intermittent dysrhythmias.
Management of Other Causes of Bradydysrhythmias: Eg, hypoxia, hyperkalemia, hypermagnesemia, preexisting acidosis, hypothermia, endocrine/neuroendocrine disorders, drug overdose/toxicity.
Temporary Cardiac Pacing: For bradydysrhythmias that fail to respond to pharmacologic therapy or as a bridge to permanent pacemaker insertion.
Invasive: Eg, temporary transvenous pacing wire, Chandler probe through appropriate thermodilution PA catheter (Swan-Ganz), epicardial pacing wires inserted during cardiac surgical procedure.
Noninvasive transcutaneous: Via skin electrodes, one on left anterior chest wall and one posteriorly between shoulder blades.
Diet: Low-fat, low-cholesterol, ↓-caffeine diet for recurrent dysrhythmias.
Pharmacotherapy: To stimulate ↑ in HR for bradydysrhythmias in order to ↑ CO and BP.
Atropine: Parasympatholytic that blocks "slowing" action of vagus nerve, resulting in ↑ HR. May be ineffective in severe second-degree type II and third-degree heart block. *Dosage:* 0.5-1.0 mg IV push q3-5min up to total of 0.04 mg/kg for bradycardia. (50 kg = 2 mg, 75 kg = 3 mg, 100 kg = 4 mg.) If ineffective, temporary cardiac pacing initiated.
Catecholamine infusions: Stimulate B_1 receptors of sympathetic nervous system, resulting in ↑ HR.
> *Epinephrine:* 2-10 μg/min continuously
> *Dopamine:* 5-20 μg/kg/min continuously
> *Isoproterenol:* 2-10 μg/min continuously; used cautiously in patients at high risk for MI

Permanent Pacemaker: Implanted SC to provide electrical impulse to heart when nl pacemakers/conduction system fail to maintain HR. AV sequential pacing may be necessary with limited/absent conduction between atria and ventricles.

PATIENT-FAMILY TEACHING

- Importance of promptly reporting chest pain, lightheadedness, SOB, activity intolerance, syncope
- Self-measuring of pulse rate/rhythm
- Causes of heart block; pacing devices used during, after hospitalization
- At-home dietary guidelines
- Safety regarding pacemakers

Nursing Diagnoses/Interventions

Decreased cardiac output r/t altered rate, rhythm, conduction; r/t negative inotropic cardiac changes secondary to cardiac disease

Desired outcome: Within 15 min of dysrhythmia onset, patient has adequate cardiac output: BP ≥90/60 mm Hg, HR 60-100 bpm, PAP 20-30/8-15 mm Hg, PAWP 6-12 mm Hg, CVP 2-6 mm Hg, CO 4-7 L/min, CI 2.5-4.0 L/min/m^2, or within 10% baseline for all.

- Monitor continuous ECG, noting response to antidysrhythmics and transcutaneous or transvenous cardiac pacing.
- Monitor VS for baseline status and prn for changes in cardiac rhythm, including PA readings if PA catheter in place.
- Document dysrhythmias by saving rhythm strips. Use 12/18-lead ECG to diagnose new symptomatic dysrhythmias.
- Note changes in SpO$_2$ with symptomatic bradycardia.
- Manage life-threatening dysrhythmias using ACLS guidelines.
- Provide supplemental O$_2$ for symptomatic bradycardia.
- Monitor lab values to assess cause of bradycardia.
- Administer medications that support cardiac output and BP if antidysrhythmics or cardiac pacing are insufficient to ↑ BP.

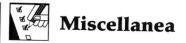

Miscellanea

CONSULT MD FOR
- Failure of bradycardia to respond to prescribed treatments
- Worsening symptoms: chest pain; SOB; dyspnea; hypotension; altered mental status; SpO$_2$ <90%; ↑ PAP, PAWP or CVP; bradycardia
- Possible complications: heart failure, cardiac arrest (PEA, asystole), hypoxemia, new dysrhythmias

RELATED TOPICS
- Antidysrhythmic therapy
- Cardiomyopathy
- Coronary artery disease
- Hyperkalemia
- Hypermagnesemia
- Myocardial infarction, acute

ABBREVIATIONS
ASD: Atrial septal defect
EF: Ejection fraction
EP: Electrophysiologic
PEA: Pulseless electrical activity

REFERENCES
American Heart Association: *Textbook of advanced cardiac life support,* Dallas, 1994, The Association.
Cheitlin MD, Sokolow M, McIlroy MB: *Clinical cardiology,* ed 6, Norwalk, Conn, 1993, Appleton & Lange.
Dracup K: *Meltzer's intensive coronary care: a manual for nurses,* ed 5, Norwalk, Conn, 1995, Appleton & Lange.
Jacobsen C: Arrhythmias and conduction disturbances. In Woods SL: *Cardiac nursing,* ed 3, Philadelphia, 1995, Lippincott.
Keen J, Baird M, Allen J: *Mosby's critical care and emergency drug reference,* ed 2, St Louis, 1996, Mosby.
Lewandowski DM, Jacobsen C: AV blocks: are you up to date? *Am J Nurs* 95(12): 26-33, 1995.
Porterfield LM: The cutting edge in arrhythmias, *Crit Care Nurse (Suppl):* June 1993.
Steuble BT: Dysrhythmias and conduction disturbances. In Swearingen PL, Keen JH (eds): *Manual of critical care nursing,* ed 3, St Louis, 1995, Mosby.

Authors: **Marianne Saunorus Baird and Barbara Tueller Steuble**

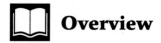 **Overview**

PATHOPHYSIOLOGY

Occurs when left ventricle is unable to maintain sufficient cardiac output to meet bodily needs. Often begins when diseased LV myocardium cannot pump blood returning from lungs into the systemic circulation. Also can occur because of ↑ afterload, eg, systemic hypertension. If LV and pulmonary vascular pressure exceed pulmonary capillary oncotic pressure (>30 mm Hg), fluid floods pulmonary interstitial spaces, resulting in pulmonary edema, which impairs O_2 and CO_2 exchange. If sustained, can precipitate RV failure.

HISTORY/RISK FACTORS
- CAD risk factors
- Age >65
- Noncompliance with low-sodium diet or medications
- Cardiomyopathy, previous MI, valvular heart disease

CLINICAL PRESENTATION

Nocturnal dyspnea, dyspnea on exertion, orthopnea, cyanosis or pallor, palpitations, weakness, fatigue, anorexia, change in mentation

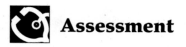 **Assessment**

PHYSICAL ASSESSMENT

Neuro: Somnolence, confusion, anxiety
Resp: Crackles, wheezing, moist cough, frothy sputum, dyspnea, tachypnea
CV: Tachycardia, S_3 or summation gallop, pulsus alternans, dysrhythmias, ↓ intensity of peripheral pulses, delayed capillary refill, peripheral edema
GU: Oliguria
Integ: Diaphoresis

VITAL SIGNS/HEMODYNAMICS
RR: ↑
HR: ↑
BP: ↓
Temp: NI
CO/CI: ↓
PAP/PAWP: ↑
SVR: ↑
ECG: Dysrhythmias, ischemic changes possible (eg, ST-segment elevation/depression)

LABORATORY STUDIES

Serum Electrolytes: May reveal hyponatremia (dilutional); hyperkalemia if glomerular filtration ↓; or hypokalemia caused by diuretics.
CBC: ↓ Hgb and Hct possible with anemia or dilution.
ABGs: To determine hypoxemia, respiratory alkalosis.
Digitalis Levels: Digitalis toxicity possible because of low CO state and ↓ renal excretion of the drug.

IMAGING

Chest X-ray: Reveals pulmonary clouding, ↑ interstitial density, engorged pulmonary vasculature, cardiomegaly.

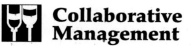 **Collaborative Management**

Treatment of Underlying Cause, Precipitating Factors: Atherosclerotic heart disease, AMI, dysrhythmias, cardiomyopathy, ↑ circulating volume, systemic hypertension, valvular or septal abnormalities, cardiac tamponade, constrictive pericarditis.
O_2: *Via* nasal cannula or other device; titrated to maintain SpO_2 ≥92%-96%. ET intubation and mechanical ventilation may be necessary.
Bed Rest: To ↓ cardiac workload and facilitate mobilization of fluid from extremities.
Stress Reduction: To ↓ endogenous catecholamine release and ↓ sympathetic tone.

Low-Calorie Diet (if weight control necessary) and Low-Sodium Diet: Extra salt and water are held in circulatory system, causing ↑ heart strain. Fluids may be limited to 1500 ml/day.

Pharmacotherapy
Morphine: To induce vasodilatation and ↓ venous return, preload, sympathetic tone, anxiety, myocardial O_2 consumption, pain.
Diuretics: To ↓ blood volume and ↓ preload.
Inotropic agents: Digitalis to strengthen contractions; dobutamine, milrinone, or amrinone to support BP and enhance contractility.
Vasodilators: Nitrates (oral, topical, IV) to dilate venous or capacitant vessels, thereby causing ↓ preload and cardiac and pulmonary congestion. Nitroprusside and nifedipine dilate arterial or resistant vessels and ↓ afterload, thus promoting forward flow.
Treatment of Acute Pulmonary Edema: Immediate interventions include O_2, possible ET intubation, diuretic therapy, inotropes, vasodilators, morphine.

PATIENT-FAMILY TEACHING
- Physiologic process of LV failure; how ↑ fluid volume is caused by poor heart functioning
- Importance of low-sodium diet and medications to help ↓ volume overload; how to read and evaluate food labels
- S&S of fluid volume excess necessitating medical attention: irregular or slow pulse, ↑ SOB, orthopnea, ↓ exercise tolerance, steady weight gain (≥1 kg/day for 2 successive days)
- If patient taking digitalis, technique for measuring HR; parameters for holding digitalis (usually for HR <60/min) and notifying physician
- Importance of avoiding activities that require straining; use of stool softeners, bulk-forming agents, laxatives as needed
- Warning signals to stop activity and rest: chest pain, SOB, dizziness or faintness, unusual weakness; use of prophylactic NTG
- Phone number for American Heart Association: 1-800-242-8721

Nursing Diagnoses/Interventions

Impaired gas exchange r/t alveolar-capillary membrane changes secondary to fluid collection in alveoli and interstitial spaces

Desired outcome: Within 24 h of treatment initiation, patient has improved gas exchange: PaO_2 ≥80 mm Hg, RR 12-20 breaths/min with eupnea, and clear breath sounds.

- Monitor respiratory rate, rhythm, and character q1-2h. Be alert to RR >20 breaths/min, irregular rhythm, use of accessory muscles, or cough.
- Auscultate breath sounds, noting crackles, wheezes, other adventitious sounds.
- Provide supplemental O_2 to maintain SpO_2 ≥92%.
- Assess ABGs; note changes in response to O_2 supplementation or treatment of altered hemodynamics.
- Suction secretions as needed.
- Encourage deep breathing, coughing, and turning q2h.
- Place in semi- or high-Fowler's position to maximize chest excursion.

Fluid volume excess r/t compromised regulatory mechanism secondary to ↓ cardiac output

Desired outcome: Within 24 h of treatment, patient becomes normovolemic: clear lung sounds, ↑ UO, weight loss, PAWP ≤18 mm Hg, SVR ≤1200 dynes/sec/cm^{-5}, CO ≥4 L/min.

- Auscultate lung fields for crackles, rhonchi, or other adventitious sounds.
- Monitor I&O closely. Report positive fluid state or ↓ in UO to <0.5 mg/kg/h.
- Weigh qd; report significant ↑ in weight.
- Note changes from baseline to detect worsening heart failure: ↑ pedal edema, JVD, S_3 gallop or new murmur, dysrhythmias.
- Monitor hemodynamic status q1-2h and prn. Note response to drug therapy as well as indicators of need for more aggressive therapy: ↑ PAWP, SVR; ↓ CO.
- Administer diuretics (furosemide), positive inotropes (dobutamine, milrinone), and vasodilators (nitroprusside).
- Limit oral fluids; offer ice chips or frozen juice pops to ↓ thirst and discomfort of dry mouth.
- Maintain bed rest or activity restrictions.

Activity intolerance r/t imbalance between O_2 supply and demand secondary to ↓ myocardial functioning

Desired outcome: Within 12-24 h before transfer from CCU, patient exhibits cardiac tolerance to ↑ levels of activity: RR <24 breaths/min, NSR on ECG, HR ≤120 bpm (or within 20 bpm of resting HR), BP within 20 mm Hg of nl for patient, absence of chest pain.

- Maintain prescribed activity level; teach rationale for activity limitation.
- Organize nursing care so that periods of activity are interspersed with extended periods of uninterrupted rest.
- Assist with active/passive ROM exercises, as appropriate. Encourage as much activity as possible within prescribed allowances.
- Note physiologic response to activity, including BP, HR, RR, and heart rhythm. Signs of activity intolerance include chest pain, ↑ SOB, excessive fatigue, ↑ dysrhythmias, palpitations, HR response >120 bpm, SBP >20 mm Hg from baseline or >160 mm Hg, and ST-segment changes.
- If activity intolerance noted, instruct patient to stop activity and to rest.
- Administer medications (eg, NTG tablets, paste, patch) to ↓ preload.
- As needed, refer patient to PT department.

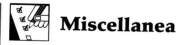 **Miscellanea**

CONSULT MD FOR

- Inability to maintain SpO_2 ≥92% despite supplemental O_2
- Deteriorating cardiac performance: new-onset S_3 or summation gallop, murmur, dysrhythmias, frothy sputum, crackles, sustained hypotension
- Unacceptable hemodynamics: CO <4 L/min, PAWP >18 mm Hg, SVR >1200 dynes/sec/cm^{-5}, MAP <70 mm Hg
- UO <0.5 mg/kg/h × 2 consecutive h
- Complications: pulmonary edema, cardiogenic shock, unrelieved chest pain, ECG evidence of ischemia

RELATED TOPICS

- Cardiomyopathy
- Hemodynamic monitoring
- Mechanical ventilation
- Myocardial infarction, acute
- Shock, cardiogenic
- Vasodilator therapy
- Vasopressor therapy

REFERENCES

Dracup K, Dunbar SB, Baker DW: Rethinking heart failure, *Am J Nurs* 95(7): 22-28, 1995.

Paul S: The pathophysiologic process of ventricular remodeling: from infarct to failure, *Crit Care Nurs Q* 18(1): 7-21, 1995.

Pratt NG: Pathophysiology of heart failure: neuroendocrine response, *Crit Care Nurs Q* 18(1): 22-31, 1995.

Steuble BT: Congestive heart failure/pulmonary edema. In Swearingen PL, Keen JH (eds): *Manual of critical care nursing,* ed 3, St Louis, 1995, Mosby.

Wright JM: Pharmacologic management of congestive heart failure, *Crit Care Nurs Q* 18(1): 32-44, 1995.

Author: **Barbara Tueller Steuble**

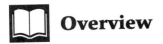 **Overview**

PATHOPHYSIOLOGY

Results most commonly from ↑ PVR, which can be caused by LV failure and pulmonary vascular congestion, certain lung disorders (eg, COPD, primary pulmonary hypertension, profound pulmonary hypoxemia), or acute RV MI. Regardless of initial cause, RV contractility is impaired, resulting in ↑ RVEDP. RV preload ↑, causing ↑ RAP and venous congestion. ↑ venous pressures result in venous stasis, hepatic congestion, peripheral edema, ascites. V/Q mismatch possible if pulmonary hypertension severe.

HISTORY/RISK FACTORS

- CAD risk factors
- Inferior wall or RV MI
- Pulmonary emboli
- Chronic bronchitis, emphysema
- Noncompliance with low-sodium diet or medications

CLINICAL PRESENTATION

Fluid retention, peripheral edema, ↓ UO, nausea, vomiting, anorexia

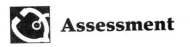 **Assessment**

PHYSICAL ASSESSMENT

Neuro: Somnolence, confusion if severe
Resp: Tachypnea; crackles usually absent unless concomitant LV heart failure present
CV: Right-sided S_3, S_4; tachycardia; dependent pitting edema; JVD; pulsus alternans; S&S of tricuspid regurgitation, including murmur at LSB and giant a waves in neck veins; Kussmaul's sign
GI: Hepatosplenomegaly, hepatojugular reflux, ascites, abdominal tenderness

VITAL SIGNS/HEMODYNAMICS

RR: ↑
HR: ↑
BP: ↓ or nl
Temp: Nl
CO/CI: ↓ or nl
CVP/RAP: ↑

PVR: ↑ if COPD, hypoxemia present
PAWP: ↑ only with biventricular failure
ECG: A-Fib common. 18-lead ECG may show injury/infarction patterns in right leads V_4-V_6 with RV infarct.

LABORATORY STUDIES

Serum Electrolytes: May reveal hyponatremia (dilutional); hyperkalemia if glomerular filtration ↓; or hypokalemia caused by diuretics.
Liver Enzymes: ↑ bilirubin level caused by hepatic venous congestion.
CBC: ↓ Hgb and Hct with anemia or dilution.
ABGs: May reveal hypoxemia caused by ↓ O_2 available from fluid-filled alveoli and respiratory alkalosis because of ↑ RR.
Digitalis Levels: Digitalis toxicity possible because of low CO state, which also causes ↓ renal excretion of the drug.

IMAGING

Chest X-ray: Will reveal pulmonary clouding, ↑ interstitial density, engorged pulmonary vasculature, and cardiomegaly.

Collaborative Management

Treatment of Underlying Cause, Precipitating Factors: LV heart failure, pulmonary edema, pulmonary hypertension, AMI, pulmonary embolism, hypoxemia, fluid overload or excess sodium intake, COPD, mitral or pulmonary valvular stenosis. Unlike LV heart failure in which the goal is to ↓ afterload, the goal in RV failure is to ↑ filling pressure and augment CO while avoiding fluid overload.
O_2: *Via* nasal cannula or other device; titrated to maintain SpO_2 ≥92%-96%. Mechanical ventilation may be necessary.
Fluid Management: Crystalloids, colloids given cautiously with ongoing assessment/hemodynamic monitoring to prevent overload.
Bed Rest: To ↓ cardiac workload and facilitate mobilization of fluid from extremities.
Stress Reduction: To ↓ endogenous catecholamine release and ↓ sympathetic tone.
Low-Calorie Diet (if weight control necessary) and Low-Sodium Diet: Excessive

sodium and water retention contribute to LV heart failure. Fluids may be limited to 1500 ml/day if there is evidence of overload, LV failure.

Pharmacotherapy

Inotropic agents: Digitalis to strengthen contractions; dopamine, dobutamine, milrinone, or amrinone to support BP and enhance contractility.
Morphine: May be given in AMI to ↓ sympathetic tone, anxiety, myocardial O_2 consumption, and pain; but also may ↓ venous return/preload and cause ↓ CO. Used with caution.
Diuretics: Generally avoided because ↑ preload necessary to promote maximal CO. May be used cautiously if crackles, other evidence of fluid volume overload or LV failure present.
Vasodilators: Nitrates (oral, topical, IV) used cautiously and in ↓ dosage to promote coronary arterial dilatation. Excessive doses ↓ preload and may ↓ RV contraction, thus reducing total CO.

PATIENT-FAMILY TEACHING

- Physiologic process of heart failure: how fluid volume ↑ because of poor heart functioning
- Importance of low-sodium diet and medications to help ↓ volume overload
- S&S of fluid volume excess that necessitate medical attention: irregular or slow pulse, ↑ SOB, orthopnea, ↓ exercise tolerance, steady weight gain (≥1 kg/day for 2 successive days)
- If patient taking digitalis, technique for measuring HR; parameters for holding digitalis (usually for HR <60/min) and notifying physician
- Activity progression; S&S of activity intolerance that signal need for rest; use of prophylactic NTG
- Importance of avoiding activities that require straining; use of stool softeners, bulk-forming agents, laxatives as needed
- Warning signals to stop activity and rest: chest pain, SOB, dizziness or faintness, unusual weakness
- Phone number for American Heart Association: 1-800-242-8721

Nursing Diagnoses/Interventions

Decreased cardiac output r/t ↓ preload and inotropic changes in heart function secondary to RV heart failure

Desired outcome: Within 24 h of treatment, patient has adequate CO: CVP/RAP 6-8 mm Hg (acceptable for this patient), PVR ≤100 dynes/sec/cm^{-5}, CO ≥4 L/min, UO ≥0.5 ml/kg/h, and orientation × 3 or baseline mental status.

- Administer fluids as necessary to optimize preload and maintain CO. Desired range for RAP is usually 6-8 mm Hg.
- Auscultate lung fields for crackles, which suggest excessive fluid volume (concommitant LV heart failure).
- Monitor I&O closely. Be alert for ↓ in UO to <0.5 mg/kg/h. Compare I&O ratio to estimate fluid status.
- Weigh qd to help monitor overall fluid status.
- Note changes from baseline to detect worsening RV heart failure: ↑ pedal edema, JVD, right-sided S_3,S_4 gallop, and atrial or other dysrhythmias. A new murmur suggests tricuspid regurgitation.
- Monitor hemodynamic status q1-2h and prn. Note response to drug therapy as well as indicators of need for more aggressive therapy. Avoid sudden or excessive ↓ in preload.
- Administer positive inotropes (dobutamine, milrinone) to optimize CO. Avoid diuretics or vasodilators unless LV heart failure is also present.
- Maintain bed rest or activity restrictions.

Impaired gas exchange r/t alveolar-capillary membrane changes secondary to fluid collection in alveoli and interstitial spaces; or secondary to altered blood flow caused by inadequate RV contractility or pulmonary hypertension

Desired outcome: Within 24 h of treatment initiation, patient has improved gas exchange: Pao$_2$ ≥80 mm Hg, RR 12-20 breaths/min with eupnea, clear breath sounds.

- Monitor respiratory rate, rhythm, and character q1-2h. Be alert to RR >20 breaths/min, irregular rhythm, use of accessory muscles of respiration, or cough.
- Auscultate breath sounds, noting crackles, wheezes, other adventitious sounds.
- Provide supplemental O$_2$ to maintain Spo$_2$ ≥92%.
- Assess ABGs; note changes in response to O$_2$ supplementation or treatment of altered hemodynamics.
- Suction secretions as needed.
- Encourage deep breathing, coughing, turning q2h.
- Place in semi- or high-Fowler's position to maximize chest excursion.
- If mechanical ventilation necessary, monitor ventilator settings, ET tube function, respiratory status.

Activity intolerance r/t imbalance between O$_2$ supply and demand secondary to ↓ myocardial functioning

Desired outcome: Within 12-24 h before transfer from CCU, patient exhibits cardiac tolerance to ↑ levels of activity: RR <24 breaths/min, NSR on ECG, HR ≥120 bpm (or within 20 bpm of resting HR), BP within 20 mm Hg of nl for patient, and absence of chest pain.

- Maintain prescribed activity level; teach rationale for activity limitation.
- Organize nursing care so that periods of activity are interspersed with extended periods of uninterrupted rest.
- Assist with active/passive ROM exercises, as appropriate. Encourage as much activity as possible within prescribed allowances.
- Note physiologic response to activity, including BP, HR, RR, and heart rhythm. Signs of activity intolerance include chest pain, ↑ SOB, excessive fatigue, ↑ dysrhythmias, palpitations, HR response >120 bpm, SBP >20 mm Hg from baseline or >160 mm Hg, and ST-segment changes.
- If activity intolerance noted, instruct patient to stop activity and to rest.
- As needed, refer patient to PT department.

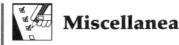

Miscellanea

CONSULT MD FOR

- Inability to maintain Spo$_2$ ≥92% despite supplemental O$_2$
- Deteriorating cardiac performance: new-onset S$_3$ or summation gallop, murmur, crackles, sustained hypotension
- Unacceptable hemodynamics: CO <4 L/min, RAP/CVP >8 mm Hg, PVR >100 dynes/sec/cm^{-5}, MAP <70 mm Hg
- UO <0.5 mg/kg/h × 2 consecutive h
- Complications: eg, cardiogenic shock, hepatic insufficiency, profound ascites, renal insufficiency

RELATED TOPICS

- Bronchitis, chronic
- Cardiomyopathy
- Emphysema
- Heart failure, left ventricular
- Hemodynamic monitoring
- Myocardial infarction, acute
- Pulmonary embolus, fat
- Pulmonary embolus, thrombotic
- Pulmonary hypertension

ABBREVIATIONS

LSB: Left sternal border
RVEDP: Right ventricular end-diastolic pressure

REFERENCES

Dahlen R, Roberts SL: Acute congestive heart failure: pathophysiologic alterations, *Intensive and Crit Care Nurs* 11(4): 210-216, 1995.

Dracup K, Dunbar SB, Baker DW: Rethinking heart failure, *Am J Nurs* 95(7): 22-28, 1995.

Proulx R et al: Detection of right ventricular myocardial infarct, *Crit Care Nurse* 12(3): 50-59, 1992.

Steward S, Kucia A, Poropat S: Early detection and management of right ventricular infarction: the role of the critical care nurse, *Dimens Crit Care Nurs* 14(6): 282-292, 1995.

Turner DM, Turner LA: Right ventricular myocardial infarction: detection, treatment, and nursing implications, *Crit Care Nurse* 15(1): 22-29, 1995.

Wright JM: Pharmacologic management of congestive heart failure, *Crit Care Nurs Q* 18(1): 32-44, 1995.

Author: **Barbara Tueller Steuble**

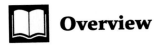 **Overview**

PATHOPHYSIOLOGY
Pregnancy-related coagulopathy in the form of severe preeclampsia-eclampsia associated with vasospastic hypertension. Accompanied by microangiopathic disease, alterations in microcirculation, endothelial dysfunction, immune or inflammatory responses, and activation of the clotting cascade. This coagulopathy resembles DIC except that coagulation assays remain nl.

INCIDENCE
2%-12% of severe preeclampsia population, with mortality rate of 2%-24%

HISTORY/RISK FACTORS
- Preeclampsia-eclampsia
- Second or third trimester of gestation
- Hypertensive disorders of pregnancy: greatly contributes to maternal and perinatal morbidity and mortality
- Endothelial cell injury of vasculature
- ↑ BP

CLINICAL PRESENTATION
Multisystem, nonspecific complaints: malaise, epigastric pain, nausea, vomiting, headaches, weakness, RUQ abdominal pain

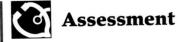 **Assessment**

PHYSICAL ASSESSMENT
Neuro: Headache, seizures, visual disturbances, ↓ LOC, generalized malaise
Resp: SOB, dyspnea
CV: ↓ pulse quality, ↑ BP, peripheral edema, possible chest discomfort
GI: Epigastric pain, nausea, vomiting, RUQ pain, hypoglycemia
GU: ↓ UO
Integ: Petechiae, ecchymoses, oozing from mucous membranes/invasive sites

VITAL SIGNS/HEMODYNAMICS
RR: ↑
HR: ↑
BP: ↑
Temp: Nl
CVP/PAWP: Nl to ↑
SVR: ↑
CO: ↓ from expected value
12/18-Lead ECG: May reveal changes r/t myocardial ischemia, including ST-segment depression or T-wave inversion. Sinus tachycardia may be present. If myocardial perfusion altered, PACs or PVCs may be noted.

LABORATORY STUDIES
Hematology: Hgb/Hct ↓ caused by hemolysis associated with HELLP. Platelets ↓ because of platelet aggregation.
Clotting Studies: To differentially diagnose coagulopathies and bleeding disorders: PT/PTT unchanged, fibrinogen ↓, FSPs unchanged, clotting time ↑.
Liver Studies: May be reflective of hepatic insufficiency: alkaline phosphatase ↑, LDH ↑, AST/ALT ↑, total bilirubin ↑.
Renal Studies: May be reflective of renal insufficiency: BUN/creatinine ↑, urine protein positive, 24-h urine protein ↑.
Creatinine Clearance: ↓

IMAGING
Liver/Gall Bladder Ultrasound: For diagnosis of abdominal pain, including assessment of hepatic hematoma, which would signal ruptured liver, a surgical emergency.

DIAGNOSTIC PROCEDURE
Fetal Assessment: Evaluates for nl baseline HR for gestational age, stability of baseline HR, short- and long-term variability. Acceleration of fetal HR ≥15 beats over baseline for 15 sec rules out acidosis; late decelerations signal uteroplacental insufficiency.

Collaborative Management

Goal of therapy: to prevent maternal and fetal complications, including seizures, shock/hypotension, and liver rupture.
Supplemental O$_2$: Promotes O$_2$ delivery to tissues.
Prevention of Seizures: Initiate MgSO$_4$ infusion.
Preparation for Delivery: Determine whether cervix favorable for induction of labor; if not, prepare for Caesarean section.
Fetal Monitoring: To assess stability of fetal HR.
Hemodynamic Monitoring: Appropriate if patient has pulmonary edema, persistent oliguria, severe hypertension unresponsive to hydralazine, or is hemodynamically unstable and requires induction of anesthesia.
Monitoring for Bleeding: Check all invasive sites, mucous membranes, and VS. Sudden ↑ in HR coupled with hypotension may signal hepatic rupture.
Pharmacotherapy
MgSO$_4$ infusion: Dosage must be titrated correctly to clinical response during infusion or seizures may develop.
Amobarbital sodium: For seizures unresponsive to MgSO$_4$.
Corticosteroids: May be used throughout pregnancy to ↓ complications.
Hydralazine: To ↓ BP.
Nitroprusside: To ↓ BP if hydralazine ineffective.
NTG: To assist with ↓ BP if nitroprusside ineffective in stabilizing overall hemodynamics.
Labetalol: To ↓ BP if hydralazine ineffective.
Calcium gluconate: Antidote for MgSO$_4$ toxicity.
Caesarean Section: For fetal delivery if maternal cervix unfavorable to labor induction.
Plasma Exchange: Considered during postpartum period for patients who do not recover in 72-96 h from anomalies.

PATIENT-FAMILY TEACHING
- Disease process, associated complications, care during L&D and postpartum
- Purpose, expected results, anticipated sensations of all nursing/medical interventions
- Relationship of factors in past hx that may affect coagulation status, including collagen vascular disorders and bleeding problems
- Medications: drug name, dosage, purpose, schedule, precautions, drug-drug and food-drug interactions, and potential side effects

Nursing Diagnoses/Interventions

Altered protection r/t to HELLP syndrome secondary to pregnancy-induced hypertension: preeclampsia-eclampsia

Desired outcomes: Within 24 h of delivery, maternal VS normalized to within 10% of baseline or: SBP ≥90 but ≤140 mm Hg, DBP <90 mm Hg, RR 12-20 breaths/min, blood glucose >70 mg/dl, platelets >100,000 μl (acceptable value for these patients), Hgb >10 g/dl, Hct >32%. No signs of overt bleeding or liver dysfunction present.

ANTEPARTUM

- Stabilize mother and fetus; prepare for delivery.
- Monitor maternal VS at least q15min.
- Fetus is at high risk. Continuously monitor fetal HR, baseline HR, periodic and nonperiodic changes, and variability for hypoxia r/t uteroplacental insufficiency.

INTRAPARTUM

- Prevent tissue hypoxia and hemorrhage.
- Initiate $MgSO_4$ infusion as prescribed and titrate to clinical effects to avoid seizures.
- $MgSO_4$ ↓ cardiac conduction; monitor mother for dysrhythmias.
- Provide IV fluid therapy as prescribed.
- Monitor for excessive vaginal bleeding at least q15min.
- Monitor maternal VS at least q15min.
- Continue fetal monitoring as described in antepartum phase.
- Be alert for maternal respiratory depression.
- Measure UO qh. Output of 30-200 ml/h desirable to maximize effect of $MgSO_4$ while avoiding toxicity.
- If hemodynamic monitoring is being used, assess CO/CI, CVP/PAWP at least q30min.
- Keep calcium gluconate at bedside in case $MgSO_4$ toxicity develops.
- If eclampsia develops, administer $MgSO_4$ boluses as prescribed.
- Administer antihypertensives as prescribed; monitor carefully to avoid causing ↑ arterial pressure too rapidly or aggressively, which would ↓ uteroplacental perfusion. Target DBP at 90-100 mm Hg.
- Monitor blood glucose qh.

POSTPARTUM

- Continue $MgSO_4$ for 12-24 h as prescribed.
- Monitor platelet counts and liver function tests. Abnormalities usually resolve in 72-96 h.
- Monitor blood glucose q4h until normalized.

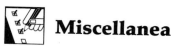 # Miscellanea

CONSULT MD FOR

- Sudden, severe abdominal pain associated with hypotension, severe SOB, chest pain, uncontrolled bleeding, seizures, Spo_2 <90%, ↑ crackles in lung bases or ↑ JVD, hypoglycemia, fetal distress, hematuria, anuria, ↓ fibrinogen
- Possible complications: ruptured liver, renal failure, uncontrollable seizures, tissue hypoxia or hemorrhage (may lead to MODS), laboratory abnormalities that persist >96 h following delivery, persistent hypoglycemia, placental abruption, respiratory failure

RELATED TOPICS

- Disseminated intravascular coagulation
- Idiopathic thrombocytopenic purpura
- Multiple organ dysfunction syndrome
- Systemic inflammatory response syndrome
- Thrombotic thrombocytopenic purpura

ABBREVIATIONS

FSPs: Fibrin split products
HELLP: Hemolysis, elevated liver enzymes, low platelets
MgSO4: Magnesium sulfate
MODS: Multiple organ dysfunction syndrome

REFERENCES

Jones KA, Abramowicz JS, Annissi D: Severe HELLP syndrome presenting with acute gum bleeding following toothbrushing at 38 wks gestation, *Am J Crit Care* 2(5): 395-396, 1993.

Koenigseder LA, Crane PB, Lucy PW: HELLP: a collaborative challenge for critical care and obstetric nurses, *Am J Crit Care* 2(5): 385-392, 1993.

Magann EF, Washburne JF, Sullivan CA: Corticosteroid-induced arrest of HELLP syndrome progression in a marginally viable pregnancy, *Eur J Obstet Gynecol Reprod Biol* 59(2): 217-219, 1995.

Magann EF, Bass D, Chauhan SP: Antepartum corticosteroids: disease stabilization in patients with the syndrome of hemolysis, elevated liver enzymes and low platelets (HELLP), *Am J Obstet Gynecol* 171(4): 1148-1153, 1994.

Martin JN Jr, Files JC, Blake PG: Postpartum plasma exchange for atypical preeclampsia-eclampsia as HELLP (hemolysis, elevated liver enzymes and low platelets) syndrome, *Am J Obstet Gynecol* 172(4): 1107-1127, 1995.

Poole J: HELLP syndrome and coagulations of pregnancy, *Crit Care Nurs Clin North Am* 5(3): 475-487, 1993.

Sauer PM, Harvey CJ: Pregnancy induced hypertension: understanding severe preeclampsia and the HELLP syndrome, *Crit Care Nurs Clin North Am* 4(4): 703-710, 1992.

Author: **Marianne Saunorus Baird**

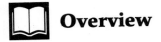

Overview

DESCRIPTION
Form of RRT involving an artificial semipermeable membrane that is used to diffuse water, electrolytes, and waste products from the blood. Blood is heparinized, passed through the dialyzer, and returned to circulation. For the acutely ill, dialysis may be needed from $3 \times$ wk to qd.

INDICATIONS FOR HEMODIALYSIS
- Volume excess
- Hyperkalemia and other electrolyte disturbances
- Metabolic acidosis
- Uremic intoxication:
    CNS (encephalopathy)
    Hematologic (bleeding as a result of platelet dysfunction)
    GI (anorexia, nausea, vomiting)
    CV (pericarditis)
- Need for removal of dialyzable substances (metabolites, drugs, toxins)

HISTORY/RISK FACTORS
- ATN
- Chronic renal failure
- Hepatorenal syndrome
- Hypertension

CLINICAL PRESENTATION
- Oliguria
- ↑ BUN/creatinine
- Edema: peripheral, periorbital, sacral
- Weakness, other evidence of electrolyte imbalance
- Bleeding tendencies

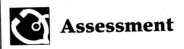

Assessment

PHYSICAL ASSESSMENT
Neuro: Altered mental status, lethargy, disorientation
Resp: SOB, Kussmaul's respirations, crackles
CV: S_3 and S_4 gallop, pericardial friction rub, JVD, dysrhythmias, hypertension
GI: Nausea, vomiting, anorexia
GU: Oliguria, anuria
MS: Weakness, muscle tenderness, asterixis
Other: Uremic frost, pallor, ecchymosis, bleeding from puncture sites also possible.

VITAL SIGNS/HEMODYNAMICS
RR: ↑
HR: ↑, irregular
BP: ↑
Temp: Nl; or slight ↑ with infection
Other: Hemodynamics usually reflect fluid volume excess with ↑ CVP/PAWP, ↑ SVR. CO may ↓ if heart failure present.

ECG: Dysrhythmias common. May show hyperkalemic changes: peaked T waves, prolonged PR interval, ST depression, widened QRS.

LABORATORY STUDIES
Chemistries: BUN, creatinine, and uric acid levels ↑ in ARF, as will K^+, PO_4^{3-}, and possibly Mg^{2+}.
Creatinine Clearance: Most reliable estimation of GFR; usually <50 ml/min.
Urinalysis: Large amounts of protein and many RBC casts common. Sediment wnl when causes are prerenal.
Hematology: Hct may be low as a result of renal failure; Hct and Hgb ↓ steadily if bleeding or hemodilution present. PT, PTT may ↑ because of ↓ platelet adhesiveness.
ABGs: Metabolic acidosis (low $Paco_2$ and plasma pH).

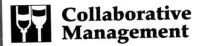

Collaborative Management

System Components
Dialyzer (artificial kidney): Consists of blood compartment, dialysate compartment, and semipermeable membrane. Small molecules, eg, electrolytes, water, and waste products, pass through this membrane; RBCs, protein, and bacteria are too large to cross.

Dialysate: Electrolyte solution similar to nl plasma. Potassium concentration varies according to patient need. Glucose may be necessary, but it can cross the semipermeable membrane, resulting in hypoglycemia. Use of a glucose bath ↓ risk of hypoglycemia.

Vascular access
AV shunt: Insertion of Silastic tube into an artery and vein, enabling blood to flow from artery to vein externally.

Subclavian, femoral, or internal jugular catheter: Temporary access placed in a large vein to enhance blood flow.

AV fistula: Anastomosis of artery and vein, resulting in dilated vessels for easy cannulation and ↑ blood flow.

Graft: Bovine, Gore-Tex, or saphenous vein that connects artery and vein internally in arm or thigh.

Hemasite: T-shaped device inserted in arterialized vein with a Gore-Tex graft. The T projects out of the skin, resulting in external entry point.

Dietary Restrictions: Between treatments, protein, potassium, and sodium accumulate because of kidneys' inability to excrete excesses of these products, necessitating their restriction. Individualized guidelines typically include protein 1.0-1.2 g/kg/day; sodium 80-100 mEq/day; and potassium 40-80 mEq/day.

Fluid Restriction: Weight gain between treatments usually caused by fluid retention. Fluid intake may be limited to 1500-1800 ml/24 h.

Phosphate Binders: To control hyperphosphatemia, which can occur because of inability to excrete excess dietary phosphates.

Vitamin D Analogs, Calcium Replacement: To prevent hypocalcemia and renal osteodystrophy. If hypocalcemia occurs, parathyroid glands release parathormone, which releases calcium from bone and may lead to bone demineralization and osteodystrophy.

Water-Soluble Vitamins and Folic Acid: Dialyzable, necessitating replacement after dialysis.

PATIENT-FAMILY TEACHING
- Necessity of vascular access; sensations that can be anticipated during cannula insertion.
- Importance of/rationale for protecting involved extremity after cannula or shunt placement.
- Importance of notifying staff members if S&S of infection occur.
- Importance of avoiding taking BP, drawing blood, or using restrictive clothing, name bands, or restraints on arm with fistula.
- Frequency of/rationale for assessment of VS and blood tests to monitor status during procedure.
- Dietary restrictions as necessary (eg, sodium, potassium).

Nursing Diagnoses/Interventions

Risk for infection r/t invasive procedure used for access for dialysis
Desired outcome: Patient infection free: normothermia, WBCs ≤11,000 μl, blood free of infective organisms, and absence of erythema, purulent drainage, access site pain.
- Assess condition of access site qd. Be alert to erythema, purulent drainage, or tenderness.
- Keep all external devices (shunts, subclavian catheters, femoral catheters) covered with dry, sterile dressing between treatments.
- Report ↑ temp, malaise, and access site drainage or pain.
- Teach patient to notify staff if S&S of infection occur.

Fluid volume excess (or risk for same) r/t dietary indiscretions of sodium and fluids and compromised regulatory mechanisms secondary to renal failure
Desired outcome: Within 24-48 h of admission, patient becomes normovolemic: balanced I&O; stable weight; HR ≤100 bpm; BP wnl for patient; RR 12-20 breaths/min; and absence of edema, crackles, and other S&S of hypervolemia.
- Monitor I&O q4h and weight qd. Be alert to weight gain of >0.5-1 kg/24 h.
- Assess for S&S of hypervolemia: crackles, tachycardia, pericardial friction rub, pulsus paradoxus, and presence of peripheral, periorbital, and sacral edema.
- Maintain prescribed fluid restrictions.

Risk for fluid volume deficit r/t active loss secondary to excess fluid removal during dialysis or bleeding secondary to heparinization
Desired outcomes: Patient remains normovolemic: balanced I&O, daily weight within 1-2 lbs of calculated dry weight, BP wnl for patient, CVP ≥2 mm Hg, and HR ≤100 bpm. Hct 20%-30% (an acceptable range with dialysis) and there is no evidence of blood loss caused by line separation or membrane rupture.
- Weigh patient qd. Monitor I&O. Be alert to output >1500 ml over intake.
- Monitor Hct results before each hemodialysis. Be alert to >2-pt drop.
- If hypotension occurs, give NS or volume expanders; notify physician.
- Secure lines and needles with tape to prevent disconnection and dislodgment.
If blood loss occurs because of line separation or dialyzer rupture, send type and screen to the laboratory as necessary.
- Maintain pressure over venipuncture sites for ≥5 min after needles have been removed.

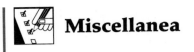 ## Miscellanea

CONSULT MD FOR
- S&S of fluid volume excess: weight gain >0.5-1 kg/24 h, crackles, tachycardia, significant edema
- S&S of fluid volume deficit: output >1500 over intake, >2-pt ↓ in Hct, ↓ BP during dialysis, blood loss caused by line separation or dialyzer rupture
- Loss of patency of dialysis access site: absence of thrill, bruit; dark strands or white serum in AV shunt and tubing
- S&S of disequilibrium syndrome: headache, nausea & vomiting, asterixis, stupor, seizures
- Complications: electrolyte imbalance, hypovolemic or hemorrhagic shock, heart failure, septicemia, access site infection

RELATED TOPICS
- Acute tubular necrosis: oliguric
- Heart failure, left ventricular
- Hyperkalemia
- Hypernatremia
- Metabolic acidosis, acute
- Pulmonary embolus, air
- Renal failure, acute

ABBREVIATIONS
GFR: Glomerular filtration rate
RRT: Renal replacement therapy

Altered peripheral tissue perfusion (or risk for same): Access site, r/t interruption of vascular flow secondary to clot formation, pressure, obstruction, or disconnection of vascular access device

Desired outcomes: Patient's access site for dialysis has adequate perfusion: presence of thrill and bruit, visualization of blood flow, and warmth of shunt tubing or AV fistula. Warmth and brisk capillary refill (<2 sec) present in the access extremity.

- Confirm patency of access site by palpating for a thrill and auscultating for bruit (buzzing sound) over shunt or AV fistula. Monitor access extremity for warmth and brisk capillary refill.
- Keep small section of shunt tubing exposed for visualization of blood flow. Ensure that blood appears uniformly red and that external tubing is warm to the touch. Dark strands or white serum in tubing can signal clotting. If patency cannot be confirmed, streptokinase or embolectomy may be indicated to save the fistula.
- Avoid taking BP, drawing blood, or using restrictive clothing, name bands, or restraints on arm with fistula.
- If using pressure dressing over access site, make sure it is snug enough to prevent bleeding but not so tight that it could stop blood flow. Remove pressure dressing after 1-2 h.
- Maintain constant infusion of heparin through subclavian or femoral line or flush with heparinized saline and cap as prescribed.
- Keep shunt clamps or rubbershod hemostats at bedside to clamp line in event of accidental disconnection.
- Always check fistula, graft, or shunt for patency after any hypotensive episode.
- If for any reason it is suspected that air has entered the vascular access, clamp the line and place patient in left side-lying Trendelenburg position, which will trap air at apex of the heart's right ventricle, away from the outflow tract. Call physician *stat,* administer O_2, and monitor VS carefully.

Altered protection (or risk for same) r/t neurosensory alterations secondary to endogenous chemical alteration (dialysis disequilibrium syndrome) occurring with rapid removal of metabolic wastes and changes in serum osmolality

Desired outcome: Patient verbalizes orientation $\times$ 3 and does not exhibit S&S of disequilibrium syndrome: headache, nausea, vomiting, restlessness, asterixis, stupor, coma, seizures.

- Monitor for S&S of disequilibrium syndrome.
- Recognize predisposing factors: BUN >150 mg/dl, hypernatremia (serum sodium >147 mEq/L), severe metabolic acidosis, and hx of neurologic problems (eg, seizures). The syndrome may be prevented by short, frequent dialysis exchanges and by $\uparrow$ dialysate osmolality by adding glucose, glycerol, urea, or mannitol or by giving IV mannitol during treatment.
- Monitor BUN levels before/after dialysis to evaluate changes occurring along with S&S of disequilibrium.
- Raise side rails, and keep an appropriately-sized oral airway at the bedside.

REFERENCES

Hansen SK: Patient assessment in acute hemodialysis, *CANNT J* 2(1): 17-19, 1992.

Keen ML, Lancaster LE, Binkly LS: Hemodialysis. In Lancaster LE (ed): *Core curriculum for nephrology nursing,* ed 3, Pitman, NJ, 1995, AJ Janetti.

Kelleher RM: Dialysis in the surgical intensive care patient: a case study, *Crit Care Nurs Q* 14(4): 72-77, 1992.

Peschman P: Acute hemodialysis: issues in the critically ill, *AACN Clin Issues in Crit Care Nurs* 3(3): 545-557, 1992.

Weiskittel PD: Renal-urinary disorders. In Swearingen PL, Keen JH (eds): *Manual of critical care nursing,* ed 3, St Louis, 1995, Mosby.

Author: **Patricia D. Weiskittel**

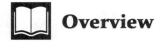

Overview

DESCRIPTION

Specialized methods of evaluating CV performance. The following major cardiac mechanisms determine CO:

Preload: Function of the volume of blood delivered to ventricle and ventricular compliance (ability to stretch) at end diastole. The greater the myocardial muscle stretch, the greater the force of contraction. However, excessive stretch ↓ contractility. Clinically, preload described as VEDP because ventricular pressure corresponds closely with volume. RV diastolic (filling) pressure reflected by RAP or CVP. LV diastolic (filling) pressure reflected by LAP, PADP, or PAWP measurements.

Afterload: Tension that develops within ventricular myocardium during systole. For heart to eject its contents, it must overcome vascular resistance. Afterload evaluated by calculating PVR for RV afterload and SVR for LV afterload. The higher the afterload, the greater the work of the heart to overcome resistance to flow.

Contractility: Inherent capacity of the myocardium to contract. Although not measured directly, a change can be inferred when there is ↓ CO while other variables that affect CO (ie, preload, afterload, HR) remain the same. Factors positively influencing contractility are sympathetic stimulation, calcium, and positive inotropic agents. Acidemia, hypoxia, β-blockers, and antidysrhythmics ↓ it.

COMPLICATIONS

With PA or CVP catheter insertion, the following may occur: carotid artery puncture, air embolism, RV perforation, hemorrhage, thoracic duct injury, pneumothorax, and cardiac tamponade. With PA catheter insertion, ventricular dysrhythmias may occur.

CLINICAL PRESENTATION

Acute or severely ill patients about whom detailed information regarding cardiac performance, tissue perfusion, blood volume, tissue oxygenation, and vascular tone is required

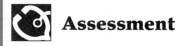

Assessment

PHYSICAL ASSESSMENT

Findings depend on individual clinical condition.

HEMODYNAMICS

Variable, according to specific patient condition; likely to be unstable. See Appendix for values and formulas used to calculate them.

DIRECT HEMODYNAMIC MANAGEMENT

Arterial Catheters: Generally inserted *via* radial artery. Waveform displayed on bedside monitor for continuous observation of SBP, DBP, and MAP. In hypertensive and hyperdynamic states, the waveform shows steep rate of ↑ and high peak systolic pressure. In shock states or severe heart failure the waveform is damped with a slow rate of ↑.

SBP: ↑ in SBP often reflects changes in vascular compliance, such as hypertension. ↓ in SBP seen with disorders that result in ↓ stroke volume or arterial vasodilation.

DBP: Important because coronary artery blood flow occurs during diastole, and any ↓ in DBP may result in subendocardial ischemia.

MAP: Average pressure within arterial tree throughout cardiac cycle. Calculated by the following formula:

$$MAP = \frac{SBP + 2\,(DBP)}{3}$$

NI is 70-105 mm Hg. Because MAP is the product of CO × SVR, ↑ CO or SVR will ↑ MAP; a ↓ in either value will ↓ MAP.

CVP Catheters: CVP is measurement of systemic venous pressure at right atrial level. NI is 2-6 mm Hg. Used to assess fluid volume excess or deficit; may not accurately assess fluid state in heart failure.

PA Catheters: Inserted *via* jugular, subclavian, or femoral vein and passed through heart's right side into pulmonary capillary bed. Data derived from these catheters include RAP, RVP, PAP, PAWP, CO, core body temp, and SvO_2. Other calculated hemodynamic and O_2 transport variables may be derived as well.

RAP: Essentially the same as CVP. NI mean RAP is 4-6 mm Hg.

RVP: Measured during catheter insertion only. NI RVP is 25/0-5 mm Hg. ↑ RV systolic pressure seen in pulmonic stenosis, pulmonary hypertension, or VSD. ↑ RV diastolic pressure may occur with constrictive pericarditis.

PAP: NI PAP is 20-30/8-15 mm Hg. With healthy pulmonary vasculature the PADP corresponds closely to the PAWP and reflects LVEDP. A significant difference (ie, >5 mm Hg) between PADP and PAWP seen with pulmonary disease or hypoxia.

PAWP: Reflects LVEDP; used to evaluate cardiac performance. NI mean PAWP is 6-12 mm Hg. PEEP/CPAP >10 cm H_2O may result in falsely ↑ PAP and PAWP. Correlation of measured pressure with the respiratory cycle may improve accuracy of measurements.

CO: Volume of blood in liters ejected by heart each min and product of stroke volume and HR. NI CO is 4-7 L/min. NI stroke volume is 55-100 ml/beat. To adjust CO for body size, CO is divided by BSA to obtain value known as *cardiac index* (CI). NI CI is 2.5-4 L/min/m².

SVR: Major factor that determines LV afterload. SVR calculated with the following formula:

$$SVR = \frac{(MAP - RAP)}{CO} \times 80$$

NI for SVR is 900-1200 dynes/sec/cm^{-5}. ↑ SVR will ↑ workload of heart; therefore measures are taken (eg, vasodilator therapy) to keep SVR wnl.

PVR: Clinical measure of RV afterload. The formula for calculating PVR is the following:

$$PVR = \frac{PAM - PAWP}{CO} \times 80$$

NI is 60-100 dynes/sec/cm^{-5}. PVR may ↑ as a result of mitral or aortic valve disease, congenital heart disease, long-standing LV heart failure, hypoxia, COPD, or pulmonary embolus.

Svo$_2$: Measured with mixed venous blood samples from distal port of PA catheter or by continuous monitoring *via* a fiberoptic PA catheter. Svo$_2$ is average percentage of Hgb bound with O$_2$ in venous blood and reflects patient's ability to balance O$_2$ supply and demand at tissue level. Four factors affect O$_2$ supply-demand relationship and Svo$_2$ values: Sao$_2$, CO, Hgb, and Vo$_2$. NI for Svo$_2$ is 60%-80%. Very low levels (<30%) usually associated with lactic acidosis and poor prognosis.

Collaborative Management

PULMONARY ARTERY PRESSURE MONITORING

PASP: NI = 20-30 mm Hg. ↑ can signal RV failure, cardiac tamponade, heart failure, pulmonary hypertension, hypoxia. ↓ can signal hypovolemia, ↓ preload.

PADP: NI = 8-15 mm Hg. ↑ can signal LV failure, mitral stenosis, left-to-right shunts, pulmonary hypertension, hypoxia. ↓ can signal hypovolemia, ↓ preload.

PAWP: NI = 6-12 mm Hg. ↑ can signal LV failure, cardiac tamponade, acute mitral regurgitation, acute VSD, volume overload. ↓ can signal hypovolemia, ↓ afterload. PAWP > PADP = mechanical problem.

Svo$_2$ MONITORING

Sao$_2$: ↑ Sao$_2$ causes ↑ Svo$_2$ as seen with supplemental O$_2$. ↓ Sao$_2$ results in ↓ Svo$_2$ as with ↓ O$_2$ supply (ie, ARDS, ET suctioning).

CO: ↑ CO causes ↑ Svo$_2$ as with ↑ contractility (eg, inotrope administration). ↓ CO results in ↓ Svo$_2$ as with dysrhythmias, MI, and ↑ SVR.

Hgb: ↓ Hgb causes ↓ Svo$_2$ as with hemorrhage, hemolysis, severe anemia.

Vo$_2$: ↑ Vo$_2$ results in ↓ Svo$_2$ as when metabolic demands exceed O$_2$ supply (eg, shivering, seizures, hyperthermia, hyperdynamic states). ↓ Vo$_2$ causes ↑ Svo$_2$ as when there is failure of peripheral tissue to extract or use O$_2$. Examples include significant peripheral AV shunting: cirrhosis, renal failure; redistribution of blood away from beds where O$_2$ extraction occurs: sepsis, acute pancreatitis, major burns; blockage of O$_2$ uptake or use: cyanide poisoning; carbon monoxide poisoning.

Mechanical Problems: Artifactitious ↑ in Svo$_2$ can occur with wedged PA catheter.

MECHANICAL PROBLEMS

Overdamping: Waveform smaller than usual with a slow rise and diminished or absent dicrotic notch; not associated with hypovolemia

Causes: Air bubbles in system, thrombus formation, lodging of catheter against vessel wall, kinking of catheter or tubing, loose connection in tubing or transducer, incorrect calibration, spontaneous PA catheter migration into near-wedged position

Catheter Whip: Waveform erratic, "noisy," with highly variable and inaccurate pressures

Cause: Excess movement of catheter tip (may require repositioning)

No Waveform

Causes: Large leak in system, usually with blood backing up into tubing; loose or defective transducer or air in transducer; stopcock turned to wrong position; catheter tip or lumen totally occluded by clot; inadequate pressure on pressure bag

Inability To Obtain PAWP: Absence of wedge waveform after balloon inflation

Causes: Balloon rupture, retrograde catheter slippage

PATIENT-FAMILY TEACHING

- Use and purpose of PA/arterial catheter
- Insertion procedure, emphasizing use of anesthetic agent, importance of not moving during procedure, frequent x-rays, application of dressing to insertion site
- Expected sensations: prick from local anesthetic, pressure as catheter advances, coldness from cleansing solution, burning of lidocaine, claustrophobia from drapes, dull pushing/pulling sensations in neck, coldness from injection of iced solution (if used)
- Importance of reporting any anxiety or discomfort during procedure

Nursing Diagnoses/Interventions

Risk for infection r/t presence of invasive hemodynamic catheters
Desired outcome: Patient infection free: normothermia, WBCs ≤11,000 μl, negative culture results, and absence of erythema, heat, swelling, or purulent drainage at insertion site.
- Monitor temp for ↑ >37° C (99° F) and WBCs for ↑.
- As prescribed, obtain culture of any suspicious drainage; report positive findings.
- Use NS rather than D_5W for hemodynamic flush solution.
- Change hemodynamic tubing, transducer, and flush solution according to hospital protocol.
- Maintain closed system to transducer and for flush solution. Keep all external openings and stopcocks securely capped at all times.
- Use closed system for cardiac output injectate.
- Change dressing per agency protocol, using aseptic technique.
- Record date of catheter insertion and ensure that catheter is changed per agency protocol.
- If infection suspected, send catheter tip for C&S.

Altered cardiopulmonary tissue perfusion (or risk for same) r/t interrupted blood flow secondary to migration of PA catheter into wedged position, overwedging of balloon, continuous wedge position, or local vascular thrombosis
Desired outcomes: Within 2 h of this diagnosis, patient has adequate pulmonary perfusion: nl PA waveform and RR 12-20 breaths/min with eupnea.
- Monitor PA waveform continuously.
- Assess for interrupted pulmonary arterial blood flow as evidenced by acute onset of pleuritic chest pain, SOB, tachypnea, and hemoptysis.
- Evaluate position of catheter *via* chest x-ray. Look for wedge-shaped infiltrate, which could signal impaired pulmonary tissue perfusion.
- Monitor PA waveform when wedging balloon. Inject enough air to obtain wedge configuration but no more than amount recommended by catheter manufacturer. Never pull back on syringe to remove air; disconnect syringe and allow passive deflation of balloon.
- Follow trends of PADP rather than those of PAWP after correlating PADP to PAWP q4-8h. Be aware that PADP may exceed PAWP by ≥5 mm Hg with acidosis, hypoxemia, pulmonary emboli, lung disease, and associated pulmonary hypertension.
- Pay special attention to PA waveform when patient moves about (eg, when being taken to x-ray department or getting up and into a chair).

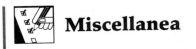 # Miscellanea

CONSULT MD FOR
- Continuously wedged PA waveform
- S&S of peripheral vascular ischemia with peripheral arterial catheter
- Hemodynamic instability unresponsive to initial interventions

RELATED TOPICS
- Heart failure, left ventricular
- Multiple organ dysfunction syndrome
- Pulmonary embolus, air
- Ventricular tachycardia

ABBREVIATIONS
LVEDP: Left ventricular end-diastolic pressure
Svo$_2$: Mixed venous oxygen saturation
VEDP: Ventricular end-diastolic pressure
Vo$_2$: Oxygen consumption
VSD: Ventricular septal defect

Altered peripheral tissue perfusion (involved extremity) r/t interrupted blood flow secondary to presence of arterial catheter or thrombosis caused by catheter

Desired outcome: Within 2 h of this diagnosis, patient has adequate perfusion to affected extremity: brisk capillary refill (<2 sec), natural color, warm skin, nl sensation, and ability to move fingers.

- On a continuous basis, monitor capillary refill, color, temp, sensation, and movement. Be alert to indicators of ischemia and teach these to patient, stressing importance of notifying staff promptly should they occur.
- Maintain arterial line on continuous flush with flush solution recommended by agency; ensure that pressure bag remains inflated at 300 mm Hg.
- Ensure tight connections of tubing throughout system.
- Support patient's wrist or appropriate extremity with arm board or other supportive device to prevent catheter flexion and movement.

Risk for injury r/t potential for insertion complications secondary to ventricular irritability, patient movement during insertion procedure, or difficult anatomy

Desired outcome: Patient has no complications from PA or CVP catheter insertion as evidenced by NSR on ECG, BP wnl for patient, HR ≤100 bpm, RR ≤20 breaths/min with eupnea, nl breath sounds, and absence of adventitious breath sounds or muffled heart sounds.

- During preprocedure teaching, caution about importance of remaining still during catheter insertion. Provide sedative as prescribed.
- Perform baseline assessment, monitoring BP, HR, RR, breath sounds, heart sounds, and ECG. Perform postprocedure assessment, comparing it with baseline findings. Be alert to ↓ BP, pulsus paradoxus, ↑ HR or RR, ↓ or absent breath sounds, muffled heart sounds, and dysrhythmias on ECG. Report significant findings.
- After procedure, obtain chest x-ray as prescribed.
- Maintain lidocaine at bedside for immediate IV injection if patient has sustained ventricular dysrhythmias.

REFERENCES

Chernow B: *The pharmacologic approach to the critically ill patient,* ed 3, Baltimore, 1994, Williams & Wilkins.

Gillman PH: Continuous measurement of cardiac output: a milestone in hemodynamic monitoring, *Focus Crit Care* 19(2): 155-158, 1992.

Hayden R: Trend-spotting with an Svo$_2$ monitor, *Am J Nurs* 93(1): 26-33, 1993.

Renner L, Meyer L: Injectate port selection affects accuracy and reproducibility of cardiac output measurements with multiport thermodilution pulmonary artery catheters, *Am J Crit Care* 3(1): 55-61, 1994.

Shinners PA, Pease MO: A stabilization period of 5 min is adequate when measuring pulmonary artery pressures after turning, *Am J Crit Care* 2(6): 474-477, 1993.

Shoemaker W: Monitoring and management of acute circulatory problems: the expanded role of the physiologically oriented critical care nurse, *Am J Crit Care* 1(1): 38-53, 1992.

Author: **Janet Hicks Keen**

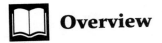 **Overview**

PATHOPHYSIOLOGY

Characterized by premature pathologic destruction (hemolysis) of RBCs, which ↓ O_2-carrying capacity of blood, resulting in reduced tissue oxygenation. This hypoxic state produces tissue ischemia and can progress to tissue infarction. May accelerate to a crisis state wherein microthrombi composed of hemolyzed blood cells precipitate organ congestion, MODS, and shock.

HISTORY/RISK FACTORS

- Emotional, physiologic stress: trauma, surgery, critical illness
- Acute infectious process
- Abnormal immune responses
- Hemolytic anemia, including G6PD deficiency, thalassemias, pyruvate kinase deficiency
- Sickle cell disease

CLINICAL PRESENTATION

Fever; abdominal, chest, joint, back pain; headache; dizziness; palpitations

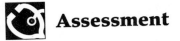 **Assessment**

PHYSICAL ASSESSMENT
Resp: SOB
GI: Splenomegaly, hepatomegaly, abdominal guarding
MS: Monoarticular or polyarticular arthritis
Integ: Jaundice, chronic skin ulcers, particularly in ankle area
Assoc Findings: Lymphadenopathy, retinal detachment; signs of peripheral nerve damage, including paresthesias, paralysis, chills, vomiting

VITAL SIGNS/HEMODYNAMICS
RR: ↑
HR: ↑
BP: Nl, ↑, or ↓
Temp: Nl, ↑, or ↓
CVP/PAP/PAWP: ↑ if coronary microthrombi and ischemia present; ↓ if in shock

LABORATORY STUDIES
RBCs: Total number ↓; ↑ premature RBCs.
Reticulocytes: RBC precursors; ↑ results from ↑ bone marrow production of RBCs.
Sickle Cell Test: Screens for Hgb S, which is indicative of sickle cell anemia.
Hgb Electrophoresis: Screens for abnormal Hgb often present in hemolytic anemias.
ESR: ↑ in hemolytic anemia more often than in other anemias.

Collaborative Management

Volume Replacement: Fluid and/or blood replacement prevents profound hypotension and can ↓ likelihood of deposition of hemolyzed RBCs in the microvasculature.
O_2 Therapy: To relieve SOB or dyspnea and facilitate tissue oxygenation.
RBC Exchange Therapy for Sickle Cell Crisis: Cytapheresis procedure used if unresponsive to other treatments for sickle cell disease.
Thrombocytapheresis: Cytapheresis procedure for symptoms of excessive thrombosis. Reduces platelets rapidly in an attempt to ↓ clotting before onset of MODS.
Corticosteroids: Used with limited success.
Pain Management: Aspirin, acetaminophen, NSAIDs, narcotics, and sedatives may be necessary for relief of pain and anxiety.
Splenectomy: Sometimes recommended for splenic sequestration crisis related to hemolytic anemia.
Antisickling Agents: Some clinical trials currently under way to evaluate efficacy of these agents in ablating sickling phenomenon.

PATIENT-FAMILY TEACHING

- S&S of impending hemolytic crisis: fever, abnormal pain, headache, dizziness, palpitations, paresthesias, paralysis
- S&S of sensorimotor impairment: unsteady gait, paresthesias, blurring of vision, weakness, paralysis
- Smoking cessation: support groups and programs that assist in stopping cigarette smoking to ↓ vasoconstriction associated with nicotine intake
- Medications: drug name, dosage, frequency, and possible side effects, especially r/t steroids
- Prevention of infection: especially important if patient on long-term steroid therapy or has had splenectomy; importance of pneumococcal vaccine and wearing Medic-Alert ID bracelet
- How to assess extremities qd for evidence of tissue breakdown or blood sequestration (ie, swelling, erythema, tenderness)

Nursing Diagnoses/Interventions

Altered peripheral, cardiopulmonary, renal, cerebral tissue perfusion r/t interruption of arterial or venous blood flow secondary to microthrombi formation
Desired outcome: Within 24 h of treatment onset, patient has adequate perfusion: warm extremities, pink nail beds, peripheral pulses ≥2+ on a scale of 0-4+, SBP >90 mm Hg, HR 60-100 bpm, RR 12-20 breaths/min with eupnea, O_2 saturation >90%, UO ≥0.5 ml/kg/h, orientation × 3.

- Initiate aggressive IV fluid volume replacement as prescribed to prevent deposition of hemolyzed RBCs in the microvasculature.
- Assess extremities for coolness, pallor, ↓ pulse intensity, and prolonged capillary refill. Use Doppler device if unable to palpate pulses.
- Monitor for impending shock: ↑ HR, RR, restlessness, and anxiety; cool and clammy skin; followed by ↓ in BP.
- Keep lower extremities elevated slightly to promote venous blood flow.
- Monitor for ↓ O_2 saturation *via* Spo_2. Be alert to sustained ↓.
- Monitor ABGs for acidosis (ie, pH <7.35 and hypercarbia/CO_2 retention [$Paco_2$ >45 mm Hg]), indicating hypoperfusion, hypoxemia, and respiratory insufficiency.
- Monitor UO for a ↓, which can signal ↓ renal perfusion.
- Monitor neurologic status q2-4h, using Glasgow Coma Scale (see Appendix).

Pain r/t tissue ischemia secondary to vessel occlusion; r/t inflammation/injury secondary to blood within the joints
Desired outcome: Within 1-2 h of initiating treatment, patient's subjective evaluation of discomfort improves as documented by pain scale; nonverbal indicators of discomfort are ↓/absent.

- Monitor for signs of discomfort, including guarded positioning, muscle spasm, and ↑ in HR, BP, and RR. Devise pain scale with patient, rating discomfort from 0 (no pain) to 10.
- Medicate for pain as prescribed; assess medication effectiveness *via* pain scale.
- Consider alternate method of pain control, such as relaxation techniques: guided imagery, controlled breathing, meditation, playing soft music.
- Use therapeutic/healing touch to relieve pain if practitioner is trained and patient agrees to participate, or consult trained practitioner.
- Apply warm compresses to joints to ↑ circulation and thereby improve tissue oxygenation.
- Apply elastic stockings to promote venous return and enhance circulation. As an alternative, apply pneumatic compression stockings.
- Encourage isometric or ROM exercises of extremities to promote circulation.
- Reassure that pain will ↓ as crisis subsides.
- Reassure that crisis is time limited. Enable significant others to be with patient, if possible, during crisis.

Risk for fluid volume deficit or excess r/t failure of renal regulatory mechanisms of fluid and electrolyte balance secondary to microthrombi occluding the nephrons
Desired outcome: Volume status maintained at/returns to baseline: UO ≥0.5 ml/kg/h, stable weight, BP wnl for patient, HR 60-100 bpm, RR 12-20 breaths/min, good skin turgor, moist mucous membranes, urine specific gravity 1.005-1.025, PAWP 6-12 mm Hg, and CVP 2-6 mm Hg.

- Monitor I&O qh. Be alert to UO <0.5 ml/kg/h for 2 consecutive h, which could signal onset of ATN secondary to ↓ renal perfusion.
- Evaluate efficacy of volume expansion by closely comparing CVP, PAWP, and PADP. Overzealous volume expansion can lead to heart failure and pulmonary edema with CVP >20%-25% nl and PAWP >16 mm Hg.
- Administer diuretics as prescribed in well-hydrated or overhydrated patient with UO <0.5 ml/kg/h.
- Assess for S&S of volume depletion: poor skin turgor; dry mucous membranes; hypotension; tachycardia; ↓ UO, PAWP, and CVP.
- Monitor electrolytes and serum osmolality. Universal ↑ in electrolytes and osmolality is indicative of dehydration. Universal ↓ signals fluid overload.
- Assess pH (nl is 7.35-7.45) before replacing electrolytes, since acidosis and alkalosis alter electrolyte values. Replace K^+ cautiously if pH is outside nl.

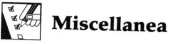 **Miscellanea**

CONSULT MD FOR
- Spo_2 <90%
- UO <0.5 ml/kg/h × 2 h
- ↑ pain or ineffective pain relief
- S&S of complications: ↓ peripheral vascular perfusion, ↓ cerebral perfusion, shock, infection

RELATED TOPICS
- Acute tubular necrosis
- Anemias
- Multiple organ dysfunction syndrome
- Pain
- Shock, hypovolemic
- Stroke: ischemic

ABBREVIATIONS
ATN: Acute tubular necrosis
ESR: Erythrocyte sedimentation rate
MODS: Multiple organ dysfunction syndrome

REFERENCES
Baird MS: Hemolytic dysfunctions. In Swearingen PL, Keen JH (eds): *Manual of critical care nursing*, ed 3, St Louis, 1995, Mosby.
Bentler E: Hemolytic anemia due to chemical and physical agents. In Bentler E et al (eds): *Williams' hematology*, ed 5, New York, 1995, McGraw-Hill.
Embury SH: Sickle cell disease. In Hoffman R et al (eds): *Hematology: basic principles and practice*, ed 2, New York, 1995, Churchill-Livingstone.
Lottman MS, Thompson KS: Management of persons with hematologic problems. In Phipps WJ et al (eds): *Medical-surgical nursing: concepts & clinical practice*, ed 5, St Louis, 1995, Mosby.
Pechet L: The hematologic anemias. In Rippe JM et al (eds): *Intensive care medicine*, ed 3, Boston, 1996, Little, Brown.

Author: **Marianne Saunorus Baird**

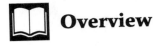 **Overview**

PATHOPHYSIOLOGY
Accumulation of blood in the pleural space. Blunt trauma and penetrating thoracic trauma, including iatrogenic causes, result in bleeding, usually from chest wall vessels, great vessels, heart, or lungs. Blood accumulation causes alveolar collapse and ventilatory compromise. If severe, can lead to hypovolemic shock and lung collapse.

HISTORY/RISK FACTORS
- Blunt or penetrating chest trauma
- Thoracic surgery
- Anticoagulant therapy
- Subclavian central catheter insertion
- Thoracoabdominal organ biopsy

CLINICAL PRESENTATION
Tachypnea, dyspnea, chest pain; chest wall contusion, abrasions, lacerations if trauma-related

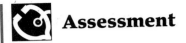 **Assessment**

PHYSICAL ASSESSMENT
Pallor, cyanosis, dullness over affected side, tachycardia, ↓/absent breath sounds, change in mental status. If blunt trauma-related, rib fractures may be palpated. If large, mediastinal shift may be present.

VITAL SIGNS/HEMODYNAMICS
RR: ↑
HR: ↑
BP: ↓
Temp: wnl
CVP/PAP: May be ↓ because of blood loss
CO: May be ↓ because of blood loss

LABORATORY STUDIES
ABGs: Hypoxemia may be accompanied by hypercarbia with resultant respiratory acidosis. SaO_2 may be ↓ initially; usually returns to nl within 24 h.
CBC: ↓ Hgb proportionate to amount of blood lost.

IMAGING
Chest X-ray: To reveal blood in pleural space, size of hemothorax, and any mediastinal shift. Blood in pleural space evidenced by haziness over affected area and loss of acute costophrenic angle.

Collaborative Management

O_2 Therapy: Necessary because of hypoxemia; ↑ to maintain $SpO_2 \geq 92\%$.
Thoracentesis: To remove blood from pleural space.
Chest Tube Placement: Large-bore (30-40 F) thoracic catheter inserted in symptomatic patients to drain fluid. Placement depends on location of hemothorax. Suction commonly used, generally 20-30 cm. Chest tube may produce pleural inflammation, causing pleuritic pain, slight temp ↑, and pleural friction rub.
Autotransfusion: Collection of shed blood, which is filtered and immediately reinfused. Used if hemothorax is acute and rapidly bleeding.
Thoracotomy: To locate source and control bleeding if loss >200 ml/h over 2 h or if hemothorax is massive (1.5-4 L).
IV Fluids/PRBCs: To replace intravascular volume.
Analgesia: Provides relief of pain from hemothorax or its treatment. Opiates used initially; NSAIDS may help relieve pain associated with pleural inflammation.

PATIENT-FAMILY TEACHING
- Purpose for chest-tube placement and maintenance
- Importance of turning, coughing, deep breathing to facilitate lung reexpansion; how to splint to ↓ pain during these activities

Nursing Diagnoses/Interventions

Impaired gas exchange r/t altered O_2 supply secondary to V/Q mismatch
Desired outcomes: Following treatment/intervention, patient exhibits adequate gas exchange and ventilatory function: RR $\geq$20 breaths/min with eupnea and orientation $\times$ 3. At a minimum of 24 h before hospital discharge, ABGs are as follows: Pao_2 $\geq$90 mm Hg and $Paco_2$ 35-45 mm Hg (or values within acceptable baseline parameters).

- Monitor serial ABGs to detect $\downarrow$ Pao_2 and $\uparrow$ $Paco_2$, which can signal respiratory failure.
- Observe for indicators of hypoxia: $\uparrow$ restlessness, anxiety, changes in mental status. Cyanosis may be a late sign.
- Assess VS and breath sounds q2h (check q15min after thoracotomy until stable) for signs of respiratory distress: $\uparrow$ RR, $\downarrow$/absent movement of chest wall on affected side, paradoxical movement of chest wall, $\uparrow$ WOB, use of accessory muscles, complaints of $\uparrow$ dyspnea, and cyanosis. Evaluate HR and BP for indications of shock.
- Position patient to enable full expansion of unaffected lung. Semi-Fowler's position usually provides comfort and allows adequate expansion of chest wall and descent of diaphragm.
- Change patient's position q2h to promote drainage and lung reexpansion and facilitate alveolar perfusion.
- Encourage deep breathing, coughing. Provide necessary analgesia to $\downarrow$ discomfort during deep-breathing exercises; teach or provide chest tube site splinting during these activities.
- Deliver and monitor O_2 as indicated. Titrate to maintain Spo_2 $\geq$90%-92%.

Ineffective breathing pattern (or risk of same) r/t $\downarrow$ lung expansion secondary to malfunction of chest-drainage system
Desired outcome: Following interventions, patient becomes eupneic.

- Monitor q2-4h (as appropriate) to assess breathing pattern while chest-drainage system is in place. Auscultate breath sounds, reporting $\downarrow$; be alert to signs of respiratory distress.
- Assess and maintain closed chest-drainage system.
  Ensure airtight system by securing all connection sites and evaluating/applying air occlusive dressing.
  Avoid kinks in or compression of tubing, and eliminate dependent loops in tubing.
  Monitor output in drainage system. Report $\uparrow$ or $\downarrow$ or change to bright red color.
  Maintain fluid in underwater-seal chamber and suction chamber at appropriate levels.
  Suction amount is determined by water level in suction control chamber. Minimal bubbling in this chamber is desirable. *Note:* Suction aids in reexpansion of the lung; briefly removing suction (eg, for transporting) will not disrupt the closed chest-drainage system.
- Follow institution's policy about chest-tube stripping. This mechanism for maintaining chest-tube patency is controversial and associated with creating high negative pressures in the pleural space, which can damage fragile lung tissue. Stripping may be indicated when bloody drainage or clots are visible in the tubing. Squeezing alternately hand over hand along drainage tube may generate sufficient pressure to move fluid along the tube. Fluctuations >6 cm could signal $\uparrow$ WOB as a result of partial occlusion of the system or $\downarrow$ lung compliance.
- Fluctuations in the long tube of the underwater-seal chamber are characteristic of a patent chest tube. Fluctuations stop when either the lung has reexpanded or there is a kink or obstruction in the chest tube. Bubbling in the underwater-seal chamber occurs on expiration and is a sign that air is leaving the pleural space. Continuous bubbling, however, may be a signal that air is leaking into the drainage system.
- Keep necessary emergency supplies at bedside: petrolatum gauze pad to apply over insertion site if the chest tube becomes dislodged, and sterile water in which to submerge the chest tube if it becomes disconnected from the underwater-seal system.

Pain r/t impaired pleural integrity, inflammation, or presence of chest tube
Desired outcomes: Within 1 h of intervention, subjective perception of pain $\downarrow$ as documented by pain scale. Objective indicators, such as grimacing, are $\downarrow$/absent.

- Assess degree of discomfort q3-4h, using verbal and nonverbal cues. Devise pain scale with patient, rating pain from 0 (no pain) to 10 (severe). Medicate with analgesics, using pain scale to evaluate and document effectiveness of the medication.
- Premedicate 30 min before initiating coughing, exercising, repositioning.
- Teach how to splint affected side when coughing, moving, repositioning.
- Provide for 90-min periods of undisturbed rest, which may $\uparrow$ pain threshold.
- Stabilize chest tube to reduce pull or drag on latex connector tubing. Tape chest tube securely to thorax.

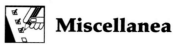

Miscellanea

CONSULT MD FOR

- S&S of hypoxemia/impending respiratory failure: restlessness, change in mental status, dyspnea, tachypnea, cyanosis, $\downarrow$ Pao_2, $\uparrow$ $Paco_2$
- Loss of chest tube patency or failure to drain hemothorax: $\downarrow$ breath sounds on affected side, sudden cessation of drainage, mediastinal shift, inability to mobilize visible clots in chest tube
- Chest tube output >200 ml/h $\times$ 2 h
- S&S of hemorrhagic shock

RELATED TOPICS

- Cardiac surgery: CABG
- Cardiac surgery: valvular disorders
- Chest trauma
- Pneumothorax
- Shock, hemorrhagic

REFERENCES

Gordon PA, Norton JM, Merrell R: Refining chest tube management: analysis of the state of practice, *Dimens Crit Care Nurs* 14(1): 6-12, 1995.

Howard C: Pneumothorax/hemothorax. In Swearingen PL: *Manual of medical-surgical nursing,* ed 3, St Louis, 1994, Mosby.

Monti CM, Rice CL, Hudson LD: Treatment of respiratory complications resulting from trauma. In Bone RC (ed): *Pulmonary and critical care medicine,* St Louis, 1995, Mosby.

Swearingen PL, Howard CA: Managing respiratory procedures. In *Photo-atlas of nursing procedures,* ed 3, Menlo Park, 1996, Addison-Wesley.

Wright JE, Shelton BK: Thoracic trauma. In *Desk reference for critical care nursing,* Boston, 1993, Jones & Bartlett.

Author: **Cheri A. Goll**

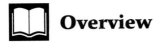 **Overview**

PATHOPHYSIOLOGY
Occurs when heparin therapy causes mild or severe ↓ in freely circulating platelets. Unusual platelet aggregation results in heparin resistance, arterial and venous thrombosis, and subsequent emboli in extreme cases. Seen in all forms of heparin therapy; incidence greater with IV therapy. Two types of HIT:
Mild: Occurs 1-3 days after heparin initiation. Generally resolves in 5 days. Mild ↓ in platelets; no treatment required.
Severe: Occurs 4-8 days after heparin initiation. Platelets ↓ to <100,000 μl. Thrombosis with subsequent embolization and bleeding apparent. *Complications:* PE, AMI, cerebral infarction, and circulatory impairment resulting in limb amputation. Mortality rate 29%. ***Heparin must be discontinued immediately.***

HISTORY/RISK FACTOR
Previous drug-induced immunologic thrombocytopenia

CLINICAL PRESENTATION
Mild: Slight ↓ in platelets without clinical symptoms
Severe: Hemorrhage, ecchymosis, and other S&S depending on location of thrombosis or embolus

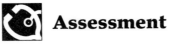 **Assessment**

PHYSICAL ASSESSMENT (Severe HIT)
Neuro: ↓ LOC, paralysis, strokelike symptoms, paresthesias
Resp: SOB, hemoptysis, tachypnea
CV: Chest pain; dysrhythmias; ↓/absent pulse; pallor in affected extremity
GI: Hematemesis; melena, other GI bleeding
Other: Petechiae, purpura, epistaxis, bruising, bleeding of mucosal surfaces and wounds

VITAL SIGNS/HEMODYNAMICS
RR: ↑ if PE or blood loss occurs
HR: ↑ if blood loss occurs
BP: ↓ if blood loss occurs
Temp: NI
CVP/PAWP: ↓ if blood loss occurs
PAP: ↑ if PE present
CO: ↓ if blood loss, AMI occurs
ECG: Dysrhythmias, ST-segment changes if myocardial ischemia present

LABORATORY STUDIES
Platelets: *Mild:* 100,000-150,000 μl; *severe:* <100,000 μl
Bleeding Time: Prolonged if platelets <100,000 μl.
Platelet Antibody Screen: Positive findings attributable to presence of IgG platelet antibodies.
PT, PTT, Thromboplastin Time: These clotting factors remain wnl.
Fibrinogen: Low nl or low as a result of ↑ consumption. NI is 200-400 mg/dl.
FDPs: ↑ to ≥40 μg/ml as a result of fibrinolysis of platelet-fibrin thrombi.
Platelet Aggregation: >100% (or high value of specific laboratory) because of release of platelet membrane antibody.

DIAGNOSTIC PROCEDURE
Bone Marrow Aspiration: NI or ↑ megakaryocytes (platelet precursors).

Collaborative Management

Heparin Therapy: If platelets >100,000 μl and patient symptom free, heparin may be continued. Oral anticoagulation begun immediately if possible. If platelets <100,000 μl and bleeding or thrombosis develops, ***all heparin discontinued immediately, including heparin "flushes."***
Monitoring Heparin Therapy: Preheparin platelet count done to establish baseline: qd × 4 days, then q2d. If ↑ amounts of heparin needed to maintain therapeutic levels (ie, PTT 40-60 sec), suspect heparin resistance, which sometimes precedes HIT.
Vena Caval Filter: Considered if thrombosis occurs with ↓/loss of perfusion to an extremity. ↓ risk of PE caused by extremity clot migration.
Platelet Transfusion: May be initiated after discontinuation of heparin therapy if bleeding fails to subside.
Plasma Exchange: In severe cases, 2-3 L plasma removed and replaced with albumin, crystalloids, or fresh frozen plasma to assist in ↓ bleeding by removing bound heparin from body.
Alternate Anticoagulant: Warfarin sodium (Coumadin), acetylsalicylic acid (aspirin), dipyridamole (Persantine), or dextran may be considered. Low-molecular-weight heparin, eg, enoxaparin (Lovenox), has been used.

PATIENT-FAMILY TEACHING
- Basic pathophysiology of HIT and importance of reporting this problem to all subsequent health care providers
- Importance of wearing Medic-Alert bracelet

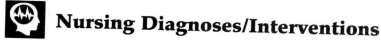 # Nursing Diagnoses/Interventions

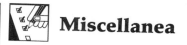 # Miscellanea

Altered protection r/t ↓ platelets with risk of bleeding and thromboembolization
Desired outcome: Within 24 h of discontinuing heparin therapy, patient exhibits no signs of new bleeding, bruising, or thrombosis: HR 60-100 bpm or within 10% of baseline; RR 12-20 breaths/min with eupnea; SBP ≥90 mm Hg; and all peripheral pulses at baseline or >2+ on 0-4+ scale.

- Assess for signs of bleeding q2h: hemoptysis, GI bleeding, hematuria, bleeding from invasive sites or mucous membranes.
- Assess for signs of thrombosis q2h: ↓ peripheral pulses, altered sensation in extremities, pallor, coolness, cyanosis, or capillary refill time >2 sec.
- Avoid IM injections and venous and arterial punctures as much as possible until bleeding time returns to nl.
- Monitor platelet count qd for significant changes. Be alert for values <150,000 μl or below baseline.
- Assess ECG, respiratory rate and pattern, and BP for active bleeding. Be alert to sustained ↑ in HR and RR or ischemic ECG changes (ST depression/elevation).
- Monitor heparin dose carefully. ↑ doses required to maintain therapeutic level (PTT 40-60 sec or 2-2½ × baseline) could signal heparin resistance, an early indicator of HIT.
- Monitor Hgb and Hct values qd in patients with recent or active bleeding.
- Assess mental status and extremity sensation and strength at least q8h.
- Monitor for signs of MODS caused by thrombosis or prolonged hypotension if patient has hemorrhaged. Be alert for respiratory distress, chest pain, ↑ temp, ↓ UO, intolerance of diet or vomiting, abdominal distention, ↓ bowel sounds, and elevated liver enzymes.

Fluid volume deficit (or risk for same) r/t active blood loss
Desired outcome: Patient becomes normovolemic within 24 h of treatment: HR wnl for patient or 60-100 bpm; RR 12-20 breaths/min with eupnea; UO ≥0.5 ml/kg/h; and absence of abdominal pain/tenderness, back pain, or pain from invasive sites.

- Monitor for signs of hypovolemia: ↑ HR, RR, restlessness, fatigue; ↓ BP, UO. If hemodynamic monitoring present, check for ↓ CVP/PAWP and CO.
- Administer supplemental O₂ if patient is bleeding actively.
- Assess for abdominal pain, tenderness, guarding, or back pain, which may signal intraabdominal bleeding.
- Replace lost volume with plasma expanders (albumin, hetastarch [Hespan]) or blood products as indicated. Use PRBCs for profound hemorrhage or possible FFP if other coagulopathy (HELLP, DIC) present. Platelet transfusions are not recommended. See Appendix for blood table.

CONSULT MD FOR

- Platelet count <150,000 μl
- Abnormal bleeding from GI tract, mucosa, venipuncture sites
- S&S of stroke, myocardial ischemia/infarction, pulmonary emboli, peripheral thrombosis
- Heparin resistance: ↑ heparin doses required to maintain therapeutic PTT levels

RELATED TOPICS

- GI bleeding: upper
- Myocardial infarction, acute
- Pulmonary embolus
- Shock, hemorrhagic

ABBREVIATIONS

FDP: Fibrin degradation product
FFP: Fresh frozen plasma
HELLP: Hemolysis, elevated liver enzymes, low platelet count
MODS: Multiple organ dysfunction syndrome
PE: Pulmonary embolus
PRBCs: Packed red blood cells

REFERENCES

Atkins PJ: Postoperative coagulopathies, *Crit Care Nurs Clin North Am* 5(3): 459-471, 1993.
Baird MS: Hematologic dysfunctions. In Swearingen PL, Keen JH (eds): *Manual of critical care nursing*, ed 3, St Louis, 1995, Mosby.
Kimbrell JD: Acquired coagulopathies, *Crit Care Nurs Clin North Am* 5(3): 453-458, 1993.
Kotschwar T: Low-molecular-weight heparins: a new class of antithrombotic agents, *Pharmacy and Therapeutics*, 34-51, 1994.
Lottman MS, Thompson KS: Assessment of the hematologic system. In Phipps WJ et al (eds): *Medical-surgical nursing: concepts & clinical practice*, ed 5, St Louis, 1995, Mosby.

Author: **Marianne Saunorus Baird**

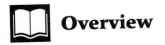 **Overview**

PATHOPHYSIOLOGY
Loss of liver's functional capacity from extensive hepatocellular damage that occurs slowly (as with cirrhosis) or suddenly (as with acute viral or drug-induced hepatitis). Preexisting liver damage usually not a factor with acute hepatic failure, thus damage may be reversible. Alcoholic liver disease presents a unique set of problems in that an acute episode of hepatic failure is superimposed on chronic failure.

Cirrhosis: Chronic liver disease associated with widespread liver tissue necrosis, fibrosis, and nodule formation. Changes in liver structure irreversible, but compensation can be achieved if liver protected from further damage by alcohol cessation or arrest of inflammatory processes.

Acute Hepatic Failure: Sudden, severe liver decompensation resulting from massive hepatocellular necrosis. May present as terminal stage of chronic liver disease, or may result from acute process such as viral hepatitis, alcoholic hepatitis, or shock.

FHF: Severe acute hepatic failure with encephalopathy develops without preexisting liver disease. HBV and HDV are the most frequent causes.

ASSOCIATED PATHOPHYSIOLOGY
Jaundice: Occurs because of inability of failing liver to metabolize bilirubin.

Encephalopathy: Attributed to metabolic derangement and diversion of portal blood flow.

↑ ICP, Cerebral Edema: Seen in acute hepatic failure but usually not in chronic form.

Bleeding Tendencies: Caused by inadequate vitamin K absorption, failure of liver to synthesize clotting factors or clear activated clotting factors, and thrombocytopenia.

Infections, Including Sepsis: Common as a result of generalized state of debilitation and failure of liver to produce immune-related proteins and filter blood from intestines.

Circulatory Abnormalities: Hyperdynamic circulation, with ↑ CO and ↓ vasomotor tone.

Hepatorenal Syndrome: Functional renal failure that develops as a result of ↑ preglomerular vascular resistance and ↓ GFR.

Fluid Retention, Ascites: Attributed to intrahepatic vascular obstruction with transudation of fluid into peritoneum, defective albumin synthesis, and hormonal disturbances.

Metabolic Abnormalities: Include hypoglycemia, dilutional hyponatremia, and hypokalemia.

Note: Prolonged jaundice, ascites, persistently ↓ albumin, prolonged PT, and severe encephalopathy associated with poor outcome.

HISTORY/RISK FACTORS
Cirrhosis
- Chronic alcohol ingestion
- HBV, HCV
- Hepatobiliary disorders

Acute Hepatic Failure
- Chronic liver disease
- Infection of liver, especially HBV, HDV
- Drug-induced hepatitis
- Poisoning
- Alcoholic hepatitis
- Prolonged shock

CLINICAL PRESENTATION
Mild confusion to delirium and sometimes deep coma. Dark urine, light stools, ascites, edema, GI bleeding are common findings.

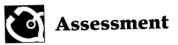 **Assessment**

PHYSICAL ASSESSMENT
- Scleral jaundice in early stages; generalized, deep-yellow skin in late/fulminant
- Fluid sequestration: edema, ascites, weight gain
- Small, bright-red spider angioma: on upper trunk, face, neck, and arms with cirrhosis; notably absent with fulminant failure
- Fixed facial expression, slowness with speech and movement, asterixis
- Multiple ecchymotic areas, purpura, bleeding of oral and nasal mucosa
- Hyperdynamic circulatory changes: tachycardia, warm extremities, active precordial impulse, soft systolic ejection murmur
- Crackles: if pleural effusion, ascites present
- Cyanosis, nail clubbing: possible with chronic liver disease r/t pulmonary AV shunting and V/Q mismatch
- Small, hard liver in chronic liver disease
- Enlarged, firm liver in fulminant failure
- JVD attributable to ↑ RAP caused by ↑ intrapleural pressures from diaphragmatic elevation
- Gynecomastia, testicular atrophy, scant body hair: common in men with chronic hepatic disease

VITAL SIGNS/HEMODYNAMICS
RR: Nl; ↑ if ascites significant
HR: Nl, bounding
BP: Nl or slight ↓
Temp: ↑ with infection
SVR: ↓
CO: ↑
Other: Expanded total blood volume

LABORATORY STUDIES
Virologic Markers: HAV, HBV, and HCV. HAV is usually mild; rarely causes FHF. HBV can cause severe acute, chronic infections. Suprainfection with HDV ↑ likelihood for FHF. HCV infection often chronic.

Biochemistry
Bilirubin: ↑ caused by failure in hepatocyte metabolism and obstruction. High/persistently ↑ levels = poor prognosis.

Alkaline phosphatase (ALP): Isoenzyme of liver origin (ALP$_1$); ↑ with liver disease.

Alanine aminotransferase (ALT/SGPT): ↑ is sensitive and specific indicator of liver dysfunction; values >300 IU/L usually present with acute hepatic failure.

Aspartate aminotransferase (AST/SGOT): Enzyme present in heart muscle, liver, and skeletal muscle. AST/ALP ratio >1.0 present with alcoholic cirrhosis and liver congestion. Ratio <1.0 with acute hepatitis and viral hepatitis.

Albumin: ↓, especially with ascites. Persistently low levels = poor prognosis.

Sodium: Retained but associated with water retention, which results in nl sodium levels or even dilutional hyponatremia. Severe hyponatremia present in terminal stage and associated with tense ascites and hepatorenal syndrome.

Potassium: Slightly ↓. Hypokalemic acidosis common.

Glucose: Hypoglycemia usually present.

BUN: ↓ because of failure of Krebs cycle enzymes in liver; ↑ because of bleeding.

Ammonia: ↑ because of inability of failing liver to convert ammonia to urea and shunting of intestinal blood *via* collateral vessels.

Hemat: Marked ↓ in Hgb, Hct with acute variceal hemorrhage. ↓ leukocytes, platelets expected partly as result of hypersplenism. If infection present, leukocytes may ↑ to nl or be ↑. PT prolonged and unresponsive to vitamin K therapy.

Urinalysis: ↑ urobilinogen, bilirubin. With ascites, 24-h urine volume ↓ and 24-h sodium ↓ (<5 mEq/day in severe cases).

IMAGING
Liver Scan: Imaging by radioisotope, ultrasound, or CT can aid in determining liver size and abnormal tissue such as tumors.

DIAGNOSTIC PROCEDURES
Liver Biopsy: Specimen of liver obtained for microscopic analysis and diagnosis. Percuta-

neous liver biopsy contraindicated with markedly prolonged PT or low platelet counts because of hemorrhage risk.

EEG: To detect or confirm early encephalopathy.

Abdominal Paracentesis: Catheter or trocar inserted into abdominal cavity to remove fluid, which is sent for analysis of protein, electrolytes, WBCs, and culture. Drainage rarely indicated because fluid is rapidly replaced from the blood and may result in intravascular depletion and hypovolemic shock.

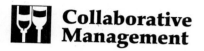 # Collaborative Management

Correction of Precipitating Factors: GI hemorrhage or blood loss from other sources requires immediate volume resuscitation. Hypoxia must be corrected immediately. Acute infections treated aggressively with appropriate antibiotics. Electrolyte disturbances resulting from diuretics, diarrhea, or other causes corrected promptly. ETOH and hepatotoxic drugs eliminated.

Fluid and Electrolyte Management: Unless hyponatremia profound, sodium-containing fluids avoided because they contribute to ascites and may potentiate renal insufficiency. Hypokalemia common and must be corrected because hypokalemic alkalosis can precipitate encephalopathy. Albumin and D_5W generally used for fluid resuscitation unless ↓ Hct signals need for PRBCs. In unstable patients, PAP monitoring initiated to ensure adequate tissue perfusion without fluid overload. Hyperdynamic circulatory state supported by fluid administration, sympathomimetic agents (eg, dopamine) as necessary.

Bed Rest: Necessary to ↓ metabolic demands placed on liver during nl daily activity.

Nutritional Therapy: High-calorie, high-protein (80-100 g) diet of high biologic value indicated for patients without encephalopathy to ensure tissue repair. Sodium moderately restricted. If GI function impaired and patient unable to tolerate enteral feedings, PN initiated. For acute hepatic encephalopathy, protein eliminated totally until recovery.

Pharmacotherapy: Drugs with hepatotoxic potential should be discontinued. These include acetaminophen, ETOH, methotrexate, NSAIDs, oral contraceptives, phenytoin, rifampin, many antibiotics, many inhaled anesthetics, chemotherapeutic agents.

Corticosteroids: Helpful in some forms of chronic active hepatitis.

Sedatives: Avoided if possible because they can precipitate or contribute to encephalopathy. If necessary, diphenhydramine (Benadryl) or oxazepam (Serax) often selected because they can be eliminated safely in hepatic disease.

Histamine H_2-receptor antagonists: To block acid secretion and prevent gastric erosions, which are common with chronic or severe hepatic failure.

Sucralfate (Carafate): Binds to gastric erosions and coats gastric/duodenal mucosa.

Dextrose: In the event of hypoglycemia, bolus of 50% dextrose or continual infusion of 10% solution indicated.

Management of Resp Failure: Intubation or mechanical ventilation may be indicated if advanced encephalopathy, aspiration of gastric contents, or impairment of ventilation secondary to ascites present. Continuous Spo_2 used with respiratory failure or if patient at high risk for same. Need for adequate tissue oxygenation cannot be overemphasized, since hepatic hypoxia a significant contributor to hepatic failure.

Management of Ascites

Restriction of fluid, sodium intake: If ascites severe, sodium limited to <500 mg/day.

Restriction of physical activity: To ↓ metabolites that must be handled by liver.

Diuretics: Spironolactone (Aldactone), amiloride, or other potassium-sparing diuretics may be used to control ascites. For severe ascites, mannitol may be added to the regimen. Goal with diuresis: 1 L/day. If diuresis too rapid, may lead to acute hypovolemia, shock, and hepatorenal syndrome.

Albumin: To ↑ intravascular colloidal pressure.

Paracentesis: Removal of ascitic fluid may be attempted for refractory ascites.

Peritoneal-venous shunt: A shunt system (eg, LeVeen or Denver) may be surgically placed for refractory ascites. Peritoneal cavity drained by long, perforated catheter that runs into intrathoracic superior vena cava. Device designed so that fluid can flow only one direction from—peritoneum into bloodstream. *Complications:* fluid overload, infection, DIC, peritonitis, shunt occlusion, and precipitation of variceal hemorrhage.

Management of Encephalopathy

Elimination, correction of precipitating factors: Variceal hemorrhage, infection, dehydration, electrolyte imbalance, sedative use, dietary protein intake, constipation.

Elimination of dietary protein: Reintroduced gradually when symptoms improve.

Early, thorough catharsis by magnesium citrate or enemas (usually tap water): To remove intestinal contents.

Administration of neomycin: To ↓ intestinal bacteria that produce ammonia; used only in acute situations.

Administration of lactulose: To create an environment unfavorable to ammonia-forming intestinal bacteria and cause osmotic diarrhea. Dose adjusted to produce two to three semiformed stools per day.

ICP monitoring: To detect cerebral edema, guide pharmacologic management (eg, mannitol, furosemide) and other therapeutic measures, eg, positioning.

Management of Bleeding Complications: FFP and platelets given to correct defects in clotting factors and thrombocytopenia. Vitamin K may be prescribed to help correct bleeding tendencies but may have little effect.

Management of Hepatorenal Syndrome: Often occurs because of overaggressive diuretic therapy, paracentesis, hemorrhage, diarrhea, or dehydration. Prevention, when possible, essential. Electrolytes corrected, and ascites mobilized slowly. Hepatic failure, the causative factor, is treated. Renal dialysis seldom employed because it does not improve survival and can lead to GI hemorrhage and shock.

Hepatic Transplantation: For irreversible, progressive liver disease if supportive therapy has failed. Only therapy available for FHF; requires highly skilled team of specialists.

PATIENT/FAMILY TEACHING

- Importance of sufficient rest and adherence to prescribed diet
- Infection control: if r/t hepatitis infection, recommended prophylaxis for sexual partners and household contacts exposed to the virus
- Alcohol, drug treatment programs if alcohol- and drug-related hepatic failure has occurred
- Importance of avoiding OTC medications without consulting health care provider
- S&S of infection: fever, unusual drainage from paracentesis/other invasive sites, warmth and erythema surrounding invasive sites, abdominal pain
- S&S of unusual bleeding, including prolonged mucosal bleeding, very large or painful bruises, dark stools
- Sodium restriction if ascites present; protein restriction if patient has residual or chronic encephalopathy
- Necessity of alcohol cessation for several mos after complete recovery from acute episode; if hepatic failure not r/t alcohol ingestion, allowance of one or two glasses of beer or wine/day after full recovery
- Necessity of weighing qd and reporting weight loss/gain ≥5 lbs

Nursing Diagnoses/Interventions

Fluid volume deficit r/t ↓ intake secondary to medically prescribed restrictions; and r/t ↓ circulating volume secondary to hypoalbuminemia, altered hemodynamics, fluid sequestration, and diuretic therapy

Desired outcome: Within 24 h of this diagnosis, patient normovolemic: MAP ≥70 mm Hg, HR 60-100 bpm, brisk capillary refill (<2 sec), distal pulses >2+ on 0-4+ scale, CVP 2-6 mm Hg, PAP 20-30/8-15 mm Hg, PAWP 6-12 mm Hg, CI ≥3.0 L/min/m^2, SVR 900-1200 dynes/sec/cm^{-5}, UO ≥0.5 ml/kg/h, and orientation × 3.

- Monitor HR, BP, ECG, and CV status qh or more frequently if unstable. Be alert to MAP ↓ ≥10 mm Hg and to ↑ in HR suggestive of hypovolemia or circulatory decompensation.
- Measure central pressures and CO q1-4h. Be alert to low/↓ CVP, PAWP, and CO. Calculate SVR q4-8h or more frequently if unstable. ↑ HR, ↓ PAWP, CO less than baseline, or CI <3.0, along with ↓ UO, suggest hypovolemia. Because of altered vascular responsiveness, SVR may not ↑ with hypovolemic hepatic failure. Be aware that a "normal" CO actually may be ↓ for these patients. Monitor Svo$_2$ as available to evaluate tissue oxygenation.
- Monitor filling pressures qh immediately after paracentesis or if patient dehydrated or hemorrhaging.
- Measure and record UO qh. Be alert to output <0.5 ml/kg/h for 2 consecutive h. If ↓ or other indicators of fluid volume deficit present, consider cautious ↑ in fluid intake; reevaluate volume status. Use caution in giving potent diuretics, since they may precipitate encephalopathy or renal insufficiency by causing rapid diuresis and electrolyte changes.
- Minimize infusion of sodium-containing fluids because they contribute to ascites and peripheral edema and may potentiate functional renal failure.
- Monitor serum and urine sodium levels. Serum sodium <120 mEq/L and urine sodium <10 mEq/L are associated with the development of hepatorenal syndrome.
- Estimate ongoing fluid losses. Measure all drainage from peritoneal or other catheters q2-4h. Weigh patient qd. Compare 24-h intake to output. Weight loss should not exceed 0.5 kg/day because more rapid diuresis can lead to intravascular volume depletion and impair renal function.
- Monitor BUN, creatinine, and potassium values. Be aware that alterations in hepatic function can cause ↓ BUN levels and GI bleeding results in ↑ values.
- Monitor serum albumin, and administer albumin replacements as indicated.
- Avoid giving NSAIDs, which can inhibit renal prostaglandin and ↓ GFR.

Fluid volume excess: Interstitial, r/t compromised regulatory mechanisms secondary to acute or chronic hepatic failure

Desired outcomes: Within 48 h of this diagnosis, patient normovolemic: CVP 2-6 mm Hg, PAWP 6-12 mm Hg, HR 60-100 bpm, RR 12-20 breaths/min with eupnea, ↓/stable abdominal girth, absence of crackles, edema, uncomfortable ascites, and other clinical indicators of fluid volume excess.

- Monitor VS, hemodynamic parameters, and CV status q1-2h. Be alert to CVP >6 mm Hg or PAWP >12 mm Hg.
- Monitor for evidence of pulmonary edema r/t fluid overload. Note presence of dyspnea, orthopnea, basilar crackles that do not clear with coughing, and tachypnea.
- Use minimal amounts of fluids necessary to administer IV medications and maintain IV catheter patency.
- If fluids restricted, offer mouth care and/or ice chips.
- Measure and record abdominal girth qd. To ensure accurate measurements, measure at widest point, and mark this level for subsequent measurement. Measure in same position each time, preferably supine.
- Monitor serum electrolyte levels, especially sodium and potassium.

Impaired gas exchange r/t altered O$_2$ supply secondary to AV shunting, V/Q mismatch, and diaphragmatic limitation associated with ascites, hydrothorax, or central respiratory depression occurring with encephalopathy

Desired outcome: Within 4 h of this diagnosis, patient has adequate gas exchange: Pao$_2$ ≥80 mm Hg, Paco$_2$ <45 mm Hg, RR 12-20 breaths/min with eupnea, O$_2$ saturation >92%, and orientation × 3.

- Monitor and document RR q1-4h. Note pattern, excursion depth, and effort.
- Administer supplemental O$_2$ to enhance cerebral and hepatic oxygenation. Consider intubation if patient obtunded. Monitor Pao$_2$, Paco$_2$, and O$_2$ saturation.

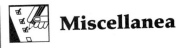 # Miscellanea

CONSULT MD FOR
- S&S of fluid volume deficit/excess
- Electrolyte imbalance: hypokalemia, severe hyponatremia (Na$^+$ <120 mEq/L)
- S&S of pulmonary infection, other respiratory complications
- S&S of GI, other hemorrhage: ↓ Hct/Hgb, ↑ BUN, occult blood in stools, gastric contents
- S&S of urinary, blood stream, other infections

- Maintain body positions that optimize ventilation. Elevate HOB ≥30 degrees, depending on patient comfort and hemodynamic status.
- Assess for atelectasis; pulmonary infection; hydrothorax (eg, ↓ breath sounds, dullness to percussion).

Sensory/Perceptual alterations r/t endogenous chemical alteration (accumulation of ammonia, other CNS toxins with hepatic dysfunction), therapeutically restricted environment, sleep deprivation, and hypoxia

Desired outcomes: By time of hospital discharge, patient exhibits stable personality pattern, age-appropriate behavior, intact intellect appropriate for level of education, distinct speech, and coordinated gross and fine motor movements.

- Avoid or minimize precipitating factors:
    Eliminate/↓ dietary protein.
    Avoid/correct constipation.
    Check gastric secretions, vomitus, and stools for occult blood.
    Evaluate Hct and Hgb for evidence of bleeding.
    Monitor for indicators of infection.
    Evaluate serum ammonia levels.
    Be alert for potential sources of electrolyte imbalance (eg, diarrhea, gastric aspiration).
    Avoid use of sedative or tranquilizing agents and hepatotoxic drugs.
    Correct hypoxemia.
- Evaluate for CNS effects such as personality changes, childish behavior, intellectual impairment, slurred speech, ataxia, asterixis.
- Administer handwriting or psychometric tests (if appropriate for LOC) qd to evaluate mild or subclinical encephalopathy.
- Administer enemas to clear colon of intestinal contents that contribute to encephalopathy. Repeat as necessary to ensure thorough colon cleansing.
- Administer neomycin to ↓ intestinal bacteria, which contribute to cerebral intoxicants. Monitor for ototoxicity and nephrotoxicity caused by neomycin. Avoid giving neomycin in renal insufficiency.
- Administer lactulose to ↓ ammonia formation in intestine. Adjust dose to produce two to three semiformed stools qd.
- Protect confused or unconscious patient from injury.
    Leave side rails up; consider padding them if patient active. Have call light within patient's reach at all times.
    Tape all catheters and tubes securely to prevent dislodgement.
- Consider possibility of seizures in severe encephalopathy; have airway management equipment readily available.
- Minimize unnecessary noise, lights, and other environmental stimuli.
- Monitor ICP and CPP. With ↑ ICP, position carefully, and avoid fluid overload, hypercarbia, and hypoxemia. Administer mannitol and furosemide (Lasix) as indicated. Sedation or coma induction may be necessary if cerebral edema does not respond to these measures.

Altered protection r/t clotting anomaly and thrombocytopenia

Desired outcome: Patient's bleeding, if it occurs, is not prolonged.

- Avoid giving IM injections. If they are necessary, use small-gauge needles and maintain firm pressure over injection sites for several min. Avoid massaging IM injection sites.
- Maintain pressure for several min over venipuncture sites. Inform laboratory personnel of patient's bleeding tendencies.
- Avoid arterial punctures. Consider use of an indwelling arterial line.
- Monitor PT levels and platelet counts qd. Consult physician for significant prolongation of PT or significant ↓ in platelets. Administer vitamin K as indicated.
- Assess for signs of bleeding. Note oral and nasal mucosal bleeding and ecchymotic areas, and test stools, vomitus, urine, and gastric drainage for occult blood. Be alert to prolonged bleeding or oozing of blood from venipuncture sites and incisions.
- Use electric rather than straight razor for patient shaving. Provide soft-bristled toothbrush or sponge-tipped applicator and mouthwash for oral hygiene.
- Avoid indwelling gastric drainage tubes as they may irritate gastric mucosa or varices, causing bleeding to occur.
- Administer FFP and platelets as indicated. Monitor carefully for fluid volume overload.
- A postshunt coagulopathy may develop in some patients after peritoneal-venous shunt surgery. Monitor these patients closely.
- Be aware that if FSPs are present in the blood and there is significant thrombocytopenia, patient may have DIC.

RELATED TOPICS
- Cirrhosis
- Disseminated intravascular coagulation
- Esophageal varices
- Hypokalemia
- Increased intracranial pressure
- Systemic inflammatory response syndrome
- Types and characteristics of viral hepatitis (see Appendix)

ABBREVIATIONS
FFP: Fresh frozen plasma
FHF: Fulminant hepatic failure
FSPs: Fibrin split products
GFR: Glomerular filtration rate
PRBCs: Packed red blood cells
Svo$_2$: Mixed venous oxygen saturation

REFERENCES
Butler R: Managing the problems of cirrhosis, *Am J Nurs* 94(3): 46-49, 1994.

Covington J: Nursing care of patients with alcoholic liver disease, *Crit Care Nurse* 13(3): 47-57, 1993.

Keen JH: Hepatic failure. In Swearingen PL, Keen JH (eds): *Manual of critical care nursing*, ed 3, St Louis, 1995, Mosby.

Kucharski S: Fulminant hepatic failure, *Crit Care Nurs Clin North Am* 5(1): 141-151, 1993.

Lancaster S, Stockbridge J: PV shunts relieve ascites, *RN* 55(8): 58-60, 1992.

Smith SL, Ciferni M: Liver transplantation for acute hepatic failure: a review of clinical experience and management, *Am J Crit Care* 2(2): 137-144, 1993.

Author: **Janet Hicks Keen**

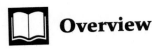

Overview

PATHOPHYSIOLOGY

Processes whereby part of the brain is displaced through openings within intracranial cavity. Occurs when there is a pressure difference between supratentorial and infratentorial compartments. When this occurs, the vascular system is compressed, destroyed, or lacerated, causing ischemia, necrosis, and ultimately death. Several herniation syndromes possible.

Cingulate: Unilateral hemispheric ↑ in ICP; causes normally midline cingulate gyrus to shift to opposite side. Compresses anterior cerebral artery and internal cerebral vein, contributing further to cerebral edema, ischemia, ↑ ICP.

Uncal: Occurs when expanding lesion of middle or temporal fossa forces tip (uncus) of temporal lobe toward midline, displacing brain downward toward spinal cord. Compression of oculomotor nerve (III) and posterior cerebral artery occurs. Herniation of brainstem through foramen magnum occurs if not treated immediately.

Transtentorial (central): Occurs with expanding lesions of frontal, parietal, or occipital lobes or with severe cerebral edema. Subcortical structures (basal ganglia, thalamus, hypothalamus) herniate, compressing midbrain and posterior cerebral arteries bilaterally. Often preceded by cingulate and uncal herniation.

Transcranial (extracranial): Occurs when intracranial contents under pressure forced through an open wound, surgical site, or cranial vault fracture. Loss of brain volume ↓ ICP and may prevent intracranial herniation. Patient at risk for infection, further brain injury, and death.

HISTORY/RISK FACTORS

- Head injury, cerebral contusion
- Ruptured cerebral aneurysm, subarachnoid hemorrhage
- Intracranial hematoma
- Encephalitis, meningitis
- ↑ ICP

CLINICAL PRESENTATION

↓ LOC, weakness/paralysis, pupil fixed and dilated on side of herniation

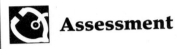

Assessment

PHYSICAL ASSESSMENT

Cingulate
Motor response: Unilateral or bilateral lower extremity weakness/paralysis

Early Uncal
Pupillary: Ipsilateral dilatation with sluggish contraction; brisk contralateral reaction
Oculocephalic response: Wnl
Oculovestibular response: Ipsilateral response
Motor response: Contralateral extensor plantar reflex

Late Uncal
Resp pattern: Sustained hyperventilation
Pupillary: Ipsilateral fixed and dilated
Oculocephalic/oculovestibular responses: Impaired or absent
Motor response: Ipsilateral hemiplegia, abnormal posturing, or absence of all responses

Early Transtentorial: Diencephalic
Resp pattern: Deep sighs, yawning
Pupillary: Small with minimal contraction to light
Oculocephalic/oculovestibular responses: Wnl
Motor response: Contralateral paresis; bilateral Babinski reflex present

Late Transtentorial: Diencephalic
Resp pattern: Cheyne-Stokes
Oculocephalic/oculovestibular responses: Unchanged
Motor responses: Abnormal flexion posturing

Transtentorial: Midbrain/Upper Pons
Resp pattern: Sustained hyperventilation
Pupillary: Midpositioned, irregularly shaped, unresponsive to light
Oculocephalic/oculovestibular responses: May be dysconjugate
Motor response: Abnormal extension posturing

Transtentorial: Lower Pons/Upper Medulla
Resp pattern: Shallow, rapid, irregular
Pupillary: Midpositioned/fixed
Oculocephalic/oculovestibular responses: Absent
Motor response: Flaccid but bilateral Babinski's reflex possible

VITAL SIGNS/HEMODYNAMICS

RR: ↑; pattern varies based on brain area compressed
HR: Nl, ↓, or ↑
BP: Nl or ↑ SBP with widened pulse pressure if there is brainstem compression
Temp: Nl or ↑
ICP: ↑
CPP: ↓

Other: Cushing's triad, a late sign of mechanical compression or severe brainstem dysfunction

ECG: ↑ ICP results in prominent U waves, ST-segment changes, notched T waves, and prolonged QT interval. Also may show sinus bradycardia, SVT, and ventricular dysrhythmias.

IMAGING

CT Scan: Gray and white matter, blood, and CSF detectable because of their radiologic densities. CT capable of diagnosing cerebral hemorrhage, infarction, hydrocephalus, edema, and structural shifts.

MRI: Identifies type, location, and extent of injury. Provides detailed spatial resolution, follows metabolic processes, and detects structural changes.

EEG: Useful in detecting areas of abnormal brain activity (irritability) and generalized brain activity, coma, or suspected brain death.

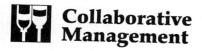 **Collaborative Management**

Focuses on treating emergent pathology and controlling ICP.

Surgical Intervention: To evacuate mass lesions (epidural, subdural, intracranial hematomas), place ICP monitoring system, elevate depressed skull fractures, débride open wounds and brain tissue, repair dural tears or scalp lacerations. Temporal lobectomy may be necessary to control severe ↑ in ICP.

Management of ICP Dynamics: Uses variety of techniques (intraventricular cannula, subarachnoid screw, epidural or intraparenchymal fiberoptic sensor). Monitoring systems provide digital display of ICP, but CPP must be calculated (CPP = MAP − ICP). Maintain ICP ≤15 mm Hg and CPP 60-80 mm Hg.

Hyperventilation via mechanical ventilation: Controls ICP by reducing $Paco_2$, thereby vasoconstricting cerebral vessels and causing ↓ cerebral blood volume.

Reduction of ICP by CSF drainage: Intraventricular or ventriculostomy systems used to drain CSF and ↓ ICP. Keep drainage collection bags at level of ear tragus or higher to prevent excessive CSF flow caused by higher-to-lower pressure gradient.

Diuresis therapy: ↓ cerebral brain volume by extracting fluid from brain's intracellular compartment. Dehydration is a major complication; strict attention to serum electrolytes and osmolality necessary.

Maintenance of BP Within Acceptable Range: Hypotension can result in ↓ cerebral perfusion, causing cerebral vessels to vasodilate. To maintain CPP, dopamine HCl may be used at doses of 3-5 μg/kg/min. Hypertension may cause ↑ capillary permeability and petechial hemorrhage. Antihypertensives, eg, labetalol HCl (Normodyne) or nitroprusside sodium (Nipride), used to control BP.

Reduction of metabolic demand: Control of seizure activity *via* sedating agents (midazolam HCl [Versed], propofol [Diprivan]) and maintenance of normothermia are important strategies in ↓ metabolic demand of cerebral tissue.

Barbiturate coma: Pentobarbital sodium (Nembutal) to ↓ metabolic demand. Continuous ICP and hemodynamic monitoring with controlled ventilation necessary because barbiturates induce profound cardiac and cerebral depression.

Modifying Nursing Care Activities That ↑ ICP: Sustained ↑ in ICP (>5 min) must be avoided. Space activities such as bathing, turning, and suctioning to prevent stair-step ↑ in ICP.

Flexion, extension, lateral movements: Maintain neck in neutral position to prevent flexion and lateral movements that can significantly ↑ ICP. Stabilize neck with towel rolls or sandbags.

Positioning: Adjust based on clinical response; desired effect is improved perfusion and ↓ ICP.

PATIENT-FAMILY TEACHING

- Signs of ↑ ICP: change in LOC, visual disturbances, dizziness, motor or behavior change
- Importance of avoiding Valsalva maneuver, agitation, continuous coughing

Nursing Diagnoses/Interventions

Decreased adaptive capacity: Intracranial, r/t compromise of pressure/volume dynamics
Desired outcome: Patient exhibits adequate intracranial adaptive capacity within 72 h of treatment: orientation $\times$ 3 (or consistent with baseline); equal and normoreactive pupils; BP wnl for patient; HR 60-100 bpm; RR 12-20 breaths/min with eupnea (or mechanically controlled ventilation); ICP 0-15 mm Hg; CPP 60-80 mm Hg.
- Assess qh for ↑ ICP and herniation (change in behavior or LOC, pupillary changes).
- Calculate CPP by means of the formula

$$CPP = MAP - ICP$$
$$\text{where } \frac{MAP = SBP + 2(DBP)}{3}$$

- Assess for ↑ ICP (ICP >15 mm Hg) or CPP <60 mm Hg.
- Assess for, treat conditions that can cause ↑ restlessness with concomitant ↑ ICP: hypoxemia, pain, fear, anxiety.
- Implement measures that help prevent ↑ ICP and herniation:
    Maintain complete bed rest.
    Keep HOB at optimal level based on clinical response.
    Avoid neck flexion, extension, or rotation.
    Maintain quiet, relaxing environment.
    Minimize agitation and restlessness.
    Maintain adequate ventilation to prevent cerebral hypoxia.
    Avoid vigorous, prolonged suctioning.
    Hyperoxygenate with 100% oxygen before/during/after suctioning.
    Maintain normovolemia.
    Monitor and record I&O.
    Teach patient measures to prevent ↑ ICP.

Miscellanea

CONSULT MD FOR
- ICP >15 mm Hg, CPP <60-80 mm Hg
- S&S of ↑ ICP: change in LOC, behavior, or motor movement; pupillary changes
- $Paco_2$ >30 mm Hg, Pao_2 <80 mm Hg

RELATED TOPICS
- Agitation syndrome
- Head injury
- Increased intracranial pressure
- Intracranial surgery
- Mechanical ventilation
- Paralytic therapy
- Subarachnoid hemorrhage
- Vasodilator therapy
- Vasopressor therapy

ABBREVIATION
CPP: Cerebral perfusion pressure

- Administer antihypertensives to prevent hypertension.
- If ↑ ICP occurs suddenly, perform hyperinflation with manual resuscitator using 100% O_2 at ≥50 breaths/min to ↓ $Paco_2$.
- If prescribed for acutely ↑ ICP, administer bolus of mannitol (ie, 1.5-2.0 g/kg as a 15%-25% solution infused over 30-60 min). Monitor carefully to avoid profound fluid/electrolyte disturbances.

Impaired gas exchange r/t ↓ O_2 supply and ↑ CO_2 production secondary to ↓ ventilatory drive occurring with pressure on respiratory center, imposed inactivity

Desired outcomes: $Paco_2$ 25-30 mm Hg during hyperventilation, 35-40 mm Hg as ICP stabilizes, and 35-45 mm Hg by time of discharge from ICU. By time of discharge, patient has adequate gas exchange: Pao_2 ≥80 mm Hg, RR 12-20 breaths/min with eupnea, no adventitious breath sounds.

- Assess respiratory rate, depth, rhythm. Auscultate lung fields for breath sounds q1-2h. Monitor for abnormal respiratory patterns.
- Deliver O_2 within prescribed limits. Assess for hypoxia: confusion, agitation, restlessness, irritability. Cyanosis is a late indicator.
- Ensure patent airway *via* proper neck positioning and suctioning as necessary. Hyperoxygenate before and after each suction pass.
- Monitor ABGs. Be alert for hypoxemia (Pao_2 <80). Monitor for $Paco_2$ ≥25-30. ↑ levels may ↑ cerebral blood flow and thus ↑ ICP. Maintain O_2 saturation at >94%.
- Assist with turning q2h to promote lung drainage/expansion and alveolar perfusion.
- Evaluate need for artificial airway in patient unable to maintain airway patency or adequate ventilatory effort.
- Monitor ICP for sustained ↑ during respiratory care activities. Modify activities to avoid sharp or sustained ↑.

REFERENCES

Davis A et al: Neurlogic dysfunctions. In Swearingen PL, Keen JH (eds): *Manual of critical care nursing,* ed 3, St Louis, Mosby.

Nussbaum ES et al: Complete temporal lobectomy for surgical resuscitation of patients with transtentorial herniation secondary to unilateral hemispheric swelling, *Neurosurgery* 29(1): 62-66, 1991.

Author: **Alice Davis**

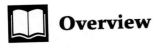 **Overview**

PATHOPHYSIOLOGY

Calcium exerts a sedative effect on nerve cells and has important intracellular functions, including development of cardiac action potential and muscle contraction. Symptoms occur because of ↑ in total serum calcium or in the percentage of free, ionized calcium (Ca^{2+}). About half of plasma calcium is free, ionized calcium. Slightly less than half is bound to protein, primarily to albumin. Only ionized calcium is physiologically important. The percentage of calcium that is ionized is affected by plasma pH and albumin level. If accompanied by nl or ↑ serum phosphorus level, calcium phosphate crystals may precipitate in the serum and deposit throughout the body. Soft tissue calcifications usually occur when the product of serum calcium and phosphorus (ie, calcium × phosphorus) >70 mg/dl.

HISTORY/RISK FACTORS

- ↑ release of calcium from bone: hyperparathyroidism, malignancies, prolonged immobilization, Paget's disease
- ↑ intake of calcium: excessive amounts given during cardiopulmonary arrest, milk-alkali syndrome
- ↑ intestinal absorption: with vitamin D overdose or hyperparathyroidism
- ↓ urinary excretion: medications (eg, thiazide diuretics), hyperparathyroidism
- ↑ ionized calcium: acidosis

CLINICAL PRESENTATION

Lethargy, weakness, anorexia, bone pain, fractures, altered mental status

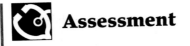 **Assessment**

PHYSICAL ASSESSMENT

Neuro: Confusion, depression, paresthesias, stupor, coma
CV: Hypertension, heart block, digitalis sensitivity, cardiac arrest
GI: Nausea, vomiting, constipation
GU: Polyuria, calculi

VITAL SIGNS/HEMODYNAMICS

RR: Nl
HR: Irregular if ventricular dysrhythmias, heart block present
BP: May be ↑; may be ↓ if patient is polyuric, hypovolemic
Temp: Nl
CO: ↓ if significant dysrhythmias present
ECG: Shortening of ST segment and QT interval, PR interval prolonged; ventricular dysrhythmias

LABORATORY STUDIES

Total Serum Calcium Level: >10.5 mg/dl. Should be evaluated with serum albumin level. For every 1.0 g/dl ↑ in serum albumin level, there will be a 0.8-1.0 mg/dl ↑ in total calcium.
Ionized Calcium Level: >5.5 mg/dl.
PTH Level: ↑ in primary or secondary hyperparathyroidism. PTH level will not be ↑ if hypercalcemia caused by malignancy.

IMAGING

X-rays: May reveal osteoporosis, bone cavitation, urinary calculi.

Collaborative Management

Treatment of Underlying Cause: Eg, antitumor chemotherapy for malignancy or partial parathyroidectomy for hyperparathyroidism; discontinuation of thiazide diuretics.
IV Isotonic Saline: Given rapidly to ↑ urinary calcium excretion. Concomitant administration of furosemide prevents fluid volume excess and causes ↑ calcium excretion.
Low-Calcium Diet, Cortisone: To ↓ intestinal absorption of calcium.
Reducing Bone Resorption: ↑ weight-bearing activity, pamidronate, mithramycin, or gallium nitrate.
Calcitonin: To ↓ bone resorption, ↑ bone deposition of calcium and phosphorus, and ↑ urinary calcium and phosphate excretion.
Partial Parathyroidectomy: To treat primary hyperparathyroidism.

PATIENT-FAMILY TEACHING

- Reassurance that altered sensorium is temporary and will improve with treatment
- Importance of weight-bearing exercise
- Necessity of low-calcium diet (when prescribed) and avoiding calcium-containing medications (eg, antacids such as Tums); emphasis on intake of fruits (eg, cranberries, prunes, or plums) that leave an acid ash in urine
- Importance of adequate fluid intake

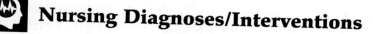

Nursing Diagnoses/Interventions

Altered protection r/t neurosensory alterations secondary to hypercalcemia
Desired outcomes: Within 24-48 h of initiating treatment, patient verbalizes orientation to time, place, and person. Patient does not exhibit evidence of injury caused by neurosensory changes.
- Monitor for worsening hypercalcemia. Assess LOC; orientation to time, place, and person; and neurologic status with each VS check.
- Use reality therapy: clocks, calendars, familiar objects; keep at bedside within patient's visual field.
- Administer fluids and diuretics. Evaluate response to therapy. Monitor serum calcium, potassium, phosphorus, and albumin levels. Observe for signs of fluid volume excess with treatment.
- Poor coordination, weakness, and altered gait may occur. Provide a safe environment. Keep side rails up and bed in lowest position with wheels locked. Assist with ambulation if it is allowed.
- Monitor patient taking digitalis for S&S of digitalis toxicity: multifocal or bigeminal PVCs, PAT with varying AV block, secondary AV block, Wenckebach (Mobitz I).
- Encourage ↑ mobility to reduce bone resorption. Ideally patient will be out of bed and up in a chair at least 6 h/day.

Altered urinary elimination r/t dysuria, urgency, frequency, and polyuria secondary to diuretics, calcium stone formation, or changes in renal function occurring with hypercalcemia
Desired outcome: Within 24 h of treatment initiation, patient exhibits voiding pattern and urine characteristics wnl for patient.
- Monitor I&O qh. Be alert for oliguria or polyuria. ↑ urinary calcium concentrations ↓ the kidneys' ability to concentrate urine, leading to polyuria and potentially to fluid volume deficit (nephrogenic DI). Renal calculi can cause obstruction resulting in hematuria or oliguria. Also monitor for volume depletion when giving diuretics: ↓ BP, CVP, PAP; ↑ HR.
- Monitor UO and BUN/creatinine values to assess renal function.
- ↑ fluid intake (at least 3 L in nonrestricted patients) to ↓ risk of renal stone formation.

Miscellanea

CONSULT MD FOR
- S&S of urinary tract obstruction: oliguria, polyuria, hematuria, ↑ BUN/creatinine, flank pain, nausea, vomiting
- S&S of complications: DI, ARF, fluid volume excess or deficit
- S&S of digitalis toxicity in patients taking digoxin

RELATED TOPICS
- Diabetes insipidus
- Hypovolemia
- Renal failure, acute

ABBREVIATION
DI: Diabetes insipidus

REFERENCES
Horne MM: Fluid and electrolyte disturbances. In Swearingen PL, Keen JH (eds): *Manual of critical care nursing,* ed 3, St Louis, 1995, Mosby.

Horne MM, Heitz UE, Swearingen PL: *Pocket guide to fluid, electrolyte, and acid-base balance,* ed 3, St Louis, 1997, Mosby.

Kaplan M: Hypercalcemia of malignancy: a review of advances in pathophysiology, *Oncol Nurs Forum* 21(6): 1039-1046, 1993.

Author: **Mima M. Horne**

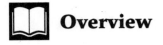 **Overview**

PATHOPHYSIOLOGY
Serum potassium level >5.0 mEq/L. Changes in serum K^+ levels reflect changes in ECF potassium, not necessarily changes in total body levels of potassium. Distribution of potassium between ECF and ICF affected by insulin levels, acid-base balance, and tissue catabolism. Potassium is excreted primarily in urine. Because K^+ affects the resting membrane potential of nerve and cardiac cells, abnormal serum K^+ levels adversely affect neuromuscular and cardiac function.

HISTORY/RISK FACTORS
Inappropriately High Intake
- Usually IV

↓ Excretion
- Renal disease (both ARF and CRF)
- Potassium-sparing diuretics, ACE inhibitors

Movement Out of Cells
- Metabolic acidosis
- Insulin deficiency, particularly in dialysis patients; common in DKA before treatment
- Tissue catabolism, eg, with fever, sepsis, trauma, surgery

CLINICAL PRESENTATION
Irritability, abdominal cramping, diarrhea, ascending weakness, paresthesias

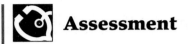 **Assessment**

PHYSICAL ASSESSMENT
Irregular pulse and abdominal distention; cardiac standstill may occur at levels >8.5 mEq/L.

VITAL SIGNS/HEMODYNAMICS
RR: NI
HR: NI or irregular
BP: NI; may be ↓ if dysrhythmias present
Temp: NI
CO: May be ↓ because of dysrhythmias
ECG: Tall, thin T waves; prolonged PR interval; ST depression; widened QRS complex; loss of P wave. Eventually, QRS complex widened further and cardiac arrest occurs.

LABORATORY STUDIES
Serum Potassium: >5.0 mEq/L
ABGs: May show metabolic acidosis

Collaborative Management

SUBACUTE
Cation Exchange Resins (eg, sodium polystyrene sulfonate [Kayexalate]): Given PO or *via* retention enema to exchange Na^+ for K^+ in the gut. Kayexalate usually combined with sorbitol to promote rapid transit through the gut, induce diarrhea, and thus promote GI potassium loss.

ACUTE
IV Calcium Gluconate: To counteract neuromuscular and cardiac effects of hyperkalemia. Serum K^+ levels will remain elevated.
IV Glucose and Insulin: To shift K^+ into the cells. ↓ serum K^+ temporarily.
Sodium Bicarbonate: To shift K^+ into the cells. ↓ serum K^+ temporarily.
Note: Effects of calcium, glucose and insulin, and sodium bicarbonate last only a few h. These medications must be followed with dialysis or cation exchange resins.
Dialysis: For rapid removal of K^+ from the body.

PATIENT-FAMILY TEACHING
- Importance of avoiding foods high in potassium, salt substitutes: eg, avocados, bananas, cantaloupes, carrots, cauliflower, dried beans/peas, dried fruit, mushrooms, nuts, oranges, peanuts, potatoes, pumpkins, spinach, tomatoes

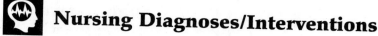 **Nursing Diagnoses/Interventions**

Decreased cardiac output (or risk for same) r/t electrical factors (ventricular dysrhythmias) secondary to severe hyperkalemia or too rapid correction of hyperkalemia with resulting hypokalemia

Desired outcomes: Within 6 h after treatment initiation, patient's cardiac output adequate: CO 4-7 L/min, HR ≤100 bpm, BP wnl for patient, and absence of heart failure or pulmonary edema. ECG shows NSR without ectopy or other electrical disturbances. Serum K^+ levels wnl: 3.5-5.0 mEq/L.

- Monitor I&O. Be alert to oliguria, which causes ↑ risk for hyperkalemia.
- Monitor for hyperkalemia: irritability, anxiety, abdominal cramping, diarrhea, ascending weakness, paresthesias, irregular pulse. Be alert to hypokalemia that may occur after treatment: muscle weakness and cramps, nausea, vomiting, ↓ bowel sounds, paresthesias, weak and irregular pulse. Assess for hidden sources of potassium: medications, banked blood, salt substitutes, GI bleeding, or conditions that cause ↑ catabolism.
- Monitor serum K^+ and other laboratory values that may affect K^+ levels (eg, BUN, creatinine, ABGs, glucose).
- Monitor ECG for signs of hypokalemia, which may result from therapy: ST-segment depression, flattened T waves, presence of U wave, ventricular dysrhythmias; or continuing hyperkalemia: tall, thin T waves; prolonged PR interval; ST depression; widened QRS complex; loss of P wave.
- Administer insulin and glucose in the order prescribed. When glucose is administered first, it stimulates endogenous insulin release and may potentiate the potassium-lowering effects of the exogenous insulin.
- Administer calcium gluconate cautiously in patients receiving digitalis because digitalis toxicity can occur. Do not add calcium gluconate to solutions containing sodium bicarbonate because precipitates may form.
- If administering cation exchange resins by enema, encourage patient to retain solution for at least 30-60 min to ensure therapeutic effects. Administer Kayexalate (without sorbitol) *via* Foley catheter inserted into rectum. Cleansing enemas are recommended before administration to enhance absorption and afterward to ↓ risk of bowel complications.

 Miscellanea

CONSULT MD FOR
- New-onset ECG changes associated with hypo/hyperkalemia
- Hemodynamically significant dysrhythmias
- UO <0.5 ml/kg/h × 2 h

RELATED TOPICS
- Hemodialysis
- Hypokalemia
- Renal failure, acute
- Renal failure, chronic

ABBREVIATIONS
ECF: Extracellular fluid
ICF: Intracellular fluid

REFERENCES
Horne MM: Fluid and electrolyte disturbances. In Swearingen PL, Keen JH (eds): *Manual of critical care nursing,* ed 3, St Louis, 1995, Mosby.
Horne MM, Heitz UE, Swearingen PL: *Pocket guide to fluid, electrolyte, and acid-base balance,* ed 3, St Louis, 1997, Mosby.
Rose BD: *Clinical physiology of acid-base and electrolyte disorders,* ed 4, New York, 1994, McGraw-Hill.

Author: **Mima M. Horne**

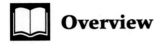 Overview

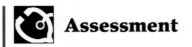 Assessment

Collaborative Management

Overview

PATHOPHYSIOLOGY
Serum magnesium levels >2.5 mEq/L; occurs almost exclusively in individuals with renal failure who have ↑ intake of magnesium-containing medications. It may also occur in acute adrenocortical insufficiency (Addison's disease) or in patients treated with parenteral magnesium. The primary symptoms of hypermagnesemia are the result of depressed peripheral and central neuromuscular transmission.

HISTORY/RISK FACTORS
- ↓ excretion of magnesium: renal failure, adrenocortical insufficiency
- ↑ intake of magnesium: excessive use of magnesium-containing antacids, enemas, and laxatives or excessive administration of magnesium sulfate

CLINICAL PRESENTATION
Symptoms usually do not occur until magnesium level >4 mEq/L. Nausea, vomiting, flushing, diaphoresis, sensation of heat, altered mental functioning, drowsiness, coma, and muscular weakness or paralysis. Paralysis of respiratory muscles may occur when level >10 mEq/L.

Assessment

PHYSICAL ASSESSMENT
Hypotension, soft tissue calcification, bradycardia, ↓ DTRs. Patellar (knee jerk) reflex lost once level >8 mEq/L.

VITAL SIGNS/HEMODYNAMICS
RR: ↑ because of muscle weakness
HR: ↓
BP: ↓
Temp: Nl
SVR: ↓ because of vasodilatation
ECG: Prolonged QT interval and AV block may occur in severe hypermagnesemia (levels >12 mEq/L).

LABORATORY STUDY
Serum Magnesium: >2.5 mEq/L

Collaborative Management

Identification/Removal of Cause
Diuretics and 0.45% NaCl Solution: To promote magnesium excretion in patients with adequate renal function.
IV Calcium Gluconate, 10 ml of 10% Solution: To antagonize neuromuscular effects of magnesium for potentially lethal hypermagnesemia.
Dialysis with Magnesium-Free Dialysate: For severely ↓ renal function.

PATIENT-FAMILY TEACHING
- Reassurance that altered mentation and muscle strength will improve with treatment
- Necessity for patients with CRF to review all OTC medications with physician before use
- List of common magnesium-containing medications (eg, Di-Gel, Gelusil, Maalox, Mylanta, Milk of Magnesia, Haley's M-O, Epsom salts)
- Necessity of avoiding combination vitamin-mineral supplements, since they usually contain magnesium

Nursing Diagnoses/Interventions

Altered protection r/t neurosensory alterations secondary to hypermagnesemia
Desired outcomes: Within 12 h of treatment initiation, patient verbalizes orientation to time, place, and person. Patient does not exhibit evidence of injury caused by complications of hypermagnesemia. Patient has no symptoms of soft tissue (metastatic) calcifications: oliguria, corneal haziness, conjunctivitis, irregular HR, papular eruptions.

- Monitor serum magnesium levels.
- Assess and document LOC, orientation, and neurologic status (eg, hand grasp) with each VS check. Assess patellar (knee jerk) reflex in patients with moderately ↑ magnesium level (>5 mEq/L). Absent reflex suggests level ≥7 mEq/L.
- Keep side rails up and bed in its lowest position with wheels locked.
- Assess for development of soft tissue calcification.
- Monitor for cardiopulmonary effects of hypermagnesemia: hypotension, flushing, bradycardia, respiratory depression.

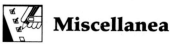 **Miscellanea**

CONSULT MD FOR
- ↓/absent patellar reflex
- Hypotension, bradycardia, respiratory depression
- S&S of soft tissue calcification

RELATED TOPICS
- Bradycardia
- Heart block: AV conduction disturbance
- Hemodialysis
- Renal failure, acute
- Renal failure, chronic

REFERENCES

Horne MM: Fluid and electrolyte disturbances. In Swearingen PL, Keen JH (eds): *Manual of critical care nursing,* ed 3, St Louis, 1995, Mosby.

Horne MM, Heitz UE, Swearingen PL: *Pocket guide to fluid, electrolyte, and acid-base balance,* ed 3, St Louis, 1997, Mosby.

Author: **Mima M. Horne**

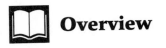 **Overview**

PATHOPHYSIOLOGY

Serum sodium level >145 mEq/L. Occurs with water loss or sodium gain. Because sodium is the major determinant of ECF osmolality, hypernatremia always causes hyperosmolality. This causes a shift of water out of the cells, leading to cellular dehydration and ↑ ECF volume. If plasma sodium ↓ too quickly via administration of water, there will be rapid and dramatic movement of water into the cells, which will affect brain cells and cause dangerous cerebral edema. Significant hypernatremia will not occur if individual can access water and has a nl thirst mechanism.

HISTORY/RISK FACTORS

- Sodium gain: IV hypertonic saline or sodium bicarbonate, ↑ oral intake, primary aldosteronism, saltwater near drowning, drugs such as sodium polystyrene sulfonate (Kayexalate)
- Water loss: diaphoresis, respiratory infection, DI, osmotic diuresis, osmotic diarrhea

CLINICAL PRESENTATION

Intense thirst, fatigue, restlessness, agitation, coma. Symptoms occur only in individuals without access to water or with altered thirst mechanism (eg, infants, elders, the comatose).

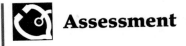 **Assessment**

PHYSICAL ASSESSMENT

Flushed skin, peripheral and pulmonary edema (sodium gain); ↓ skin turgor, postural hypotension (water loss)

VITAL SIGNS/HEMODYNAMICS

RR: ↑ with sodium gain
HR: ↑
BP: slight ↓ with water loss
Temp: ↑
Sodium Excess: ↑ CVP/PAP
Water Loss: ↓ CVP/PAP

LABORATORY STUDIES

Serum Sodium: >145 mEq/L
Serum Osmolality: ↑ caused by elevated serum sodium.
Urine Specific Gravity or Urine Osmolality: ↑ caused by kidneys' attempt to retain water; ↓ in DI and osmotic diuresis (eg, hyperglycemia).

Collaborative Management

Treatment of Underlying Cause: Eg, DI.
IV/Oral Water Replacement: For water loss. If sodium >160 mEq/L, IV D_5W or hypotonic saline given to replace pure water deficit. Correct gradually to avoid too great a shift of water into brain cells.
Diuretics, Oral/IV Water Replacement: For sodium gain.

PATIENT-FAMILY TEACHING

Reassurance that altered sensorium is temporary and will improve with treatment

Nursing Diagnoses/Interventions

Altered protection r/t neurosensory alterations secondary to hypernatremia or cerebral edema occurring with too rapid correction of hypernatremia

Desired outcomes: Within 48 h after treatment, patient verbalizes orientation to time, place, and person and does not exhibit evidence of injury caused by altered sensorium or seizures.

- Cerebral edema may occur if hypernatremia is corrected too rapidly. Monitor serial serum sodium levels to check for too rapid reduction of serum sodium.
- Assess for cerebral edema: lethargy, headache, nausea, vomiting, ↑ BP, widening pulse pressure, ↓ HR, altered sensorium, seizures.
- Assess and document LOC, orientation, and neurologic status with each VS check. Reorient as necessary.
- Keep side rails up and bed in lowest position with wheels locked.
- Use reality therapy, such as clocks, calendars, and familiar objects; keep these items at bedside within patient's visual field.
- If seizures anticipated, keep an airway at bedside.
- Provide comfort measures to ↓ thirst.

FOR ↓ ECF VOLUME

Fluid volume deficit r/t abnormal loss of body fluids or ↓ intake

Desired outcomes: Within 24 h of initiation of fluid therapy, patient normovolemic: UO ≥0.5 ml/kg/h, specific gravity 1.010-1.030, stable weight, no clinical evidence of hypovolemia, BP wnl for patient, CVP 2-6 mm Hg, PAP 20-30/8-15 mm Hg, CO 4-7 L/min, MAP 70-105 mm Hg, HR 60-100 bpm, and SVR 900-1200 dynes/sec cm^{-5}.

- Monitor I&O qh. Initially, intake should exceed output during therapy. Monitor urine specific gravity; expect ↓ with therapy.
- Monitor VS and hemodynamic pressures for signs of continued hypovolemia: ↓ BP, CVP, PAP, CO, MAP; and ↑ HR and SVR.
- Weigh patient qd. Acute weight changes usually indicate fluid changes. If individual is not being fed, a 1-kg ↓ in daily weight equals a 1-L fluid loss.
- Administer PO and IV fluids as prescribed. Ensure adequate intake, especially in elders because of ↑ risk of volume depletion in this population. Document response to fluid therapy.
- Monitor for fluid overload or too rapid fluid administration: crackles, SOB, tachypnea, tachycardia, ↑ CVP, ↑ PAP, JVD, edema.
- Monitor for hidden fluid losses: eg, measure and document abdominal girth or limb size, if indicated.

FOR ↑ ECF VOLUME

Fluid volume excess r/t excessive fluid or sodium intake or compromised regulatory mechanism

Desired outcomes: Within 24 h after treatment initiation, patient normovolemic: absence of edema, BP wnl for patient, HR 60-100 bpm, CVP 2-6 mm Hg, PAP 20-30/8-15 mm Hg, MAP 70-105 mm Hg, and CO 4-7 L/min.

- Monitor I&O qh. UO should be ≥0.5 ml/kg/h. If patient is receiving diuretic therapy, specific gravity should be <1.010-1.020.
- Observe for and document presence of edema: pretibial, sacral, periorbital; rate pitting on 0-4+ scale.
- Weigh patient qd. Daily weight is the single most important indicator of fluid status. A 2-kg acute weight gain usually indicates a 2-L fluid gain. Weigh patient at same time each day.
- Limit oral, enteral, and parenteral sodium intake as prescribed. Be aware that many antibiotics and some other parenteral medications contain significant amounts of sodium. Consult pharmacist as necessary.
- Provide oral hygiene at frequent intervals to keep oral mucous membrane moist and intact.
- Document response to diuretic therapy (eg, status of UO, CVP/PAP, adventitious breath sounds, edema). Many diuretics cause hypokalemia, as evidenced by muscle weakness, PVCs, ECG changes such as flattened T wave, presence of U waves. Potassium-sparing diuretics (eg, spironolactone, triamterene) may cause hyperkalemia: weakness, ECG changes (eg, peaked T wave, prolonged PR interval, widened QRS complex).
- Monitor overcorrection and dangerous volume depletion secondary to therapy: vertigo, weakness, syncope, thirst, confusion, poor skin turgor, flat neck veins, acute weight loss.

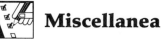

Miscellanea

CONSULT MD FOR

- Rapid ↓ in serum sodium levels >0.5 mEq/L/h or 12 mEq/L/day in severely hypernatremic patients
- S&S of cerebral edema: headache, altered mental status, nausea and vomiting, widened pulse pressure, seizures

RELATED TOPICS

- Diabetes insipidus
- Hyperosmolar hyperglycemic nonketotic syndrome
- Hypokalemia
- Pulmonary edema

ABBREVIATIONS

DI: Diabetes insipidus
ECF: Extracellular fluid

REFERENCES

Horne MM: Fluid and electrolyte disturbances. In Swearingen PL, Keen JH (eds): *Manual of critical care nursing,* ed 3, St Louis, 1995, Mosby.

Horne MM, Heitz UE, Swearingen PL: *Pocket guide to fluid, electrolyte, and acid-base balance,* ed 3, St Louis, 1997, Mosby.

Rose BD: *Clinical physiology of acid-base and electrolyte disorders,* ed 4, New York, 1994, McGraw-Hill.

Author: **Mima M. Horne**

Overview

PATHOPHYSIOLOGY

Life-threatening emergency resulting from insulin deficiency. Endogenous insulin insufficient to control blood glucose, but usually adequate to prevent lipolysis and formation of ketone bodies, thereby avoiding ketoacidosis. Severe hyperglycemia results in significant serum hyperosmolality and pronounced osmotic diuresis. Serious dehydration and electrolyte loss occur, especially Na^+ and K^+. PO_4^{3-} and Mg^{2+} deficiencies also common. Blood becomes more viscous, impeding flow, which ↑ risk of thromboemboli. ↑ cardiac workload and ↓ renal and cerebral blood flow may result in MI, renal failure, and stroke, contributing to high mortality rate. The severely ill may present with mixed syndrome of HHNS and DKA.

HISTORY/RISK FACTORS

- NIDDM (type II DM): Primary cause, most often in elders
- Acute exacerbation of chronic illness, particularly renal or CV
- Ingestion of high-caloric enteral or parenteral feedings
- Stressors, such as trauma or infection
- Use of diabetogenic drugs: eg, glucocorticoids, some diuretics, phenytoin, thyroid preparations

CLINICAL PRESENTATION

Polyuria, polydipsia, weight loss, weakness, orthostatic hypotension. Seizures, altered mental status common; 50% of patients comatose. Symptoms may be ignored by elders and their families, thus delaying diagnosis and treatment.

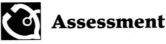 **Assessment**

PHYSICAL ASSESSMENT

Neuro: Lethargy, confusion, coma
Resp: Tachypnea, shallow respirations, absence of fruity breath odor
CV: Tachycardia, dysrhythmias, hypotension
Integ: Dry skin, mucous membranes; poor skin turgor

VITAL SIGNS/HEMODYNAMICS

RR: ↑
HR: ↑
BP: ↓
Temp: May be ↑, since infection potential cause.
CVP/PAPs: ↓ reflecting dehydration; may be 3-4 mm Hg < baseline.
Note: Patients usually >50 yrs and have pre-existing cardiac or pulmonary disorders; hemodynamic factors should be evaluated based on nl or optimal values for each individual.
ECG: Dysrhythmias associated with *hypokalemia* possible: depressed ST segments, flat or inverted T waves, ↑ ventricular dysrhythmias.

LABORATORY STUDIES

Serum Glucose: 800-2000 mg/dl
Serum Ketones: Nl or slightly ↑
Urine Glucose: Positive
Urine Acetone: Negative
Serum Osmolality: >350 mOsm/L
ABGs: HCO_3^- nl or slightly ↓ if lactic acidosis present; pH nl or mildly acidotic (<7.4)
Serum Electrolytes: K^+ nl or ↓ (<3.5 mEq/L); Na^+ ↑, nl, or ↓
Hct: ↑ because of hemoconcentration
BUN/Creatinine: ↑
WBCs: ↑ because of stress, dehydration, possible infection
Triglycerides: ↑

Collaborative Management

Replacement of Electrolytes and ECF Volume: 0.45% saline or isotonic saline used; potassium, phosphate, and magnesium supplements may be added. Half the estimated fluid deficit replaced during first 12 h and remainder over next 24 h. Dextrose added once blood glucose ≤200-300 mg/dl to prevent rebound hypoglycemia.
Rapid-Acting Insulin: Usually administered in low doses. IV route preferred. In most cases, continuous drips used and titrated based on serum glucose levels. Blood glucose should not drop >100 mg/dl/h because of risk of too rapid ↓ in serum osmolality.
Insertion of PA Flow-Directed Catheter: To assess fluid status, since many patients have underlying cardiopulmonary disease.
Treatment of Underlying Cause: Eg, infection treated with appropriate antibiotics.

PATIENT-FAMILY TEACHING

- Causes, prevention, and treatment of HHNS and the common early symptoms of worsening DM: polyuria, polydipsia, polyphagia, dry and flushed skin, irritability.
- Importance of testing blood glucose levels qd as prescribed, reporting blood glucose >250 mg/dl to physician.
- Importance of taking oral hypoglycemic agents as prescribed. Caution that exogenous insulin may be required during periods of physical and emotional stress and that blood glucose levels should be monitored closely during these times, as well as during illness or injury.
- Hospital and community resources (eg, diabetes educator, dietitian, social worker, local American Diabetes Association [ADA], and support groups).
- Address for ADA: American Diabetes Association, Inc., 1660 Duke St., Alexandria, VA 22314. Toll-free phone number: 800-232-3472.

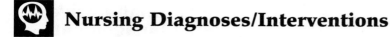 # Nursing Diagnoses/Interventions

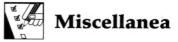 # Miscellanea

Fluid volume deficit r/t ↓ circulating volume secondary to hyperglycemia and induced osmotic diuresis

Desired outcomes: Within 12 h of initiating treatment, patient normovolemic: BP ≥90/60 mm Hg (or wnl for patient), MAP ≥70 mm Hg, HR 60-100 bpm, CVP 2-6 mm Hg, PAWP 6-12 mm Hg, balanced I&O, UO ≥0.5 ml/kg/h, firm skin turgor, pink and moist mucous membranes, NSR on ECG.

- Monitor VS q15min until condition stable for 1 h. Be alert to tachycardia, dysrhythmias, hypotension, ↓ CVP/PAWP.
- Monitor for S&S of dehydration: poor skin turgor, dry mucous membranes, sunken and soft eyeballs, tachycardia, orthostatic hypotension.
- Measure I&O accurately. ↓ UO may signal diminishing intravascular fluid volume or impending renal failure. Weigh patient qd.
- Administer IV fluids to rehydrate. Be alert to S&S of fluid overload: JVD, dyspnea, crackles, CVP >6 mm Hg.
- Monitor laboratory tests for abnormalities. Be alert for hypokalemia, a common complication of treatment.
- Use continuous cardiac monitor. Observe for ECG changes typical of hypokalemia.
- Monitor neurologic function for S&S of cerebral edema, which may develop with overly aggressive treatment.
- Observe for S&S of electrolyte imbalance associated with HHNS and its treatment.
    Hypokalemia: ECG changes, muscle weakness, hypotension, drowsiness, hypoactive bowel sounds
    Hypophosphatemia: Muscle weakness, respiratory failure, ↓ cardiac function
    Hypomagnesemia: Nausea, vomiting, lethargy, weakness, personality changes, tetany, tremor or muscle fasciculations, seizures, confusion progressing to coma

Risk for injury r/t altered cerebral function secondary to hyperosmolality, dehydration, cerebral edema associated with HHNS, or hypoglycemia

Desired outcome: Patient verbalizes orientation × 3; nl breath sounds auscultated over airways; and oral cavity and musculoskeletal system remain intact and free of injury.

- Monitor orientation, LOC, and respiratory status, especially airway patency, at frequent intervals. Keep oral airway, manual resuscitator and mask, and supplemental O₂ at bedside.
- Reduce likelihood of injury caused by falls; maintain bed in lowest position with side rails up; use soft restraints as necessary.
- Place gastric tube to intermittent suction in comatose patients to ↓ likelihood of aspiration.
- Elevate HOB to 45 degrees to minimize risk of aspiration.
- Initiate seizure precautions and keep an oral airway at bedside.
- Initially, monitor blood glucose qh. Be alert to blood glucose that drops faster than 100 mg/dl/h or <250-300 mg/dl.

CONSULT MD FOR

- HR >120 bpm or BP <90/60 mm Hg or ↓ ≥20 mm Hg from baseline, MAP ↓ ≥10 mm Hg from baseline, CVP <2 mm Hg, and PAWP <6 mm Hg.
- UO <0.5 ml/kg/h for 2 consecutive h.
- Blood glucose <250-300 mg/dl or ↓ in blood glucose >100 mg/dl/h
- S&S of fluid overload: ↑ CVP, crackles, JVD, dyspnea
- Serum values and S&S of electrolyte abnormalities, especially K^+, PO_4^{3-}, and Mg^{2+}
- Evidence of infection
- ↓/absent peripheral pulses, S&S of DVT
- Altered LOC or worsening neurologic function

RELATED TOPICS

- Diabetic ketoacidosis
- Hyperkalemia
- Hypokalemia
- Hypomagnesemia
- Hypophosphatemia
- Metabolic acidosis, acute
- Shock, hypovolemic

ABBREVIATION
ECF: Extracellular fluid

REFERENCES

Horne MM: Endocrinologic dysfunctions. In Swearingen PL, Keen JH (eds): *Manual of critical care nursing*, ed 3, St Louis, 1995, Mosby.

Jones TL: From diabetic ketoacidosis to hyperglycemic hyperosmolar nonketotic syndrome, *Crit Care Nurs Clin North Am* 6(4): 703-721, 1994.

Lorber D: Nonketotic hypertonicity in diabetes mellitus, *Med Clin North Am* 79(1): 39-52, 1995.

Sauve DO, Kessler CA: Hyperglycemic emergencies, *AACN Clin Issues in Crit Care Nurs* 3(2): 350-360, 1992.

Reising DL: Acute hyperglycemia: Putting a lid on the crisis, *Nursing* 25(2): 33-40, 1995.

Author: **Mima M. Horne**

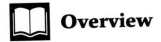 **Overview**

PATHOPHYSIOLOGY

Serum phosphorus levels >4.5 mg/dl. As serum levels ↑, serum Ca^{2+} levels often ↓, which may cause hypocalcemia to develop. Hypocalcemia is most likely to occur in sudden, severe hyperphosphatemia (eg, after IV administration of phosphates) or when patient is prone to hypocalcemia (eg, with CRF). The primary complication is metastatic calcification (ie, precipitation of calcium phosphate in the soft tissue, joints, arteries).

HISTORY/RISK FACTORS

- ARF, CRF
- ↑ intake: phosphorus supplements, vitamin D excess with ↑ GI absorption, phosphorus-containing laxatives or enemas, massive transfusion
- Extracellular shift: respiratory acidosis, DKA
- Cellular destruction: chemotherapy, ↑ tissue catabolism, rhabdomyolysis
- ↓ urinary losses: hypoparathyroidism, volume depletion

CLINICAL PRESENTATION

Usually, few symptoms experienced. Anorexia, nausea, vomiting, muscle weakness, hyperreflexia, tetany, tachycardia may occur. Possible S&S of hypocalcemia, soft tissue calcification.

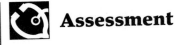 **Assessment**

PHYSICAL ASSESSMENT

Metastatic Calcification: Oliguria, corneal haziness, conjunctivitis, irregular HR, papular eruptions

Hypocalcemia

Positive Trousseau's Sign: Ischemia-induced carpopedal spasm

Positive Chvostek's Sign: Unilateral contraction of facial and eyelid muscles

VITAL SIGNS/HEMODYNAMICS

RR: Nl

HR: Nl; may be irregular if myocardial soft tissue calcification present

BP: Nl; may be ↓ if dysrhythmias present

Temp: Nl

CO: ↓ if dysrhythmias present

ECG: Dysrhythmias possible. Prolonged QT interval caused by elongation of ST segment.

LABORATORY STUDIES

Serum Phosphate Level: >4.5 mg/dl (2.6 mEq/L)

PTH Level: ↓ in hypoparathyroidism

IMAGING

X-ray: May show skeletal changes of osteodystrophy.

Collaborative Management

Identification/Elimination of Cause Aluminum, Magnesium, or Calcium Gels or Antacids: To bind phosphorus in the gut, thus ↑ GI elimination of phosphorus.

Dialytic Therapy: May be necessary for acute, severe hyperphosphatemia accompanied by symptoms of hypocalcemia.

PATIENT-FAMILY TEACHING

- Purpose of phosphate binders and need to take them as prescribed with or after meals to maximize effectiveness
- Possibility of constipation because of binder use and preventive measures for same, eg, bulk-building supplements or stool softener; importance of avoiding phosphate-containing laxatives and enemas
- Necessity to avoid or limit foods high in phosphorus: eg, dried beans, eggs, fish, meats, milk, poultry, whole grains
- Importance of avoiding phosphorus-containing OTC medications: certain laxatives, enemas, mixed vitamin-mineral supplements

Nursing Diagnoses/Interventions

Risk for injury r/t internal factors associated with precipitation of calcium phosphate in the soft tissue (eg, cornea, lungs, kidney, gastric mucosa, heart, blood vessels) and periarticular region of the large joints (eg, hips, shoulders, and elbows) or development of hypocalcemic tetany
Desired outcome: Patient does not exhibit S&S of physical injury caused by precipitation of calcium phosphate in the soft tissue or joints or hypocalcemic tetany.

- Monitor serum phosphorus and calcium levels. Calculate calcium-phosphorus product (calcium × phosphorus). Values ≥70 mg/dl are associated with precipitation of calcium phosphate in the soft tissues. Be aware that phosphorus values may be kept slightly higher (4-6 mg/dl) to ensure adequate levels of 2,3-DPG in CRF, thereby minimizing effects of chronic anemia on O_2 delivery to the tissues.
- Avoid vitamin D products and calcium supplements until serum phosphorus level approaches nl.
- Assess for S&S of metastatic calcification: oliguria, corneal haziness, conjunctivitis, irregular HR, papular eruptions.
- Monitor for evidence of ↑ hypocalcemia: numbness and tingling of fingers and circumoral region, hyperactive reflexes, muscle cramps. In addition, check for positive Trousseau's or Chvostek's signs, since these S&S signal latent tetany. If present, consult physician stat.
- Because hyperphosphatemia can impair renal function, monitor renal function carefully: UO, BUN/creatinine values.

Miscellanea

CONSULT MD FOR

- Calcium-phosphorus product ≥70 mg/dl
- S&S of metastatic calcification
- S&S of severe hypocalcemia, including positive Trousseau's, Chvostek's signs.
- ↓ UO; ↑ BUN/creatinine.

RELATED TOPICS

- Hemodialysis
- Hypocalcemia
- Renal failure, acute
- Renal failure, chronic

REFERENCES

Horne MM: Fluid and electrolyte disturbances. In Swearingen PL, Keen JH (eds): *Manual of critical care nursing*, ed 3, St Louis, 1995, Mosby.
Horne MM, Heitz UE, Swearingen PL: *Pocket guide to fluid, electrolyte, and acid-base balance*, ed 3, St Louis, 1997, Mosby.

Author: **Mima M. Horne**

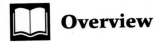 **Overview**

PATHOPHYSIOLOGY
Seen in about 1% of the hypertensive population. There is threat of immediate vascular necrosis, which can occur if DBP >120 mm Hg or MAP ≥150 mm Hg. The extreme pressure can cause arteriolar damage (ie, fibrinoid necrosis of the intima and media of vessel wall). Hypertensive encephalopathy possible as ↑ cerebral blood flow and pressure cause cerebral edema. Although any organ is vulnerable, damage to eyes and kidneys most likely, leading to blindness and renal failure.
Pheochromocytoma: Chromaffin-cell tumor of the adrenal medulla causing a surge of catecholamines (epinephrine and norepinephrine) resulting in episodic ↑ of BP, ↑ metabolism, and hyperglycemia. Although found in only 0.5% of all new cases of hypertension, it is seen in much greater incidence with hypertensive crisis.

COMPLICATIONS
Nephrosclerosis, aortic dissection, stroke, CAD, heart failure, PVD

HISTORY/RISK FACTORS
- Psychologic stress, diet high in sodium, cigarette smoking
- Genetic factors
- Renal disease: eg, acute glomerulonephritis, chronic pyelonephritis
- Endocrine disorders: eg, Cushing's syndrome, pheochromocytoma, primary aldosteronism
- Drug-induced disorders: eg, from cyclosporine, oral contraceptives, steroids

CLINICAL PRESENTATION
General: Although most patients are symptom free, vague discomfort, fatigue, dizziness, and headache can occur.
Pheochromocytoma: Palpitations, headache, diaphoresis, pallor, warmth or flushing, tremor, excitation, feelings of impending doom, tachypnea, abdominal pain, nausea, and vomiting. Postural hypotension and paradoxical response to antihypertensive medications may occur.

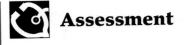 **Assessment**

PHYSICAL ASSESSMENT
Neuro: Irritability, cognitive alterations, confusion, somnolence, stupor, visual loss, focal deficits, coma, positive Babinski's reflex, hemiparesis, hemiplegia, ataxia
Resp: Dyspnea, orthopnea, and crackles
CV: LV heave at mitral valve, S_4 gallop, pulsus alternans

VITAL SIGNS/HEMODYNAMICS
RR: ↑
HR: ↑
BP: ↑
Temp: Nl
SVR: Greatly ↑
CO: ↑ unless heart failure ensues; with heart failure, ↓
ECG: LV hypertrophy demonstrated by ↑ voltage in V_{5-6}. Strain pattern of ST-segment depression and T-wave inversion reflects repolarization abnormalities caused by endocardial fibrosis.

LABORATORY STUDIES
Urinalysis/Urine Culture: Specific gravity may be low (<1.010) and proteinuria present. Glomerulonephritis suspected if urine contains granular or red cell casts or if patient has hematuria. Pyelonephritis suspected with bacterial growth in urine.
Chemistries: If renal parenchymal disease present, may have serum creatinine >1.3 mg/dl and BUN >20 mg/dl.

IMAGING
Echocardiogram: Will show LV hypertrophy with or without dilatation.
Chest X-ray: If LV dilatation present, cardiac silhouette will be enlarged. If failure present, pulmonary congestion and pleural effusions will appear. If widening of aorta seen, dissection suspected.
Radiographic Studies to Detect Pheochromocytoma: Angiography, IVP, CT scan may identify the tumor.

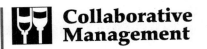 **Collaborative Management**

PHARMACOTHERAPY
Nifedipine: Given SL by piercing capsule and extruding contents; provides rapid onset of antihypertensive effects.
Nitroprusside: Drug of choice because of its almost immediate vasodilatation effects. Usual initial dose is 10-25 μg/min, with ↑ of 5-10 μg q5min. Direct arterial pressure monitoring essential for titration, with constant vigilance to prevent hypotension. Serum thiocyanate levels drawn after 48 h and regularly thereafter. Levels <10 mg/dl considered safe.
Labetalol Hcl: Fast-acting α and β blocker. Dose of 20-80 mg given by slow IV push. Monitor for bronchospasm, heart block, orthostatic hypotension.
NTG: Coronary and peripheral vasodilator. Administered starting at 5 μg/min. Onset of action rapid, so BP must be monitored closely.
Enalapril: ACE inhibitor. Usual dose is 0.625-1.25 mg IV bolus. Peak effect from first dose observed at 4 h, but for subsequent doses, peak effect occurs 1 h after administration. Used with caution in renal failure or bilateral renal artery stenosis.
Phentolamine: α-Adrenergic blocking agent; most effective when used for secondary hypertension caused by pheochromocytoma. Use with caution in CAD.
Oral Antihypertensives: Added once patient able to take oral medications. Medications used include diuretics, β blockers, ACE inhibitors, calcium blockers, adrenergic inhibitors.

LIFE-STYLE ALTERATIONS
Weight reduction if indicated, alcohol consumption <1 oz ETOH/day, daily intake of sodium modified to 2 or 3 g, smoking cessation, and regular aerobic program.

SURGERY
Forms of secondary hypertension respond well to surgical correction of primary problem. Coarctation of the aorta repaired. Renal artery stenosis corrected by grafting or renal artery angioplasty. Pheochromocytoma excised.

PATIENT-FAMILY TEACHING
- Life-style modification: weight reduction, moderation of alcohol intake, regular physical exercise, ↓ sodium intake, smoking cessation
- Relaxation, stress-reduction techniques to use in conjunction with medications: guided imagery, meditation, progressive muscle relaxation, and music therapy

Nursing Diagnoses/Interventions

Altered cardiopulmonary, cerebral, and renal tissue perfusion r/t interruption of arterial flow secondary to vasoconstriction; or interruption of venous flow secondary to vasodilatation or tissue edema that occurs with loss of autoregulation

Desired outcome: Tissue perfusion established within 24 h: systemic arterial BP 110-160/70-110 mm Hg (or wnl for patient), MAP 70-105 mm Hg, equal and normoreactive pupils, strength and tone of extremities bilaterally equal and nl for patient, orientation × 3, UO ≥0.5 ml/kg/h.

- Monitor BP and MAP q1-5min during titration of medications; as condition stabilizes, q15min-1h. When oral medications begin to affect BP, wean nitroprusside and other potent vasodilators gradually to prevent hypotensive episodes. Continuous monitoring by arterial cannulation or automatic BP apparatus recommended.

    Correlate cuff pressure with direct arterial pressure.

    Determine ideal range for BP control and maximal nitroprusside dose with physician.

    Usual guidelines: SBP <140-160 mm Hg, MAP <110 mm Hg, or DBP <90 mm Hg.

    If hypotension develops, ↓ or stop nitroprusside infusion until pressure ↑.

- Assess for neurologic deficit qh. Be alert to sensorimotor deficit if MAP >140 mm Hg. As condition stabilizes, perform neurostatus checks at least q4h.
- Assess for ↓ renal perfusion by monitoring I&O and weighing patient qd. Also be alert to azotemia (↑ BUN), ↓ creatinine clearance, and ↑ serum creatinine.

Pain r/t headache secondary to cerebral edema occurring with high perfusion pressures

Desired outcomes: Within 6 h after treatment initiation, subjective evaluation of pain improves, as documented by pain scale. Nonverbal indicators, such as grimacing, are ↓/absent.

- Monitor for headache pain, rating discomfort from 0 (no pain) to 10 (severe).
- Provide pain medications, eg, use acetaminophen with codeine for moderate pain and morphine for severe pain. Assess effectiveness of pain medication, using pain scale.
- Maintain quiet, low-lit environment free of extensive distraction and stimulation. Limit visitations as indicated.

Sensory/Perceptual alterations r/t ↓ visual acuity secondary to retinal damage occurring with high perfusion pressures; r/t pain secondary to cerebral edema

Desired outcome: Within 24-48 h of this diagnosis, patient reads print, recognizes objects or people, and demonstrates coordination of movement.

- Assess for ↓ visual acuity by monitoring ability to read and recognize objects or people; or use hand-held Snellen chart. Evaluate coordination of movement to determine depth perception.
- If patient has ↓ visual acuity, assist with feeding and other ADL and keep personal effects within patient's visual field.
- Reassure that visual problems usually resolve when BP is lowered sufficiently.

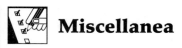

Miscellanea

CONSULT MD FOR
- MAP >140 mm Hg
- UO <0.5 ml/kg/h × 2 h
- Weight gain ≥1 kg/day
- New onset focal deficit or altered mental status

RELATED TOPICS
- Aortic aneurysm/dissection
- Heart failure, left ventricular
- Renal failure, acute
- Stroke: hemorrhagic and ischemic

REFERENCES
Baas LS, Steuble BT: Cardiovascular dysfunctions. In Swearingen PL, Keen JH (eds): *Manual of critical care nursing,* ed 3, St Louis, 1995, Mosby.

Foley JJ: Pharmacologic management of hypertensive crisis in the emergency department, *J Emerg Nurs* 20(2): 134-135, 1994.

Lip GY, Beevers M, Beevers DG: Complications and survival of 315 patients with malignant-phase hypertension, *J Hypertens* 13(8): 915-924, 1995.

Rorsche R: Hypertension: diagnosis, acute antihypertension therapy, and long-term management, *AACN Clin Issues* 6(4): 515-525, 1995.

Varon J, Fromm RE: Hypertensive crises: the need for urgent management, *Postgrad Med* 99(1): 189-200, 1996.

Author: **Linda S. Baas**

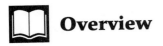 **Overview**

PATHOPHYSIOLOGY
Caused by excessive circulating thyroid hormone, which exaggerates nl body functions and produces a hypermetabolic state. *Graves' disease* (diffuse toxic goiter) accounts for ≈85% of reported cases; characterized by spontaneous exacerbations and remissions that appear to be unaffected by therapy. *Thyrotoxic crisis* or *thyroid storm* results from sudden surge of large amounts of thyroid hormone into the bloodstream, causing even greater ↑ in body metabolism characterized by marked CNS and CV stimulation. This results in profound tachycardia, hypertension, and ↑ SVR. Excessive cardiac workload may lead to LV heart failure.

HISTORY/RISK FACTORS
Graves' Disease
- Family hx
- Autoimmune disorder

Thyrotoxic Crisis
- Infection
- Trauma
- Emotional stress
- Thyroid surgery

CLINICAL PRESENTATION
Palpitations, menstrual irregularities, weight loss, fatigue, heat intolerance, ↑ perspiration, frequent defecation, anxiety, restlessness, tremor, insomnia

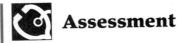 **Assessment**

PHYSICAL ASSESSMENT
Hyperthyroidism: Tachycardia, widened pulse pressure, hyperpyrexia, thyroid gland enlargement, muscle weakness, hyperreflexia, fine tremor, fine hair, thin skin, hypercholesterolemia, impaired glucose tolerance, stare and/or lid drag

Thyrotoxic Crisis (thyroid storm): Acute exacerbation of some or all the above signs: marked tachycardia, hyperpyrexia, CNS irritability, coma; possible S&S of hyperdynamic LV heart failure: crackles, summation gallop, ↓ peripheral pulses, hypotension

VITAL SIGNS/HEMODYNAMICS
RR: ↑
HR: ↑
BP: ↑; ↓ later if LV heart failure present as a result of thyrotoxic crisis
Temp: ↑
CVP/PAP: ↑ if LV failure present; ↓ if dehydration present
SVR: ↑ as a result of catecholamine excess
CO/CI: ↑ initially; later ↓ if thyrotoxic crisis with LV failure occurs
ECG: Tachydysrhythmias, ventricular irritability; ischemic/injury patterns in susceptible individuals (eg, with underling CAD, profound anemia)

LABORATORY STUDIES
TSH: ↓
Free Thyroxine Index and T$_3$: ↑
Thyrotropin-Releasing Hormone Stimulation Test: Failure of expected ↑ in TSH.
Radioiodine (^{123}I) Uptake and Thyroid Scan: Clarifies size of gland and detects presence of uptake *via* "hot" nodules.

Collaborative Management

Pharmacotherapy
Antithyroid agents: PTU and methimazole (Tapazole) the first line of treatment.
Iodides: Reserved for failure to respond to antithyroid drugs and relapse or other severe or unusual situation. Radioactive iodine (^{131}I) commonly used and usually results in hypothyroidism, which is controlled with replacement therapy.
β-Blocking agent (eg, propranolol [Inderal]): To relieve tachycardia, anxiety, heat intolerance, tremor.
Mild tranquilizers: To minimize anxiety and promote rest.
Diet: If significant weight loss has occurred, a diet high in calories, protein, carbohydrates, and vitamins recommended.
Subtotal Thyroidectomy: Surgical removal of part of the gland used for patients with extremely enlarged glands or multinodular goiter. Most frequent postop complication is hemorrhage at operative site. The following complications are rare but can be extremely serious: hypoparathyroidism, laryngeal nerve injury, tetany (owing to damage to parathyroid glands).

PATIENT/FAMILY TEACHING
- Rationale/importance for a diet high in calories, protein, carbohydrates, vitamins
- Changes that can occur as a result of therapy: weight gain, normalized bowel function, ↑ skeletal muscle strength, return to nl activity levels
- Indicators that necessitate medical attention: fever, rash, sore throat (side effects of thioamides), symptoms of hypothyroidism or worsening hyperthyroidism
- Importance of avoiding physical and emotional stress early in recuperative stage and maximizing coping mechanisms for dealing with stress

Nursing Diagnoses/Interventions

Altered protection r/t potential for thyrotoxic crisis (thyroid storm) secondary to emotional stress, trauma, infection, or surgical manipulation of the gland
Desired outcomes: Patient free of symptoms of thyroid storm: normothermia, BP within 10 mm Hg baseline, HR ≤100 bpm, and orientation × 3. If thyroid storm occurs, it is noted promptly and immediate treatment is initiated.
- For patients in whom thyroid storm may occur, monitor VS qh for hypertension, ↑ HR, and fever >38.3° C (10° F), since these are often the first signs of thyroid storm.
- Ensure good hand washing and sterile technique for dressing changes and invasive procedures. Advise visitors who have contracted or been exposed to a communicable disease to wear a surgical mask or defer the visit.

IN THE PRESENCE OF THYROID STORM
- Monitor for effects of thyroid storm: summation gallop, crackles, and, ultimately, heart failure (↓ amplitude of peripheral pulses, hypotension).
- Administer IV fluids as indicated to provide adequate hydration and prevent vascular collapse. Fluid volume deficit may occur as a result of ↑ fluid excretion by the kidneys or excessive diaphoresis. Monitor I&O qh to prevent fluid overload or inadequate fluid replacement.
- Administer PTU to prevent further synthesis and release of thyroid hormones.
- Administer propranolol to block SNS effects.
- Administer sodium iodide as prescribed, 1 h *after* administering PTU. If given before PTU, sodium iodide can exacerbate symptoms in susceptible persons.
- Administer small doses of insulin to control hyperglycemia, which can occur as a result of hypermetabolic state.
- O_2 demands ↑ because of hypermetabolism; administer supplemental O_2. Monitor Svo_2 as available.

Hyperthermia r/t ↑ metabolic rate associated with thyrotoxic crisis
Desired outcomes: Patient's temp remains within acceptable limits (36°-38.9° C [97°-102° F]) or returns to acceptable limits within 4-6 h of this diagnosis. An open airway is secured in the event of hyperthermic seizures.
- Monitor rectal or core temp q1-2h.
- Administer acetaminophen to ↓ temp. *Caution:* Aspirin is contraindicated because it releases thyroxine from protein-binding sites and ↑ free thyroxine levels.
- Provide cool sponge baths, or apply ice packs to axillae and groin to ↓ fever.
- If high temp continues, use a hypothermia blanket. Be sure to protect skin in contact with blanket and inspect skin q2h for tissue damage caused by local vasoconstriction. Massage skin q2h to promote circulation and minimize tissue damage.
- Check temp at frequent intervals to ensure that sudden ↓ (along with shivering) does not occur, which could ↑ metabolic demand.
- Have oral airway and suction equipment readily available in the event of seizure activity.

Anxiety r/t SNS stimulation
Desired outcome: Within 24 h of admission, patient is free of harmful anxiety: HR ≤100 bpm, RR 12-20 breaths/min with eupnea, and ↓/absent irritability and restlessness.
- Reassure patient and explain all procedures before performing them.
- Assess for signs of anxiety; administer short-acting sedatives (eg, alprazolam [Xanax] or lorazepam [Ativan]).
- Provide cool, calm, stress-free environment away from loud noises or excessive activity.
- Limit number of visitors and amount of time they spend with patient. Advise significant others to avoid arguments and discussion of stressful topics.
- Give propranolol as indicated to ↓ symptoms of anxiety, tachycardia, heat intolerance.
- Reassure that anxiety symptoms are r/t disease process and treatment will ↓ severity.
- Inform significant others that patient's behavior is physiologic and should not be taken personally.

Impaired corneal tissue integrity r/t dryness that can occur with exophthalmos in persons with Graves' disease
Desired outcome: Within 24 h of admission, patient's corneas are moist and intact.
- Teach patient to wear dark glasses to protect corneas.
- Administer eyedrops as indicated to supplement lubrication and ↓ SNS stimulation, which can cause lid retraction.
- If appropriate, apply eye shields or tape eyes shut at hs.
- Administer thioamides to maintain nl metabolic state and halt progression of exophthalmos.

 # Miscellanea

CONSULT MD FOR
- S&S of thyroid storm: temp >101° F, BP changed ≥10 mm Hg from baseline, ↑ HR, summation gallop, crackles
- Hemodynamically significant tachydysrhythmias: eg, HR >150 bpm, runs of VT
- Complications: eg, fluid volume deficit, severe anxiety, hyperglycemia

RELATED TOPICS
- Anxiety
- Heart failure, left ventricular
- Hypothyroidism
- Hypovolemia

ABBREVIATIONS
PTU: Propylthiouracil
SNS: Sympathetic nervous system
TSH: Thyroid-stimulating hormone
T_3: Triiodothyronine

REFERENCES
Dillman WH: The thyroid. In Bennett JC, Plum F: *Cecil textbook of medicine,* ed 20, Philadelphia, 1996, Saunders.
Gill GN: Principles of endocrinology. In Bennett JC, Plum F: *Cecil textbook of medicine,* ed 20, Philadelphia, 1996, Saunders.
Hall R: Hyperthyroidism and Graves' disease. In Besser GM, Thorner MO (eds): *Clinical endocrinology,* ed 4, London, 1994, Mosby-Wolfe.
Loriaux TC, Drass JA: Endocrine and diabetic disorders. In Kinney M, Packa D, Dunbar S: *AACN's clinical reference for critical care nursing,* ed 3, St Louis, 1993, Mosby.

Author: **Marianne Saunorus Baird**

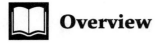 **Overview**

PATHOPHYSIOLOGY
Expansion of ECF volume. Can lead to heart failure and pulmonary edema, especially in patients with cardiovascular dysfunction.

HISTORY/RISK FACTORS
- Retention of sodium and water: heart failure, hepatic failure, nephrotic syndrome, glucocorticosteroid therapy
- Abnormal renal function: acute or CRF with oliguria or anuria
- Excessive administration of IV fluids
- Interstitial-to-plasma fluid shift: fluid remobilization after burns, major trauma or surgery, excessive administration of hypertonic or colloid oncotic solutions

CLINICAL PRESENTATION
SOB, orthopnea, weight gain, edema

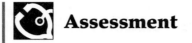 **Assessment**

PHYSICAL ASSESSMENT
Resp: Crackles, rhonchi, wheezes
CV: Bounding pulses, tachycardia, S_3/S_4 gallop
Assoc Findings: Edema, weight gain, ascites, JVD, moist skin

VITAL SIGNS/HEMODYNAMICS
RR: ↑
HR: ↑
BP: ↑; ↓ with heart failure
Temp: Nl
CVP/PAWP: ↑
MAP: ↑; ↓ with heart failure

LABORATORY STUDIES
Hct Levels: ↓ results from hemodilution.
BUN: ↑ with renal failure.
ABGs: May reveal hypoxemia and respiratory alkalosis in the presence of pulmonary edema. Respiratory acidosis may be present in severe pulmonary edema.
Serum Sodium and Osmolality: ↓ if hypervolemia caused by excessive retention of water (eg, in CRF).
Urinary Sodium: ↑ if kidneys attempt to excrete excess sodium. Will not be ↑ in conditions with secondary hyperaldosteronism (eg, heart failure, cirrhosis, nephrotic syndrome).
Urine Specific Gravity: ↓ if kidneys attempt to excrete excess volume. May be fixed at ≈ 1.010 in ARF.

IMAGING
Chest X-ray May reveal pulmonary vascular congestion.

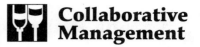 **Collaborative Management**

Restriction of Sodium and Water: Oral, enteral, or parenteral
Diuretics: IV or PO; loop diuretics (eg, furosemide) for severe hypervolemia or renal failure
Dialysis or CAVH: In renal failure or life-threatening fluid overload

PATIENT-FAMILY TEACHING
- Need for adherence to low-sodium diet, as indicated
- Importance of fluid restriction and how to measure fluid volume

Nursing Diagnoses/Interventions

 # Miscellanea

Fluid volume excess r/t excessive fluid or sodium intake or compromised regulatory mechanism

Desired outcomes: Within 24 h after treatment initiation, patient normovolemic: absence of edema, BP wnl for patient, HR 60-100 bpm, CVP 2-6 mm Hg, PAP 20-30/8-15 mm Hg, MAP 70-105 mm Hg, and CO 4-7 L/min.

- Monitor I&O qh. UO should be ≥0.5 ml/kg/h. If patient is receiving diuretic therapy, specific gravity should be <1.010-1.020.
- Observe for and document presence of edema: pretibial, sacral, periorbital; rate pitting on 0-4+ scale.
- Weigh patient qd. Daily weight is the single most important indicator of fluid status. A 2-kg acute weight gain usually indicates a 2-L fluid gain. Weigh patient at same time each day.
- Limit oral, enteral, and parenteral sodium intake as prescribed. Be aware that many antibiotics and some other parenteral medications contain significant amounts of sodium. Consult pharmacist as necessary.
- Limit fluids as prescribed. Offer a portion of allotted fluids as ice chips to minimize thirst.
- Provide oral hygiene at frequent intervals to keep oral mucous membrane moist and intact.
- Document response to diuretic therapy (eg, status of UO, CVP/PAP, adventitious breath sounds, edema).
- Many diuretics cause hypokalemia. Monitor accordingly for muscle weakness, PVCs, ECG changes (eg, flattened T wave, presence of U waves). Potassium-sparing diuretics (eg, spironolactone, triamterene) may cause hyperkalemia as evidenced by weakness, ECG changes (eg, peaked T wave, prolonged PR interval, widened QRS complex).
- Monitor for overcorrection and dangerous volume depletion secondary to therapy: vertigo, weakness, syncope, thirst, confusion, poor skin turgor, flat neck veins, acute weight loss.

Impaired gas exchange (or risk for same) r/t alveolar-capillary membrane changes secondary to pulmonary vascular congestion occurring with ECF expansion

Desired outcomes: Within 12 h of treatment initiation, patient has adequate gas exchange: RR ≤20 breaths/min with eupnea, HR ≤100 bpm, PaO_2 ≥80 mm Hg, pH 7.35-7.45, $PaCO_2$ 35-45 mm Hg, and SpO_2 ≥92%. Patient does not exhibit crackles, gallops, or other clinical indicators of pulmonary edema. PAWP ≤12 mm Hg.

- Monitor for indicators of pulmonary edema: air hunger, anxiety, cough with production of frothy sputum, crackles, rhonchi, tachypnea, tachycardia, S_3 gallop, and ↑ PAP and PAWP. Administer diuretics such as furosemide or other medications (eg, morphine, NTG) that reduce venous return to the heart.
- Monitor ABGs and SpO_2 for evidence of hypoxemia. Administer O_2 as prescribed to maintain SpO_2 at ≥92%. ↑ O_2 requirements may indicate ↑ pulmonary vascular congestion.
- Keep in semi-Fowler's or position of comfort. Avoid restrictive clothing.

Impaired skin and tissue integrity (or risk for same) r/t edema secondary to fluid volume excess

Desired outcome: Patient's skin and tissue remain intact.

- Assess color, temp, capillary refill, and peripheral pulses of all extremities q8h. Use Doppler device if necessary.
- Turn and reposition at least q2h.
- Check tissue areas at risk with each position change.
- Use pressure-relief mattress.
- Support arms and hands on pillows and elevate legs to ↓ dependent edema.
- Treat early pressure ulcers with occlusive dressings per unit protocol. Consult physician if areas of tissue breakdown are present in patients with ↑ risk for infection (eg, DM, renal failure, immunosuppressed).
- Consult skin/wound care nurse specialist, as available, for advanced tissue breakdown or any alteration in tissue integrity in high-risk patients.

CONSULT MD FOR
- UO <0.5 ml/kg/h × 2 h or failure to respond to parenteral diuretics after 2 h
- ↓/absent peripheral pulses
- S&S of pulmonary edema: frothy sputum, crackles, dyspnea, tachypnea, ↑ PAWP, SpO_2 ≤92%

RELATED TOPICS
- Continuous arteriovenous hemofiltration/Continuous venovenous hemofiltration
- Heart failure, left ventricular
- Hemodialysis
- Pressure ulcers
- Pulmonary edema
- Renal failure, acute
- Renal failure, chronic

ABBREVIATIONS
CAVH: Continuous arteriovenous hemofiltration
ECF: Extracellular fluid

REFERENCES
Horne MM: Fluid and electrolyte disturbances. In Swearingen PL, Keen JH (eds): *Manual of critical care nursing,* ed 3, St Louis, 1995, Mosby.
Horne MM, Heitz UE, Swearingen PL: *Pocket guide to fluid, electrolyte, and acid-base balance,* ed 3, St Louis, 1997, Mosby.
Rose BD: *Clinical physiology of acid-base and electrolyte disorders,* ed 4, New York, 1994, McGraw-Hill.

Author: **Mima M. Horne**

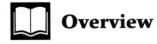 **Overview**

PATHOPHYSIOLOGY

Calcium exerts a sedative effect on nerve cells and has important intracellular functions, including development of cardiac action potential and muscle contraction. About half of plasma calcium is free, ionized calcium (Ca^{2+}). Slightly less than half is bound to protein, primarily to albumin. Only ionized calcium is physiologically important. The percentage of calcium that is ionized is affected by plasma pH and albumin level. Total calcium levels may ↓ as a result of ↑ calcium loss, ↓ intestinal absorption, or altered regulation (eg, hypoparathyroidism).

HISTORY/RISK FACTORS

↓ Ionized Calcium
- Alkalosis
- Rapid administration of citrated blood. Citrate added to blood to prevent clotting may bind with calcium, causing hypocalcemia.
- Hemodilution

↑ Calcium Loss in Body Fluids: As with loop diuretics

↓ Intestinal Absorption
- ↓ intake
- Impaired vitamin D metabolism: as in renal failure, especially chronic
- Chronic diarrhea
- Postgastrectomy

Hypoparathyroidism

Hyperphosphatemia: As in renal failure

Hypomagnesemia

Acute Pancreatitis

CLINICAL PRESENTATION

Numbness with tingling of fingers and circumoral region, alterations in mental status. In chronic hypocalcemia, fractures may be present as a result of ↑ bone porosity. Sudden drops in plasma Ca^{2+} levels may cause hypotension as a result of vasodilatation and heart failure caused by ↓ myocardial contractility.

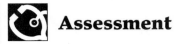 **Assessment**

PHYSICAL ASSESSMENT

Positive Trousseau's Sign: Ischemia-induced carpopedal spasm

Positive Chvostek's Sign: Unilateral contraction of facial and eyelid muscles

Neuro: Anxiety, depression, psychosis, hyperreflexia, tetany, convulsions

Resp: Crackles if heart failure present

CV: Vasodilatation, hypotension, S_3, JVD if calcium level severely ↓

VITAL SIGNS/HEMODYNAMICS

RR: Nl

HR: Nl

BP: ↓ if calcium level ↓ suddenly or hypocalcemia is severe

Temp: Nl

ECG: Prolonged QT interval caused by elongation of ST segment

LABORATORY STUDIES

Total Serum Calcium Level: <8.5 mg/dl. Should be evaluated with serum albumin. For every 1.0 g/dl ↓ in serum albumin level, there is a 0.8-1.0 mg/dl ↓ in total calcium level. This ↓, however, has little impact on ionized calcium level. Symptomatic hypocalcemia can occur with nl total calcium levels when there is a sudden ↑ in serum pH.

Ionized Serum Calcium Level: <4.5 mg/dl.

PTH Level: ↓ levels occur in hypoparathyroidism; ↑ levels may occur with other causes of hypocalcemia.

Magnesium and Phosphorus Levels: ↑ phosphorus levels and ↓ magnesium levels may precipitate hypocalcemia.

Collaborative Management

Treatment of Underlying Cause

Calcium Replacement: PO or IV. Always clarify type of IV calcium to be given. Both calcium chloride and calcium gluconate come in 10 ml ampules. One ampule of calcium chloride contains 13.6 mEq calcium, whereas one ampule of calcium gluconate contains 4.5 mEq calcium. Tetany is treated with 10-20 ml of 10% calcium gluconate IV. Hypomagnesemia-induced hypocalcemia is often refractory to calcium therapy alone and requires magnesium replacement.

Vitamin D Therapy (eg, dihydrotachysterol, calcitriol): To ↑ calcium absorption from the GI tract.

Aluminum- or Calcium-Containing Antacids: To ↓ elevated phosphorus level by binding phosphorus in the GI tract.

PATIENT-FAMILY TEACHING

- Importance of taking oral calcium supplements ac and at hs
- Necessity of taking phosphorus-binding antacids with meals
- Reassurance that neurosensory symptoms of hypocalcemia improve with treatment

Nursing Diagnoses/Interventions

Altered protection (risk of tetany and seizures) r/t neurosensory alterations secondary to severe hypocalcemia

Desired outcome: Patient does not exhibit evidence of injury caused by complications of severe hypocalcemia.

- Monitor for worsening hypocalcemia: numbness and tingling of fingers and circumoral region, hyperactive reflexes, and muscle cramps. Check for positive Trousseau's or Chvostek's signs; they signal latent tetany. Monitor total and ionized calcium levels as available.
- Rapid administration of IV calcium can cause hypotension. Administer at rate ≥0.5-1 ml/min. Observe IV insertion site for infiltration because calcium will slough tissue. Use central line for concentrated calcium solutions. Do not add calcium to solutions that contain sodium bicarbonate or sodium phosphate because precipitates will form.
- Calcium replacement therapy may cause toxicity in patients taking digitalis because calcium potentiates effects of digoxin. Monitor for S&S of digitalis toxicity: lethargy, confusion, nausea, vomiting, visual disturbances.
- For patients with chronic hypocalcemia, administer oral calcium 30 min ac or at hs for maximal absorption. Give aluminum hydroxide antacids with meals.
- Consult physician if response to calcium therapy is ineffective. Tetany that does not respond to IV calcium may be caused by hypomagnesemia.
- Maintain seizure precautions for patients with symptoms; ↓ environmental stimuli.
- Avoid hyperventilation, since respiratory alkalosis may precipitate tetany resulting from ↑ pH with a reduction in ionized calcium.
- Monitor for calcium loss (eg, with loop diuretics, renal tubular dysfunction) or conditions that place patient at risk (eg, acute pancreatitis).

Decreased cardiac output r/t altered conduction or negative inotropy secondary to hypocalcemia or digitalis toxicity occurring with calcium replacement therapy

Desired outcomes: Within 12 h of treatment initiation, patient's cardiac output adequate: PAP 20-30/8-15 mm Hg, CVP ≤6 mm Hg, CO 4-7 L/min, HR ≤100, BP wnl for patient, and absence of clinical signs of heart failure or pulmonary edema. ECG shows NSR.

- Monitor ECG for signs of worsening hypocalcemia (prolonged QT interval) or digitalis toxicity with calcium replacement: multifocal or bigeminal PVCs, PAT with varying AV block, Wenckebach (Mobitz I) heart block.
- Hypocalcemia may ↓ cardiac contractility. Monitor for S&S of heart failure or pulmonary edema: crackles, rhonchi, SOB, ↓ BP; and ↑ HR, PAP, CVP.

Ineffective breathing pattern r/t laryngeal spasm occurring with severe hypocalcemia

Desired outcome: Within 1 h of treatment initiation, patient has effective breathing pattern: eupnea, RR 12-20 breaths/min, and absence of laryngeal spasm: laryngeal stridor, dyspnea, crowing.

- Assess respiratory rate, character, and rhythm. Be alert to laryngeal stridor, dyspnea, and crowing, which occur with laryngeal spasm, a life-threatening complication of hypocalcemia.
- Keep an emergency tracheostomy tray at bedside.

Miscellanea

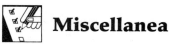

CONSULT MD FOR
- S&S of worsening hypocalcemia: numbness and tingling of fingers and circumoral region, hyperactive reflexes, and muscle cramps, which precede overt tetany
- Positive Trousseau's or Chvostek's sign
- S&S of heart failure, pulmonary edema, or digitalis toxicity

RELATED TOPICS
- Renal failure, chronic
- Heart failure, left ventricular
- Hypercalcemia
- Pancreatitis, acute

REFERENCES
Horne MM: Fluid and electrolyte disturbances. In Swearingen PL, Keen JH (eds): *Manual of critical care nursing,* ed 3, St Louis, 1995, Mosby.

Horne MM, Heitz UE, Swearingen PL: *Pocket guide to fluid, electrolyte, and acid-base balance,* ed 3, St Louis, 1997, Mosby.

Author: **Mima M. Horne**

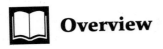

Overview

PATHOPHYSIOLOGY

Lowering of blood glucose caused by excessive dose of insulin or oral hypoglycemic agents, skipping meals, or too much exercise without concomitant ↑ in food intake. Typically occurs during peak action of insulin/hypoglycemic agent, particularly at night when asleep and having not eaten adequate bedtime snack. Symptoms usually occur when blood glucose <50 mg/dl or has dropped significantly (eg, to 90 mg/dl from 180-200 mg/dl in elderly). Alcohol consumption another cause because it depletes glycogen stores, resulting in ↑ insulin levels. Mentation changes caused by severe hypoglycemia can be indistinguishable from those caused by alcoholic stupor. Misdiagnosis can be fatal.

HISTORY/RISK FACTORS
- IDDM (type I), NIDDM (type II)
- ETOH abuse/alcoholism
- Anorexia nervosa
- Poorly constructed weight control program
- Use of anabolic steroids for body building
- Prolonged vomiting, diarrhea
- Insulinoma

CLINICAL PRESENTATION
- Erratic behavior, confusion
- Cool, clammy skin; diaphoresis
- Syncope

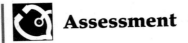

Assessment

PHYSICAL ASSESSMENT
Neuro: Tremors, seizures, altered thought process, stupor, coma
Resp: Tachypnea
CV: Diaphoresis, tachycardia, weak pulses, hypotension
GI: Hunger, nausea, eructation

VITAL SIGNS/HEMODYNAMICS
RR: ↑
HR: ↑
BP: ↓
Temp: Wnl
Hemodynamics: If available, reflect hypovolemia, distributive shock with ↓ CVP/PAP, ↓ SVR, ↓ CO.
ECG: Sinus tachycardia; possible PAT, PVCs; possible VT in severe cases, especially with underlying CAD or hx of dysrhythmias. May see ST-segment depression in cardiac compromised patients.

LABORATORY STUDIES
Serum Glucose: <50 mg/dl
ABGs: May show acute respiratory alkalosis resulting from tachypnea.
Other: Usually not applicable unless complications ensue.

Collaborative Management

Rapid-Acting Sugar: 10-15 g (eg, 4-6 oz fruit juice, 2-3 tsp honey or table sugar, 5 small hard candies) given PO. If symptoms persist for >15 min, treatment repeated. After resolution, patient consumes protein/complex carbohydrate snack, such as milk with crackers/bread.
Glucagon: If unable to swallow, 1 mg glucagon injected SC or IM. Glucagon stimulates the liver to break down stored glycogen into glucose and usually results in regaining of consciousness in 15-30 min; used rarely in hospital setting.
D50: IV injection of 25-50 ml D50, which usually revives unconscious individual in <10 min. Hyperglycemia and headache may occur after D50, particularly if 50 ml given. Protein or complex carbohydrate snack may be given once consciousness is regained unless blood glucose has been ↑ to >200 mg/dl.

PATIENT/FAMILY TEACHING
- Explanations about DM, including diagnostic testing and management, with emphasis on use of insulin/oral hypoglycemics
- Review of S&S and immediate interventions for hypoglycemia
- Evaluation of current diet for adequate nutritional requirements, caloric content, patient satisfaction; referral to dietitian as needed
- Review of onset, peak action, duration of hypoglycemic medication; avoidance of drugs that contribute to hypoglycemia (salicylates, sulfonamides, methyldopa, anabolic steroids, acetaminophen, ETOH, haloperidol, marijuana)
- Importance of testing blood glucose when symptoms of hypoglycemia occur
- Explanation that injection of insulin into site about to be exercised heavily (eg, jogger's thigh) results in quicker absorption of insulin and possibly hypoglycemia
- Explanation that a change in medication type may require change in dose to prevent hypoglycemia; explanation of need to follow prescription directions precisely

Nursing Diagnoses/Interventions

Altered protection r/t potential for brain damage or death secondary to hypoglycemia
Desired outcome: Within 10-30 min of intervention, patient is alert and verbalizes orientation to time, place, and person.

- Be aware that hypoglycemia requires immediate intervention because, if severe, it can lead to brain damage and death.
- Administer fast-acting carbohydrate: sugar, fruit juice, or hard candy. Consult physician if patient incoherent, unresponsive, or incapable of taking carbohydrates PO. If any of these indicators occur, IV access is required. Prepare to administer 50 ml D_{50} by IV push.
- Continue to monitor blood glucose levels q30-60min to identify recurrence of hypoglycemia.
- Once patient is alert, ask about most recent food intake. Any situation preventing food intake, such as nausea, vomiting, dislike of hospital food r/t cultural preferences, or fasting for a scheduled test, should be determined and addressed immediately.
- If food intake has been adequate, consult with physician about ↓ in daily dose of antihyperglycemic medication.
- Be aware that hypoglycemia may lead to rebound hyperglycemia (Somogyi phenomenon). Suspect Somogyi phenomenon if there are wide fluctuations in blood glucose over several h or if patient is experiencing nocturnal hypoglycemia.

Risk for trauma r/t oral, musculoskeletal, and airway vulnerability secondary to seizure activity
Desired outcome: Within 4 h of hypoglycemic event, patient verbalizes orientation to time, place, and person and is free of signs of trauma caused by seizures or altered LOC. If a seizure occurs, it is detected, reported, and treated promptly.

- Monitor LOC at frequent intervals. Anticipate seizure potential with severe hypoglycemia, and have airway, protective padding, and suction equipment at bedside. Keep side rails raised.
- Place call light within patient's reach. Keep patient near nurses' station for close monitoring.
- Keep potentially harmful objects (eg, sharp items, hot beverages) out of patient's reach.

DURING SEIZURE

- Remain with patient. Note type, duration, and characteristics of seizure activity and any post-seizure response. This should include, as appropriate, precipitating event, aura, initial location and progression, automatisms, type and duration of movement, changes in LOC, eye movement (eg, deviation, nystagmus), pupil size and reaction, bowel and bladder incontinence, head deviation, tongue deviation, teeth clenching.
- Prevent or break fall, and ease patient to floor if seizure occurs while patient is out of bed. Keep in bed if seizure occurs while there, and lower HOB to a flat position.
- If jaws are clenched, do not force object between teeth, because this can break teeth or lacerate oral mucous membrane. If able to do so safely and without damage to oral tissue, insert an airway. Avoid use of tongue depressor, which may splinter.
- Protect patient's head from injury during seizure activity. A towel folded flat may be used to cushion head from striking the ground. Position head to maintain open airway. Remove or pad objects (eg, chairs) patient may strike. Remove patient's glasses.
- Do not restrain patient but rather guide movements gently to prevent injury.
- Roll into side-lying position to promote drainage of secretions and maintain patent airway. Use head tilt, chin lift maneuver. Provide O_2 and suction as needed.
- Loosen belts, other tight clothing.

AFTER SEIZURE

- Reassure and reorient patient. Check neurologic status and VS; ask if an aura preceded seizure activity. Record this information and postictal characteristics.
- Provide quiet, calm environment because sounds and stimuli can be confusing to the awakening patient. Keep talk simple and to a minimum. Speak slowly and with pauses between sentences. Repeating may be necessary. Use room light that is behind, not above, patient to prevent additional seizures and for comfort. Do not offer food or drink until patient is fully awake.
- Check tongue for lacerations and body for injuries. Monitor urine for red or cola color, which may signal rhabdomyolysis or myoglobinuria from muscle damage. Monitor for weakness or paralysis, dysphasia, or visual disturbances.

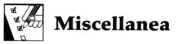

Miscellanea

CONSULT MD FOR

- S&S of hypoglycemia that do not respond to rapid-acting sugar
- Severe hypoglycemia: unresponsiveness or incoherence; seizure activity

RELATED TOPIC

- Diabetes mellitus

ABBREVIATION

D_{50}: 50% dextrose

REFERENCES

Baird MS: Hypoglycemia. In Swearingen PL (ed): *Pocket guide to medical-surgical nursing,* ed 2, St Louis, 1996, Mosby.

Flier JS: Hypoglycemia/pancreatic islet cell disorder. In Bennett JC, Plum F (eds): *Cecil textbook of medicine,* ed 20, Philadelphia, 1996, Saunders.

Horne MM, Heitz UE, Swearingen PL: *Pocket guide to fluid, electrolyte, and acid-base balance,* ed 3, St Louis, 1996, Mosby.

Marks V: Hypoglycemia and insulinomas. In Besser GM, Thorner MO (eds): *Clinical endocrinology,* ed 2, London, 1994, Mosby-Wolfe.

Author: **Marianne Saunorus Baird**

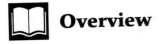 **Overview**

PATHOPHYSIOLOGY

Serum potassium level <3.5 mEq/L. Occurs as a result of loss of K^+ from the body or movement of K^+ into the cells. K^+ is lost from the body via kidneys, GI tract, and skin or may be lost from ECF as a result of intracellular shift. Distribution of K^+ between ECF and ICF maintained via sodium-potassium pump. Because K^+ affects the resting membrane potential of nerve and cardiac cells, abnormal serum K^+ levels adversely affect neuromuscular and cardiac function.

HISTORY/RISK FACTORS
Reduction in Total Body Potassium
- Hyperaldosteronism
- Abnormal urinary losses (eg, diuretics, hypomagnesemia)
- GI losses
- ↓ intake: eg, NPO status, TPN
- Dialysis

Intracellular Shift
- ↑ exogenous insulin
- Acute alkalosis
- Physical or emotional stress (caused by ↑ epinephrine)

CLINICAL PRESENTATION

Muscle weakness and cramps, nausea, vomiting, ileus, paresthesias, enhanced digitalis effect, dysrhythmias (eg, PACs, PVCs)

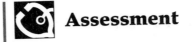 **Assessment**

PHYSICAL ASSESSMENT

↓ bowel sounds, weak and irregular pulse, ↓ reflexes, ↓ muscle tone

VITAL SIGNS/HEMODYNAMICS
RR: Nl; ↓ in sudden, severe hypokalemia
HR: Irregular
BP: Nl; may be ↓ if dysrhythmias present
Temp: Nl
CO: May be ↓ because of dysrhythmias
ECG: ST-segment depression, flattened T wave, presence of U wave, ventricular dysrhythmias; *with severe hypokalemia:* ↑ amplitude of P wave, prolonged PR interval, widened QRS complex

LABORATORY STUDIES
Serum Potassium Levels: <3.5 mEq/L
ABGs: May show metabolic alkalosis because hypokalemia usually associated with this condition. Hypokalemia also associated with metabolic acidosis (eg, occurring with treatment of DKA, diarrhea, renal tubular acidosis).

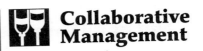 **Collaborative Management**

Treatment of Underlying Cause
Replacement of Potassium: With mild hypokalemia, usual dosage is 40-80 mEq/day IV or PO. Potassium never administered by IV push. It *must* be diluted in concentrations of ≤30-40 mEq/L of IV solution. Rapid administration could result in life-threatening hyperkalemia. If immediate repletion necessary it may be given at rates up to 10-20 mEq/h. However, these patients should be on a continuous cardiac monitor. Development of peaked T waves suggests hyperkalemia; infusion should be slowed or stopped until patient stabilizes.
Potassium-Sparing Diuretics: May be given in place of oral potassium supplements.

PATIENT-FAMILY TEACHING
- Foods high in K^+: eg, avocados, bananas, cantaloupes, carrots, cauliflower, dried beans/peas, dried fruit, mushrooms, nuts, oranges, peanuts, potatoes, pumpkins, spinach, tomatoes
- Need to take K^+ supplements with full glass of water or juice

Nursing Diagnoses/Interventions

Decreased cardiac output (or risk for same) r/t altered conduction secondary to hypokalemia or too rapid correction of hypokalemia with resulting hyperkalemia

Desired outcome: Within 2 h of treatment, patient has adequate cardiac conduction: nl T-wave configuration and NSR without ectopy on ECG.

- Administer potassium supplement as prescribed. Avoid giving IV KCl at a rate $\geq$10-20 mEq/h. Potassium supplementation for symptomatic hypokalemia usually is given in isotonic saline because D_5W will $\uparrow$ insulin-induced intracellular shift of K^+. If hypokalemia severe, concentrated solutions of potassium may be hung in limited volumes (eg, 20 mEq in 100 ml of isotonic NaCl), but it should be administered no more rapidly than 40 mEq/h.
- Do not add KCl to IV solution containers in the hanging position; this can cause layering of medication. Invert solution container before adding medication, and mix well.
- Be aware that IV KCl can cause local irritation of veins and chemical phlebitis. Assess IV insertion site for erythema, heat, or pain. Phlebitis may necessitate changing of IV site. Oral supplements may cause GI irritation. Administer with full glass of water or fruit juice. Oral potassium supplements are not equivalents and should not be interchanged.
- Monitor I&O qh. Potassium supplements should not be given if patient has inadequate UO because hyperkalemia can develop rapidly in patients with oliguria (<15-20 ml/h).
- Monitor ECG for signs of continuing hypokalemia (ST-segment depression, flattened T wave, presence of U wave, ventricular dysrhythmias) or hyperkalemia (tall, thin T waves; prolonged PR interval; ST depression; widened QRS complex; loss of P wave), which may develop during potassium replacement.
- Administer potassium cautiously in patients receiving potassium-sparing diuretics (eg, spironolactone or triamterene) or ACE inhibitors (eg, captopril) because of potential for development of hyperkalemia.
- Because hypokalemia can potentiate effects of digitalis, monitor patients receiving digitalis for $\uparrow$ digitalis effect: PVCs, PAT with varying AV block, (second degree AV block, Wenckebach [Mobitz I]).

Ineffective breathing pattern (or risk for same) r/t weakness or paralysis of respiratory muscles secondary to sudden severe hypokalemia (K^+ <2-2.5 mEq/L)

Desired outcome: Within 2 h of treatment, patient has effective breathing pattern: nl respiratory depth, pattern and rate of 12-20 breaths/min.

- Be aware that severe hypokalemia can lead to weakness of respiratory muscles and eventually to apnea. If rapid and shallow respirations occur, respiratory arrest may follow.
- Keep manual resuscitator at bedside.
- Reposition patient q2h to prevent stasis of secretions; suction airway as needed.
- Encourage deep breathing (and coughing if indicated) q2h in conscious patients.

Miscellanea

CONSULT MD FOR

- Hemodynamically significant PVCs, other dysrhythmias
- Chemical phlebitis associated with potassium infusion
- UO $\leq$0.5 ml/kg/h $\times$ 2 h
- Rapid, shallow respirations (signal severe hypokalemia; may precede arrest)
- New-onset ECG changes associated with hypo/hyperkalemia

RELATED TOPICS

- Diabetic ketoacidosis
- Hyperkalemia
- Ventricular tachycardia

ABBREVIATIONS

ECF: Extracellular fluid
ICF: Intracellular fluid

REFERENCES

Horne MM: Fluid and electrolyte disturbances. In Swearingen PL, Keen JH (eds): *Manual of critical care nursing,* ed 3, St Louis, 1995, Mosby.

Horne MM, Heitz UE, Swearingen PL: *Pocket guide to fluid, electrolyte, and acid-base balance,* ed 3, St Louis, 1997, Mosby.

Rose BD: *Clinical physiology of acid-base and electrolyte disorders,* ed 4, New York, 1994, McGraw-Hill.

Author: **Mima M. Horne**

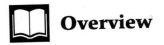 **Overview**

PATHOPHYSIOLOGY
Serum magnesium level <1.5 mEq/L. Because magnesium is a major intracellular ion, it plays a vital role in nl cellular function by activating enzymes involved in metabolism of carbohydrates and protein and triggering the sodium-potassium pump, thus affecting intracellular K^+ levels. Dysrhythmias and sudden death ↑ when ↓ magnesium levels occur in combination with MI, heart failure, or digitalis toxicity. ↓ magnesium intake identified as a risk factor for hypertension, cardiac dysrhythmias, ischemic heart disease, and sudden cardiac death. Hypomagnesemia usually associated with hypocalcemia and hypokalemia.

HISTORY/RISK FACTORS
- Chronic alcoholism: because of poor dietary intake, ↓ GI absorption, ↑ UO
- ↓ GI absorption: caused by cancer, colitis, pancreatic insufficiency, surgical resection of the GI tract, diarrhea
- ↑ GI loss: prolonged vomiting or gastric suction
- Low-magnesium or magnesium-free parenteral solutions, especially with refeeding after starvation
- Hyperaldosteronism: because of volume expansion
- DKA: result of movement of magnesium out of the cell and loss in urine because of osmotic diuresis
- Diuresis: resulting from medications, diuretic phase of ATN
- Protein-calorie malnutrition
- Cardiopulmonary bypass

CLINICAL PRESENTATION
Lethargy, weakness, fatigue, mood changes, hallucinations, confusion, anorexia, nausea, vomiting, paresthesias

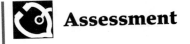 **Assessment**

PHYSICAL ASSESSMENT
↑ reflexes, tremors, convulsions, tetany, and positive reactions for Chvostek's and Trousseau's signs in part caused by accompanying hypocalcemia. Skeletal and respiratory muscle weakness may be present, as well as tachycardia, hypertension, and coronary spasm.

Positive Trousseau's Sign: Ischemia-induced carpopedal spasm
Positive Chvostek's Sign: Unilateral contraction of facial and eyelid muscles

VITAL SIGNS/HEMODYNAMICS
RR: ↑ but shallow
HR: ↑
BP: ↑
Temp: Nl
CVP/PAWP: ↑ if heart failure or hypervolemia present
SVR: ↑
CO: May be ↓ because of ↓ myocardial contractility, dysrhythmias
ECG: Reflects magnesium deficiencies: ventricular ectopy, torsades de pointes, and A-fib. Also may reveal calcium and potassium deficiencies, including tachydysrhythmias, prolonged PR and QT intervals, widening of QRS complex, ST-segment depression, and flattened T waves. ↑ digitalis effect possible: multifocal or bigeminal PVCs, PAT, AV heart blocks.

LABORATORY STUDIES
Serum Magnesium: <1.5 mEq/L. Hypomagnesemia is the most frequently undiagnosed electrolyte imbalance in hospitalized patients.
Serum Albumin: ↓ level may cause ↓ magnesium level because of reduction in protein-bound magnesium. Amount of free ionized magnesium may be unchanged, and it is that level which is physiologically important.
Serum Potassium: May be ↓ as a result of failure of cellular sodium-potassium pump to move K^+ into the cell and accompanying loss of K^+ in urine; may be resistant to potassium replacement until magnesium deficit has been corrected.
Serum Calcium: Hypocalcemia may occur as a result of ↓ in PTH.

Collaborative Management

Identification/Elimination of Cause: Eg, treat diarrhea, remove factors causing excessive diuresis, improve nutrition.
IV or IM MgSO₄: For severe hypomagnesemia or its symptoms.
Oral Magnesium: Magnesium-containing antacids (eg, Mylanta, Maalox, Gelusil, Milk of Magnesia) or magnesium chloride (Slow-Mag).

PATIENT-FAMILY TEACHING
- Explanation that oral magnesium supplements may cause diarrhea and that antidiarrheal medications may be necessary
- Importance of intake of foods high in magnesium (bananas, green and leafy vegetables, oranges, seafood)
- Importance of avoiding hyperventilation for patient in whom hypocalcemia suspected, since metabolic alkalosis may precipitate tetany as a result of ↑ calcium binding
- Reassurance that altered mood and sensorium are temporary and will improve with treatment

Nursing Diagnoses/Interventions

Altered protection r/t neurosensory alterations secondary to hypomagnesemia
Desired outcomes: Within 8 h of treatment initiation, patient verbalizes orientation to time, place, and person. Patient does not exhibit evidence of injury caused by complications of severe hypomagnesemia.

- Monitor serum magnesium levels. Be especially vigilant for patients who are chronic alcohol users or who have heart failure, recent MI, or digitalis toxicity.
- Be aware that symptoms of hypomagnesemia may be mistakenly attributed to delirium tremens of chronic alcoholism.
- Administer IV MgSO$_4$ with caution; if given too rapidly, it may lead to cardiac or respiratory arrest. Patients receiving IV magnesium should be monitored for ↓ BP, labored respirations, and diminished patellar reflex (knee jerk). Absent patellar reflex signals hyporeflexia caused by dangerous hypermagnesemia. Should any of these changes occur, stop the infusion and consult physician stat. Keep calcium gluconate at bedside in the event of hypocalcemic tetany or sudden hypermagnesemia.
- For chronic hypomagnesemia, administer oral magnesium supplement cautiously in patients with reduced renal function. Caution patient that oral magnesium supplements may cause diarrhea. Administer antidiarrheal medications as needed.
- Encourage intake of foods high in magnesium.
- Maintain seizure precautions for patients with symptoms (ie, those who have hyperreflexia). ↓ environmental stimuli.
- For patients in whom hypocalcemia suspected, caution against hyperventilation. Metabolic alkalosis may precipitate tetany as a result of ↑ calcium binding.
- Dysphagia may occur. Test ability to swallow water before giving food or medications.
- Assess and document LOC, orientation, and neurologic status with each VS check. Reorient as necessary.

Decreased cardiac output r/t electrical alterations associated with tachydysrhythmias or digitalis toxicity secondary to hypomagnesemia
Desired outcomes: Within 24 h of treatment initiation, patient's cardiac output adequate: CO ≥4 L/min, CI ≥2.5 L/min/m^2, NSR on ECG, and HR wnl for patient. Patient has UO ≥0.5 ml/kg/h.

- Monitor heart rate and regularity with each VS check. Be alert to ↓ CO and CI.
- Assess ECG for evidence of hypomagnesemia. Consider hypomagnesemia as a cause in patients who develop sudden ventricular dysrhythmias.
- Because hypomagnesemia (and hypokalemia) potentiates cardiac effects of digitalis, monitor patients taking digitalis for digitalis-induced dysrhythmias.
- Monitor UO qh. Be alert to output ≤0.5 ml/kg/h.

Altered nutrition: Less than body requirements of magnesium r/t hx of poor intake or anorexia, nausea, and vomiting secondary to hypomagnesemia or starvation
Desired outcome: Within 24 h of resumption of oral feedings, patient receives diet adequate in magnesium.

- Encourage intake of small, frequent meals.
- Administer antiemetics as prescribed.
- Include patient, significant others, and dietitian in meal planning as appropriate.
- Provide oral hygiene before meals to enhance appetite.
- As with the other major intracellular electrolyte levels, magnesium depletion may develop with refeeding after starvation. Anticipate hypomagnesemia with refeeding, and ensure ↑ dietary intake or supplementation.
- Consult physician for patients receiving magnesium-free solutions (eg, TPN) for prolonged periods of time.

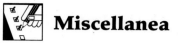 **Miscellanea**

CONSULT MD FOR
- Hemodynamically significant dysrhythmias
- Seizure activity
- S&S of hypermagnesemia in patients receiving IV MgSO$_4$
- S&S of ↓ CO or digitalis toxicity

RELATED TOPICS
- Hypermagnesemia
- Nutrition support, parenteral
- Status epilepticus

ABBREVIATIONS
ATN: Acute tubular necrosis
PTH: Parathyroid hormone

REFERENCES
Horne MM: Fluid and electrolyte disturbances. In Swearingen PL, Keen JH (eds): *Manual of critical care nursing,* ed 3, St Louis, 1995, Mosby.
Horne MM, Heitz UE, Swearingen PL: *Pocket guide to fluid, electrolyte, and acid-base balance,* ed 3, St Louis, 1997, Mosby.
Workman ML: Magnesium and phosphorus: the neglected electrolytes, *AACN Clin Issues in Crit Care Nurs* 3(3): 655-663, 1992.

Author: **Mima M. Horne**

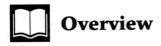 **Overview**

PATHOPHYSIOLOGY

Serum sodium <135 mEq/L. Can occur as a result of net gain of water or loss of sodium-rich fluids that are replaced by water. Clinical indicators and treatment depend on cause and whether hyponatremia is associated with nl, ↓, or ↑ ECF volume. Pseudohyponatremia may be caused by hyperglycemia, in which osmotic action of the elevated glucose causes a shift of water out of the cells and into ECF, thus diluting existing sodium. For every 100 mg/dl ↑ in glucose, sodium is diluted by 1.6 mEq/L.

HISTORY/RISK FACTORS

↓ ECF Volume

- GI losses: diarrhea, vomiting, fistulas, NG suction
- Renal losses: diuretics, salt-wasting kidney disease, adrenal insufficiency
- Skin losses: burns, wound drainage

NI/↑ ECF Volume

- SIADH: excessive production of antidiuretic hormone
- Edematous states: heart failure, cirrhosis, nephrotic syndrome
- Excessive administration of hypotonic IV fluids or excessively dilute enteral feedings
- Oliguric renal failure
- Primary polydipsia

CLINICAL PRESENTATION

Neurologic symptoms occur if serum sodium level ↓ to 120-125 mEq/L, especially if ↓ is sudden. Seizures, coma, and permanent neurologic damage may occur when sodium level <115 mEq/L.

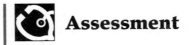 **Assessment**

PHYSICAL ASSESSMENT

Hyponatremia with ↓ ECF Volume: Irritability, apprehension, dizziness, personality changes, postural hypotension, dry mucous membranes, cold and clammy skin, tremors, seizures, coma

Hyponatremia with NI/↑ ECF Volume: Headache, lassitude, apathy, confusion, weakness, edema, weight gain, ↑ BP, hyper-reflexia, muscle spasms, seizures, coma

VITAL SIGNS/HEMODYNAMICS

↓ ECF VOLUME

RR: NI
HR: ↑
BP: ↓
Temp: NI
Hemodynamics: Evidence of hypovolemia (↓ CVP, PAP, CO, MAP; ↑ SVR)

NL/↑ ECF VOLUME

RR: NI
HR: NI
BP: NI; occasionally ↑
Temp: NI
Hemodynamics: Evidence of hypervolemia (↑ CVP, PAP, MAP)

LABORATORY STUDIES

Serum Sodium: <135 mEq/L
Serum Osmolality: ↓, except in cases of pseudohyponatremia.
Urine Specific Osmolality: Usually >100 mOsm/kg but < plasma level. In SIADH, urine is inappropriately concentrated.
Urine Sodium: ↓ (usually <20 mEq/L) except in SIADH, salt-wasting kidney disease, and adrenal insufficiency.

Collaborative Management

HYPONATREMIA WITH ↓ ECF VOLUME

Replacement of Sodium and Fluid Losses: Essential to *turn off* physiologic stimulus to ADH release and enable kidneys to restore balance between sodium and water.
Replacement of Other Electrolyte Losses: Eg, potassium, bicarbonate.
IV Hypertonic Saline: If serum sodium dangerously low or patient has extreme symptoms.

HYPONATREMIA WITH ↑ ECF VOLUME

Treatment of Underlying Cause: Eg, SIADH, oliguric renal failure.
Diuretics
Water Restriction: 1000 ml/day will establish negative water balance and ↑ serum sodium levels in most adults.

PATIENT-FAMILY TEACHING

Reassurance that altered sensorium is temporary and will improve with treatment

Nursing Diagnoses/Interventions

Fluid volume deficit r/t abnormal fluid loss
Fluid volume excess r/t excessive intake of hypotonic solutions, or ↑ retention of water
Desired outcome: Within 24 h of initiating treatment, patient normovolemic: HR 60-100 bpm, RR 12-20 breaths/min, BP wnl for patient, CVP 2-6 mm Hg, and PAP 20-30/8-15 mm Hg.
- If patient is receiving hypertonic saline, assess carefully for intravascular fluid overload: tachypnea, tachycardia, SOB, crackles, ↑ CVP, ↑ PAWP, S_3 gallop.
- Monitor I&O qh. Monitor urine specific gravity.
- Weigh patient qd. Acute weight changes usually indicate fluid changes. If individual is not being fed, a 1-kg ↓ in daily weight equals a 1-L fluid loss.
- Administer PO and IV fluids as prescribed. Provide frequent mouth care for patients on fluid restriction. Document response to fluid therapy.
- Monitor for fluid overload if patient is receiving hypertonic saline: crackles, SOB, tachypnea, tachycardia, ↑ CVP, ↑ PAP, JVD, edema.
- Monitor for hidden fluid losses: eg, measure and document abdominal girth or limb size, if indicated.

Altered protection r/t neurosensory alterations secondary to sodium level <120-125 mEq/L
Desired outcomes: Within 48 h of treatment, patient verbalizes orientation to time, place, and person and does not exhibit signs of physical injury caused by altered sensorium.
- Assess LOC, orientation, and neurologic status with each VS check. Reorient as necessary.
- Keep side rails up and bed in lowest position with wheels locked.
- Use reality therapy, such as clocks, calendars, and familiar objects; keep these items at bedside within patient's visual field.
- If seizures expected, keep appropriate-size airway at bedside.
- Monitor serum sodium levels. The level should not be corrected too rapidly because of risk of neurologic damage.

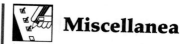 ## Miscellanea

CONSULT MD FOR
- Significant alterations in neurologic status or seizures, which may signal worsening hyponatremia or neurologic damage caused by too rapid correction of hyponatremia
- Serum sodium levels ↑ faster than 0.5 mEq/L/h during initial day of treatment for severe hyponatremia
- S&S of fluid overload: tachypnea, dyspnea, crackles, ↑ CVP/PAWP, S_3 gallop

RELATED TOPICS
- Burns
- Cirrhosis
- Heart failure, left ventricular
- Hypovolemia
- Renal failure, acute
- Renal failure, chronic
- Syndrome of inappropriate antidiuretic hormone

ABBREVIATIONS
ADH: Antidiuretic hormone
ECF: Extracellular fluid

REFERENCES
Horne MM: Fluid and electrolyte disturbances. In Swearingen PL, Keen JH (eds): *Manual of critical care nursing*, ed 3, St Louis, 1995, Mosby.
Horne MM, Heitz UE, Swearingen PL: *Pocket guide to fluid, electrolyte, and acid-base balance*, ed 3, St Louis, 1997, Mosby.
Rose BD: *Clinical physiology of acid-base and electrolyte disorders*, ed 4, New York, 1994, McGraw-Hill.

Author: **Mima M. Horne**

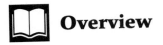 **Overview**

PATHOPHYSIOLOGY

Serum phosphorus <2.5 mg/dl. Phosphorus has many vital functions: formation of adenosine triphosphate and RBC 2,3-DPG; metabolism of carbohydrates, protein, and fat; and maintenance of acid-base balance. Phosphorus is also critical to nl nerve and muscle function, and it provides structural support to bones and teeth.

HISTORY/RISK FACTORS

- Intracellular shifts: carbohydrate load, respiratory alkalosis, treatment of DKA
- ↑ utilization resulting from tissue repair: TPN with inadequate phosphorus; recovery from malnutrition
- ↑ urinary losses: hypomagnesemia, ECF volume expansion, hyperparathyroidism, thiazide diuretics, diuretic phase of ATN, glucosuria
- ↓ intestinal absorption or ↑ intestinal loss: phosphorus-binding medications (eg, aluminum hydroxide antacids, sucralfate); vomiting and diarrhea; malabsorption; prolonged gastric suction
- Dialysis
- Mixed causes: chronic alcohol abuse, DKA, severe burns, mechanical ventilation, postsurgery, sepsis

CLINICAL PRESENTATION

Acute: Confusion, seizures, coma, chest pain, muscle pain and weakness, ↑ susceptibility to infection, numbness and tingling of fingers and circumoral region, incoordination, respiratory failure
Chronic: Memory loss, lethargy, weakness, bone pain

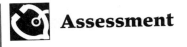 **Assessment**

PHYSICAL ASSESSMENT

Acute: Difficulty with speaking, weakness of respiratory muscles, weakening hand grasp. Bruising and bleeding may occur because of platelet dysfunction. Rhabdomyolysis, hemolysis, and S&S of impaired myocardial oxygenation may occur in severe hypophosphatemia. Hypoxia may cause ↑ RR and metabolic alkalosis as a result of hyperventilation.
Chronic: Joint stiffness, arthralgia, osteomalacia, cyanosis, pseudofractures.

VITAL SIGNS/HEMODYNAMICS

RR: ↑ caused by hypoxia
HR: ↑ caused by hypoxia
BP: May be ↓ if myocardial function ↓
Temp: Nl
Hemodynamics: Severely depleted patients may show signs of ↓ myocardial function, including ↑ PAWP, and ↓ CO, BP. Response to pressor agents poor until corrected.

LABORATORY STUDIES

Serum Phosphorus Level: <2.5 mg/dl (1.7 mEq/L)
Mild hypophosphatemia: 1.0-2.5 mg/dl
Severe hypophosphatemia: <1.0 mg/dl
PTH Level: ↑ in hyperparathyroidism
Serum Magnesium Level: ↓ caused by ↑ urinary excretion of magnesium in hypophosphatemia.

IMAGING

X-rays: May reveal skeletal changes of osteomalacia.

Collaborative Management

Identification/Elimination of Cause
Phosphorus Supplementation: ↑ intake of high-phosphorus foods (dried beans, eggs, fish, meats, milk, poultry, whole grains). Oral phosphate supplements such as Neutra-Phos (sodium and potassium phosphate) or Phospho-Soda (sodium phosphate). IV sodium phosphate or potassium phosphate necessary in severe hypophosphatemia or when GI tract nonfunctional.

PATIENT-FAMILY TEACHING

- Reassurance that altered sensorium is temporary and will improve with treatment
- Foods high in phosphorus, which should be incorporated into diet: eg, dried beans, eggs, fish, meats, milk, poultry, whole grains

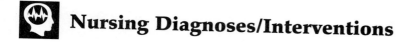 **Nursing Diagnoses/Interventions**

Altered protection r/t neurosensory alterations secondary to hypophosphatemia
Desired outcomes: Within 24 h of treatment initiation, patient verbalizes orientation to time, place, and person. Patient does not exhibit evidence of injury caused by neurosensory changes.
- Monitor serum phosphorus levels and for associated electrolyte and acid-base imbalances: hypokalemia, hypomagnesemia, respiratory alkalosis, metabolic acidosis.
- Apprehension, confusion, and paresthesias signal developing hypophosphatemia. Assess LOC, orientation, and neurologic status with each VS check. Reorient as necessary.
- Administer IV phosphate at prescribed rate. Potential complications of IV phosphorus include *tetany* resulting from hypocalcemia (serum calcium levels may ↓ suddenly if serum PO_4^{3-} levels ↑ suddenly), *soft tissue calcification,* and *hypotension* caused by too rapid delivery. When administered as potassium phosphate, the infusion rate should not exceed 10 mEq/h. Monitor IV site for infiltration because potassium phosphate can cause necrosis and tissue sloughing.
- Keep side rails up and bed in its lowest position with wheels locked.
- Use reality therapy, such as clocks, calendars, familiar objects. Keep these articles at bedside, within patient's visual field.
- If patient is at risk for seizures, keep an appropriate-size airway at bedside.

Impaired gas exchange r/t altered O_2-carrying capacity of the blood secondary to ↓ 2,3-DPG with consequent left shift of the oxyhemoglobin dissociation curve (ie, at a given Pao_2 level, more O_2 will be bound to Hgb and less will be available to the tissues).
Desired outcome: Within 12 h of treatment initiation, patient has adequate gas exchange: RR 12-20 breaths/min with eupnea, orientation × 3, Spo_2 ≥92%, and absence of hypoxia.
- Assess for signs of hypoxia: restlessness, confusion, ↑ RR, chest pain, and cyanosis (a late sign).
- Monitor Spo_2. Administer O_2 as prescribed to maintain Spo_2 at ≥92%.

Ineffective breathing pattern r/t ↓ strength of respiratory muscles secondary to hypophosphatemia
Desired outcome: Within 8 h of treatment initiation, nonventilated patient becomes eupneic. For ventilated patient, improved weaning is noted within 24 h.
- Monitor rate, depth of respirations. Assess for ↓ tidal volume or ↓ minute ventilation.
- Assess patient and monitor ABGs for evidence of hypoxemia or hypercapnia. Administer O_2; adjust ventilator settings as indicated.
- Incidence of hypophosphatemia ↑ in artificially ventilated patients. Hypophosphatemia may contribute to difficulty in weaning from ventilators. Monitor for and correct hypophosphatemia before weaning.

Decreased cardiac output r/t negative inotropic changes associated with ↓ myocardial functioning secondary to severe phosphorus depletion
Desired outcome: Within 12 h of treatment initiation, patient's cardiac output adequate: CI ≥2.5 L/min/m², CVP <6 mm Hg, PAP 20-30/8-15 mm Hg, HR ≤100 bpm, BP wnl for patient, and absence of clinical signs of heart failure or pulmonary edema.
- Monitor for signs of heart failure or pulmonary edema: crackles, rhonchi, SOB, ↓ BP; and ↑ HR, PAP, CVP.
- As necessary, use pressor or inotropic agents (eg, dobutamine, milrinone) to ↑ CO. Be aware that response to pressor/inotropic agents may be poor until hypophosphatemia corrected.
- Prevent hyperventilating, since metabolic alkalosis causes ↑ movement of phosphorus into the cells, which negatively affects cardiac output.
- Auscultate lung sounds q1-2 h and monitor UO. ↑ in crackles and ↓ in UO suggest heart failure, and thus diuretics may be necessary.
- Monitor ECG continuously. Be alert for dysrhythmias; treat according to type and agency protocol.

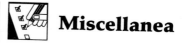 **Miscellanea**

CONSULT MD FOR
- Altered mental status
- S&S of heart failure, pulmonary edema
- Hemodynamically significant dysrhythmias
- S&S of respiratory muscle fatigue, hypoxemia, hypercarbia

RELATED TOPICS
- Diabetic ketoacidosis
- Heart failure, left ventricular
- Mechanical ventilation
- Pulmonary edema
- Respiratory alkalosis, acute

ABBREVIATIONS
ECF: Extracellular fluid

REFERENCES
Horne MM: Fluid and electrolyte disturbances. In Swearingen PL, Keen JH (eds): *Manual of critical care nursing,* ed 3, St Louis, 1995, Mosby.
Horne MM, Heitz UE, Swearingen PL: *Pocket guide to fluid, electrolyte, and acid-base balance,* ed 3, St Louis, 1997, Mosby.
Workman ML: Magnesium and phosphorus: the neglected electrolytes, *AACN Clin Issues in Crit Care Nurs* 3(3): 655-663, 1992.

Author: **Mima M. Horne**

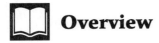 ## Overview

PATHOPHYSIOLOGY

Profound body heat loss resulting in core (rectal, esophageal, PA) temp <35° C (95° F). Compensatory mechanisms (eg, vasoconstriction, shivering) fail, and internal body temp drops. Metabolic rate ↓ affects all organ systems. Profound vasoconstriction and hypoventilation impair O_2 delivery. If severe or prolonged, coma, apnea, and metabolic derangements ultimately lead to death.

HISTORY/RISK FACTORS

- Environment: prolonged exposure or inadequate protection in cool, wet, or snowy climates
- Failure of thermoregulatory control: intoxicant, head injury
- Multisystem injury: exposed body surface or viscera, cold resuscitation fluids, cool ambient temp, prolonged scene time, major blood loss
- Altered mental status, including intoxication
- Inadequate fatty insulation/malnutrition
- Cardiovascular disease
- Advanced age

CLINICAL PRESENTATION

Mild (34°-35° C)
- Cold skin, shivering
- Slurred speech, impaired coordination
- Peripheral vasoconstriction
- Tachycardia, tachypnea
- Diuresis

Moderate (31°-33° C)
- ↑ DTRs, muscle rigidity
- Confusion, delirium
- Hypotension
- A-fib, bradycardia

Profound (≤30° C)
- Fixed, dilated pupils
- Deep coma
- Absent DTRs
- VF, asystole
- Apnea

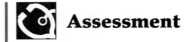 ## Assessment

PHYSICAL ASSESSMENT

Variable, depending on degree
Integ: Early, pallor; later, cyanosis
Neuro: Mild confusion→delirium→profound coma
Resp: Tachypnea→hypoventilation→apnea
CV: Tachycardia→dysrhythmias, hypotension

VITAL SIGNS/HEMODYNAMICS

RR: Initially ↑, then ↓
HR: Initially ↑, then ↓
BP: Initially ↑, then ↓
Temp: ↓
CVP/PAWP: Initially nl, then ↓
CO: Initially nl, then ↓
SVR: ↑
Other: Cold-induced diuresis may cause hypovolemia.
ECG: Sinus tachycardia; then A-fib, bradycardia, PVCs, VF, asystole. T wave inversion, Q-T prolongation possible. Possible Osborne or J waves with moderate to severe hypothermia.

LABORATORY STUDIES

Hgb/Hct: ↑ as a result of hemoconcentration caused by cold-induced diuresis
Electrolytes: Derangements likely according to degree of metabolic acidosis
PT/PTT: Prolonged if coagulopathy develops from pooled circulation/capillary sludging
Fibrinogen: ↑ with coagulopathy
ABGs: Initial respiratory alkalosis; later, pH <7.35 and HCO_3^- <22 mEq/L as a result of metabolic acidosis and excess lactate production; ↓ PaO_2 because of left shift in oxyhemoglobin dissociation curve; O_2 unloading to peripheral tissue impaired
Blood Alcohol, Toxicology Screen: Checks presence of intoxicant(s)

Collaborative Management

Oxygenation: Secure airway by intubation if necessary. Humidify supplemental O_2 and warm to 42°-46° C. Mechanical ventilation may be necessary.
Fluid Management: Warm all IV fluids to 43° C. Store crystalloids in blanket warmer. NS preferred over LR because of impaired lactate metabolism.
Rewarming: Remove wet garments, dressings, linens. Rewarm by 1°-2° C/h. More rapid warming causes VF, hypovolemic shock. If patient alert and swallowing, give warm PO liquids.
Active external: Use radiant heat sources, heating blankets, hot water bottles for mild hypothermia or after core temp ≥35° C. Premature surface rewarming leads to return of cold blood to heart, causing myocardial irritability and creating afterdrop in core temp.
Core: Use PD; gastric, colonic, bladder lavage with warm fluids. In extreme cases extracorporeal blood warming may be necessary.
Treatment of Dysrhythmias: Sinus tachycardia, A-fib, bradycardias usually resolve with rewarming. Transient ventricular dysrhythmias do not require treatment. VF or symptomatic VT requires defibrillation per ACLS guidelines.
Pharmacotherapy: Use all medications cautiously and in small incremental doses to avoid bolus dose effect with release of drugs from periphery during rewarming.

PATIENT-FAMILY TEACHING

- High-risk activities; prevention measures
- Medications: drug name, purpose, dosage, schedule, precautions, food-drug and drug-drug interactions, potential side effects
- Purpose, expected results, anticipated sensations of all nursing/medical interventions

Nursing Diagnoses/Interventions

Hypothermia r/t temporary loss of temp regulatory mechanisms resulting from shock, CNS ischemia, or ↓ body heat production

Desired outcomes: Core temp >35° C within 24 h. Complications are avoided: NSR on ECG; oriented × 3; Pao_2 ≥80; balanced acid-base; absence of prolonged bleeding.

- Administer warm humidified O_2. If alkalotic, avoid hyperventilation.
- Maintain warm ambient room temp.
- Keep patient dry, and cover head to reduce heat loss. Keep patient covered with warmed blankets whenever possible.
- Monitor core temp *via* rectal or esophageal probe, urinary catheter attachment, or PA catheter.
- Be aware that vasodilatation during rewarming can cause intravascular fluid volume deficit and necessitate frequent titration of vasoactive infusions.
- Monitor for and promptly report serious dysrhythmias (ie, A-fib with rapid ventricular response, ventricular dysrhythmias, and AV conduction block).
- If CPR necessary, continue until core temp reaches 30° C before concluding patient cannot be resuscitated. Defibrillation may not be successful with profound hypothermia.
- Monitor neurologic status q15-30min. Confusion, disorientation, somnolence make evaluation of concurrent head injury difficult.
- Check ABG values at frequent intervals for hypoxemia and metabolic acidosis. Hypothermia causes shift to left in oxyhemoglobin dissociation curve and may impair O_2 unloading to peripheral tissue. Ask lab to correct gases for patient's temp.
- DIC may develop several days after hypothermic episode. Monitor for excessive bleeding from wounds, surgical incisions, venipuncture sites.
- As rewarming occurs, monitor peripheral circulation and extremities for gangrene.

Fluid volume deficit r/t active loss secondary to cold-induced diuresis; vasodilatation during rewarming

Desired outcomes: Patient normovolemic within 12 h of treatment: MAP ≥70 mm Hg, HR 60-100 bpm, CVP 2-6 mm Hg, PAWP 6-12 mm Hg, CI ≥2.5 ml/min/m², UO ≥0.5 ml/kg/h.

- Initially monitor BP q5-15min until stable. Watch changes in MAP >10 mm Hg.
- Monitor HR, ECG, CV status q15min until volume restored and VS stable.
- With volume depletion or active blood loss, administer warm pressurized fluids. Warm all crystalloids to 43° C until patient approaches normothermia. Use blood warmers or rapid-volume infusers, if necessary, for immediate warming of large volumes (ie, 800-1200 ml/min) of blood and fluids as they are infused.
- During resuscitation monitor for circulatory overload and pulmonary edema caused by impaired myocardial contractility occurring with hypothermia.
- Measure UO q1-2h. UO <0.5 ml/kg/h for 2 consecutive h suggests inadequate intravascular volume.
- Administer O_2 to maximize tissue delivery.

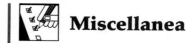 # Miscellanea

CONSULT MD FOR
- A-fib with rapid ventricular response, CV instability
- VT/VF
- Deteriorating mental status
- Hypotension that fails to respond to fluid challenge
- UO <0.5 ml/kg/h for 2 consecutive h

RELATED TOPICS
- Bradycardia
- Disseminated intravascular coagulation
- Hypoglycemia
- Metabolic acidosis
- Multiple organ dysfunction syndrome
- Shock, hypovolemic
- Ventricular fibrillation

ABBREVIATIONS
DTR: Deep tendon reflex
PA: Pulmonary artery
PD: Peritoneal dialysis

REFERENCES
Cardona VC et al: *Trauma nursing: from resuscitation through rehabilitation,* ed 2, Philadelphia, 1994, Saunders.

Keen JH: Major trauma. In Swearingen PL, Keen JH (eds): *Manual of critical care nursing,* ed 3, St Louis, 1995, Mosby.

Neff JA, Kidd PS: *Trauma nursing: the art and science,* St Louis, 1993, Mosby.

Author: **Janet Hicks Keen**

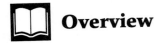 **Overview**

PATHOPHYSIOLOGY
Condition in which there is inadequate circulating thyroid hormone causing ↓ metabolic rate that affects all body systems. When untreated or a stressor such as infection affects an individual with hypothyroidism, a life-threatening condition known as *myxedema coma* can occur. Coma and seizures also can occur. Myxedema coma usually develops slowly, has a >50% mortality rate, and requires prompt and aggressive treatment.

HISTORY/RISK FACTORS
Primary Hypothyroidism
- Accounts for >90% of cases; caused by pathologic thyroid changes
- Dietary iodine deficiency, thyroiditis, thyroid atrophy, radiation therapy to the neck, surgical removal of all or part of the gland, drugs that suppress thyroid activity

Secondary Hypothyroidism
- Caused by dysfunction of the anterior pituitary gland, which results in ↓ release of TSH
- Pituitary tumors, postpartum pituitary gland necrosis, or hypophysectomy

CLINICAL PRESENTATION
Early fatigue, weight gain, anorexia, lethargy, cold intolerance, menstrual irregularities, depression, muscle cramps

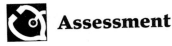 **Assessment**

PHYSICAL ASSESSMENT
Hypothyroidism: Possible goiter, bradycardia, hypothermia, deepened voice or hoarseness, hypercholesterolemia, obesity, non–pitting peripheral edema (myxedema). Skin may be dry, cool, and coarse; hair may be thin, coarse, and brittle. Tongue may be enlarged (macroglossia), and reflexes slowed.
Myxedema Coma: Hypoventilation, hypoglycemia, hypothermia, hypotension, bradycardia, shock.

VITAL SIGNS/HEMODYNAMICS (for severe hypothyroidism/myxedema coma)
RR: Nl or ↓
HR: ↓
BP: ↓
Temp: ↓
CVP/PAP: ↓
CO/CI: ↓
SVR: ↓
ECG: Sinus bradycardia

LABORATORY STUDIES
TSH: ↑ unless disease is longstanding or severe.
TRH Stimulation Test: ↑ basal; exaggerated ↑ in early hypothyroidism.
FTI and T_4 Levels: ↓
^{131}I Scan and Uptake: <10% in 24 h. In secondary hypothyroidism, uptake ↑ with administration of exogenous TSH.
Antimicrosomal Antibodies: Positive test represents Hashimoto's thyroidism.

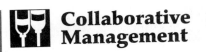 **Collaborative Management**

Oral Thyroid Hormone: Given early in treatment for primary hypothyroidism. For secondary hypothyroidism, thyroid supplements can promote acute symptoms and therefore are contraindicated.
Stool Softeners: To minimize constipation.
Diet: High in fiber to help prevent constipation; restriction of sodium to ↓ edema; and reduction in calories to promote weight loss.
TREATMENT OF MYXEDEMA COMA
Oxygenation: Supplemental O_2 *via* nasal cannula or mask to compensate for ↓ ventilatory drive. Intubation and mechanical ventilation may be necessary.
IV Thyroid Supplements: Corrects thyroid hormone deficiency. Rapid IV administration can precipitate hyperadrenalism. Can be avoided by concomitant administration of IV hydrocortisone.
Treatment of Hypotension: *Via* IV fluids, NS, and LR. Hypotonic solutions, such as D_5W, contraindicated because they can ↓ serum sodium levels further. Because of altered metabolism, response to vasopressors is poor.
Treatment of Hypoglycemia: *Via* IV D_{50}.
Treatment of Hyponatremia: Fluids restricted or hypertonic (3%) saline administered.
Treatment of Associated Illnesses: Eg, infections.
Caution: Because of alterations in metabolism, patients do not tolerate sedatives, CNS depressants. Also, external warming measures are contraindicated because they can produce vasodilation and vascular collapse.

PATIENT/FAMILY TEACHING
- Medications: drug name, purpose, dosage, schedule, precautions, drug-drug and food-drug interactions, and potential side effects
- Expected changes that can occur with hormone replacement therapy: ↑ energy level, weight loss, ↓ peripheral edema, improvement in neuromuscular problems
- Importance of avoiding physical and emotional stress; ways for patient to maximize coping mechanisms for dealing with stress
- S&S that necessitate medical attention: fever or other symptoms of upper respiratory, urinary, or oral infections and S&S of hyperthyroidism, which may result from excessive hormone replacement

Nursing Diagnoses/Interventions

Ineffective breathing pattern r/t upper airway obstruction occurring with enlarged thyroid gland and/or ↓ ventilatory drive caused by greatly ↓ metabolism

Desired outcome: Within 7 days of treatment initiation, patient has effective breathing pattern: RR 12-20 breaths/min with eupnea, nl skin color, SaO_2 ≥95%, and absence of adventitious breath sounds.

- Assess rate, depth, and quality of breath sounds, and be alert to adventitious sounds (eg, from developing pleural effusion) or ↓/crowing sounds (eg, from swollen tongue or glottis).
- Be alert to signs of inadequate ventilation: changes in respiratory rate or pattern and circumoral or peripheral cyanosis.
- Administer supplemental humidified O_2. Monitor SpO_2.
- Teach coughing, deep breathing, use of incentive spirometer. Suction upper airway prn.
- For patient with respiratory insufficiency, be prepared for intubation and mechanical ventilatory assistance.

Fluid volume excess r/t compromised regulatory mechanisms occurring with adrenal insufficiency

Desired outcome: By a minimum of 24 h before hospital discharge, patient becomes normovolemic: UO ≥0.5 ml/kg/h, stable weight, nondistended jugular veins, presence of eupnea, and peripheral pulse amplitude ≥2+ on 0-4+ scale.

- Monitor I&O qh for ↓ output. Weigh qd and note ↑ trends.
- Monitor for signs of heart failure: ↑ PAWP/CVP, ↓ CO, presence of S_3/S_4, JVD, crackles, SOB, and ↓ amplitude of peripheral pulses.
- Restrict fluid and sodium intake as indicated for dilutional hyponatremia. If restriction of fluid/sodium intake is ineffective, administration of hypertonic (3%) saline and loop diuretics may be necessary.
- Monitor serum electrolytes closely, especially sodium and potassium.
- Use infusion control device to maintain accurate infusion rate of IV fluids.

Risk for infection r/t compromised immunologic status secondary to alterations in adrenal function

Desired outcome: Patient free of infection: normothermia, absence of adventitious breath sounds, nl urinary pattern and characteristics, and well-healing wounds.

- Be alert to early indicators of infection: fever, erythema, swelling, discharge from wounds or IV sites; urinary frequency, urgency, dysuria; cloudy or malodorous urine; adventitious sounds on auscultation of lung fields; changes in color, consistency, amount of sputum.
- Minimize risk of UTI by providing meticulous care of indwelling catheters.
- Use sterile technique when performing dressing changes and invasive procedures.
- Provide good skin care to maintain skin integrity and prevent pressure ulcers.
- Advise visitors who have contracted or been exposed to a communicable disease not to enter room or to wear a surgical mask, if appropriate.

Altered protection (risk of myxedema coma) r/t inadequate response to treatment of hypothyroidism or stressors such as infection

Desired outcome: Patient free of symptoms of myxedema coma: HR ≥60 bpm, BP ≥90/60 mm Hg (or wnl for patient), RR ≥12 breaths/min with eupnea, orientation × 3.

- Monitor VS at frequent intervals and be alert to bradycardia, hypotension, ↓ RR.
- Monitor for signs of hypoxemia: restlessness, ↓ LOC, ↓ PaO_2, ↓ SpO_2.
- Monitor serum electrolytes and glucose levels. Be especially alert to ↓ sodium and glucose.
- In the presence of myxedema coma, restrict fluids or administer hypertonic saline; administer IV thyroid replacement hormones with IV hydrocortisone and IV glucose to treat hypoglycemia; monitor for onset of heart failure; and keep oral airway and manual resuscitator at bedside in the event of seizure, coma, or need for ventilatory assistance.

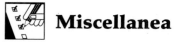 ## Miscellanea

CONSULT MD FOR
- S&S of hypoxemia
- S&S of heart failure: crackles, ↑ PAWP, dependent edema, ↓ peripheral pulses
- S&S of impending myxedema coma: SBP <90 mm Hg, HR <60 bpm, RR <12 breaths/min

RELATED TOPICS
- Heart failure, left ventricular
- Heart failure, right ventricular
- Hyperthyroidism
- Hypervolemia
- Hyponatremia
- Myxedema coma

ABBREVIATIONS
D_{50}: 50% dextrose
FTI: Free thyroxine index
TRH: Thyrotropin-releasing hormone
TSH: Thyroid-stimulating hormone
T_4: Thyroxine

REFERENCES
DeGroot LJ: Thyroid physiology and hypothyroidism. In Besser GM, Thorner MO (eds): *Clinical endocrinology,* ed 4, London, 1994, Mosby-Wolfe.

Dillman WH: The thyroid. In Bennett JC, Plum F: *Cecil textbook of medicine,* ed 20, Philadelphia, 1996, Saunders.

Gill GN: Principles of endocrinology. In Bennett JC, Plum F: *Cecil textbook of medicine,* ed 20, Philadelphia, 1996, Saunders.

Loriaux TC, Drass JA: Endocrine and diabetic disorders. In Kinney M, Packa D, Dunbar S: *AACN's clinical reference for critical care nursing,* ed 3, St Louis, 1993, Mosby.

Author: **Marianne Saunorus Baird**

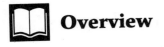 Overview

PATHOPHYSIOLOGY

Depletion of ECF volume. Depending on type of fluid lost, may be accompanied by acid-base, osmolar, or electrolyte imbalance. Compensatory mechanisms include ↑ SNS stimulation (↑ HR, ↑ cardiac contractility, ↑ SVR), thirst, ↑ release of ADH and aldosterone. Prolonged hypovolemia may lead to ARF or shock.

HISTORY/RISK FACTORS

- Abnormal GI losses: vomiting, NG suctioning, diarrhea, intestinal drainage
- Abnormal skin losses: burns, excessive diaphoresis
- Abnormal renal losses: diuretic therapy, DI, polyuric renal disease, adrenal insufficiency, osmotic diuresis (eg, uncontrolled DM, postdye study)
- Third spacing or plasma-to-interstitial fluid shift: peritonitis, intestinal obstruction, burns, ascites
- Hemorrhage: major trauma, GI bleeding, obstetric complications
- Altered intake: coma, fluid deprivation

CLINICAL PRESENTATION

Dizziness, weakness, fatigue, syncope, anorexia, nausea, vomiting, thirst, confusion, constipation

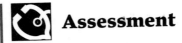 Assessment

PHYSICAL ASSESSMENT

CV: Orthostatic hypotension, ↑ HR
GU: ↓ UO (unless polyuric renal disease or DI present); poor skin turgor; dry, furrowed tongue; dry mucous membranes
Assoc Findings: Sunken eyeballs, flat neck veins, ↑ temp, acute weight loss (except with third spacing)

VITAL SIGNS/HEMODYNAMICS

RR: Nl or ↑
HR: ↑
BP: Orthostatic changes; ↓
Temp: Nl or ↑
CVP/PAP: ↓
MAP: ↓
SVR: ↑
CO: ↓

LABORATORY STUDIES

BUN: ↑ because of dehydration, ↓ renal perfusion, or ↓ renal function. BUN/plasma creatinine ratio of >20:1 suggests hypovolemia.
Hct: ↑ with dehydration; ↓ with bleeding.
Serum Electrolytes: Variable, depending on type of fluid lost.
Hyponatremia: Most types of hypovolemia; ADH triggers ↑ water intake/retention, thus diluting serum sodium.
Hypokalemia: Abnormal GI or renal losses.
Hyperkalemia: Adrenal insufficiency.
Hypernatremia: ↑ insensible or sweat losses, DI.
ABGs: Metabolic acidosis (pH <7.35 and HCO_3^- <22 mEq/L) may occur with lower GI losses, shock, or DKA. Metabolic alkalosis (pH >7.45 and HCO_3^- >26 mEq/L) may occur with upper GI losses and diuretic therapy.
Urine Specific Gravity: Usually ↑ as a result of kidneys' attempt to conserve water. May be ↓ with abnormal renal losses.
Urine Sodium: Kidneys will attempt to conserve sodium in response to ↑ aldosterone. In absence of renal disease, osmotic diuresis, or diuretic therapy, value should be <20 mEq/L.
Serum Osmolality: Often ↑, but varies depending on type of fluid lost and compensatory responses.
Urine Osmolality: ↑ (usually >450 mOsm/kg) as kidneys attempt to conserve water.

Collaborative Management

Treatment of Underlying Cause: Eg, surgery to correct hemorrhage, bowel obstruction; antibiotic therapy for peritonitis.
Restoration of Normal Fluid Volume/Correction of Electrolyte Disturbances: Fluid administered at rate that induces positive fluid balance (eg, 50-100 ml in *excess* of sum of all hourly losses).
Dextrose and water solutions: Provide free water only; distributed evenly through ICF and ECF; used to treat water deficit.
Isotonic saline: Expands ECF only; does not enter ICF. Appropriate for rapid volume replacement in shock.
Blood and albumin: Expand only intravascular portion of ECF.
Mixed saline/electrolyte solutions: Provide additional electrolytes (eg, K^+ and Ca^{2+}) and a buffer (lactate or acetate).
Dextran or hetastarch: Colloid solutions that expand intravascular portion of ECF.

PATIENT-FAMILY TEACHING

- Necessity for adequate oral intake
- Reassurance that altered sensorium will improve with therapy

Nursing Diagnoses/Interventions

Fluid volume deficit r/t abnormal loss of body fluids or ↓ intake

Desired outcomes: Within 24 h of initiation of fluid therapy, patient normovolemic: UO ≥ 0.5 ml/kg/h, specific gravity 1.010-1.030, stable weight, no clinical evidence of hypovolemia, BP wnl for patient, CVP 2-6 mm Hg, PAP 20-30/8-15 mm Hg, CO 4-7 L/min, MAP 70-105 mm Hg, HR 60-100 bpm, and SVR 900-1200 dynes/sec cm^{-5}.

- Monitor I&O qh. Initially, intake should exceed output. Monitor urine specific gravity; expect ↓ with therapy.
- Monitor VS and hemodynamics for signs of continued hypovolemia: ↓ BP, CVP, PAP, CO, MAP; ↑ HR and SVR.
- Place patient who is in shock in supine position with legs elevated to 45 degrees to ↑ venous return.
- Weigh patient qd. Acute weight changes usually indicate fluid changes. If individual is being fed, a 1-kg ↓ in daily weight equals a 1-L fluid loss.
- Administer PO and IV fluids as prescribed. Ensure adequate intake, especially in elders because of ↑ risk of volume depletion in this population.
- Monitor for fluid overload or too rapid fluid administration: crackles, SOB, tachypnea, tachycardia, ↑ CVP, ↑ PAP, JVD, and edema.
- Monitor for hidden fluid losses: eg, measure and document abdominal girth or limb size, if indicated.
- Remember that Hct will ↓ as patient becomes rehydrated. ↓ in Hct associated with rehydration is accompanied by ↓ in sodium and BUN values.

Altered cerebral, renal, and peripheral tissue perfusion r/t hypovolemia

Desired outcome: Within 12 h after therapy initiation, patient has adequate perfusion: alertness, warm and dry skin, BP wnl for patient, HR ≤100 bpm, UO ≥0.5 ml/kg/h, and capillary refill <2 sec.

- Monitor for ↓ cerebral perfusion: vertigo, syncope, confusion, restlessness, anxiety, agitation, excitability, weakness, nausea, and cool, clammy skin.
- Protect patients who are confused, dizzy, or weak. Keep side rails up and bed in lowest position with wheels locked. Raise to sitting or standing positions slowly. Assist with ambulation. Monitor for orthostatic hypotension: ↓ BP, ↑ HR, dizziness, diaphoresis. If symptoms occur, return to supine position.
- To avoid unnecessary vasodilatation, treat fevers promptly. Cover with a light blanket to maintain body temp.
- Reassure patient, significant others that sensorium changes improve with therapy.
- Palpate peripheral pulses bilaterally in arms and legs. Use Doppler device if unable to palpate pulses.
- Monitor UO. Be alert to output <0.5 ml/kg/h for 2 consecutive h.

 # Miscellanea

CONSULT MD FOR
- Development of orthostatic changes in BP and HR
- SBP <90 mm Hg while fluid and blood replacement active
- Weight loss >2 kg/day
- UO <0.5 ml/kg/h × 2 h
- Complications such as ARF, fluid overload, worsening tissue perfusion

RELATED TOPICS
- Diabetes insipidus
- Diabetic ketoacidosis
- Metabolic acidosis, acute
- Metabolic alkalosis, acute
- Renal failure, acute
- Shock, hypovolemic

ABBREVIATIONS
ADH: Antidiuretic hormone
ARF: Acute renal failure
DI: Diabetes insipidus
ECF: Extracellular fluid
ICF: Intracellular fluid
SNS: Sympathetic nervous system

REFERENCES
Horne MM: Fluid and electrolyte disturbances. In Swearingen PL, Keen JH (eds): *Manual of critical care nursing,* ed 3, St Louis, 1995, Mosby.

Horne MM, Heitz UE, Swearingen PL: *Pocket guide to fluid, electrolyte, and acid-base balance,* ed 3, St Louis, 1997, Mosby.

Rose BD: *Clinical physiology of acid-base and electrolyte disorders,* ed 4, New York, 1994, McGraw-Hill.

Author: **Mima M. Horne**

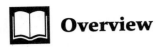 **Overview**

PATHOPHYSIOLOGY
Characterized by premature platelet destruction, resulting in ↓ platelet count to <100,000 μl. Platelet life span averages 1-3 days as a result of antiplatelet IgG and IgM antibodies, which destroy platelets in spleen's reticuloendothelial system. Believed to be an autoimmune response.

COMPLICATION
Intracranial hemorrhage the most serious complication (<1% of cases).

HISTORY/RISK FACTORS
Acute ITP: Viral infection occurring about 3 wks before hemorrhagic episode.
Chronic ITP
- Age 20-50
- Female
- Other hematologic disorders: autoimmune hemolytic anemia, hemophilia, Hodgkin's lymphoma, chronic lymphocytic leukemia
- Immune system disorders: HIV, SLE

CLINICAL PRESENTATION
Petechiae, purpura, prolonged bleeding common. Occasionally, epistaxis, GI and gingival bleeding, and ↑ menstrual flow occur.

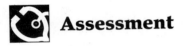 **Assessment**

PHYSICAL ASSESSMENT
Neuro: Altered LOC, other S&S of intracranial hemorrhage
Integ: Petechiae, purpura, most commonly on distal upper and lower extremities; ecchymosis; generalized bruising
Other: Joint tenderness, visual (retinal) disturbances resulting from bleeding into these areas

VITAL SIGNS/HEMODYNAMICS (if blood loss occurs)
RR: ↑
HR: ↑

BP: ↓
CVP/PAWP: ↓
CO: ↓
Other: Bradycardia, widened pulse pressure, irregular respirations if ICP ↑ result of hemorrhage

LABORATORY STUDIES
Platelets: ↓ to <50,000-75,000 μl.
Bleeding Time: Prolonged when platelets <100,000 μl.
Screening Coagulation Tests (PT, PTT, thrombin time): Nl; these tests measure nonplatelet components of coagulation pathway.
Platelet Antibody Screen: Positive findings attributable to presence of IgG and IgM antiplatelet antibodies.
CBC with Differential: Hgb and Hct may be ↓ because of blood loss or simultaneous hemolytic anemia (Evans syndrome); WBCs usually nl.

DIAGNOSTIC PROCEDURES
Bone Marrow Aspiration: Reveals megakaryocytes (platelet precursors) in nl or ↑ numbers with a "nonbudding" appearance, indicating defective platelet production.
Capillary Fragility Test: >1+ signals that >11 petechiae present in a 2.5 cm radial area on the skin, following prolonged application of BP cuff. Nl is 1+ or <10 petechiae.

Collaborative Management

Platelet Transfusion: Given for life-threatening hemorrhage only. Presence of antiplatelet antibodies renders prophylactic transfusions ineffective.
Glucocorticoid Therapy: Adrenocorticosteroids (eg, prednisone 1-2 mg/kg/day) effective to ↑ platelet count in 3-14 days after treatment initiation. If no improvement within 2-3 wks or excessive steroid doses required, splenectomy considered.
Splenectomy: Treatment of choice if refractory to glucocorticoids. Condition stabilizes in 70%-90% of splenectomies. Positive results attributed to removal of site of destruction of antibody-sensitized platelets.

IV Infusions of Gamma Globulin: Given 400 mg/kg/day for 5 days, resulting in ↑ platelets in 60%-70% of patients. Less effective with long-standing, chronic ITP.
Immunosuppression: Various drugs, including azathioprine, cyclophosphamide, vincristine, and cyclosporine, given alone or in combination with prednisone may be indicated in patients failing to respond to splenectomy or too unstable to be surgical candidates.
Other Pharmacotherapeutics: Anti-Rh immunoglobin, vinca "alkaloid-loaded" platelets, colchicine, danazol.
Plasmapheresis: Several days of plasma exchange transfusion to remove ≈ 1.0-1.5 × plasma volume and replace it with a suitable solution (eg, colloids, crystalloids, plasma). Reserved for life-threatening hemorrhage that is unresponsive to other measures.

PATIENT-FAMILY TEACHING
- Importance of avoiding all medications that may ↓ platelet aggregation, especially aspirin, ibuprofen
- During acute (bleeding) phase of ITP, how to perform oral hygiene using sponge-tipped applicators soaked in water or diluted mouthwash to help prevent gum bleeding
- Use of electric razor for shaving during and after bleeding phase of ITP
- S&S of impending bleeding: ↑ pulse rate, rapid breathing, ↑ bruising, painful joints, "spitting up" blood, blood in urine, and tarry stools
- Importance of avoiding Valsalva's maneuver (eg, straining at stool, lifting, forceful coughing or nose blowing), which could cause intracranial bleeding
- Necessity of avoiding tobacco products (particularly cigarettes) and excessive caffeine, which may cause vasoconstriction and thus impede platelet circulation through capillary network
- Importance of wearing Medic-Alert bracelet and obtaining pneumococcal vaccination if splenectomy has been performed

Nursing Diagnoses/Interventions

Altered protection r/t ↓ platelet count resulting in ↑ risk of bleeding
Desired outcomes: Within 72 h of treatment onset, patient exhibits no clinical signs of new bleeding or bruising episodes. Secretions and excretions negative for blood, and VS within 10% of nl for patient.

- Monitor for signs of bleeding: ↑ HR and RR; ↓ BP; oozing from invasive sites; bleeding mucous membranes; new or ↑ petechiae, purpura, bruising; hematuria; GI bleeding (ie, vomitus, gastric aspirate, stool with frank or occult blood). As available, monitor for ↓ CVP/PAWP, CO.
- Assess for abdominal pain, tenderness, guarding, or back pain, any of which may signal intraabdominal bleeding.
- Avoid IM injections and all venous and arterial punctures, which may cause intradermal bleeding. Hold pressure on invasive sites for ≥5 min, and subsequently apply a small pressure dressing or collagen-coated adhesive dressing (ie, Tipstop) over sites from which needles or IV catheters have been removed.
- Monitor platelet count qd for significant changes. Be alert for sustained low values (<100,000 μl).
- Avoid administering NSAIDs (eg, aspirin, ibuprofen).
- If severe menorrhagia present, confer with physician regarding need for progestational hormones for suppression of menses. If active bleeding occurs, administer supplemental O_2; replace lost volume with plasma expanders (eg, albumin, PPF, and/or blood products.)

Decreased adaptive capacity (or risk for same): Intracranial, r/t potential for intracranial hemorrhage (<1% of patients) secondary to ↓ platelet level
Desired outcomes: Throughout hospitalization, patient remains free of intracranial hemorrhage: orientation × 3; normoreactive pupils and reflexes; nl visual acuity, motor strength, coordination; absence of headache.

- Assess for signs of ↑ ICP: ↓ LOC, impaired pupillary responses (unequal or sluggish/absent response to light), weakness and paralysis, slow HR, and change in respiratory rate/pattern.
- Monitor for headache, visual disturbances, or motor dysfunction, which are symptoms of ↑ ICP.
- If signs of ↑ ICP are noted, take immediate measures to ↓ ICP and promote cerebral perfusion: eg, reduce stimulation, provide supplemental O_2, and optimize BP. Be aware that ICP can ↑ rapidly with severe bleeding, sometimes causing death within 1 h of onset. Signs of impending herniation include unconsciousness, failure to respond to deeply painful stimuli, decorticate or decerebrate posturing, Cushing's triad, nonreactive/fixed pupils.
- Optimize volume status. As indicated, use osmotic or other diuretic for ↑ ICP.
- Position with HOB slightly elevated (30-40 degrees) and neck in neutral position to ↓ ICP.
- Confer with physician regarding use of stool softeners or cough suppressants as necessary.

Pain r/t joint inflammation and injury secondary to bleeding into synovial cavity of the joint(s) or postop after splenectomy
Desired outcomes: Within 4 h of treatment onset, patient's subjective evaluation of discomfort improves as documented by a pain scale; nonverbal indicators are absent/↓. HR, RR, and BP are within 10% of baseline.

- Devise pain scale with patient, rating discomfort from 0 (no pain) to 10.
- Monitor for fatigue and malaise. As much as possible, eliminate activities that cause fatigue and malaise.
- Elevate legs to ↓ joint pain in lower extremities. Avoid knee flexion.
- ↓ stress on joints by supporting extremities with pillows, making sure bed is not "gatched" at knee.
- Consult with physician as necessary to adjust analgesics. Avoid meperidine for pain relief in elders because adverse effects are common.
- Evaluate anxiety level, and provide emotional support to control fear and anxiety. If patient becomes agitated, evaluate possible causes, including hypoxemia, poor pain or anxiety control, fluid and electrolyte imbalance, alcohol or drug withdrawal; intervene appropriately.

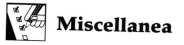 # Miscellanea

CONSULT MD FOR
- Platelet count <100,000 μl
- S&S of ↑ ICP: headache, visual disturbances
- S&S of bleeding: frank or occult blood in vomitus, stool, urine; new or ↑ petechiae, purpura, or bruising; ↑ HR, RR; ↓ BP

RELATED TOPICS
- GI bleeding: upper
- Herniation syndromes
- Immobility, prolonged
- Increased intracranial pressure
- Pain
- Shock, hemorrhagic

ABBREVIATION
PPF: Plasma protein fraction

REFERENCES
Baird MS: Hematologic dysfunctions. In Swearingen PL, Keen JH (eds): *Manual of critical care nursing,* ed 3, St Louis, 1995, Mosby.
Kimbrell JD: Acquired coagulopathies, *Crit Care Nurs Clin North Am* 5(3): 453-458, 1993.
Lottman MS, Thompson KS: Assessment of the hematologic system. In Phipps WJ et al (eds): *Medical-surgical nursing: concepts & clinical practice,* ed 5, St Louis, 1995, Mosby.
Secor VH: Mediators of coagulation and inflammation: relationship and clinical significance, *Crit Care Nurs Clin North Am* 5(3): 411-434, 1993.
Williams WJ: Approach to the patient. In Bentler E et al (eds): *Williams' hematology,* ed 5, New York, 1995, McGraw-Hill.

Author: **Marianne Saunorus Baird**

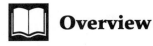 **Overview**

PATHOPHYSIOLOGY
Results in physiologic deconditioning with multiple body systems affected.
CV: ↑ HR and BP for submaximal workload, ↓ in functional capacity, ↓ in circulating volume, orthostatic hypotension, reflex tachycardia, ↑ risk of thromboemboli
Resp: Modest ↓ in pulmonary function, stasis of secretions, and possible atelectasis
MS: Loss of muscle mass, contractile strength; disuse joint contractures

HISTORY/RISK FACTORS
- Chronic or critical illness, debilitation
- Musculoskeletal, neurologic disorders
- Advanced age
- Glasgow Coma Score ≤12
- Multisystem injury
- Sensory/perceptual alterations

CLINICAL PRESENTATION
Generalized weakness, flaccidity, spasticity of extremities

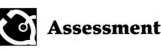 **Assessment**

PHYSICAL ASSESSMENT
Neuro: Variable, according to underlying condition
Resp: At rest, slight ↓ in tidal volume, possible ↓ breath sounds in bases and/or scattered crackles; with modest activity, ↑ rate and depth or dyspnea
CV: Orthostatic hypotension, reflex tachycardia, activity intolerance, dysrhythmias
GI: Dry oral mucous membranes, constipation, abdominal distention
MS: Muscle mass wasting, ↓ strength, ↓ ROM

VITAL SIGNS/HEMODYNAMICS
RR: ↑ with modest activity
HR: ↑ with modest activity
BP: Orthostatic hypotension
Temp: Nl
Other: Low-level activity may stress deconditioned cardiopulmonary system leading to evidence of heart failure: pulmonary congestion, ↑ PAWP, right → left shunt, ↓ BP, dysrhythmias, inadequate perfusion

LABORATORY STUDIES
Hct/Hgb: Checks for ↓, which could negatively impact oxygenation and activity tolerance.
ESR: May be ↑ if DVT develops.
Protein Status: Evaluated *via* serum albumin (3.5-5.5 g/dl), transferrin (180-260 mg/dl), thyroxine-binding prealbumin (20-30 mg/dl), and retinol binding protein (4-5 mg/dl). If hydration status nl and anemia absent, albumin and transferrin levels used as baseline indica-

tors of adequacy of protein intake and synthesis. Values for short turnover proteins (thyroxine-binding prealbumin and retinol binding protein) most useful for determining response to therapy.

Nitrogen Status: If more N taken in than excreted, N state is positive and an anabolic state exists. If more N excreted than taken in, N state is negative and a catabolic state exists. Accurate measurement of 24-h food intake and UO required to determine N state.

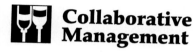 **Collaborative Management**

Oxygenation: Supplemental O_2, especially with initial activity, to ↑ cellular oxygenation impaired by cardiopulmonary deconditioning

Fluids: To optimize volume status and prevent orthostasis, since ↓ circulating volume likely

Nutrition: Enteral or parenteral nutrition to rebuild and prevent mobilization of protein stores and loss of muscle mass

Antiembolism Hose: To minimize orthostatic hypotension

Pneumatic Sequential Compression Stockings: To promote venous return and prevent DVT

Dietary Consultation: For nutritional assessment, protein supplementation

PT/OT Consultation: For complex cases (eg, active RA, spasticity, existing contractures)

Pharmacotherapy

For constipation: Bulk-building additives (psyllium), milk of magnesia, stool softeners (eg, docusate sodium), strong laxatives (eg, bisacodyl) as needed

For DVT prophylaxis: Aspirin, heparin, low-molecular-weight heparins (eg, enoxaparin, dalteparin), or warfarin as indicated in high-risk individuals

PATIENT-FAMILY TEACHING

- Importance of and procedure for ROM exercises
- Interventions for preventing deconditioning
- Importance of participation in self-care activities
- Indicators of DVT
- Calf-pumping and ankle-circling exercises
- Measures to prevent orthostatic hypotension

Nursing Diagnoses/Interventions

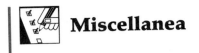 # Miscellanea

CONSULT MD FOR
- Evidence of DVT: positive Homans' sign, fever, tachycardia, ↑ ESR

RELATED TOPICS
- Nutrition, enteral and parenteral
- Pressure ulcers
- Pulmonary embolus, thrombotic

ABBREVIATIONS
ESR: Erythrocyte sedimentation rate
PVD: Peripheral vascular disease
RA: Rheumatoid arthritis
RPE: Rate (d) perceived exertion

Activity intolerance r/t prolonged bed rest, generalized weakness, and imbalance between O_2 supply and demand
Desired outcome: Within 48 h of discontinuing bed rest, patient exhibits cardiac tolerance to low-intensity exercise: HR ≤20 bpm over resting HR, SBP ≤20 mm Hg over or under resting SBP, RR ≤20 breaths/min, warm and dry skin, and absence of chest pain.
- Perform ROM exercises bid-qid on each extremity. Individualize exercise plan as follows:
    Type of exercise: Begin with passive exercises; progress to active assisted exercises. When patient able, supervise active isotonic exercises, during which patient contracts a selected muscle group, moves the extremity at a slow pace, and then relaxes the muscle group. Avoid isometric exercises in cardiac patients.
    Intensity: Begin with 3-5 reps. Assess tolerance by measuring HR and BP at rest, peak exercise, and 5 min after exercise. If HR or SBP ↑ >20 bpm or mm Hg over resting level, ↓ number of reps. If HR or SBP ↓ >10 bpm or mm Hg at peak exercise, this could be a sign the heart cannot meet this workload.
    Duration: Begin with 5 min or less. Gradually ↑ to 15 min.
    Frequency: Begin exercises bid-qid. As duration ↑, frequency can ↓.
    Assessment of exercise tolerance: Be alert to S&S that CV, Resp systems are unable to meet demands during exercise: ↑ SOB, ↓ SBP, diaphoresis, dysrhythmias, crackles.
- Ask patient to RPE during exercise, using 1-10 scale: RPE >3 should not be present with weak or light effort. ↓ intensity and ↑ frequency until RPE ≤3 attained.
- As condition improves, ↑ activity to include sitting in chair. Assess for orthostatic hypotension. ↑ amount of time spent in high-Fowler's position and move patient slowly.
- ↑ activity level by having patient perform self-care activities as tolerated.

Risk for disuse syndrome r/t mechanical, prescribed immobilization; severe pain; altered LOC
Desired outcome: Patient displays full ROM without verbal or nonverbal indicators of pain.
Note: Modification may be required for flaccidity (ie, immediately following stroke or SCI) to prevent subluxation; or for spasticity (ie, during recovery period for stroke or SCI) to prevent ↑ spasticity. Consult with PT or OT for these patients. ROM exercises contraindicated with rheumatologic disease during inflammatory phase and for dislocated or fractured joints.
- Be alert to areas prone to joint contracture: shoulder, wrist, fingers, hips, knees, feet.
- Change position at least q2h. Post a turning schedule at bedside.
    Place in position that achieves proper standing alignment: head neutral or slightly flexed on neck, hips extended, knees extended or minimally flexed, and feet at right angles to legs. Maintain this position with pillows, towels, or other positioning aids.
    To prevent hip flexion contractures, ensure prone or side-lying position, with hips extended for same amount of time as supine.
    When HOB must be ↑ 30 degrees, extend patient's shoulders and arms, using pillows to support position; allow fingertips to extend over pillows' edges.
    When able to place prone, move patient to end of bed and allow feet to rest between mattress and footboard. Put thin pads under angles of axillae, lateral aspects of clavicles.
- To maintain joints in neutral position, use pillows, rolled towels, blankets, sandbags, antirotation boots, splints, orthotics. Monitor involved skin at frequent intervals for altered integrity.
- Assess for footdrop: inspect for plantarflexion and evaluate ability to pull toes upward. To prevent footdrop, foam boots or "high top" tennis shoes may be used to support feet.
- For noncardiac patients needing greater help with muscle strength, assist with resistive exercises (eg, moderate weightlifting) to ↑ muscle size, endurance, and strength.
- If joints require rest, isometric exercises can be used for noncardiac patients. Teach how to contract a muscle group and hold contraction for a count of 5 or 10.
- Provide periods of uninterrupted rest between exercises/activities to help replenish energy.

Self-care deficit r/t cognitive, neuromuscular, or musculoskeletal impairment; or r/t activity intolerance attributable to prolonged bed rest
Desired outcome: Physical needs met by patient, nursing staff, or significant others.
- Assess self-care ability based on functional status (eg, hemiplegia, sensory/motor deficit).
- If patient comatose, meet all physical needs. Involve significant others in plan of care.
- For patient who is not comatose, promote as much self-care as patient is capable of providing. Assess for activity tolerance during self-care activities.
- If patient alert, keep toiletries and other necessary items within reach.
- Provide adequate time for performance of self-care activities.

- If visual impairment exists, place all objects within visual field. If diplopia present, apply an eye patch and alternate it between eyes q2-3h.
- Provide adjuncts that facilitate self-care, eg, built-up eating utensils, long-handled shoe horns, pick-up sticks, and similar aids.

Altered peripheral tissue perfusion r/t interrupted arterial and venous flow secondary to prolonged immobility

Desired outcomes: By discharge from ICU, patient has adequate peripheral circulation: nl skin color and temp and capillary refill >2 sec in peripheral extremities.

- Identify DVT risk: chronic infection, hx of PVD, smoking; advanced age, obesity, anemia.
- Assess for DVT: pain, redness, swelling, warmth in involved area; coolness; unnatural color or pallor; ↓ capillary refill; superficial venous dilatation distal to involved area; fever, ↑ HR, ↑ ESR.
- If asymptomatic for DVT, assess for positive Homans' sign: flex knee 30 degrees and dorsiflex foot. Posterior leg pain elicited with dorsiflexion may be a sign of DVT.
- Teach calf-pumping and ankle-circling exercises. Instruct patient to repeat each movement 10 times, performing each exercise qh, provided patient free of symptoms of DVT.
- Encourage deep breathing hourly.
- If not contraindicated by PVD, apply antiembolic or pneumatic sequential compression stockings. Remove stockings, and inspect underlying skin for irritation, breakdown q8h.
- Teach not to cross feet at ankles, knees. Raise foot of bed 10 degrees to ↑ venous return.
- Patients at risk for DVT may require anticoagulant therapy, eg, aspirin, sodium warfarin, heparin. Teach how to self-monitor for and report bleeding (epistaxis, bleeding gums, hematemesis, hemoptysis, melena, hematuria, ecchymoses).
- If patient prone to DVT, acquire and record bilateral baseline measurements of midcalf, knee, midthigh. Monitor these measurements qd.

Altered cerebral tissue perfusion (orthostatic hypotension) r/t interrupted arterial flow to brain secondary to prolonged bed rest

Desired outcome: Immediately after position change, cerebral perfusion adequate: HR <120 bpm and BP ≥90/60 mm Hg (or within 20 mm Hg of nl for patient), dry skin, nl skin color, no vertigo and syncope. HR, BP return to resting levels within 3 min.

- Assess for factors that ↑ risk of orthostatic hypotension (recent diuresis, diaphoresis, change in vasodilator therapy), altered autonomic control (diabetic cardiac neuropathy, denervation after heart transplant, Parkinson's disease, advanced age), or severe LV dysfunction.
- Apply antiembolic hose to help prevent orthostatic hypotension once patient mobilized. As necessary, supplement hose with elastic wraps to groin when patient is out of bed.
- Prepare for getting out of bed by urging position changes, calf pumping, ankle circles to ↑ venous return before rising. Consider use of tilt table to reacclimate to upright positions.
- Before mobilization: (1) check BP; (2) have patient dangle legs at bedside; ask about light-headedness or dizziness; (3) ↓ in SBP of 20 mm Hg and ↑ in HR, with vertigo or impending syncope, signal need for return to supine position; (4) if leg dangling tolerated, have patient stand at bedside; if no adverse S&S, begin ambulation.

Constipation r/t less than adequate fluid or dietary intake and bulk, immobility, lack of privacy, positional restrictions, and use of narcotic analgesics

Desired outcomes: Within 24 h of this diagnosis, patient verbalizes measures that promote bowel elimination and relates return of nl bowel pattern, character within 3-5 days.

- Assess patient's bowel hx: monitor bowel movements, diet, and I&O. Fecal impaction may result in oozing of liquid stool and be confirmed *via* digital examination. Use gentle digital examination for patients with cardiac disease.
- Auscultate for bowel sounds, which may be ↓/absent with paralytic ileus. High-pitched rushing sounds may be heard during abdominal cramping, suggesting early intestinal obstruction.
- If impaction suspected, use a gloved, lubricated finger to remove stool from rectum. Oil-retention enemas may presoften impacted stool.
- Unless contraindicated, encourage high-roughage diet and fluid intake of at least 2-3 L/day.
- Maintain patient's nl bowel habits whenever possible. Provide warm fluids before breakfast, and encourage toileting afterward to gain advantage of gastrocolic reflexes.
- Promote peristalsis: maximize activity level within limitations of endurance, therapy, pain.
- Use pharmacologic interventions as necessary. A suggested hierarchy of interventions: (1) bulk-building additives (psyllium), (2) mild laxatives (milk of magnesia), (3) stool softeners (docusate sodium), (4) potent laxatives and cathartics (bisacodyl), (5) medicated suppositories, and (6) enemas.
- Evaluate narcotic agents, calcium channel blockers, anticholinergics, and other medications that may cause constipation.

REFERENCES

Baas LS, Ross DG: Caring for patients on prolonged bed rest. In Swearingen PL, Keen JH (eds): *Manual of critical care nursing,* ed 3, St Louis, 1995, Mosby.

Hunt AH, Civitelli R, Halstead L: Evaluation of bone resorption: a common problem during impaired mobility, *Sci Nurs* 12(3): 90-94, 1995.

Lathers CM, Charles JB: Orthostatic hypotension in patients, bed rest subjects, and astronauts, *J Clin Pharmacol* 34(5): 403-417, 1994.

St. Pierre BA, Slaskerud JH: Clinical nursing implications for the recovery of atrophied skeletal muscle following bed rest, *Rehabil Nurs* 20(6): 314-317, 1995.

Von Rueden KT, Harris JR: Pulmonary dysfunction related to immobility in the trauma patient, *AACN Clin Issues (CDM)* 6: 212-28, 1995.

Authors: **Linda S. Baas and Dennis G. Ross**

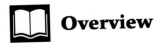 **Overview**

DESCRIPTION
May be used to treat lethal cardiac dysrhythmias; recommended for patients at risk for sudden cardiac death because of VT or VF that cannot be suppressed with pharmacologic therapy. In addition, sophisticated ICDs may be programmed to provide antitachycardic pacing, cardioversion/defibrillation, bradycardic pacing, and tiered therapy (multiple-staged responses to patient's precise rate/rhythm). The pulse generator, which is powered by lithium batteries, is surgically inserted into a "pocket" formed in the umbilical region.

HISTORY/RISK FACTORS
- CAD, recent MI
- Cardiomyopathy
- CABG or valvular heart surgery

CLINICAL PRESENTATION
Alterations in LOC, vertigo, syncope, activity intolerance, SOB, chest pain, palpitations, sensation of "skipped beats," anxiety, restlessness, sudden cardiac death

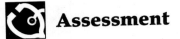 **Assessment**

PHYSICAL ASSESSMENT
Neuro: May experience altered mentation, weakness, fatigue, seizures
Resp: Crackles, dyspnea, tachypnea if LV failure present
CV: Irregular HR; paradoxical splitting of S_1, S_2; apical-radial pulse deficit; paradoxical pulse

VITAL SIGNS/HEMODYNAMICS
RR: May be ↑
HR: ↑, ↓, irregular
BP: ↓ during dysrhythmic episode
Temp: wnl
PAWP: May be ↑ as a result of heart failure
CO: ↓
ECG: Refractory VT, VF, bradycardia, heart block, other dysrhythmias

LABORATORY STUDIES
Serum Electrolytes: To identify electrolyte abnormalities that can precipitate dysrhythmias, most commonly hyperkalemia, hypokalemia, hypomagnesemia.
Drug Levels: To identify toxicities (eg, of digoxin, quinidine, procainamide, aminophylline, amiodarone) that can precipitate dysrhythmias.

DIAGNOSTIC PROCEDURES
Ambulatory Monitoring (eg, 24-h Holter monitor or cardiac event recorder): To identify subtle dysrhythmias and associated abnormal rhythms *via* patient's symptoms.
12/18-Lead ECG: To detect dysrhythmias and identify possible etiology.
EP Study: Invasive test in which two to three catheters placed in the heart, giving pacing stimuli at varying sites and voltages. Determines origin of dysrhythmia, inducibility, and effectiveness of drug therapy in dysrhythmia suppression.

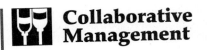 **Collaborative Management**

Antidysrhythmic Therapy: Various antidysrhythmic drugs, ablation therapy usually attempted before ICD placement.
Implantable Cardioverter/Defibrillator
Surgical approach: Median sternotomy incision usually performed if ICD concurrent with other cardiac procedures. Lateral thoracotomy may be used if there are adhesions from a previous CABG. Transvenous approach involves lead placement *via* subclavian cutdown.
Postop complications: Seroma at the generator "pocket," atelectasis, pneumothorax, thrombosis, and surgical site infection. Lead migration and lead fracture are the two most common structural problems.

PATIENT-FAMILY TEACHING
- S&S of dysrhythmias that necessitate medical attention: unrelieved and prolonged palpitations, chest pain, SOB, rapid pulse (>150 bpm), dizziness, and syncope.
- Posthospital discharge medications. Stress that it could be life-threatening to stop or skip these medications without prescribing physician's approval.
- Availability of support groups and counseling. Patients who survive sudden cardiac arrest may experience nightmares or other sleep disturbances at home. Explain that anxiety and fear, along with periodic feelings of denial, depression, anger, and confusion, are nl following this experience.
- Importance of leading nl and productive life, even though patient may fear breakthrough of life-threatening dysrhythmias.
- Advise patient and significant others to take CPR classes; provide addresses of community programs.
- Explanation of general low-fat and low-cholesterol diet and ↓ intake of products containing caffeine.
- Relaxation and stress-reduction techniques to ↓ sympathetic tone.
- Importance of wearing Medic-Alert bracelet/ID card with specific ICD information.

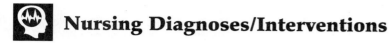 **Nursing Diagnoses/Interventions**

Decreased cardiac output r/t altered rate, rhythm, or conduction secondary to cardiac disease
Desired outcomes: Within 15 min of development of serious dysrhythmias, patient has adequate cardiac output: BP ≥90/60 mm Hg, HR 60-100 bpm, and NSR on ECG. PAP 20-30/8-15 mm Hg; PAWP ≤18 mm Hg (a reasonable outcome for these patients); RAP ≤7 mm Hg; and CO 4-7 L/min.

- Monitor heart rhythm continuously; note BP and symptoms if dysrhythmias occur or ↑ in occurrence.
- Document dysrhythmias with a rhythm strip or 12-lead ECG. Documentation of start of dysrhythmia may be important in diagnosing origin.
- If PA catheter present, note PAP, PAWP, and RAP; and monitor for ↓ cardiac output in response to dysrhythmias.
- Monitor laboratory data, particularly potassium, magnesium, and digoxin levels.
- Administer antidysrhythmias as prescribed; note response to therapy.
- Provide humidified O_2 as indicated.
- Maintain quiet environment, and administer pain medications promptly to prevent excessive sympathetic response.
- If life-threatening dysrhythmias occur, initiate immediate unit protocols or ACLS algorithms as necessary.
- When dysrhythmias occur, stay with patient; provide support and reassurance while performing assessments and administering treatment.
- Administer inotropes as prescribed to support BP and CO. Be aware that many inotropes are dysrhythmogenic.

Knowledge deficit: ICD procedure and follow-up care
Desired outcomes: Within 24-h period before procedure, patient and significant others describe rationale for procedure and method of insertion. Within 24-h period before discharge from hospital, patient and significant others describe postinsertion care and need for continued follow-up.

- Assess understanding of dysrhythmias and amount of detailed information desired.
- Discuss the following:
  Type of dysrhythmia, using rhythm strip and heart model to promote understanding.
  Need for temporary transvenous pacemaker insertion before ICD procedure, ie, to induce VT or VF or for emergency use should pacing be necessary before ICD insertion.
  Use of general anesthesia throughout procedure.
  Testing of ICD ability to terminate lethal dysrhythmias, which will occur in OR after implantation, before incision is closed. Explain that extra systoles will be given *via* temporary pacemaker to induce clinical rhythm.
  Reassurance that should the mechanism fail to terminate the dysrhythmia, patient can be paced in overdrive mode to abort the dysrhythmia.
  Importance of deep breathing, coughing (as necessary), and incentive spirometry exercises, which will be implemented immediately after surgery.
- Describe the procedure should ICD device deliver a "shock": the patient should be taken to emergency department *via* ambulance and physician notified at once. Teach patient to record number of "shocks" experienced.
- Explain that "shocks" during sinus rhythm may indicate a lead fracture in the ICD system. Usually this is detected while being monitored.

Risk for infection r/t invasive procedure into thorax
Desired outcome: Patient infection free: normothermia, WBC count ≤11,000 μl, negative cultures, and no S&S of infection at incision site or in the respiratory tract.

- Encourage deep breathing, coughing, and incentive spirometry exercises q2h, and encourage early ambulation. Provide analgesics before scheduled breathing exercises.
- Assess incision site for warmth, erythema, swelling, and drainage. The presence of a seroma, which has the same symptoms as incision site infection, may be confirmed by chest x-ray or CT scan.
- Monitor temp q2-4h, being alert to ↑ >38.6° C (101.5° F).
- Monitor CBC count for ↑ WBCs.
- Teach patient and significant others S&S of infection, both of incision site and respiratory tract. Explain that confusion, disorientation, and low-grade fevers may be the first S&S of respiratory tract infection in elders.

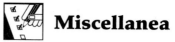 **Miscellanea**

CONSULT MD FOR
- Serious or sustained dysrhythmias
- Suspected lead fracture in ICD system: shocks during NSR
- Evidence of infection: warmth, erythema, swelling at ICD insertion site, temp >38.6° C (101.5° F), change in sputum production, cough, altered mentation

RELATED TOPICS
- Antidysrhythmic therapy
- Ventricular fibrillation
- Ventricular tachycardia

ABBREVIATION
EP: Electrophysiologic

REFERENCES
Cardiac Pacemakers, Inc: Caring for patients with AICD™ Automatic Implantable Cardioverter Defibrillator Systems, 1991.
Davidson T et al: Implantable cardioverter defibrillators: a guide for clinicians, *Heart Lung* 23(3): 205-215, 1994.
Steuble B: Dysrhythmias and conduction disturbances. In Swearingen PL, Keen JH (eds): *Manual of critical care nursing*, ed 3, St Louis, 1995, Mosby.

Author: **Cheryl L. Bittel**

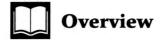 **Overview**

PATHOPHYSIOLOGY

ICP dynamics based on cranial volume/pressure relationship. Three volumes exist: brain, blood, and CSF, which normally exert a pressure <15 mm Hg. With any volume ↑ there is pressure ↑. Compensatory mechanisms, eg, shunting of CSF or vasoconstriction, activate to ↓ volume. With brain injury, compensatory mechanisms overwhelmed and extrinsic measures become necessary to maintain nl volume/pressure relationship. Treatment based on relationship between ICP and CPP. CPP = MAP − ICP. Goal: to maintain CPP >60 mm Hg and ↓ ICP to ≤15 mm Hg.

HISTORY/RISK FACTORS

- Head injury
- Ruptured cerebral aneurysm, subarachnoid hemorrhage
- Cerebral contusion
- Encephalitis, meningitis
- Stroke, ischemic or hemorrhagic

CLINICAL PRESENTATION

Deteriorating LOC, headache, rapid or irregular RR, sluggish or absent pupillary reaction to light, pupil dilatation, change in behavioral response to stimuli (motor deficits, abnormal posturing, agitation, somnolence).

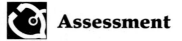 **Assessment**

PHYSICAL ASSESSMENT

Baseline data include assessment of mental status, cranial nerves, motor status, sensory status, reflexes. Thereafter, neurologic assessment based on clinical status, including Glasgow Coma Score (see Appendix) and baseline/ongoing assessment of CV, Resp, GI, GU, and Integ status for changes.

Early Findings: Headache, dizziness, vomiting, memory loss, ↓ attention and concentration skills, mental confusion, lethargy, sluggish/unequal pupillary response to light, respiratory changes if not mechanically ventilated

Later Findings: Deteriorating LOC, stupor, coma; fixed, dilated pupils; bradycardia, widening pulse pressure; abnormal posturing; absence of all responses

VITAL SIGNS/HEMODYNAMICS

RR: Varies based on compression of midbrain or brainstem structures

HR: Nl, ↓, or ↑

BP: Nl or ↑ SBP with widened pulse pressure if brainstem compression present

Temp: Nl or ↑

ICP: ↑

CPP: ↓

Other: Cushing's triad is a late sign of mechanical compression or severe brainstem metabolic dysfunction.

ECG: Prominent U waves, ST-segment changes, notched T waves, and prolonged QT interval. Also will show bradycardia, SVT, and ventricular dysrhythmias.

LABORATORY STUDIES

CSF Analysis: Useful in determining infection. Analysis includes color, turbidity/cloudiness, RBC/WBC counts, protein, glucose, electrolytes, Gram's stain, and C&S. Sample taken from ventriculostomy; LP not done while pressure ↑.

IMAGING

Skull X-ray: Detects structural deficits caused by head injury.

CT Scan: Gray and white matter, blood, and CSF detectable because of their radiologic densities. CT capable of diagnosing cerebral hemorrhage, infarction, hydrocephalus, cerebral edema, and structural shifts.

MRI: Identifies type, location, and extent of injury. Provides detailed spatial resolution, follows metabolic processes, and detects structural changes.

Cerebral Angiography: Adjunct study in diagnosing brain injury; also used if CT scan unavailable.

DIAGNOSTIC PROCEDURE

EEG: Useful in detecting areas of abnormal brain activity (irritability) and generalized brain activity, coma, or suspected brain death.

Collaborative Management

Focuses on treating emergent pathology and controlling ICP.

Management of ICP Dynamics: Monitoring systems provide digital display of ICP, but CPP must be calculated (CPP = MAP − ICP). Maintain ICP ≤15 mm Hg and CPP 60-80 mm Hg. Variety of monitoring types:

Intraventricular cannula: Placed in lateral ventricles *via* burr hole for CSF drainage, drug administration. Rapid CSF drainage can result in collapsed ventricles or subdural hematoma.

Subarachnoid screw: Placed into SAS *via* drill hole. Has less risk of infection than cannula. Cannot drain CSF.

Epidural sensor: Placed into epidural space. Has lowest risk of infection; easy to insert. Cannot directly measure CSF or drain it.

Intraparenchymal: Placed into intraparenchyma *via* twist drill. Easy to insert; measures pressure directly. Risk of intracerebral bleeding and infection; cannot drain CSF.

Reduction of ICP by CSF Drainage: Intraventricular or ventriculostomy systems used to drain CSF and ↓ ICP. Keep drainage collection bags at level of ear tragus or higher to prevent excessive CSF flow caused by higher-to-lower pressure gradient.

Hyperventilation: Controls ICP by ↓ $Paco_2$, thereby vasoconstricting cerebral vessels and causing ↓ cerebral blood volume. Accomplished *via* mechanical ventilation. $Paco_2$ maintained at 30-35 mm Hg and Pao_2 at >80 mm Hg.

Diuresis Therapy: ↓ cerebral brain volume by extracting fluid from brain's intracellular compartment. Dehydration is a major complication; strict attention to serum electrolytes and osmolality necessary.

Reduction of Metabolic Demand: Important because cerebral blood supply must match demand in order to maintain cerebral function.

$AVDo_2$ and jugular bulb O_2 saturation: Monitored to help determine if blood flow to brain matches metabolic requirements. Differentiates ischemia vs hyperemia.

Sedating agents: Use of continuous drips of midazolam HCl (Versed), propofol (Diprivan), and narcotic analgesics, such as fentanyl citrate (Sublimaze) or morphine sulfate, common. Nondepolarizing agents, eg, vecuronium bromide (Norcuron), also used.

Seizure control: Seizures greatly ↑ brain's metabolic demand; prophylaxis used as necessary. Phenytoin (Dilantin) commonly used, as well as diazepam (Valium) and phenobarbital.

Barbiturate coma: Pentobarbital sodium (Nembutal) is drug of choice. Continuous ICP, hemodynamic monitoring, and controlled ventilation necessary because barbiturates induce profound cardiac and cerebral depression.

Maintaining body temp: For every 1° C ↑, there is a 10%-13% ↑ in metabolic rate. Fever etiology important because it influences treatment choice.

Central fever: Directly attributed to brain injury; reflects derangement in hypothalamic function. Characterized by lack of sweating, no diurnal variation, plateaulike elevation up to 41° C (105.8° F), absence of tachycardia, persistence for days/wks. Controlled with external cooling rather than with antipyretics. Hypothermia therapy may ↑ metabolic demand *via* shivering. Distal extremities wrapped in bath towels or chlorpromazine (Thorazine) given to control shivering.

Peripheral fever: Associated with wound or CNS infections, other bacterial invasion. Characterized by sweating, diurnal variation, response to antipyretic agents, and tachycardia.

Cytokine release: Associated with brain injury; responds to ASA instead of acetaminophen.

BP Control: Hypotension causes ↓ cerebral perfusion. Dopamine HCl used at doses of 3-5 μg/kg/min to maintain CPP. Hypertension causes ↑ capillary permeability and petechial hemorrhage. Managed with labetalol HCl (Normodyne) or nitroprusside sodium (Nipride).

Modifying Nursing Care Activities That ↑ ICP: Sustained ↑ in ICP (>5 min) must be avoided. Space activities such as bathing, turning, and suctioning to prevent stair-step ↑ in ICP.

Suctioning: Only as needed; preoxygenate with 100% O_2; limit 2 passes of ≤10 sec each; follow each pass with 60 sec hyperventilation using 100% O_2; use suction catheter with outer-to-inner diameter ratio of 2:1.

Flexion, extension, and lateral movements: Maintain neck in neutral position to prevent flexion and lateral movements that can significantly ↑ ICP. For patients with poor neck control, stabilize neck with towel rolls or sandbags.

HOB positioning: Adjust based on clinical response. Desired effect is improvement in perfusion and ↓ in ICP.

Surgical Intervention: To evacuate mass lesions (epidural, subdural, intracranial hematomas), place ICP monitoring system, elevate depressed skull fractures, débride open wounds and brain tissue, and repair dural tears or scalp lacerations. Frontal lobectomy may be necessary to control severe ↑ in ICP.

PATIENT-FAMILY TEACHING

- Signs of ↑ ICP: headache (new, worsening), vomiting, confusion, sleepiness, visual disturbances, dizziness
- Importance of avoiding Valsalva maneuver, agitation, continuous coughing

Nursing Diagnoses/Interventions

Decreased adaptive capacity: Intracranial, r/t compromise of pressure/volume dynamics
Desired outcome: Patient exhibits adequate intracranial adaptive capacity within 72 h of treatment: orientation × 3 (or consistent with baseline); equal and normoreactive pupils; BP wnl for patient; HR 60-100 bpm; RR 12-20 breaths/min with eupnea (or controlled ventilation); ICP 0-15 mm Hg; CPP 60-80 mm Hg.

- Assess qh for ↑ ICP and herniation (altered mentation, ↑ BP with widening pulse pressure, irregular respirations, ↑ headache, pupillary changes).
- Calculate CPP by means of the formula

$$CPP = MAP - ICP$$
$$where \quad MAP = \frac{SBP + 2(DBP)}{3}$$

- Assess for ↑ ICP (ICP >15 mm Hg) or CPP <60 mm Hg.
- Assess for, treat conditions that can cause ↑ restlessness with concomitant ↑ ICP: hypoxia, hypoxemia, pain, fear, anxiety.
- Implement measures that help prevent ↑ ICP and herniation:
  Maintain complete bed rest.
  Maintain HOB in position that keeps ICP ≤15 mm Hg and CPP >60 mm Hg.
  Avoid neck hyperflexion, hyperextension, or hyperrotation.
  Maintain quiet, relaxing environment.
  Minimize vigorous activity; assist with ADL.
  Maintain adequate ventilation to prevent cerebral hypoxia.
  Avoid vigorous, prolonged suctioning.
  Hyperoxygenate with 100% O_2 before/during/after suctioning.
  Maintain normovolemia.
  Monitor and record I&O.
- Administer antihypertensives to prevent hypertension.
- If ↑ ICP occurs suddenly, perform hyperinflation with a manual resuscitator at 100% O_2 at ≥50 breaths/min to ↓ $Paco_2$.
- If prescribed for acutely ↑ ICP, administer bolus of mannitol (ie, 1.5-2.0 g/kg, as a 15%-25% solution infused over 30-60 min). Monitor carefully to avoid profound fluid/electrolyte disturbances.

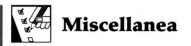 ## Miscellanea

CONSULT MD FOR
- ICP >15 mm Hg, CPP <60-80 mm Hg
- S&S of ↑ ICP: change in LOC, behavior, or motor movement; pupillary changes
- $Paco_2$ >30 mm Hg, Pao_2 <80 mm Hg
- Potential complications: meningitis, wound site infection, URI, UTI, seizures, stress ulcers, herniation

RELATED TOPICS
- Agitation syndrome
- Diabetes insipidus
- Head injury
- Herniation syndrome
- Immobility, prolonged
- Intracranial surgery
- Syndrome of inappropriate antidiuretic hormone
- Vasodilator therapy
- Vasopressor therapy

ABBREVIATIONS
$AVDo_2$: Arterial venous difference in O_2
CPP: Cerebral perfusion pressure
SAS: Subarachnoid space
URI: Upper respiratory infection

Impaired gas exchange r/t $\downarrow$ O_2 supply and $\uparrow$ CO_2 production secondary to $\downarrow$ ventilatory drive occurring with pressure on respiratory center, imposed inactivity

Desired outcomes: $Paco_2$ 25-30 mm Hg during hyperventilation, 35-40 mm Hg as ICP stabilizes, and 35-45 mm Hg by time of discharge from ICU. By time of discharge, patient has adequate gas exchange: Pao_2 $\geq$80 mm Hg, RR 12-20 breaths/min with eupnea, no adventitious breath sounds.

- Assess respiratory rate, depth, rhythm. Auscultate lung fields for breath sounds q1-2h. Monitor for abnormal respiratory patterns.
- Deliver O_2 within prescribed limits. Assess for hypoxia: confusion, agitation, restlessness, irritability. Cyanosis is a late indicator.
- Ensure patent airway *via* proper neck positioning and suctioning as necessary. Hyperoxygenate before and after each suction pass.
- Monitor ABGs. Be alert for hypoxemia (Pao_2 <80). Monitor for $Paco_2$ $\geq$25-30. $\uparrow$ levels may $\uparrow$ cerebral blood flow and thus $\uparrow$ ICP. Maintain O_2 saturation >94%.
- Assist with turning q2h to promote lung drainage/expansion and alveolar perfusion.
- Evaluate need for artificial airway in patients unable to maintain airway patency or adequate ventilatory effort.
- Monitor ICP for sustained $\uparrow$ during respiratory care activities. Modify activities to avoid sharp or sustained $\uparrow$.

Ineffective thermoregulation r/t hypothalamic injury or compression

Desired outcome: Patient becomes normothermic (or temp controlled as much as possible).

- Monitor for signs of hyperthermia: temp >38.33° C (101° F), pallor, absence of perspiration, torso warm to touch.
- Obtain specimens for blood, urine, sputum cultures as indicated for fever, suspected infection.
- Be alert to signs of meningitis: fever, chills, nuchal rigidity, Kernig's sign, Brudzinski's sign.
- Assess wounds for S&S of infection: erythema, tenderness, purulent drainage.
- If patient hyperthermic, remove excess clothing and administer tepid baths, hypothermic blanket, or ice bags to axilla or groin.
- Administer antipyretics such as acetaminophen or ASA, depending on fever etiology.
- Administer chlorpromazine to treat or prevent shivering.
- Keep environmental temp at optimal range.
- Assess for possible drug fever reaction, which can occur with antimicrobial therapy.

Impaired corneal tissue integrity (or risk for same) r/t irritation associated with corneal drying and $\downarrow$ lacrimal production secondary to altered consciousness or cranial nerve damage

Desired outcome: Patient's corneas remain moist and intact.

- Assess for corneal irritation: red and itching eyes, ocular pain, foreign body sensation.
- Lubricate eyes q2h with isotonic eye drops or ointment.

REFERENCES

Colice G: How to ventilate patients when ICP elevation is a risk, *J Crit Ill* 8(9): 1003-1020, 1993.

Davis A et al: Neurologic dysfunctions. In Swearingen PL, Keen JH (eds): *Manual of critical care nursing,* ed 3, St Louis, 1995, Mosby.

German K: Intracranial pressure monitoring in the 1990's, *Crit Care Nurs Q* 17(1): 21-32, 1994.

Prendergast V: Current trends in research and treatment of intracranial hypertension, *Crit Care Nurs Q* 17(1): 1-8, 1994.

Author: **Alice Davis**

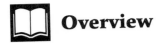 **Overview**

DESCRIPTION

A counterpulsation device that temporarily assists the failing heart by ↓ afterload and ↑ coronary artery perfusion. Phase one involves balloon inflation, termed "diastolic augmentation," causing ↑ blood flow to coronary arteries and other vital organs such as the kidneys. Phase two is systolic unloading or balloon deflation. Aortic pressure ↓ rapidly, reducing afterload and resistance to flow. With reduced afterload, ventricle empties more completely, stroke volume ↑, and myocardial O_2 consumption ↓.

Benefits
- ↑ BP, CO, UO
- Improved mental alertness, warm extremities, palpable peripheral pulses, ↓ chest pain
- Improvement of ischemic ECG changes

Complications
- Aortic dissection, thrombus formation, ↓ circulation to involved leg
- Obstruction to left subclavian artery blood flow and to renal and mesenteric arteries
- Paraplegia (from spinal artery thrombosis)
- Pneumonia and dermal ulcers caused by prolonged immobility

HISTORY/RISK FACTORS

Indicated for patients with:
- Cardiogenic shock, LV failure, unstable angina, cardiomyopathy
- Precardiac and postcardiac surgery, post-PTCA complications
- Refractory ventricular dysrhythmias caused by ischemia

CLINICAL PRESENTATION

- Severe LV failure or cardiogenic shock: dyspnea at rest, extreme weakness, activity intolerance, ↓ mental acuity, lethargy, chest pain, ↓ UO
- May have pallor, diaphoresis, cyanosis

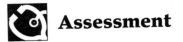 **Assessment**

PHYSICAL ASSESSMENT

Will show S&S of cardiogenic shock
Neuro: Agitation, restlessness, confusion, lethargy, unresponsiveness
Resp: Hyperventilation, dyspnea at rest
CV: Pulses weak and often irregular, pulsus alternans, S_3 or S_4 sounds
GU: Oliguria
Integ: Cold, clammy, mottled skin

VITAL SIGNS/HEMODYNAMICS

RR: ↑
HR: ↑
BP: ↓ with narrow pulse pressure
Temp: Nl or ↓
RAP: ↑
PAP: ↑
PAWP: ↑
SVR: >1200/dynes/sec/cm^{-5}
CO: <4 L/min
CI: <2.0 L/min/m^2
Svo$_2$: $<50\%$
ECG: Dysrhythmias may occur as a result of infarction, injury to areas of the conduction system or myocardium, or electrolyte imbalance. ST-segment change may denote ischemia or injury patterns.

Collaborative Management

IABP: Introducer sheath inserted through femoral artery, and balloon passed through sheath into thoracic aorta. Catheter placed so that balloon is below left subclavian artery and above renal artery. If the balloon migrates in either direction, arterial flow can be obstructed. Balloon is then connected to pump console. Pumping timed according to ECG or arterial pressure waveform. Balloon inflation occurs with diastole; deflation occurs with systole.

Pharmacotherapy: Treatment with positive inotropes, diuretics, and afterload reduction continued during IABP therapy. IV dextran or heparin given to prevent clot formation on balloon.

Supplemental O_2: Necessary to optimize tissue oxygenation.

Hemodynamic Monitoring: Arterial and PA catheters inserted to guide therapy. Also useful to evaluate progress toward myocardial tissue healing, evidenced by improved CO. If continuous Svo$_2$ monitoring available, it is used to evaluate effectiveness of IABP by reflecting tissue oxygenation. ↓ values or those $<50\%$ signal ↑ tissue extraction of O_2 and suggest poor tissue perfusion.

PATIENT-FAMILY TEACHING

- Purpose, expected results, anticipated sensations of IABP insertion
- Need to keep affected leg straight and remain on complete bed rest
- Passive foot exercises without hip flexion
- Importance of notifying staff member if pain, numbness, or tingling occurs in involved leg

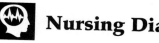 **Nursing Diagnoses/Interventions**

Decreased cardiac output (or risk for same) r/t negative inotropic changes and rate, rhythm, and conduction alterations secondary to ischemia or injury

Desired outcomes: Within 24 h of this diagnosis, patient has adequate cardiac output: BP within acceptable range, NSR on ECG, HR 60-100 bpm, peripheral pulses >2+ on 0-4 + scale, UO ≥0.5 ml/kg/h, CI ≥2.5 L/min/m^2, Svo$_2$ 60%-80%.

- Monitor BP, PAP, RAP, Svo$_2$, and heart rate and rhythm continuously. Monitor PAWP, SVR, and CO qh. Be alert to the following: ↑ PAWP, ↓ CO, ST-segment changes, ectopic heartbeats, ↓ Svo$_2$, or ↑ SVR.
- Monitor UO qh and BUN and creatinine values qd. ↑ BUN (>20 mg/dl) and serum creatinine (>1.5 mg/dl) can occur with low UO and ATN.
- Monitor bilateral peripheral pulses and extremity color and temp q2h.
- Provide humidified O$_2$ therapy or maintain ventilator settings to maintain Spo$_2$ >92%.
- Regulate IV inotropic agents, such as dobutamine, dopamine, and amrinone, to maintain CI ≥2.5-4 L/min/m^2. Monitor for side effects: tachydysrhythmias, ventricular ectopy, headache, and angina.
- Regulate afterload-reducing agents such as nitroprusside and NTG to maintain SVR <1200 dynes/sec/cm^{-5}. Monitor for drug side effects: hypotension, headache, dizziness, nausea, vomiting, and cutaneous flushing.
- Administer diuretic agents for ↑ PAWP (>16-18 mm Hg). Monitor for S&S of hypokalemia (eg, weakness, dysrhythmias), a potential side effect of diuretics.
- Minimize sympathetic response, which could ↑ SVR/afterload: administer analgesics, anxiolytics; provide quiet environment; limit other stressful stimuli.

Altered peripheral tissue perfusion (or risk for same): Involved leg, r/t compromised arterial blood flow secondary to arterial wall dissection by sheath or thrombus formation

Desired outcome: Throughout duration of hospitalization, patient has adequate perfusion in the involved leg: peripheral pulses >2+ on 0-4+ scale, nl color and sensation, warmth, full motor function; and absence of bleeding and tingling in the involved leg.

- Monitor circulation in affected leg q30min × 4 and q2h thereafter. Assess pulses, temp, color, sensation, and mobility of toes in the involved leg.
- Protect heel of involved foot, using sheepskin, occlusive opaque dressing, or heel protector.
- Have patient perform passive foot exercises without bending leg at hip: foot flexion/extension, foot circles, quadriceps setting. A pneumatic compression device may be beneficial.
- Administer IV dextran or heparin to prevent clots from forming on the balloon. Monitor for signs of bleeding, including ↓ Hct, abdominal pain, hematuria, oral bleeding, or blood-tinged mucus.
- Keep HOB at ≤30 degrees to prevent catheter kinking and to avoid catheter migration, which would occlude subclavian artery.
- Assess for the following signs of balloon migration: ↓ left radial pulse, sudden ↓ in UO (<0.5 ml/kg/h), flank pain, dizziness, ↓/absent bowel sounds, ↓ balloon augmentation.
- When the balloon is no longer needed, maintain regular balloon inflation to prevent clot formation until balloon can be removed.

Altered protection r/t risk of bleeding/hemorrhage secondary to mechanical coagulopathy and IV anticoagulants

Desired outcome: Throughout hospitalization, patient has no symptoms of bleeding: secretions and excretions negative for blood; absence of abdominal pain or ecchymoses.

- Monitor PTT, ACT, and platelet level qd. Be alert to levels outside of therapeutic range. Anticoagulation and platelet destruction *via* IABP ↑ risk of bleeding and hemorrhage.
- Monitor Hct and Hgb qd. ↓ levels may signal presence of bleeding.
- Test GI drainage and stool prn for blood.
- Maintain bleeding precautions: avoid peripheral sticks, injury; provide gentle mouth care.
- Test gastric pH prn. Administer gastric acid–neutralizing drugs, such as antacids or histamine H$_2$-receptor antagonists.
- Monitor groin and any other puncture site(s) q8h and prn.

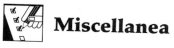 **Miscellanea**

CONSULT MD FOR
- PAWP >16-18 mm Hg or other established range
- CI <2.5 L/min/m^2
- Svo$_2$ progressively ↓ or <50%
- ECG changes: hemodynamically significant dysrhythmias, ST-segment elevation or depression
- UO <0.5 ml/kg/h × 2 h
- ↓ peripheral pulses, pallor, paresthesias, coolness of involved leg
- Signs of balloon migration: ↓ left radial pulse, sudden ↓ UO, flank pain, dizziness

RELATED TOPICS
- Acute tubular necrosis: oliguric
- Cardiac surgery: CABG
- Cardiac surgery: valvular disorders
- Cardiomyopathy
- Heart failure, left ventricular
- Hemodynamic monitoring

ABBREVIATION
ATN: Acute tubular necrosis

REFERENCES

Datascope Corp: *Mechanics of intraaortic balloon counterpulsation,* 1989, Montvale, NJ, Datascope Corp.

Goran S: From counterpulsation to paralysis: a case presentation, *Crit Care Nurse* 16(2): 54-57, 1996.

Quaal SJ: *Comprehensive intraaortic balloon pumping,* ed 2, St Louis, 1993, Mosby.

Shinn A, Joseph D: Concepts of intraaortic balloon counterpulsation, *J Cardiovasc Nurs* 8(2): 45-60, 1994.

Tueller BT: Cardiogenic shock. In Swearingen PL, Keen JH (eds): *Manual of critical care nursing,* ed 3, St Louis, 1995, Mosby.

Author: **Cheryl L. Bittel**

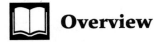

Overview

DESCRIPTION
Performed for removal of space-occupying lesion such as tumor, hematoma, or abscess; repair of vascular abnormality such as aneurysm or AVM; drainage of CSF from ventricular system; correction of skull fractures; tissue biopsy; seizure control; and pain reduction.

POSTSURGICAL COMPLICATIONS
↑ ICP: Some cerebral edema expected; usually peaks at 72 h.
Stroke: Occurs as result of BP fluctuations that lead to cerebral ischemia and infarction or as result of cerebral arterial vasospasm.
Hydrocephalus: Usually caused by slowing or complete stoppage of CSF flow through ventricular system attributable to edema, bleeding, scarring, or obstruction.
DI and SIADH: DI results from ↓ ADH production, which leads to excessive UO. SIADH results from ↑ release of ADH, which leads to reabsorption of large amounts of water *via* renal tubules, with concurrent loss of large amounts of sodium. Both conditions can cause serious fluid and electrolyte problems.
Intracranial Bleeding: May be intracerebral, intracerebellar, subarachnoid, subdural, extradural, or intraventricular.

Seizures: Occur because of surgical trauma, blood irritating cerebral tissue, edema, hypoxia, hypoglycemia, preexisting seizure disorder.
CNS Infection: Meningitis, encephalitis, ventriculitis.
CSF Leak: Results from tear or rupture of dura mater.
DVT, Pulmonary Emboli: Result of prolonged bed rest and immobility.
GI Bleeding/Cushing's Ulcer: Result of stress from surgery, ↑ SAS activity.

CLINICAL PRESENTATION
Preop and postop neurologic deficits should be noted and documented, including ↓ LOC, communicative and cognitive deficits, motor and sensory impairment, and cranial nerve deficit.

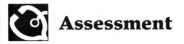

Assessment

PHYSICAL ASSESSMENT
Neuro
LOC: ↓; improves as anesthesia effects and cerebral edema subside.
Communicative and cognitive deficits
  Broca's (expressive, motor, nonfluent) dysphasia: Patient comprehends situation and follows commands appropriately but cannot articulate wishes and needs.

  Wernicke's (receptive, sensory, fluent) dysphasia: Patient does not understand situation and cannot follow commands appropriately.
Motor and sensory deficits: Motor deficits caused by weakness or paralysis resulting from injury to or edema of primary motor cortex and corticospinal (pyramidal) tracts. Sensory deficits caused by injury to or edema of primary sensory cortex or sensory association areas of the parietal lobe. Improvement seen as cerebral edema subsides.
Cranial nerve impairment: Surgery for brainstem and cerebellar lesions may involve significant cranial nerve manipulation, with considerable postop cranial nerve deficit (see Appendix).
Resp: Hyperventilation or irregular RR with ↑ ICP; crackles with atelectasis, neurogenic pulmonary edema.
CV: Possible dysrhythmias, bradycardia, ↑ SBP. Positive Homans' sign if DVT present.
GI: Paralytic ileus possible. Hyperacidity and bleeding may occur.

VITAL SIGNS/HEMODYNAMICS
RR: ↑, ↓; irregularly irregular
HR: Possible ↓ with brainstem compression
BP: Possible ↑ SBP and ↓ DBP (widened pulse pressure); ↓ if hemorrhage associated with SCI

Temp: ↓ or ↑ with thermoregulatory failure caused by injury or irritation of hypothalamic temperature-regulating centers. ↑ temp may signal infection; detrimental because of ↑ in brain's metabolic needs, potentially leading to ↑ in cerebral blood flow.

Resp Patterns: Apneustic, cluster, ataxic (see Appendix)

Other: ↓ SVR, ↓ PAWP if hemorrhagic

LABORATORY STUDIES

CSF Analysis: Useful in determining infection or blood in CSF.

Hct/Hgb: To check for blood loss caused by GI bleeding.

Electrolytes: Checks for imbalance attributable to DI, SIADH.

IMAGING

CT Scan: Gray and white matter, blood, and CSF detectable. CT can diagnose cerebral hemorrhage, infarction, hydrocephalus, cerebral edema, and structural shifts.

MRI: Provides detailed spatial resolution, follows metabolic processes, and detects structural changes.

Collaborative Management

Surgical Approach

Supratentorial: To remove or correct problems in frontal, temporal, or occipital lobes.

Infratentorial (suboccipital): To remove cerebellar and brainstem lesions.

Transsphenoidal: Gains access to pituitary gland to remove tumors, control bone pain associated with metastatic cancer.

Resp Support: O_2, mechanical ventilation provided as indicated to maintain oxygenation and prevent ↑ $Paco_2$.

ICP Monitoring: Uses variety of techniques (intraventricular cannula, subarachnoid screw, epidural or intraparenchymal fiberoptic sensor). Monitoring systems provide digital display of ICP, but CPP must be calculated. Maintain CPP between 60-80 mm Hg.

CSF Drainage: Intraventricular or ventriculostomy systems used to drain CSF and ↓ ICP. Keep drainage collection bags at level of ear tragus or higher to prevent excessive CSF flow.

Positioning: HOB elevated 30 degrees to promote venous drainage, thereby ↓ ICP.

- With infratentorial approach, supporting neck muscles altered. Patient requires support of head, neck, and shoulders when turning.
- After craniectomy do not position on side on which bone has been removed.
- After extensive surgery in which there is a large intracranial space, do not position on operative side immediately after surgery; this may cause a sudden shift in intracranial contents, with subsequent hemorrhage, herniation.

Pharmacotherapy

Corticosteroids: To ↓ cerebral edema.

Osmotic diuretics (eg, mannitol, urea): To control cerebral edema causing ↑ ICP.

Anticonvulsants (eg, phenytoin, phenobarbital): To prevent seizures.

Antibiotics: To prevent or treat postop infection.

Antipyretics: For elevated temp.

Analgesics: To treat or control pain caused by headache. Drugs of choice are acetaminophen alone or with codeine sulfate.

Acid suppression therapy (eg, antacids, histamine H_2-receptor antagonists): To prevent gastric erosion, ulceration, bleeding.

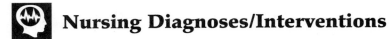 **Nursing Diagnoses/Interventions**

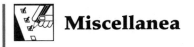 **Miscellanea**

Decreased adaptive capacity: Intracranial, r/t ↓ CPP associated with postop cerebral edema or complications of intracranial hemorrhage or infection

Desired outcomes: Within 12-24 h of treatment/interventions, patient has adequate intracranial adaptive capacity: equal/normoreactive pupils; RR 12-20 breaths/min with eupnea; HR 60-100 bpm; ICP 0-15; CPP 60-80. No clinical indicators of ↑ ICP: headache, vomiting, altered mentation, pupillary changes. By time of transfer from ICU, patient oriented × 3 with bilaterally equal extremity strength and tone or a stable deficit.

- Assess neurologic status at least qh. Monitor pupils, LOC, and motor activity; perform cranial nerve assessments as indicated. Changing LOC is an early indicator of ↑ ICP. Changes in size/reaction of pupils, ↓ in motor function (eg, hemiplegia, abnormal flexion posturing), and cranial nerve palsies all indicate deterioration and possible impending herniation.
- Monitor VS at frequent intervals. Changes in respiratory pattern, fluctuations in BP and pulse, widening pulse pressure, and slow HR could herald impending herniation. Measures must be taken to ↓ ICP (see list below).
- Monitor for ↑ ICP: restlessness, confusion, irritability, lethargy, irregularly irregular respiratory pattern, abnormal posturing, seizures, pupillary changes, bradycardia, widening pulse pressure.
- Maintain CPP at 60-80 mm Hg. Be alert to ↓ MAP (<80) or excessive ↑. Record ICP and CPP qh until stable. Consult physician if pressure changes significantly.
- Prevent fluid volume excess, which could ↑ cerebral edema, by precise delivery of IV fluids at consistent rates. Administer mannitol and furosemide at prescribed intervals to promote diuresis and ↓ intracranial brain volume.
- Treat ↑ in ICP immediately. Implement the following for ↑:
    Elevate HOB to 30 degrees.
    Loosen constrictive objects around neck.
    If recently repositioned, return to original position.
    Maintain head in neutral position.
    Assess for factors contributing to ↑ ICP: distended bladder, fear, anxiety.
    Evaluate activities (eg, suctioning, bathing, dressing changes) that ↑ pressure; reorganize care plan accordingly.
    Hyperoxygenate before and after suctioning.

Impaired gas exchange r/t ↓ O_2 supply and ↑ CO_2 production secondary to ↓ ventilatory drive occurring with pressure on respiratory center, imposed inactivity, and possible neurologic pulmonary edema

Desired outcomes: $Paco_2$ 25-30 mm Hg during hyperventilation, 35-40 as ICP stabilizes, and 35-45 by time of transfer from ICU. By time of transfer, patient has adequate gas exchange: orientation × 3, Pao_2 ≥80 mm Hg, RR 12-20 breaths/min with eupnea, no adventitious breath sounds.

- Assess respiratory rate, depth, rhythm. Auscultate lung fields for breath sounds q1-2h. Monitor for irregularly irregular respiratory patterns.
- Deliver O_2 within prescribed limits. Assess for hypoxia: confusion, agitation, restlessness, irritability. Cyanosis is a late indicator.
- Ensure patent airway *via* proper neck positioning and suctioning as necessary. Hyperoxygenate before/after each suction pass.
- Monitor ABGs. Be alert for hypoxemia (Pao_2 <80). Monitor for $Paco_2$ ≥25-30. ↑ levels may ↑ cerebral blood flow and thus ↑ ICP.

CONSULT MD FOR
- ICP >15 mm Hg, CPP <60-80 mm Hg
- S&S of ↑ ICP: altered mentation, ↑ SBP with widening pulse pressure, pupillary changes, irregular respirations
- $Paco_2$ >30 mm Hg, Pao_2 <80 mm Hg
- Potential complications: DI (excessive UO), SIADH (hyponatremia, water intoxication, ↓ BP), GI bleeding, meningitis, encephalitis, ventriculitis, DVT, pulmonary emboli.

RELATED TOPICS
- Cerebral aneurysm
- Diabetes insipidus
- GI bleeding: upper
- Head injury
- Immobility, prolonged
- Increased intracranial pressure
- Mechanical ventilation
- Status epilepticus
- Subarachnoid hemorrhage
- Syndrome of inappropriate antidiuretic hormone

ABBREVIATIONS
ADH: Antidiuretic hormone
AVM: Arteriovenous malformation
CPP: Cerebral perfusion pressure
DI: Diabetes insipidus
SAS: Subarachnoid space
SIADH: Syndrome of inappropriate antidiuretic hormone

- Assist with turning q2h, within limits of patient's injury, to promote lung drainage/expansion and alveolar perfusion. Unless contraindicated, raise HOB to 30 degrees to promote gas exchange.
- Encourage deep breathing at frequent intervals to promote oxygenation. Perform chest physiotherapy as indicated. Chest physiotherapy may ↑ ICP.
- Evaluate need for artificial airway if patient unable to maintain airway patency or adequate ventilatory effort.

Risk for infection (CNS) r/t inadequate primary defenses secondary to skull fracture, penetrating wounds, craniotomy, intracranial monitoring, or bacterial invasion resulting from pneumonia or iatrogenic causes

Desired outcome: Patient remains infection free: normothermia, WBCs ≤11,000 μl, negative culture results, HR ≤100 bpm, BP wnl for patient, and no agitation, purulent drainage, and other clinical indicators of infection.

- Assess VS for indicators of CNS infection: ↑ temp, ↑ RR, possible ↓ BP.
- Monitor for systemic infection: discomfort, malaise, agitation, restlessness. Monitor WBCs for ↑ or shift to left.
- Inspect cranial wounds for erythema, tenderness, swelling, purulent drainage. Obtain culture as indicated.
- Apply loose sterile dressing (sling) to collect CSF drainage. Do not pack. Record drainage amount, color, character.
- Caution against coughing, sneezing, nose blowing, or other Valsalva-type maneuvers, since these activities can further damage the dura.
- Use orogastric tubes with basilar skull fractures or severe frontal sinus fracture.
- Ensure timely administration of antibiotics. Reschedule any delayed by >1 h.
- Apply basic principles for care of invasive device used with ICP monitoring:
    Good hand washing technique before caring for patient.
    If patient not comatose, discourage from touching device; apply restraints *only* if necessary to keep patient from harm. Restraints can ↑ ICP by causing straining.
    Maintain aseptic technique during care of device, following agency protocol.

Risk for injury r/t potential for development of gastric ulcer (Cushing's) or gastritis secondary to hyperacidic state

Desired outcomes: Result of gastric pH test >5. Patient has no symptoms of gastric ulcer and gastritis: gastric secretions and stool negative for blood; HR ≤100 bpm; BP wnl for patient; absence of midepigastric discomfort.

- Monitor for GI bleeding or ulceration: midepigastric discomfort, occult or frank blood in stool or gastric secretions, ↓ BP, ↑ HR.
- Monitor Hct or Hgb results qd for ↓ values.
- Test gastric drainage pH q4h. Administer H₂-receptor antagonists and/or antacids as prescribed to maintain pH >5.
- Implement measures to prevent ulceration and hemorrhage:
    Give steroids, aspirin, phenytoin, other medications that irritate gastric mucosa with meal or snack.
    Limit patient's intake of acidic or spicy foods, as well as caffeine-containing substances.

REFERENCES

Arbour R: What you can do to reduce i.c.p. . . . intracranial pressure, *Nursing* 23(11): 41-46, 1993.
Davis M, Lucatorto M: Mannitol revisited, *J Neurosci Nurs* 26(3): 170-174, 1994.
Guy J, Gelb AW: Perioperative management of intracranial aneurysms, *Curr Rev Post Anesth Care Nurses* 15(10): 78-84, 1993.
Stowe AC: Care of the patient following intracranial surgery. In Swearingen PL, Keen JH (eds): *Manual of critical care nursing*, ed 3, St Louis, 1995, Mosby.

Author: **Ann Coghlan Stowe**

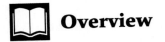 **Overview**

DESCRIPTION
Required when disease processes cause impaired alveolar ventilation, V/Q mismatch, or gas diffusion disturbances that lead to respiratory failure.

INDICATIONS
- Inability to maintain $Pao_2 \geq 60$ mm Hg despite supplemental O_2
- $Paco_2 \leq 60$ mm Hg during spontaneous ventilation
- $Svo_2 < 50\%$: associated with impaired tissue oxygenation

COMPLICATIONS
Barotrauma: Occurs when ventilatory pressures ↑ intrathoracic pressure.
Tension Pneumothorax: Develops when pressurized air enters thoracic cavity, resulting in sudden and sustained ↑ in peak inspiratory pressure. If pneumothorax suspected, disconnect ventilator and ventilate manually using 100% O_2. Prepare for immediate emergency chest tube placement.
GI Complications: Peptic ulcers with profound hemorrhage. Prophylactic acid-suppression therapy routinely initiated. Gastric dilatation can occur as a result of large amounts of swallowed air. If left untreated, vomiting, aspiration, and paralytic ileus may develop.

Hypotension with ↓ CO: May develop because of ↓ venous return secondary to ↑ intrathoracic pressure. PEEP, especially at levels >20 cm H_2O, ↑ severity of this phenomenon.
↑ ICP: Occurs as a result of ↓ venous return, which causes intracranial pooling of blood.
Fluid Imbalance: ↑ production of ADH occurs as a result of ↑ pressure on baroreceptors in thoracic aorta causing water retention. Diuretics may be necessary.
Anxiety: R/t discomfort, loss of control, and perception that health status is threatened. Hypoxemia and air hunger contribute to anxiety.

CLINICAL PRESENTATION
Varies according to underlying disease process and severity of respiratory failure. May include difficult/labored breathing, headache, anxiety, confusion, palpitations, diaphoresis, coma, respiratory arrest.

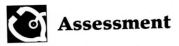 **Assessment**

PHYSICAL ASSESSMENT
Neuro: Mental status alterations, anxiety, agitation
Resp: Dyspnea, tachypnea, crackles, wheezes, rhonchi; cyanosis if respiratory compromise advanced
CV: Tachycardia, dysrhythmias

VITAL SIGNS/HEMODYNAMICS
RR: ↑
HR: ↑

BP: ↑ initially; ↓ results from vasodilatation if respiratory failure advanced
Temp: Nl; ↑ with infection
CVP/PAWP: ↓ with dehydration; ↑ with cor pulmonale
PAP: ↑ caused by hypoxic pulmonary vasoconstriction
CO: Depends on hydration, presence of heart failure; ↓ if PEEP >20 cm H_2O
SVR: ↑ initially; ↓ with advanced respiratory failure

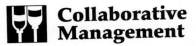 **Collaborative Management**

VENTILATOR TYPES
Volume-Cycled: Delivers preset volume of gas (tidal volume) independent of changes in airway resistance or lung compliance. Equipped with safety valves that terminate inspiration when peak pressures excessive.
Pressure-Cycled: Terminates inspiration once preset pressure reached, at which time patient exhales passively. When airway resistance ↑ because of mucous secretions or bronchospasm, inspiratory cycle may terminate before adequate tidal volume delivered. Used only for stable patients with nl lung compliance.
Negative Pressure: Generates subatmospheric pressure to thorax and trunk to initiate respiration; does not require intubation for use. Iron lung, chest cuirass shell, and poncho chest shell are examples.

MODES OF MECHANICAL VENTILATION

Controlled Mechanical Ventilation: Delivers preset tidal volume at preset rate, ignoring patient's own ventilatory drive. Use restricted to CNS dysfunction, drug-induced sedation, or severe chest trauma when inspiratory effort contraindicated.

Assist-Control Ventilation: Delivers preset tidal volume when patient initiates negative pressure respiratory effort (inspiration). Machine sensitivity adjusted to prevent hyperventilation when RR ↑.

Synchronized Intermittent Mandatory Ventilation: Standard mode of ventilation. Delivers preset tidal volume at preset rate. Patient can breathe spontaneously between ventilator breaths. Ventilator synchronized to deliver breath when patient initiates inspiration.

PEEP: Applies pressure at end of expiration. This pressure counteracts small airway collapse so that gas exchange can occur. Poorly ventilated lung areas can then participate in adequate gas exchange, thereby ↓ shunting. Does not improve lung function if problem is poor perfusion. Generally, PEEP pressures range from 2.5-10 cm H_2O. Higher pressures (>35 cm H_2O) may be used. Using this pressure can ↑ intrathoracic pressure and ↓ venous return, RV filling pressures, and CO. May cause or potentiate hypotension and shock, particularly with volume depletion.

CPAP: Similar to PEEP but used independently of mechanically delivered breaths and continuously throughout ventilatory cycle.

High-Frequency Ventilation and Oscillation: Small tidal volumes delivered at high rates. Resulting lower airway and intrathoracic pressures may ↓ risk of complications caused by barotrauma and circulatory depression. Ideal for major airway disruption. Techniques include high-frequency positive pressure ventilation, high-frequency jet ventilation, and high-frequency oscillation.

Inverse-Ratio Ventilation: Inspiratory phase prolonged and expiratory phase shortened. Nl I/E ratio = 1:2-4. During IRV the I/E ratio ↑ to >1:1 (eg, 2:1), thereby promoting alveolar recruitment, which improves oxygenation at lower levels of PEEP. A paralyzing agent and sedation may be necessary to minimize discomfort.

CAUSES OF HIGH-PRESSURE ALARM SITUATIONS

Factors That ↑ Airway Resistance
- Coughing or need for suctioning
- Exhaling against ventilator breaths
- Kinks in ventilator circuitry
- Water or expectorated secretions in circuitry

- Bronchospasm
- Change in position that restricts chest wall movement
- Breath stacking

Factors That ↓ Lung Compliance
- Pneumothorax
- Pulmonary edema
- Atelectasis
- COPD
- Worsening of underlying disease process

CAUSES OF LOW-PRESSURE ALARM SITUATIONS

- Patient disconnected from machine
- Leak in airway cuff or circuitry
- Displacement of airway above vocal cords
- Loss of compressed air source

PATIENT-FAMILY TEACHING

- Purpose, expected results, and anticipated duration of mechanical ventilation
- Nonverbal system of communication (eg, communication board, erasable marker board)
- Function of alarm system and means for alerting staff in event of dysfunction
- Progressive muscle relaxation techniques

Nursing Diagnoses/Interventions

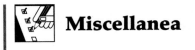 # Miscellanea

Impaired gas exchange (or risk for same) r/t altered O_2 supply secondary to nonphysiologic tidal volume distribution associated with mechanical ventilation

Desired outcome: Patient has adequate gas exchange: PaO_2 >60 mm Hg, $PaCO_2$ 35-45 mm Hg, SpO_2 ≥92%, SvO_2 ≥60%, and RR 12-20 breaths/min.

- Position to enable maximal alveolar ventilation and comfort. During mechanical ventilation the lung's dependent portion receives less tidal volume than do nondependent areas. Follow body positioning protocol:

    Analyze SpO_2, SvO_2, and ABG results in different positions to determine adequacy of ventilation.

    In unilateral lung disease, position with healthy lung down.

    In bilateral lung disease, position in right lateral decubitus position, since right lung has more surface area. If ABGs show tolerance of left lateral decubitus position, alternate positions.

- Turn q2h or more frequently according to tolerance.
- Auscultate over artificial airway to assess for leaks.
- Assess ventilator for proper functioning and settings. Ensure that circuits are tight and alarms are set.
- Keep ventilator circuitry free of condensed water and expectorated secretions.
- Monitor ABGs for ↓ PaO_2 or ↑ $PaCO_2$, which indicates inadequate gas exchange. ↓ $PaCO_2$ (<35 mm Hg) with ↑ pH (>7.35) may signal mechanical hyperventilation. Even modest alkalosis may cause dysrhythmias with heart disease or administration of inotropic medications.
- Keep manual resuscitator at bedside in case of malfunctioning equipment.

Ineffective airway clearance (or risk for same) r/t altered anatomic structure secondary to presence of ET or tracheostomy tube

Desired outcome: Patient maintains patent airway: clear breath sounds and absence of respiratory distress.

- Assess breath sounds q2h.
- Monitor for restlessness and anxiety.
- Suction secretions prn, based on presence of coughing, adventitious breath sounds, or ↑ airway resistance signaled by high-pressure alarm.
- Maintain humidification of inspired gas to prevent drying of tracheal mucosa and thickening of tracheobronchial secretions.
- Maintain artificial airway in secure and proper alignment using tape straps or other device.
- Maintain correct temp (32°-36° C) of inspired gas. Cold air irritates airways; hot air may burn lung tissue.

Ineffective breathing pattern (or risk for same) r/t anxiety secondary to use of mechanical ventilation

Desired outcome: Patient exhibits stable RR of 12-20 breaths/min (synchronized with ventilator) and absence of restlessness, anxiety, lethargy, and/or sounding of high-pressure alarm.

- Reassure that ventilatory support may be temporary until underlying pathophysiologic process has resolved.

CONSULT MD FOR

- Suspected tension pneumothorax: ↑ RR, agitation, sustained ↑ in peak inspiratory pressures, ↓ breath sounds on affected side, tracheal deviation, cyanosis
- Change in color, character of tracheobronchial secretions
- Failure to maintain PaO_2 >60 mm Hg, $PaCO_2$ <45 mm Hg, SpO_2 ≥90%-92%, and SvO_2 ≥60% at prescribed FiO_2 and ventilator settings
- Positive sputum cultures, temp ≥38.33° C (101° F), purulent tracheobronchial secretions

RELATED TOPICS

- Adult respiratory distress syndrome
- Agitation syndrome
- Mechanical ventilation, weaning
- Pneumothorax
- Respiratory failure, acute

ABBREVIATIONS

ADH: Antidiuretic hormone
I/E: Inspiration to expiration
IRV: Inverse-ratio ventilation
SvO₂: Mixed venous oxygen saturation

- Explain all procedures before initiating them. Keep patient informed of progress.
- Provide reliable means of signaling need for assistance (eg, call light) to minimize anxiety.
- Monitor for resistance to mechanical ventilation: frequent sounding of high-pressure alarm when patient breathes against mechanical inspiration or mismatch of patient's RR and ventilator cycle.
- Monitor respiratory rate and quality for signs of respiratory distress.
- When initiating mechanical ventilation, stay with patient until respirations are under control. Reassure that synchronized respirations will be possible with relaxation. Encourage progressive muscle relaxation.
- Give pain medication or sedative for restlessness, after ensuring that restlessness is not caused by ↓ Pao_2 or ↑ $Paco_2$.

Risk for infection r/t ↑ environmental exposure, tissue destruction (during intubation or suctioning), and invasive procedures

Desired outcome: Patient infection free: normothermia, WBCs <11,000 μl, clear sputum, and negative sputum culture.

- Assess for infection: temp >38° C (100.4° F), tachycardia, purulent sputum.
- Wash hands before/after contact with respiratory secretions of any patient and before/after contact with patient undergoing intubation.
- Recognize that bacteria and spores are introduced easily during suctioning. Follow standard techniques:

    Use sterile technique during suctioning.

    Suction tracheobronchial tree before oropharynx.

    Consider use of closed system for suctioning.

    Change suction canisters and tubing q24h or according to agency policy.

    Use single-use saline for suctioning. If not available, tightly recap bottle; dispose of unused portion within 24 h.

- To ↓ risk of infection caused by trauma or cross-contamination, suction prn only.
- Provide oral hygiene at least q4-8h to prevent overgrowth of nl flora and aerobic gram-negative bacilli.
- Recognize water reservoirs and ventilator equipment as potential sources of contamination by following these precautions:

    Use sterile fluids in all humidifiers and nebulizers.

    Change all ventilatory circuitry within established time frame or sooner if soiled with secretions.

    Avoid emptying condensed water or expectorated secretions back into patient.

    Empty water traps on tubing during each ventilator check.

    When disconnecting ventilatory circuits, keep ends sterile by placing on sterile gauze pads.

    Keep connectors on manual resuscitator bags clean and free of secretions between use. Change according to agency policy.

- Maintain seal on artificial airway cuff to prevent aspiration of oral secretions.
- Keep cuff sealed and HOB elevated 30-45 degrees for continuous gastric feedings. Monitor for intolerance (abdominal distention, residual feedings >100 ml).

REFERENCES

Bizek KS: Optimizing sedation in critically ill, mechanically ventilated patients, *Crit Care Nurs Clin North Am* 7(2): 315-325, 1995.

Frederick C: Noninvasive mechanical ventilation with the iron lung, *Crit Care Nurs Clin North Am* 6(4): 831-840, 1994.

Howard C: Respiratory dysfunctions. In Swearingen PL, Keen JH (eds): *Manual of critical care nursing,* ed 3, St Louis, 1995, Mosby.

Knebel A, Strider VC, Wood C: The art and science of caring for ventilator-assisted patients: learning from our clinical practice, *Crit Care Nurs Clin North Am* 6(4): 819-829, 1994.

Mee CL: Ventilator alarms: how to respond with confidence, *Nursing* 25(7): 60-64, 1995.

Author: **Cheri A. Goll**

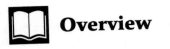 **Overview**

DESCRIPTION
Can involve any of the following: O_2, PEEP, mechanical ventilation, and artificial airway. Successful weaning depends more on overall patient status than on technique. Physiologic factors include CV status, hydration, electrolyte and acid-base status, and nutrition. Other factors must also be considered: comfort, sleep pattern, emotional state, and ability to cooperate. In addition, pulmonary function parameters must be met before weaning is initiated.

GOALS FOR WEANING
RR: <25 breaths/min
Tidal Volume: At least 3-5 ml/kg
HR/BP: Within 15% baseline
Pao_2: ≥60 mm Hg
$Paco_2$: ≤45 mm Hg
pH: 7.35-7.45
O_2 Saturation: ≥90%

CLINICAL PRESENTATION
Before weaning, patient must be able to accomplish the following:
- Initiate spontaneous respirations and move adequate volumes of air for sustained periods of time
- Have sufficient muscle strength to expel tracheobronchial secretions

Patient not ready for weaning if the following present:
- Shallow, rapid respirations or use of accessory muscles

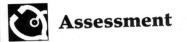 **Assessment**

PHYSICAL ASSESSMENT (optimal findings before weaning)
Neuro: Awake, oriented; evidence of intact brainstem without impairment of medullary breathing centers
Resp: Regular breathing rate, rhythm; clear, minimal tracheobronchial secretions
CV: Absence of hemodynamically significant dysrhythmias

VITAL SIGNS/HEMODYNAMICS (optimal findings before weaning)
RR: 12-20 spontaneous breaths/min
HR: 60-110 bpm or within baseline
BP: Nl
CVP/PAWP: Nl
CO: Nl or within baseline
SVR: Nl

PULMONARY FUNCTION PARAMETERS FOR WEANING
- Minute ventilation (tidal volume × RR): ≤10 L/min
- Negative inspiratory force: ≥20 cm H_2O
- Maximum voluntary ventilation: ≥2 × resting minute ventilation
- Tidal volume: 5-10 ml/kg
- ABGs: baseline; or Pao_2 ≥60 mm Hg, $Paco_2$ ≤45 mm Hg, pH 7.35-7.45
- Fio_2: ≤0.40

Collaborative Management

METHODS EMPLOYED FOR WEANING
T-piece: When patient taken off ventilator, spontaneous respiratory effort initiated for ↑ periods of time, thereby building strength and endurance for independent respiratory effort. CPAP may be added to prevent alveolar collapse, thus enabling more efficient gas exchange.
Intermittent Mandatory Ventilation: Ventilator-generated breaths ↓ gradually while patient builds strength and endurance. Most widely accepted method. If multiple failures at weaning occur, T-piece method may be used, starting with 1-2 min off ventilator, followed by 58-59 min on, with gradual reversal of this ratio until patient breathes independently.
Pressure Support Ventilation: Assists nl breathing pattern with positive airway pressure applied during inspiration; 3-5 cm H_2O pressure support added, causing significantly ↓ WOB. Patient controls rate, inspiratory time, tidal volume, and inspiratory flow rate. When inspirations stop, positive pressure stops. Gradually ↓ amount of pressure support.

PATIENT-FAMILY TEACHING
- Purpose, procedure, expected results, anticipated sensations for weaning
- Coughing, deep-breathing exercises
- Progressive muscle relaxation techniques

Nursing Diagnoses/Interventions

Impaired gas exchange (or risk for same) r/t altered O_2 supply secondary to weaning from mechanical ventilation

Desired outcomes: Patient has adequate gas exchange: Pao_2 >60 mm Hg, $Paco_2$ <45 mm Hg, Spo_2 ≥92%, Svo_2 ≥60%, and pH 7.35-7.45 (or values within 10% of baseline).

- Maintain a comfortable position to promote ventilation. Semi-Fowler's position often promotes effective respirations.
- Observe for indicators of hypoxia: tachycardia, tachypnea, cardiac dysrhythmias, anxiety, restlessness.
- Assess and record VS q15min for first h of weaning, then qh if stable. Consult physician for significant findings.
- Check tidal volume after first 15 min of weaning and prn. Within 5-10 ml/kg optimal.
- Obtain specimen for ABG analysis 20 min after weaning has been initiated. Monitor Spo_2 and Svo_2 for abnormal or ↓ values.

Anxiety r/t perceived threat to health status secondary to weaning

Desired outcome: Within 4 h of initiation of weaning process, patient expresses attainment of emotional comfort and is free of signs of harmful anxiety as evidenced by HR ≤100 bpm, RR ≤20 breaths/min, and BP wnl for patient.

- Before initiating weaning, discuss weaning plans with patient and significant others. Explain that patient's condition will be assessed at frequent intervals during the process. Provide time for questions and answers.
- Stay with patient during initial phase of weaning, keeping patient informed of progress. Provide positive feedback for positive efforts.
- Teach progressive muscle relaxation technique, which may ↓ anxiety and fear and thus relax chest muscles.
- Instruct patient to take deep breaths. This may provide confidence of knowing that he/she can initiate and sustain respirations independently.
- Leave call light within reach before leaving bedside. Reassure that help is nearby.

Miscellanea

CONSULT MD FOR
- ↑ WOB during weaning
- Deteriorating Spo_2 or inability to maintain Spo_2 ≥90%-92%; Pao_2 <60 mm Hg; $Paco_2$ >45 mm Hg
- Deteriorating mental status: agitation, lethargy
- Cyanosis

RELATED TOPICS
- Mechanical ventilation
- Psychosocial needs, patient
- Respiratory failure, acute

ABBREVIATION
Svo_2: Mixed venous oxygen saturation

REFERENCES
Arbor R: Weaning a patient from a ventilator, *Nursing* 23(2): 52-56, 1993.
Bouley G: The experience of dyspnea during weaning, *Heart Lung* 21(5): 471-476, 1992.
Bridges E: Transition from ventilatory support: knowing when the patient is ready to wean, *Crit Care Nurs Q* 15(1): 14-20, 1992.
Cason CL, DeSalvo SK, Ray WT: Changes in oxygen saturation during weaning from short term ventilator support after coronary artery bypass graft surgery, *Heart Lung* 23(5): 368-375, 1994.
McConnell E: Performing pulse oximetry, *Nursing* 24(10): 23, 1994.

Author: **Cheri A. Goll**

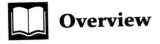 **Overview**

PATHOPHYSIOLOGY

Inflammation of brain and spinal cord, which involves the meninges (dura, arachnoid, pia), invades brain surface, and damages cranial nerves.

Bacterial: Most common form; associated with previous/ongoing infection, injury such as open/penetrating skull fracture.

Streptococcus pneumoniae: Leading cause of adult meningitis.

Neisseria meningitidis: Likely to occur with complement component deficiencies.

Haemophilus influenzae: Most common cause in children.

Listeria monocytogenes: Occurs in immuno-compromised states. Outbreaks associated with consumption of contaminated dairy products.

Gram-negative species: *Escherichia coli, Klebsiella, Proteus,* and *Pseudomonas;* especially in elders, immunocompromised, and head-injured patients.

Fungal: Most common infection, often caused by *Cryptococcus neoformans,* an opportunistic infection seen in hematologic malignancies, organ transplantation, sarcoidosis, AIDS.

HISTORY/RISK FACTORS

- Open/penetrating or basilar/facial skull fracture
- Shunt occlusion/malfunction
- Craniotomy
- Otitis media, sinusitis
- Bacteremia
- Immunocompromise (hematologic malignancies, organ transplantation, AIDS)
- Complement component deficiency (nephrotic syndrome, hepatic failure, SLE)
- Diabetes mellitus
- Alcoholism
- Advanced age

CLINICAL PRESENTATION

Fever, altered mental status, nausea & vomiting, and positive meningeal signs (stiff neck or nuchal rigidity, Brudzinski's, Kernig's)

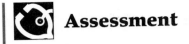 **Assessment**

PHYSICAL ASSESSMENT

Streptococcus pneumoniae: Altered mental status progressing quickly to coma; positive meningeal signs. Possible profuse sweats, myalgia, seizures, cranial nerve palsies.

Neisseria meningitides: Early macular erythematous rash progressing rapidly to petechial and purpuric states, conjunctival petechiae, aggressive behavior. Possible dysfunctions of cranial nerves VI, VII, and VIII (see Appendix) and aphasia.

Haemophilus influenzae: Early development of deafness. Possible petechial rash.

Listeria monocytogenes: Seizures and focal deficits such as ataxia, cranial nerve palsies, nystagmus seen early.

Gram-negative species: In elders, fever may be absent and headache may not be reported. Confusion and pneumonia common.

Cryptococcus neoformans: Persistent fever and headache lasting wks. Positive meningeal signs, alterations in mental status, photophobia possible.

VITAL SIGNS

RR: ↑
HR: ↑
BP: NI, ↑, or ↓
Temp: ↑
Other: If ↑ ICP present, the following may occur: irregular respirations, bradycardia, ↑ SBP, widened pulse pressure.

LABORATORY STUDIES

CSF Analysis: Obtained *via* intraventricular catheter, ventriculostomy, LP. LP contraindicated with ↑ ICP (eg, head injury, focal neurologic deficits, papilledema). Antibiotic therapy should not be delayed if CSF samples cannot be obtained. CSF analyzed for cell count, glucose, protein, Gram's stain, acid-fast stain, C&S.

Blood, Urine, Sputum Cultures: Help identify infecting organisms.

Serum WBCs: To check for infection.

IMAGING

CT Scan with Contrast and MRI: To r/o hydrocephalus; detect exudate, abscesses, and intracranial pathology, including tumors.

Collaborative Management

PHARMACOTHERAPY
Antimicrobial Therapy

Bacterial: Cefotaxime or ceftriaxone, penicillin G or ampicillin, or dexamethasone. For *Staphylococcus aureus:* nafcillin or oxacillin (if methicillin-resistant, use vancomycin). For *Mycobacterium tuberculosis:* isoniazid, rifampin, ethambutol, and pyrazinamide.

Fungal: For *C. neoformans:* Fluconazole or amphotericin B with or without flucytosine.

Anticonvulsant Therapy: Initiated if seizures observed; may be given prophylactically. Phenytoin, benzodiazepines, barbiturates may be used.

Adjunctive Therapies: Dexamethasone to ↓ inflammation; controversial. If given, administered 15-20 min before antimicrobial medications and for 4 days. Monoclonal antibodies have been investigated because of their ability to ↓ inflammation.

GENERAL

Nutritional Support: Patients who are able continue oral feeding along with IV therapy. Enteral or parenteral feeding may be initiated.

Maintenance of Normothermia: ↓ risks (↑ cerebral blood flow and ICP) associated with ↑ metabolic rate. Controlled by antipyretics such as acetaminophen or other cooling measures such as tepid baths or hypothermia treatments.

Infection Prevention: According to agency guidelines (see "Recommendations for isolation precautions in hospitals," Appendix).

PATIENT-FAMILY TEACHING

- Importance of avoiding Valsalva-like activities and those that ↑ ICP: coughing, straining, bending over
- Indicators of ↑ ICP: worsening headache, vomiting, confusion, visual disturbances, motor and sensory deficits

Nursing Diagnoses/Interventions

Decreased adaptive capacity: Intracranial, r/t compromised fluid dynamic mechanisms secondary to brain and spinal cord inflammation

Desired outcomes: Within 72 h of initiating antimicrobial therapy, patient's ICP returns to nl: orientation × 3, bilaterally equal and normoreactive pupils, bilaterally equal strength and tone of extremities, absence of cranial nerve palsies, RR 12-20 breaths/min with eupnea, HR 60-100 bpm, BP wnl for patient, and absence of S&S of ↑ ICP.

- Assess neurologic status at least qh during acute phase. Monitor pupils, LOC, and motor activity; perform cranial nerve assessments. ↓ in consciousness is an early indicator of ↑ ICP and impending herniation. Changes in pupillary size and reaction, ↓ in motor function (ie, hemiplegia, abnormal posturing), and cranial nerve palsies are other signs.
- Monitor for S&S of ↑ ICP: ↑ headache, vomiting, ↓ LOC, irregular or very rapid respirations, fluctuations in BP and pulse, widening pulse pressure, slow HR.
- Optimize cerebral perfusion by maintaining patent airway and delivering O_2 as prescribed. Be sure neck is free of constricting objects such as tracheostomy ties and O_2 tubing. Maintain neck, HOB, and body in position that keeps ICP wnl.
- Maintain normovolemia by ensuring precise delivery of IV fluids at consistent, prescribed rates.
- Ensure timely delivery of medications prescribed for prevention of sudden ↑ or ↓ in BP, HR, or RR.
- If patient shows S&S of ↑ ICP, implement measures to ↓ ICP.
  Elevate HOB to 30 degrees or elevation known to ↓ ICP.
  Maintain head in neutral position.
  Assess for factors that may be contributing to ↑ ICP: agitation, hypoxia, pain, fear, anxiety.
  Evaluate activities (eg, suctioning, bathing, dressing changes) that can ↑ pressure; reorganize care plan accordingly.
  Hyperoxygenate before/after suctioning.

Pain r/t headache, photophobia, and fever secondary to meningeal irritation

Desired outcome: Within 2 h of therapy initiation, patient's subjective evaluation of discomfort improves as documented by pain scale.

- Monitor for pain and discomfort. Devise pain scale with patient, rating discomfort from 0 (no pain) to 10. Administer analgesics as prescribed.
- Monitor temp q2h and prn. Administer tepid baths or cooling blanket and prescribed antipyretics/antibiotics to ↓ temp.
- Maintain quiet environment.
- Cluster patient care and organize visiting hours to ensure uninterrupted periods (at least 90 min) of rest.
- Darken room to minimize discomfort of photophobia. Provide blindfolds if darkening room not possible.

Risk for infection r/t potential for cross-contamination secondary to communicable nature of some types of meningitis

Desired outcome: Other patients, staff members, and significant others do not exhibit evidence of meningitis: change in LOC, fever.

FOR PATIENTS WITH BACTERIAL MENINGITIS

- May be transmitted *via* airborne droplets and contact with oral secretions. Provide private room for 24 h after start of effective therapy.
- Initiate Transmission-Based Precautions: Droplet, on admission and maintain for 24 h after start of antimicrobial therapy.
  Ensure that masks are worn by those in close contact with patient.
  As with touching *any* patient's secretions or excretions, ensure that gloves are worn during contact with oral secretions.
  Ensure careful hand washing technique after contact with patient and potentially contaminated articles and before coming into contact with another patient.

FOR PATIENTS WITH VIRAL OR NONBACTERIAL MENINGITIS

- May be transmitted *via* stool or oral secretions. Follow Standard Precautions:
  Ensure that gowns are worn if soiling of clothing likely.
  Ensure that gloves are worn for touching infective material.
  Enforce strict hand washing technique after touching patient or articles that may be contaminated and before caring for another patient.

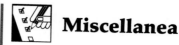 # Miscellanea

CONSULT MD FOR

- S&S of ↑ ICP: worsening headache, vomiting, confusion, visual disturbances
- Complications: SIADH, seizures, septic shock

RELATED TOPICS

- Agitation syndrome
- Antimicrobial therapy
- Increased intracranial pressure
- Recommendations for isolation precautions in hospitals (see Appendix)
- Shock, septic
- Status epilepticus

ABBREVIATION

SIADH: Syndrome of inappropriate antidiuretic hormone

REFERENCES

Davis A et al: Neurologic dysfunctions. In Swearingen PL, Keen JH (eds): *Manual of critical care nursing*, ed 3, St Louis, 1995, Mosby.

Mickles LI, Mickles DP: Listerial meningitis, *Crit Care Nurse* 14(4): 22, 25-30, 1994.

Payling KL: Meningitis: causes, treatment, and care, *Prof Nurse* 9(5): 310-313, 1994.

Author: **Alice Davis**

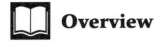 **Overview**

PATHOPHYSIOLOGY

Caused by a primary ↓ in plasma bicarbonate as reflected by serum HCO_3^- <22 mEq/L and pH <7.40. ↓ in pH stimulates respirations, as manifested by ↓ $Paco_2$. The most important mechanism for ridding excess H^+ is the ↑ in acid excretion by the kidneys. However, nonvolatile acids (eg, those occurring with DKA, lactic acidosis, renal failure) may accumulate more rapidly than they can be neutralized by buffers, compensated for by the respiratory system, or excreted by the kidneys.

HISTORY/RISK FACTORS

- Ketoacidosis: DM, alcoholism, starvation
- Lactic acidosis: respiratory or circulatory failure, drugs and toxins, septic shock
- Renal disease
- Poisonings and drug toxicity: salicylates, methanol, ethylene glycol
- Loss of alkali: draining wounds (eg, pancreatic fistulas), diarrhea, ureterostomy

CLINICAL PRESENTATION

Depends on underlying disease states. Mild metabolic acidosis (HCO_3^- 15-18 mEq/L) may result in no symptoms, but with pH <7.2, symptoms will develop. May exhibit changes in LOC that range from fatigue and confusion to stupor and coma.

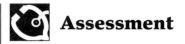 **Assessment**

PHYSICAL ASSESSMENT

Tachycardia (until pH <7.0, then bradycardia), tachypnea leading to alveolar hyperventilation (Kussmaul's respirations), dysrhythmias, shock state. With mild to moderate acidosis, skin will be cold and clammy; with severe acidosis, it will be flushed, warm, and dry.

VITAL SIGNS/HEMODYNAMICS

RR: ↑
HR: ↑
BP: ↓
Temp: ↑ if infection present
ECG: Dysrhythmias, including VF, caused by acidosis or hyperkalemia. *Hyperkalemic changes:* peaked T waves, depressed ST segment, ↓ size of R waves, ↓/absent P waves, widened QRS complex.

LABORATORY STUDIES

ABGs: pH usually <7.35; respiratory compensation reflected by ↓ $Paco_2$ (usually <35 mm Hg).
Serum Bicarbonate: Determines presence of metabolic acidosis (HCO_3^- <22 mEq/L).
Serum Electrolytes: ↑ K^+ may be present as H^+ moves into the cells to buffer and K^+ moves out to maintain electroneutrality. If K^+ nl or ↓ in the presence of metabolic acidosis, this signals low body stores of K^+.
Anion Gap: Nl anion gap is 12 (±2) mEq/L. Nl anion gap acidosis results from direct loss of HCO_3^- (eg, diarrhea, renal tubular acidosis, pancreatic fistulas) or addition of chloride-containing acids, some hyperalimentation fluids, and oral calcium chloride. ↑ anion gap acidosis (>12-14 mEq/L) results from accumulation of nonvolatile acids.

Collaborative Management

NaHCO₃: Controversial because of its potentially negative effects. May be indicated when arterial pH ≤7.2. Usual mode of delivery is IV drip but may be given IV push in emergencies. Given cautiously to avoid metabolic alkalosis and pulmonary edema caused by the sodium load.
Potassium Replacement: If potassium deficit exists, it must be corrected before NaHCO₃ is administered. When acidosis corrected, K^+ shifts back to intracellular spaces, potentially resulting in serum hypokalemia with fatal dysrhythmias.
Mechanical Ventilation: If mechanical ventilation required, compensatory hyperventilation must be allowed to continue in order to prevent acidosis from becoming more severe.
Treatment of Underlying Disorder
DKA: Insulin and fluids needed.
Alcoholism-related ketoacidosis: Glucose and saline needed.
ARF: Dialysis to maintain adequate level of HCO_3^-.
Renal tubular acidosis: May require modest amounts (<100 mEq/day) of bicarbonate.
Poisoning and drug toxicity: Depends on drug ingested or infused. Hemodialysis or PD may be necessary.
Lactic acidosis: Mortality associated with lactic acidosis is high. Treatment with NaHCO₃ is only transiently helpful.

PATIENT-FAMILY TEACHING

- Reassurance that confusion is r/t underlying pathology and will resolve with treatment; importance and types of reorientation techniques
- Medications: drug name, route, dose, schedule, precautions, food-drug and drug-drug interactions, and potential side effects (especially important for patients with DKA)

Nursing Diagnoses/Interventions

Nursing diagnoses/interventions are specific to the pathophysiologic process. If patient has septic shock or lactic acidosis, the following may apply:

Fluid volume deficit r/t active loss from vascular compartment secondary to ↑ capillary permeability and shift of intravascular volume into interstitial spaces

Desired outcomes: Within 4 h of treatment initiation, patient normovolemic: peripheral pulses >2+ on 0-4+ scale, stable body weight, UO ≥0.5 ml/kg/h, SBP ≥90 mm Hg or wnl for patient, and absence of edema and adventitious lung sounds. PAWP 6-12 mm Hg, CO 4-7 L/min, and SVR 900-1200 dynes/sec/cm^{-5}.

- Assess fluid volume by monitoring BP and peripheral pulses qh.
- Weigh qd; monitor I&O every shift and UO qh, noting 24-h trends. Weight actually may ↑ with fluid volume deficit because of shift of intravascular volume into interstitial spaces.
- Assess for interstitial edema as evidenced by pretibial, sacral, ankle, and hand edema, as well as crackles on lung field auscultation.
- Position patient supine with legs elevated to ↑ venous return and preload.
- Monitor hemodynamic pressures, particularly PAWP, CO, and SVR. Early PAWP usually ↓ to <6 mm Hg but ↑ to >12 mm Hg in the late stage. CO usually >7 L/min in the early stage and ↓ to <4 L/min in the late stage. SVR can be <900 dynes/sec/cm^{-5} in the early stage but usually ↑ to >1200 dynes/sec/cm^{-5} in the late stage.
- Administer crystalloids and colloids to maintain PAWP of 6-12 mm Hg. Assess PAWP and lung sounds at frequent intervals during fluid replacement to detect fluid overload: crackles and ↑ PAWP.
- Administer NaHCO$_3$ as prescribed for severe acidosis (pH ≤7.2). Administer cautiously to avoid metabolic alkalosis and pulmonary edema. Correct K$^+$ deficit before NaHCO$_3$ administration.
- Administer vasopressors and positive inotropes as prescribed to maintain adequate cardiac output in the presence of massive vasodilatation. Be aware that correction of severe acidosis may be necessary to optimize response to epinephrine and similar catecholamine-stimulating agents.

Miscellanea

CONSULT MD FOR
- Nl or ↓ serum K$^+$, which suggests total body K$^+$ deficit
- Hyperkalemic ECG changes
- Hemodynamically significant dysrhythmias

RELATED TOPICS
- Diabetic ketoacidosis
- Hypokalemia
- Mechanical ventilation
- Multiple organ dysfunction syndrome
- Renal failure, acute
- Shock, septic

ABBREVIATION
PD: Peritoneal dialysis

REFERENCES
Heitz UE: Acid-base imbalances. In Swearingen PL, Keen JH (eds): *Manual of critical care nursing,* ed 3, St Louis, 1995, Mosby.

Horne MM, Heitz U, Swearingen PL: *Pocket guide to fluid, electrolytes, and acid-base balance,* ed 3, St Louis, 1997, Mosby.

Lovenstein J: *Acid and basics: a guide to understanding acid-base disorders,* New York, 1993, Oxford University Press.

Rose BD: *Clinical physiology of acid-base and electrolyte disorders,* ed 4, New York, 1994, McGraw-Hill.

Author: **Ursula Heitz**

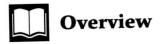 **Overview**

PATHOPHYSIOLOGY

Seen with CRF in which the kidneys' ability to excrete acids is exceeded by acid production and ingestion. Acidosis is usually mild in initial stage, with HCO_3^- 18-22 mEq/L and pH of 7.35. Treatment indicated when serum HCO_3^- levels reach 15 mEq/L. A limited degree of respiratory compensation occurs. A modest ↓ in $Paco_2$ will be noted on ABGs.

HISTORY/RISK FACTORS

- CRF
- Renal tubular acidosis
- Loss of alkaline fluid: eg, with diarrhea or pancreatic or biliary drainage

CLINICAL PRESENTATION

Process usually gradual and patient symptom free until serum $HCO_3^- \leq 15$ mEq/L. Fatigue, malaise, and anorexia may occur.

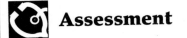 **Assessment**

PHYSICAL ASSESSMENT
Specific to underlying disorder.

VITAL SIGNS/HEMODYNAMICS
RR: ↑
HR, BP, Temp: According to underlying disorder.
ECG: Dysrhythmias, including VF, caused by acidosis or hyperkalemia. *Hyperkalemic changes:* peaked T waves, depressed ST segment, ↓ size of R waves, ↓/absent P waves, and widened QRS complex.

LABORATORY STUDIES
ABGs: $Paco_2$ <35 mm Hg; pH <7.35
Serum Bicarbonate: <22 mEq/L (usually 18-21 mEq/L); *with severe acidosis,* <15 mEq/L
Serum Electrolytes
Calcium: Checked before treatment of acidosis to prevent tetany induced by hypocalcemia (caused by ↓ in ionized calcium).
Phosphate: To determine presence of hyperphosphatemia, a common complication of CRF.
Potassium: Monitored during acidosis to determine presence of life-threatening hyperkalemia requiring emergency treatment. Monitored after acidosis has been corrected to detect hypokalemia. K^+ shifts back into the cells after correction of acidosis.

Collaborative Management

Alkalizing Agents: Oral alkalis (eg, $NaHCO_3$ tablets or sodium citrate and citric acid oral solution [Shohl's solution]) given for serum HCO_3^- levels <15 mEq/L. Used cautiously to prevent fluid overload and tetany caused by hypocalcemia. Be alert to potential for pulmonary edema if IV $NaHCO_3$ given.
Treatment of Life-Threatening Hyperkalemia: IV calcium gluconate, IV glucose and insulin, and/or IV $NaHCO_3$; cation exchange resins (sodium polystyrene sulfonate [Kayexalate]); hemodialysis. Monitoring K^+ in CRF is especially important in critical illness and postsurgery.
Hemodialysis or PD: If indicated by CRF or other disease processes.

PATIENT-FAMILY TEACHING

- Medications: drug name, purpose, dose, schedule, precautions, drug-drug and food-drug interactions, and potential side effects, particularly of alkalinizing agents
- Importance of notifying physician if drainage ↑ in volume or changes consistency *via* biliary or pancreatic drains; instruction in methods of quantifying drainage (eg, how many dressings saturated, how many dressing changes required in 24 h)
- Prescribed diet for patients with CRF
- S&S of hyperkalemia, which often accompany acidosis: abdominal cramping, diarrhea, weakness (especially of lower extremities), paresthesias

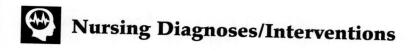

Nursing Diagnoses/Interventions

Nursing diagnoses/interventions are specific to the underlying pathophysiologic process. Some patients may have the following:

Altered protection (risk of tetany and seizures) r/t neurosensory alterations secondary to severe hypocalcemia

Desired outcome: Patient does not exhibit evidence of injury caused by complications of severe hypocalcemia.

- Monitor for worsening hypocalcemia: numbness and tingling of fingers and circumoral region, hyperactive reflexes, and muscle cramps. Check for positive Trousseau's or Chvostek's signs; they signal latent tetany. Monitor total and ionized calcium levels as available.
- Maintain seizure precautions for patients with symptoms; ↓ environmental stimuli.
- Avoid rapid administration of IV $NaHCO_3$ or hyperventilation in patients in whom hypocalcemia suspected. Alkalosis may precipitate tetany because of ↑ pH with a reduction in ionized calcium.

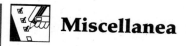

Miscellanea

CONSULT MD FOR
- New-onset electrolyte imbalance, especially hypocalcemia, hyperphosphatemia, hyper/hypokalemia
- Hemodynamically significant dysrhythmias

RELATED TOPICS
- Hyperkalemia
- Hyperphosphatemia
- Hypocalcemia
- Hypokalemia

ABBREVIATIONS
CRF: Chronic renal failure
PD: Peritoneal dialysis

REFERENCES
Heitz UE: Acid-base imbalances. In Swearingen PL, Keen JH (eds): *Manual of critical care nursing,* ed 3, St Louis, 1995, Mosby.

Horne MM, Heitz U, Swearingen PL: *Pocket guide to fluid, electrolytes, and acid-base balance,* ed 3, St Louis, 1997, Mosby.

Lovenstein J: *Acid and basics: a guide to understanding acid-base disorders,* New York, 1993, Oxford University Press.

Rose BD: *Clinical physiology of acid-base and electrolyte disorders,* ed 4, New York, 1994, McGraw-Hill.

Author: **Ursula Heitz**

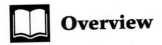 **Overview**

PATHOPHYSIOLOGY

↑ serum HCO_3^- (up to 45-50 mEq/L) resulting from H^+ loss or excess alkali intake. Compensatory ↑ in $Paco_2$ (up to 50-60 mm Hg) will be seen. Respiratory compensation limited because of hypoxemia, which develops as a result of ↓ alveolar ventilation. Severe alkalosis (pH >7.60) associated with high morbidity and mortality.

HISTORY/RISK FACTORS

- Clinical circumstances associated with volume/chloride depletion: vomiting or gastric drainage; cystic fibrosis in hot weather
- Diuretic use: usually mild metabolic alkalosis occurs, but will be more severe if potent diuretic (ie, furosemide) used
- Posthypercapnic alkalosis: after rapid correction of chronic hypercapnia (eg, in COPD)
- Excessive alkali intake: overcorrection of metabolic acidosis

CLINICAL PRESENTATION

Muscular weakness, neuromuscular instability, hyporeflexia resulting from accompanying hypokalemia. ↓ GI tract motility may result in ileus. Severe alkalosis can cause apathy, confusion, stupor.

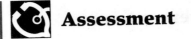 **Assessment**

PHYSICAL ASSESSMENT

↓ respiratory rate and depth, periods of apnea, tachycardia (atrial or ventricular)

VITAL SIGNS/HEMODYNAMICS

RR: ↓
HR: ↑
BP: ↓ possible as a result of dysrhythmias, impaired contractility
Temp: R/t underlying process
ECG: Atrial or ventricular dysrhythmias as a result of cardiac irritability secondary to hypokalemia; prolonged QT interval

LABORATORY STUDIES

ABGs: To determine severity of alkalosis and response to therapy.
Serum Bicarbonate Levels: ↑ to >26 mEq/L.
Serum Electrolytes: Usually, low K^+ (<4.0 mEq/L) and Cl^- (<95 mEq/L).
Urinalysis: Chloride level <15 mEq/L if hypovolemia and hypochloremia present and >20 mEq/L with excess retained HCO_3^-. Test not reliable if diuretics used within previous 12 h.

Collaborative Management

Depends on underlying disorder. Mild or moderate metabolic alkalosis usually does not require specific therapeutic interventions.
Saline Infusion: NS infusion may correct volume (chloride) deficit in patients with gastric losses. Metabolic alkalosis difficult to correct if hypovolemia and chloride deficit not corrected.
Potassium Chloride: Indicated for low K^+ levels. KCl preferred over other potassium salts because Cl^- losses replaced simultaneously.
Sodium and Potassium Chloride: Effective for posthypercapnic alkalosis, which occurs when chronic CO_2 retention is corrected rapidly (eg, *via* mechanical ventilation). If adequate amounts of Cl^- and K^+ are not available, renal excretion of excess HCO_3^- is impaired and metabolic alkalosis continues.
IV Isotonic Hydrochloride Solution, Ammonium Chloride, or Arginine Hydrochloride: Cautious administration may be warranted if severe metabolic alkalosis (pH >7.6 and HCO_3^- >40-45 mEq/L) exists, especially if chloride or potassium salts contraindicated. Delivered *via* continuous IV infusion at slow rate, with frequent monitoring of IV insertion site for signs of infiltration.

PATIENT-FAMILY TEACHING

- Importance of taking prescribed medications: drug name, dosage, purpose, schedule, precautions, drug-drug and food-drug interactions, and potential side effects
- S&S of hypokalemia: fatigue, muscle weakness, leg cramps, soft and flabby muscles, nausea, vomiting

Nursing Diagnoses/Interventions

Nursing diagnoses/interventions are specific to the underlying pathophysiologic process. Many patients will have the following:

Fluid volume deficit r/t abnormal loss of body fluids or ↓ intake

Desired outcomes: Within 24 h of initiation of fluid therapy, patient normovolemic: UO ≥0.5 ml/kg/h, specific gravity 1.010-1.030, stable weight, no clinical evidence of hypovolemia, BP wnl for patient, CVP 2-6 mm Hg, PAP 20-30/8-15 mm Hg, CO 4-7 L/min, MAP 70-105 mm Hg, HR 60-100 bpm, and SVR 900-1200 dynes/sec/cm^{-5}.

- Monitor I&O qh. Initially, intake should exceed output during therapy. Monitor urine specific gravity; expect ↓ with therapy.
- Monitor VS and hemodynamics for signs of continued hypovolemia: ↓ BP, CVP, PAP, CO, MAP; ↑ HR and SVR.
- Place shock patient in supine position with legs elevated to 45 degrees to ↑ venous return.
- Weigh patient qd. Acute weight changes usually indicate fluid changes. If individual is being fed, a 1-kg ↓ in daily weight equals a 1-L fluid loss.
- Administer PO and IV fluids as prescribed. Ensure adequate intake, especially in elders because of ↑ risk of volume depletion in this population.
- Monitor for fluid overload or too rapid fluid administration: crackles, SOB, tachypnea, tachycardia, ↑ CVP, ↑ PAP, JVD, and edema.
- Monitor for hidden fluid losses: eg, measure and document abdominal girth or limb size, if indicated.
- Remember that Hct will ↓ as patient becomes rehydrated. ↓ in Hct associated with rehydration is accompanied by ↓ in sodium and BUN values.

Miscellanea

CONSULT MD FOR
- Hemodynamically significant dysrhythmias
- Hypokalemia, hypochloremia

RELATED TOPICS
- Bronchitis, chronic
- Emphysema
- Hypokalemia

REFERENCES

Heitz UE: Acid-base imbalances. In Swearingen PL, Keen JH (eds): *Manual of critical care nursing,* ed 3, St Louis, 1995, Mosby.

Horne MM, Heitz U, Swearingen PL: *Pocket guide to fluid, electrolytes, and acid-base balance,* ed 3, St Louis, 1997, Mosby.

Lovenstein J: *Acid and basics: a guide to understanding acid-base disorders,* New York, 1993, Oxford University Press.

Rose BD: *Clinical physiology of acid-base and electrolyte disorders,* ed 4, New York, 1994, McGraw-Hill.

Author: **Ursula Heitz**

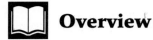 **Overview**

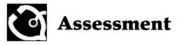 **Assessment**

Collaborative Management

PATHOPHYSIOLOGY

Results in pH >7.45 and HCO_3^- >26 mEq/L. $Paco_2$ will ↑ (>45 mm Hg) to compensate for loss of H^+ or excess serum HCO_3^-.

HISTORY/RISK FACTORS

- Hyperadrenocorticism: Cushing's syndrome, primary aldosteronism can lead to total body depletion of K^+ with profound hypokalemia (K^+ ≤2.0 mEq/L).
- Diuretic use: thiazide diuretics and furosemide cause loss of Cl^-, K^+, and H^+. Up to 1/3 of total body K^+ may be lost, causing profound hypokalemia (K^+ ≤ 2.0).
- GI loss: chronic vomiting or GI suction.
- Hypercalcemic nephropathy and alkalosis develop because of excessive intake of absorbable alkali (antacids containing calcium carbonate).

CLINICAL PRESENTATION

Patient may be symptom free.

PHYSICAL ASSESSMENT

With severe potassium depletion and profound alkalosis, patient may exhibit weakness, neuromuscular instability, and ↓ GI tract motility, which can result in ileus.

VITAL SIGNS/HEMODYNAMICS

HR: ↑
BP/CO: ↓ r/t dysrhythmias associated with hypokalemia
Others: According to underlying condition
ECG: Frequent PVCs or U waves with hypokalemia and alkalosis

LABORATORY STUDIES

ABGs: $Paco_2$ ↑ (>45 mm Hg) and pH >7.40
Serum Bicarbonate Levels: >26 mEq/L
Serum Electrolytes
K^+: Usually profoundly low (may be ≤2.0 mEq/L).
Cl^-: May be <95 mEq/L.
Mg^{2+}: May be <1.5 mEq/L if renal system involved.

Fluid Management: If volume depletion exists, NS infusions given.
Potassium Replacement: If Cl^- deficit also present, KCl is the drug of choice. If a Cl^- deficit does not exist, other potassium salts acceptable. IV doses (>40 mEq/L) require administration through central venous line because of blood vessel irritation. Continuous cardiac monitoring required if dose >10-20 mEq/L.
Potassium-Sparing Diuretics: May be added to treatment if thiazide diuretics are the cause of hypokalemia and metabolic alkalosis.
Identify and Correct Cause of Hyperadrenocorticism

PATIENT-FAMILY TEACHING

- Prescribed medication (usually thiazide diuretic): drug name, purpose, dose, schedule, precautions, drug-drug and food-drug interactions, and potential side effects
- Importance of taking only prescribed amount of diuretic; higher concentrations ↑ risk of hypokalemia and alkalosis
- Necessity of following prescribed diet (eg, if on sodium-restricted diet, explanation of rationale: ↑ sodium consumption ↑ risk of alkalosis and hypokalemia)
- Explanation regarding prescribed potassium supplements:
  Oral potassium has an unpleasant taste and is most palatable when mixed with tomato or orange juice.
  Slow-release tablets should not be chewed.
  Take with meals.
  Do not substitute foods high in potassium for prescribed supplements.

Nursing Diagnoses/Interventions

Nursing diagnoses/interventions are specific to the underlying pathophysiologic process. Many patients may experience the following:

Decreased cardiac output (or risk for same) r/t altered conduction secondary to hypokalemia
Desired outcome: Within 2 h of treatment, patient has adequate cardiac conduction: nl T-wave configuration and NSR (or baseline rhythm) without ectopy on ECG.

- Administer potassium supplement as prescribed. Avoid giving IV KCl at a rate ≥10-20 mEq/h because of potential for life-threatening hyperkalemia. Potassium supplementation usually is given in isotonic saline because D_5W will ↑ insulin-induced intracellular shift of K^+. If hypokalemia severe, concentrated IV solutions of potassium may be administered in limited volumes (eg, 20 mEq in 100 ml of isotonic NaCl), but it should be administered no more rapidly than 40 mEq/h. Concentrated solutions and infusion rates >10 mEq/h are used only with severe hypokalemia.
- Be aware that IV KCl can cause local irritation of veins and chemical phlebitis. Assess IV insertion site for erythema, heat, or pain. Oral potassium supplements may cause GI irritation. Give with full glass of water or fruit juice; encourage patient to sip slowly.
- Monitor I&O qh. Potassium supplements should not be given if patient has inadequate UO because hyperkalemia can develop rapidly in patients with oliguria (<15-20 ml/h).
- Monitor ECG for signs of continuing hypokalemia (ST-segment depression, flattened T wave, presence of U wave, ventricular dysrhythmias) or hyperkalemia (tall, thin T waves; prolonged PR interval; ST depression; widened QRS complex; loss of P wave), which may develop during potassium replacement.
- Administer potassium cautiously in patients receiving potassium-sparing diuretics (eg, spironolactone or triamterene) or ACE inhibitors (eg, captopril) because of potential for development of hyperkalemia.

Miscellanea

CONSULT MD FOR
- ECG evidence of hypokalemia
- Hemodynamically significant dysrhythmias

RELATED TOPICS
- Hypokalemia
- Hypomagnesemia
- Hypovolemia

REFERENCES
Heitz UE: Acid-base imbalances. In Swearingen PL, Keen JH (eds): *Manual of critical care nursing*, ed 3, St Louis, 1995, Mosby.

Horne MM, Heitz U, Swearingen PL: *Pocket guide to fluid, electrolytes, and acid-base balance*, ed 3, St Louis, 1996, Mosby.

Lovenstein J: *Acid and basics: a guide to understanding acid-base disorders*, New York, 1993, Oxford University Press.

Rose BD: *Clinical physiology of acid-base and electrolyte disorders*, ed 4, New York, 1994, McGraw-Hill.

Author: **Ursula Heitz**

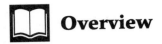 **Overview**

PATHOPHYSIOLOGY

Occurs when penicillinase-producing *S. aureus* becomes resistant to or loses responsiveness to methicillin and other semisynthetic penicillins, which under nl circumstances are used to treat this bacteria. Serious infections, including overwhelming septicemia leading to death, are possible because of ineffectiveness of traditional antimicrobial therapy. When resistant strains colonize (microorganisms present without S&S of infection), patients may harbor them for months or longer. Health care workers can be colonized in the nose or on the skin.

PREVENTION AND CONTROL METHODS

- Timely reporting of MRSA positive cultures to physicians, infection control practitioners, patient care units
- Prompt initiation of infection control practices when MRSA suspected/identified
- Controlling overuse or injudicious use of antibiotics

INCIDENCE

15% of all *S. aureus* are resistant to methicillin.

HISTORY/RISK FACTORS

- Underlying disease: malignancy, dermatitis, DM
- Invasive devices or procedures: IV catheters, surgery
- Extrinsic exposure: antimicrobials, steroids
- Hospitalization: in large teaching or referral hospitals, frequent transfers
- Suboptimal hygiene: lack of soap and water bathing, unclean environment

CLINICAL PRESENTATION

Colonization: No S&S; laboratory-confirmed culture (nares, axilla)
Infection: Laboratory-confirmed MRSA culture isolated from specific body site
Likely sites: Surgical wounds (most likely), urine, burn wounds, respiratory tract, blood, bone, chest tubes, IV catheter tips, intraabdominal abscesses, skin and soft tissue wounds (eg, leg ulcer)

 Assessment
(for infection)

PHYSICAL ASSESSMENT

Variable, depending on infection site
Neuro: Confusion, change in LOC
Resp: Thick, purulent sputum; coughing; adventitious breath sounds
GU: Cloudy, foul-smelling urine; frequency of urination, burning
Integ: Incision or open wound with erythema, edema, tenderness, pain, warmth, irritation, presence of drainage

VITAL SIGNS/HEMODYNAMICS

RR: ↑
HR: ↑
BP: Nl; ↓ if septicemic
Temp: ↑
CVP/PAWP: Usually ↓ from insensible fluid loss or SIRS
CO: ↑ early; ↓ late septicemia
SVR/MAP: ↓ if septicemic
ECG: Nl or sinus tachycardia

LABORATORY STUDIES

C&S: Of sites suspected of infection/colonization. Frequently transiently carried (here today, gone tomorrow, back again next day).
WBCs: ↑ with ↑ number of band neutrophils on differential (shift to left).

IMAGING

X-ray: To r/o abscess, collection of purulent material
CT: To r/o abscess

DIAGNOSTIC PROCEDURES

Needle Aspiration of Fluid Collection, Abscess: Aspirate sent for culture
Biopsy of Suspected Infective Material: Eg, heart valve, burn wound

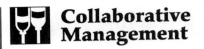 **Collaborative Management**

Infection Control

- Practice hand washing, aseptic technique, appropriate wound drainage precautions at all times for all patients.
- Keep patient care environment and equipment clean and disinfected.
- Follow Isolation Precautions per policy for MRSA colonization/infection.
- Monitor incidence of MRSA (usually *via* microbiology laboratory and infection control department).
- Institute system of flagging/tracking readmissions of MRSA patients.

Pharmacotherapy: Treatment options limited with resistance to antimicrobials. Vancomycin used for serious MRSA infections.
Surgery
I&D: To open wound, allow it to drain, and enable cleaning out of purulent material.
Repair/grafts: Possible débridement with split-thickness skin graft or free-flap graft.
Consultation with Local/State Health Departments: Initiated when developing discharge plan for MRSA patient to nursing home, other hospitals, or home health care.

PATIENT-FAMILY TEACHING

- Purpose, need for good hand washing, hygiene, aseptic (clean) wound care at home; other infection control measures
- CDC telephone: 404-329-1819; 404-329-3286

Nursing Diagnoses/Interventions

Risk for infection r/t inadequate primary defenses secondary to interruption in skin integrity; invasive lines, drains, catheters; immunocompromised status

Desired outcome: No nosocomial colonization/infection with MRSA by cross-contamination from personnel as evidenced by patient remaining infection free: normothermia, WBCs <11,000 μl, negative C&S results, no S&S of infection.

- CDC Isolation Precautions recommend that in addition to Standard Precautions, the following conditions warrant additional Contact Precautions:

  Hx of infection/colonization with multidrug-resistant organisms (eg, MRSA).

  Skin, wound, urinary tract infection with recent hospital or nursing home stay in a facility where multidrug-resistant organisms are prevalent.

FOR PATIENTS INFECTED/COLONIZED WITH MRSA

- Place in private room or in same room as other patients with MRSA.
- Wear clean, nonsterile gloves when entering room. Change gloves after contact with wound drainage/other material that may contain high concentrations of MRSA. Remove gloves before leaving room; wash hands with antimicrobial agent or waterless antiseptic agent. After removing gloves and washing hands, do not touch potentially contaminated environmental surfaces or other items.
- Wear clean, nonsterile gown when entering room if you anticipate clothing will have substantial contact with patient, environmental surfaces, or items in room, or if wound drainage or infected material (eg, sputum, urine, stool) is not contained by dressing. Remove gown before leaving. After gown removal, do not allow clothing to contact potentially contaminated surfaces.
- Take measures to contain wound drainage *via* semipermeable dressing, pouch, or other means as indicated. Consider consult with enterostomal or skin care specialist if copious wound drainage present.
- Limit movement and transport of patient from room to essential purposes only. If patient is transported out of room, maintain Precautions to minimize risk of MRSA transmission to other patients.
- When possible, dedicate use of noncritical patient care equipment to a single patient (or cohort of patients infected/colonized with MRSA) to avoid sharing among patients. If sharing is unavoidable, adequately clean and disinfect before use for another patient.

Social isolation r/t altered health status, inability to engage in satisfying personal relationships, altered mental status, or altered physical appearance

Desired outcome: Within 24 h of informing patient of resistance organism and/or implementing Isolation Precautions, patient demonstrates interaction and communication with others.

- Assess factors contributing to social isolation:

  Visitor restriction; visitors implementing special precautions.

  Absence of/inadequate support system.

  Inability to communicate (eg, mask use, door closed).

  Physical changes that affect self-concept (drainage, foul odor).

  Denial, withdrawal.
- Recognize patients at higher risk for social isolation: elders, disabled, chronically ill, economically disadvantaged, those with cultural or language barriers.
- Correct factors contributing to social isolation (eg, encourage visitation by friends, family, clergy).
- Set aside extra time to enable patient to express feelings, concerns.

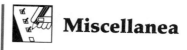

Miscellanea

CONSULT MD FOR

- MRSA positive culture results
- New-onset symptoms: erythema, tenderness, induration, purulent drainage of wounds; change in color, appearance of sputum; temp >38.33° C (101° F); WBCs >11,000 μl

RELATED TOPICS

- Antimicrobial therapy
- Enterocutaneous fistulas
- Multiple organ dysfunction syndrome
- Pneumonia
- Psychosocial needs, patient
- Recommendations for isolation precautions in hospitals (see Appendix)
- Shock, septic
- Systemic inflammatory response syndrome

ABBREVIATION

SIRS: Systemic inflammatory response syndrome

REFERENCES

Benenson AS: *Control of communicable diseases manual*, ed 16, Washington DC, 1995, American Public Health Association.

Bisno AL: Molecular aspects of bacterial colonization, *Infect Control Hosp Epidemiol* 16: 648-657, 1995.

Garner JS, Hospital infection control practices advisory committee, Guidelines for isolation precautions in hospitals, *Am J Infect Control* 24: 24-52, 1996.

Jarvis WR: The epidemiology of colonization, *Infect Control Hosp Epidemiol* 17: 47-52, 1996.

Wenzel RP: *Prevention and control of nosocomial infections*, ed 2, Baltimore, 1993, Williams & Wilkins.

Author: **Janice Speas**

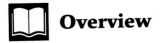 **Overview**

PATHOPHYSIOLOGY

Result of incomplete mitral valve closure during systole, causing blood to back into left atrium. ↓ ventricular outflow results in ↓ CO. When acute, ↑ LA volume and pressure ↑ pulmonary vascular pressure and may result in pulmonary edema. When chronic, ↑ LVEDV results in LV hypertrophy and failure.

HISTORY/RISK FACTORS

- Rheumatic fever
- Rheumatoid arthritis
- AMI with papillary muscle ischemia
- Infective endocarditis
- Mitral valve prolapse
- Advanced age
- Trauma

CLINICAL PRESENTATION

Fatigue, debilitation, activity intolerance, palpitations

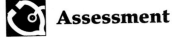 **Assessment**

PHYSICAL ASSESSMENT

Neuro: Weakness, ↓ mental acuity
Resp: Tachypnea, dyspnea (especially with exertion), crackles
CV: Systolic murmur at fifth ICS, MCL with radiation to apex; rapid upstroke with fall-off of carotid pulse

VITAL SIGNS/HEMODYNAMICS

RR: ↑
HR: ↑
BP: ↓
Temp: N/a
PAP: ↑ systolic PAP; MPAP may be nl
PAWP: Giant V waves possible
CO: ↓
ECG: LA hypertrophy with sinus tachycardia, A-fib; if advanced, LV hypertrophy with associated ST-segment, T-wave changes

IMAGING

Chest X-ray: ↑ size of cardiac silhouette suggests pulmonary congestion.
Echocardiography: Determines enlarged left atrium, ↑ LVEDV, changes in ventricular wall motion.

DIAGNOSTIC PROCEDURE

Cardiac Catheterization: Evaluates degree of regurgitation, LVEF, CAD.

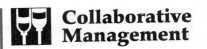 **Collaborative Management**

O₂: *Via* nasal cannula or other device; titrated to maintain SpO₂ ≥92%-96%. Mechanical ventilation may be necessary.
Diuretics: To ↓ intravascular volume and ↓ preload.
Treatment of A-fib: Digitalis glycosides to ↓ rate. Cardioversion may be used. Anticoagulants necessary to prevent embolism r/t fibrillation.
Vasodilators: In severe cases to ↓ preload and afterload.
Inotropic Agents: Dopamine, dobutamine to ↑ arterial diastolic pressure; used cautiously because ↑ SVR may worsen myocardial ischemia, mitral regurgitation.

SURGICAL PROCEDURES

Valve Replacement: Performed for moderate to severe disease; mortality rate ≈ 6%. Heterograft (pig, cow tissue) or mechanical valve used. Valve surgery ↑ risk for thrombosis and embolism (particularly with mechanical mitral valves and in patients with A-fib) and for valvular endocarditis.
IABP: May be necessary with severe mitral regurgitation and profound LV failure.

PATIENT-FAMILY TEACHING

- Physiologic process of heart failure; how fluid volume ↑ because of poor heart functioning
- S&S of fluid volume excess necessitating medical attention: irregular or slow pulse, ↑ SOB, orthopnea, ↓ exercise tolerance, steady weight gain (≥1 kg/day for 2 successive days)
- If taking digitalis, technique for measuring HR; parameters for holding digitalis (usually for HR <60/min) and notifying physician
- Purpose/procedure/expected results for valve replacement surgery, IABP as applicable
- Importance of avoiding activities that require straining; use of stool softeners, bulk-forming agents, laxatives as needed
- Warning signals to stop activity and rest: chest pain, SOB, dizziness or faintness, unusual weakness; use of prophylactic NTG
- Need for antibiotic prophylaxis
- Phone number for American Heart Association: 1-800-242-8721

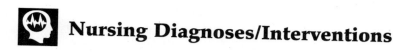

Nursing Diagnoses/Interventions

Decreased cardiac output r/t negative inotropic changes in the heart secondary to myocardial cellular destruction and dilatation

Desired outcomes: Within 24-h period before discharge from CCU, patient has adequate cardiac output: SBP $\geq$90 mm Hg; CO 4-7 L/min; CI 2.5-4 L/min/m^2; RR 12-20 breaths/min; HR $\leq$100 bpm; UO $\geq$0.5 ml/kg/h; I = O + insensible losses; warm and dry skin; orientation $\times$ 3; PAWP $\leq$18 mm Hg; and RAP 4-6 mm Hg.

- Assess for these factors associated with $\downarrow$ CO and LV congestion: JVD, dependent edema, hepatomegaly, fatigue, weakness, $\downarrow$ activity level, SOB with activity. Additional S&S include:
  Mental status: Restlessness, $\downarrow$ responsiveness
  Lung sounds: Crackles, rhonchi, wheezes
  Heart sounds: Gallop, murmur, $\uparrow$ HR
  Urinary output: UO <0.5 ml/kg/h $\times$ 2 consecutive h
  Skin: Pallor, mottling, cyanosis, coolness, diaphoresis
  Vital signs: SBP <90 mm Hg, HR >100 bpm, RR >20 breaths/ min, $\uparrow$ temp
- Be alert to PAWP >18 mm Hg and RAP >6 mm Hg. Although nl PAWP is 6-12 mm Hg, these patients usually need $\uparrow$ filling pressures for adequate preload, with PAWP at 15-18 mm Hg.
- Measure CO/CI q2-4h and prn. Adjust therapy to maintain CO within 4-7 L/min and CI at 2.5-4 L/min/m^2.
- Monitor I&O and weigh patient qd, noting trends. Strict fluid restriction (eg, 1000 ml/day) often prescribed.
- Minimize cardiac workload by assisting with ADL when necessary.
- Monitor for compensatory mechanisms ($\uparrow$ HR, BP) resulting from sodium, water retention.
- Administer medications as prescribed. Observe for the following desired effects:
  Vasodilators: $\downarrow$ BP, $\downarrow$ SVR, $\uparrow$ CO/CI
  Diuretics: $\downarrow$ PAWP
  Inotropes: $\uparrow$ CO/CI, $\uparrow$ BP
- Be alert to the following undesirable effects:
  Vasodilators: Hypotension, headache, nausea, vomiting, dizziness
  Diuretics: Weakness, hypokalemia
  Inotropes: Dysrhythmias, headache, angina

Fluid volume excess r/t compromised regulatory mechanism secondary to $\downarrow$ cardiac output

Desired outcome: Within 24 h of treatment, patient normovolemic: clear lung sounds, $\uparrow$ UO, weight loss, RAP/CVP $\leq$8 mm Hg, PVR $\leq$100 dynes/sec/cm^{-5}, and CO $\geq$4 L/min.

- Auscultate lung fields for crackles, rhonchi, other adventitious sounds.
- Monitor I&O closely. Report positive fluid state or $\downarrow$ in UO to <0.5 mg/kg/h.
- Weigh patient qd; report significant $\uparrow$ in weight.
- Note changes from baseline to detect worsening heart failure: $\uparrow$ pedal edema, JVD, S$_3$ heart sound or new murmur, dysrhythmias.
- Monitor hemodynamic status q1-2h and prn. Note response to drug therapy as well as indicators of need for more aggressive therapy: $\uparrow$ PAWP, SVR; $\downarrow$ CO.
- Administer diuretics (furosemide), positive inotropes (dobutamine, milrinone), vasodilators (nitroprusside).
- Limit oral fluids; offer ice chips or frozen juice pops to $\downarrow$ thirst and discomfort of dry mouth.
- Maintain bed rest or activity restrictions.

Activity intolerance r/t imbalance between O$_2$ supply and demand secondary to $\downarrow$ myocardial functioning

Desired outcome: Within 12-24 h before transfer from CCU, patient exhibits cardiac tolerance to $\uparrow$ levels of activity: RR <24 breaths/min, NSR on ECG, HR $\leq$120 bpm (or within 20 bpm of resting HR), BP within 20 mm Hg of nl for patient, absence of chest pain.

- Maintain prescribed activity level; teach rationale for activity limitation.
- Organize care so that activity is interspersed with extended periods of uninterrupted rest.
- Assist with active/passive ROM exercises, as appropriate. Encourage as much activity as possible within prescribed allowances.
- Note physiologic response to activity, including BP, HR, RR, heart rhythm. Signs of activity intolerance include chest pain, $\uparrow$ SOB, excessive fatigue, $\uparrow$ dysrhythmias, palpitations, HR response >120 bpm, SBP >20 mm Hg from baseline or >160 mm Hg, ST-segment changes.
- If activity intolerance noted, instruct patient to stop the activity and rest.
- Administer medications (eg, NTG tablets, paste, patch) to $\downarrow$ preload.
- As needed, refer to PT department.

Miscellanea

CONSULT MD FOR

- Inability to maintain Spo$_2$ $\geq$92% despite supplemental O$_2$
- Deteriorating cardiac performance: new onset S$_3$ or summation gallop, murmur, dysrhythmias, frothy sputum, crackles, sustained hypotension
- A-fib with rapid ventricular response
- Unacceptable hemodynamics: CO <4 L/min, PAWP >18 mm Hg, SVR >1200 dynes/sec/cm^{-5}, MAP <70 mm Hg
- UO <0.5 mg/kg/h $\times$ 2 consecutive h
- Complications: pulmonary edema, cardiogenic shock, unrelieved chest pain, ECG evidence of ischemia

RELATED TOPICS

- Atrial fibrillation
- Cardiac surgery: valvular disorders
- Endocarditis, infective
- Heart failure, left ventricular
- Intraaortic balloon pump

ABBREVIATIONS

IABP: Intraaortic balloon pump
ICS: Intercostal space
LVEDV: Left ventricular end-diastolic volume
LVEF: Left ventricular ejection fraction
MCL: Midclavicular line

REFERENCES

Hancock EW: Deep T waves and premature beats in mitral valve prolapse, *Hosp Pract* 28(5): 28-29, 1993.

Roelandt JRT, Meeter K: Diagnosis and management of valvular heart disease in the elderly, *Cardiol in the Elderly* 1(3): 235-243, 1993.

Steuble BT: Valvular heart disease. In Swearingen PL, Keen JH (eds): *Manual of critical care nursing,* ed 3, St Louis, 1995, Mosby.

Vitello-Cicciu J, Lapsley DP: Valvular heart disease. In Kinney M, Packa D, Dunbar S: *AACN's clinical reference for critical care nursing,* ed 3, 1993, St Louis, Mosby.

Wilson JS, Harrison JK, Bashore TM: Mitral stenosis, *Emerg Med* 25(15): 82-95, 1993.

Author: **Barbara Tueller Steuble**

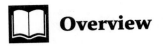 **Overview**

PATHOPHYSIOLOGY

Obstruction to forward blood flow (stenosis) across mitral valve. May be caused by sclerosing, thickening, or calcification of valve leaflets. Leads to ↑ LA volume and pressure and causes atrial hypertrophy. If acute, results in ↑ PAP with pulmonary congestion and edema. If chronic, PA resistance ↑, causing pulmonary hypertension and ↓ lung compliance. V/Q imbalance results in debilitation, easy fatigability, limited activity. If severe, RV failure ultimately develops.

HISTORY/RISK FACTORS

- Advanced age
- Infective endocarditis
- Rheumatic fever
- Rheumatoid arthritis
- Atherosclerotic heart disease

CLINICAL PRESENTATION

Chronic: Fatigue, debilitation, activity intolerance
Acute: Dyspnea, SOB, cough with frothy sputum

 Assessment

PHYSICAL ASSESSMENT

Neuro: Weakness, ↓ mental acuity
Resp: Tachypnea, dyspnea (especially with exertion), crackles
CV: Loud, long diastolic rumbling murmur at fifth ICS, MCL; may radiate to axilla; S_1 loud; opening snap with S_2; palpitations

VITAL SIGNS/HEMODYNAMICS

RR: ↑
HR: ↑
BP: NI or ↓
Temp: ↑ if infection present
PAP: ↑
PAWP: ↑
CO: ↓
ECG: Widened P wave in Lead II caused by LA enlargement; A-fib; right axis shift with LV hypertrophy

IMAGING

Chest X-ray: Will show pulmonary congestion.
Echocardiography: To determine ventricular function, chamber size, and valve function.
  Doppler flow studies: To determine blood flow.
  Color flow mapping studies: Use of colors to enhance image of blood flowing through heart.
  Transesophageal echocardiography: Uses endoscope to produce clear and undisturbed images unimpeded by chest wall.

DIAGNOSTIC PROCEDURE

Cardiac Catheterization: Ventriculogram may assist in visualizing blood flow. Measurement of chamber pressures assists in determining type of disorder present and degree of severity.

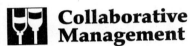 **Collaborative Management**

O₂: *Via* nasal cannula or other device; titrated to maintain Spo_2 ≥92%-96%. Mechanical ventilation may be necessary.
Diuretics: To ↓ blood volume and ↓ preload.
Low-Calorie Diet (if weight control necessary) and Low-sodium Diet: Sodium limited to ↓ fluid retention. Fluids may be limited to 1500 ml/day.
Treatment of A-fib: Digitalis glycosides to ↓ rate. Cardioversion may be used. Anticoagulants necessary to prevent embolism r/t fibrillation.
Treatment of Acute Pulmonary Edema: Immediate interventions include O₂ and possible ET intubation, diuretic therapy, inotropic agents, vasodilators, and morphine.
Antibiotic Prophylaxis: Penicillin or other antibiotic taken before dental, surgical, other invasive procedure to prevent valvular infection, endocarditis, septicemia.

SURGICAL PROCEDURES

Valve Replacement: Performed for moderate to severe disease; mortality rate ≈ 6%. Heterograft (pig, cow tissue) or mechanical valve used. Valve surgery patients at ↑ risk for thrombosis and embolism (particularly with mechanical mitral valves and in patients with A-fib) and for valvular endocarditis.
PBV: For dilatation of stenotic heart valves when surgery is an unacceptable alternative. Catheter passed *via* femoral vein through atrial septum to mitral valve opening. Series of three inflations given for 12-30 sec. If successful, results in significant improvement in valve gradient and blood flow across the valve.
Complications: Cerebral embolization, disruption of valve ring, acute valve regurgitation, valvular restenosis, hemorrhage at catheter insertion site, LV perforation by guidewire, dysrhythmias.
Commissurotomy: Stenotic valve opened by a dilating instrument. When performed early in disease course, chances of success good, but may cause valve regurgitation and recurrent stenosis.

PATIENT-FAMILY TEACHING

- Physiologic process of heart failure; how fluid volume ↑ because of poor heart functioning
- Importance of a low-sodium diet and medications to help ↓ volume overload; how to read and evaluate food labels
- S&S of fluid volume excess necessitating medical attention: irregular or slow pulse, ↑ SOB, orthopnea, ↓ exercise tolerance, steady weight gain (≥1 kg/day for 2 successive days)
- If taking digitalis, technique for measuring HR; parameters for holding digitalis (usually for HR <60/min) and notifying physician
- Purpose/procedure/expected results for valve replacement surgery, PBV, commissurotomy as applicable
- Importance of avoiding activities that require straining; use of stool softeners, bulk-forming agents, laxatives as needed
- Warning signals to stop activity and rest: chest pain, SOB, dizziness or faintness, unusual weakness; use of prophylactic NTG
- Need for antibiotic prophylaxis
- Phone number for American Heart Association: 1-800-242-8721

Nursing Diagnoses/Interventions

Fluid volume excess r/t compromised regulatory mechanism secondary to ↓ cardiac output
Desired outcome: Within 24 h of treatment, patient normovolemic: clear lung sounds, ↑ UO, weight loss, RAP/CVP ≤8 mm Hg, PVR ≤100 dynes/sec/cm^{-5}, and CO ≥4 L/min.
- Auscultate lung fields for crackles, rhonchi, or other adventitious sounds.
- Monitor I&O closely. Report positive fluid state or ↓ UO to <0.5 mg/kg/h.k
- Weigh patient qd; report significant ↑ in weight.
- Note changes from baseline to detect worsening of heart failure: ↑ pedal edema, JVD, S$_3$ heart sound or new murmur, and dysrhythmias.
- Monitor hemodynamic status q1-2h and prn. Note response to drug therapy as well as indicators of need for more aggressive therapy: ↑ PAWP, SVR; ↓ CO.
- Administer diuretics (furosemide), positive inotropes (dobutamine, milrinone), vasodilators (nitroprusside).
- Limit oral fluids; offer ice chips or frozen juice pops to ↓ thirst and discomfort of dry mouth.
- Maintain bed rest or activity restrictions.

Impaired gas exchange r/t alveolar-capillary membrane changes secondary to fluid collection in alveoli and interstitial spaces or secondary to altered blood flow caused by pulmonary hypertension
Desired outcome: Within 24 h of treatment initiation, patient has improved gas exchange: Pao$_2$ ≥80 mm Hg, RR 12-20 breaths/min with eupnea, and clear breath sounds.
- Monitor respiratory rate, rhythm, and character q1-2h. Be alert to RR >20 breaths/min, irregular rhythm, use of accessory muscles, cough.
- Auscultate breath sounds, noting crackles, wheezes, other adventitious sounds.
- Provide supplemental O$_2$ to maintain Spo$_2$ ≥92%.
- Assess ABGs; note changes in response to O$_2$ supplementation or treatment of altered hemodynamics.
- Suction secretions as needed.
- Encourage deep breathing, coughing, and turning q2h.
- Place in semi- or high-Fowler's position to maximize chest excursion.
- If mechanical ventilation necessary, monitor ventilator settings, ET tube function, respiratory status.

Activity intolerance r/t imbalance between O$_2$ supply and demand secondary to ↓ myocardial functioning
Desired outcome: Within 12-24 h before transfer from CCU, patient exhibits cardiac tolerance to ↑ levels of activity: RR <24 breaths/min, NSR on ECG, HR ≤120 bpm (or within 20 bpm of resting HR), BP within 20 mm Hg of nl for patient, absence of chest pain.
- Maintain prescribed activity level; teach rationale for activity limitation.
- Organize nursing care so that periods of activity are interspersed with extended periods of uninterrupted rest.
- Assist with active/passive ROM exercises, as appropriate. Encourage as much activity as possible within prescribed allowances.
- Note physiologic response to activity, including BP, HR, RR, and heart rhythm. Signs of activity intolerance include chest pain, ↑ SOB, excessive fatigue, ↑ dysrhythmias, palpitations, HR response >120 bpm, SBP >20 mm Hg from baseline or >160 mm Hg, and ST-segment changes.
- If activity intolerance noted, instruct patient to stop activity and rest.
- Administer medications (eg, NTG tablets, paste, patch) to ↓ preload.
- As needed, refer to PT department.

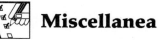 # Miscellanea

CONSULT MD FOR
- Inability to maintain Spo$_2$ ≥92% despite supplemental O$_2$
- Deteriorating cardiac performance: new onset S$_3$ or summation gallop, murmur, crackles, sustained hypotension
- New onset A-fib or A-fib with rapid ventricular response
- Unacceptable hemodynamics: CO <4 L/min, RAP/CVP >8 mm Hg, PVR >100 dynes/sec/cm^{-5}, MAP <70 mm Hg
- UO <0.5 mg/kg/h × 2 consecutive h
- Complications: cardiogenic shock, hepatic insufficiency, profound ascites, renal insufficiency

RELATED TOPICS
- Angioplasty/atherectomy, percutaneous transluminal coronary
- Cardiac surgery: valvular disorders
- Endocarditis, infective
- Heart failure, right ventricular
- Pulmonary hypertension

ABBREVIATIONS
ICS: Intercostal space
MCL: Midclavicular line
PBV: Percutaneous balloon valvuloplasty
PTCA: Percutaneous transluminal coronary angioplasty/atherectomy

REFERENCES
Roelandt J, Meeter K: Diagnosis and management of valvular heart disease in the elderly, *Cardiol in the Elderly* 1(3): 235-243, 1993.
Steuble BT: Valvular heart disease. In Swearingen PL, Keen JH (eds): *Manual of critical care nursing,* ed 3, St Louis, 1995, Mosby.
Vitello-Cicciu J, Lapsley DP: Valvular heart disease. In Kinney M, Packa D, Dunbar S: *AACN's clinical reference for critical care nursing,* ed 3, St Louis, 1993, Mosby.
Wilson JS, Harrison JK, Bashore TM: Mitral stenosis, *Emerg Med* 25(15): 82-95, 1993.

Author: **Barbara Tueller Steuble**

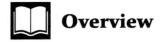 **Overview**

PATHOPHYSIOLOGY

Altered function of two or more organ systems in the acutely ill necessitating intervention in order to maintain tissue perfusion and homeostasis. Characterized by ARDS, DIC, ARF, and failure of cardiopulmonary, hepatic, GI, and other body systems. Usually the result of direct body injury or insult; develops rapidly. Can occur secondary to SIRS, which may be triggered by insults from mechanical, ischemic, chemical, or microbial sources.

HISTORY/RISK FACTORS

- Infection
- Low perfusion, shock states
- Multisystem injury
- Presence of necrotic tissue
- Immune deficiency
- Chronic illnesses
- Advanced age

CLINICAL PRESENTATION

Early Findings (reflect compensatory hypermetabolic state): Restlessness, confusion, SOB, tachypnea, tachycardia, ileus
Late Findings (consistent with impaired perfusion): Coma, respiratory failure requiring mechanical ventilation, heart failure refractory to inotropes, stress ulcers, jaundice, oliguria/anuria, bruising/uncontrolled bleeding

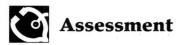 **Assessment**

PHYSICAL ASSESSMENT

Neuro: ↓ cerebral blood flow with CNS depression, stupor, coma
Resp: ↑ lung water, crackles, hyperventilation; later, hypoventilation caused by fatigue/CNS depression
CV: Pallor, edema, ↓/absent peripheral pulses, S_3/S_4 gallops, hypoperfusion, third spacing
GI: ↓/absent bowel sounds, bleeding, hepatocellular dysfunction with resultant ↑ bilirubin/liver enzymes and ↓ lactate clearance/metabolic acidosis
GU: ↓ renal perfusion, oliguria, anuria
Other: S&S of SNS activation, abnormal bleeding, acid-base imbalance

VITAL SIGNS/HEMODYNAMICS

RR: ↑
HR: ↑
BP: ↓
Temp: Initially ↑; then ↓ as thermoregulatory center fails
CVP: ↓ initially caused by relative fluid deficit; later ↑ caused by heart failure
PAP: ↑ caused by pulmonary vasoconstriction occurring with hypoxemia
PAWP: Often ↑ because of heart failure
SVR: ↓ in early stages as a result of hypermetabolic state; later ↓ results from heart failure
CO/CI: Early ↑ reflects hypermetabolic state; later ↓ caused by heart failure
Svo_2: <60% as a result of abnormally high tissue extraction; >60%-80%, reflecting precapillary shunting; <50% requires immediate intervention
CPP: ↓ as direct effect of chemical mediators and ↓ cerebral blood flow

LABORATORY STUDIES

Hematology: ↑ WBCs with ↑ number of bands (left shift). In late stages, WBCs ↓ as a result of organ sequestration, bone marrow exhaustion. Platelets ↓; PT/PTT ↑. Hgb/Hct ↓ as a result of uncontrolled bleeding. FDPs >40μg/ml = critical value; ≤10 = nl.
Chemistry
Venous lactate: Levels ↑ because of inadequate tissue perfusion/anaerobic metabolism (arterial levels may be nl because of precapillary shunting, heart failure).
Hepatic enzymes, bilirubin: ↑
BUN/creatinine: ↑
Urine creatinine clearance: ↓
Glucose: ↑ early results from gluconeogenesis; ↓ later results from hepatic failure.
Electrolytes: Multiple abnormalities present.
C&S: Blood, sputum, urine, surgical or other site; obtained if infection suspected.
ABGs: pH <7.35 and HCO_3^- <22 mEq/L as a result of metabolic acidosis. Pao_2 ↓ and $Paco_2$ ↑, reflecting acute respiratory failure.

IMAGING

X-rays: Of chest to check for ARDS; others according to underlying condition.
CT Scan: To check for intraabdominal abscess, other abnormalities.

Collaborative Management

Oxygenation: Mechanical ventilation necessary because of ↑ lung water, ARDS. Fio_2 >50% and PEEP >10 cm H_2O usually required. Inverse I/E ratio and other forms of pressure control ventilation used.
Fluids: Crystalloids, colloids (eg, albumin, PPF) given to sustain adequate intravascular volume. Sustained use of NS can lead to hyperchloremic metabolic acidosis; LR used if large volumes required. Hyperdynamic state supported until patient stable.
Blood Products: Clotting factors and inhibitors replaced *via* FFP. PT used to guide plasma replacement. Markedly ↓ fibrinogen levels may require cryoprecipitate, which contains 5-10 × more fibrinogen than plasma. Platelet transfusions rarely needed unless there is impaired platelet production and profuse bleeding.
Hemodynamic/Flow Monitoring: To maximize Do_2, Vo_2, and CI. Goal: to maintain supradynamic values by adjusting fluids, inotropes, and vasopressors and ensuring adequacy of O_2-carrying capacity *via* optimal Hct and O_2 administration.
Pharmacotherapy
Antibiotics: Broad-spectrum antibiotics if infection suspected.
Analgesia, sedation: To relieve pain and agitation, which ↑ O_2 consumption.
Positive inotropes (eg, dopamine, dobutamine): To augment cardiac contractility and CO. If SVR ↑, may be given along with *vasodilators,* such as nitroprusside and NTG. See Appendix for "Inotropic and Vasoactive Agents."
Vasopressors (eg, dopamine, norepinephrine): For refractory hypotension. See Appendix for "Inotropic and Vasoactive Agents."
Nutritional Support: Enteral nutrition optimal, but often not possible because of ischemic bowel injury. Parenteral nutrition may be necessary. Protein and caloric needs ↑ to promote healing, meet ↑ carbohydrate demand.

PATIENT-FAMILY TEACHING

- Need for early discharge planning, since posthospitalization subacute/rehabilitation/home health care often necessary
- Availability of hospital and community support systems: social worker, chaplain, psychiatric consultation

Nursing Diagnoses/Interventions

Altered cerebral, renal, and GI tissue perfusion r/t hypovolemia secondary to vasodilatation (early stage) or interruption of arterial/venous blood flow secondary to sludging of blood
Desired outcomes: Within 24 h of initiating therapy, patient has adequate perfusion: orientation $\times$ 3, peripheral pulses >2+ on 0-4+ scale, brisk capillary refill (<2 sec), UO $\geq$0.5 ml/kg/h, and $\geq$5 bowel sounds/min. BP 110-120/70-80 mm Hg (or wnl for patient), Svo_2 60%-80%, SVR 900-1200 dynes/sec/cm^{-5}, CO 4-7 L/min, and CI 2.5-4 L/min/m^2.
- Assess for $\downarrow$ cerebral perfusion: $\downarrow$ LOC, restlessness.
- Assess for $\downarrow$ renal perfusion: UO <0.5 ml/kg/h and $\uparrow$ BUN/creatinine and serum K^+ levels.
- Monitor BP continuously for $\downarrow$ SBP, nl or $\uparrow$ DBP, $\downarrow$ pulse pressures, occurring with $\downarrow$ perfusion.
- Assess for hypoperfusion: $\downarrow$ pulses, coolness, pallor/mottling, delayed capillary refill.
- Monitor Svo_2 as an indicator of tissue perfusion. Cellular O_2 delivery $\downarrow$ because of precapillary vasoconstriction and thus cellular O_2 use $\downarrow$. This may result in abnormally high Svo_2.
- Give fluids, inotropes, vasodilators, vasopressors to optimize SVR and CO/CI. $\uparrow$ filling pressures may be needed for optimal CO with ischemic myocardium/heart failure.
- Assess for $\downarrow$ splanchnic (visceral) circulation, including $\downarrow$/absent bowel sounds, $\uparrow$ amylase, $\uparrow$ bilirubin/liver enzymes, and $\downarrow$ platelet count.

Fluid volume deficit r/t active loss from vascular compartment secondary to $\uparrow$ capillary permeability and shift of intravascular volume into interstitial spaces
Desired outcomes: Within 8 h, patient normovolemic: peripheral pulses >2+ on 0-4+ scale, stable body weight, UO $\geq$0.5 ml/kg/h, SBP $\geq$90 mm Hg or wnl, and absence of edema and adventitious lung sounds. PAWP 6-12 mm Hg, CO 4-7 L/min, SVR 900-1200 dynes/sec/cm^{-5}.
- Assess fluid volume by monitoring BP, HR, and peripheral perfusion qh or more often if unstable. Continuous direct arterial pressure monitoring is optimal.
- During acute hypotension, position patient supine with legs elevated to enhance stroke volume.
- Give crystalloids, colloids to maintain PAWP of 6-12 mm Hg or $\leq$18 mm Hg with LV failure. Assess PAWP and lung sounds frequently during fluid replacement to detect fluid overload: crackles and $\uparrow$ PAWP. As indicated, give PRBCs to $\uparrow$ O_2-carrying capacity of the blood.
- Monitor hemodynamic pressures and Svo_2 as available.
- Anticipate $\downarrow$ BP, PAWP, SVR and $\uparrow$ CO/CI. Support with fluids, inotropes as necessary.
- If advanced, anticipate $\downarrow$ BP, $\uparrow$ PAWP, $\uparrow$ SVR, and $\downarrow$ CO/CI. In general, use vasodilators if MAP >100 mm Hg or vasopressors if MAP <70 mm Hg. Fluids, inotropes, vasopressors, and vasodilators all may be necessary because of desensitization to endogenous catecholamines. Titrate carefully to optimize CI and maintain Svo_2 of 60%-80%.
- Weigh qd; monitor I&O every shift and UO qh, noting 24-h trends. Weight may $\uparrow$ despite actual fluid volume deficit as a result of shift of intravascular volume into interstitial spaces.
- Assess for interstitial edema as evidenced by pretibial, sacral, ankle, and hand edema, as well as lung crackles. Take measures to protect skin integrity.

Impaired gas exchange r/t alveolar-capillary membrane changes secondary to interstitial edema, alveolar destruction
Desired outcome: Within 4 h, patient's Pao_2 $\geq$80 mm Hg; $Paco_2$ $\leq$45 mm Hg; pH 7.35-7.45; lungs clear.
- Administer high-flow supplemental O_2 to maximize O_2 available to tissues.
- If patient exhibits inadequate gas exchange (eg, Pao_2 <60 mm Hg on 100% oxygen *via* nonrebreathing mask), prepare for probability of ET intubation and mechanical ventilation.
- Assess for and maintain patent airway by assisting with coughing or suctioning as necessary.
- Assess ABGs. Be alert to $\downarrow$ Pao_2, $\uparrow$ $Paco_2$, acidosis. Monitor for dyspnea, SOB, crackles, restlessness. Adjust supplemental O_2, ventilator settings as indicated.
- Closely monitor PAWP; keep as low as possible to avoid contributing to excess lung water. Be aware that a narrow range of optimal PAWP exists because of complex pathophysiology, including intravascular fluid volume deficit, $\uparrow$ capillary permeability, possible LV failure.
- If patient is on mechanical ventilation, monitor for evidence of ARDS: $\uparrow$ peak inspiratory pressures (eg, $\downarrow$ lung compliance), Fio_2 >0.50, $\uparrow$ PEEP necessary to maintain adequate Pao_2, and diffuse bilateral pulmonary infiltrates ("white out") on chest x-ray.
- Turn q2h to maintain optimal V/Q ratios and prevent atelectasis.

Altered protection r/t clotting factor alterations or $\downarrow$ Hgb level
Desired outcomes: No bleeding; coagulation profiles nl by time of transfer from ICU.
- Obtain blood for coagulation profile.
- Check for bleeding at venipuncture sites, mucous membranes, catheter insertion sites, incisions, GI tract. Test gastric drainage, vomitus, stool for occult blood.
- Administer acid suppression therapy to $\downarrow$ gastric acid, prevent mucosal erosion.
- Avoid IM injection/multiple venipunctures; use IV route instead.

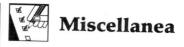 # Miscellanea

CONSULT MD FOR
- S&S of inadequate tissue perfusion: altered mental status, restlessness; $\downarrow$ BP, peripheral pulses; UO <0.5 ml/kg/h $\times$ 2 h; Svo_2 <60% or >80%; $\downarrow$/absent bowel sounds
- New-onset S&S of organ system dysfunction: ARDS, DIC, shock, ARF, mesenteric infarction ($\downarrow$/absent bowel sounds, abdominal distention, enteral feeding intolerance), GI or other unusual bleeding, seizures, hemodynamically significant dysrhythmias, profound acid-base imbalance, electrolyte abnormalities, UO <0.5 ml/kg/h $\times$ 2 h

RELATED TOPICS
- Adult respiratory distress syndrome
- Disseminated intravascular coagulation
- Hemodynamic monitoring
- Mechanical ventilation
- Renal failure, acute
- Shock, septic
- Systemic inflammatory response syndrome
- Vasopressor therapy

ABBREVIATIONS
Do_2: Oxygen delivery
FDPs: Fibrin degradation products
FFP: Fresh frozen plasma
I/E Ratio: Inspiratory-to-expiratory ratio
PPF: Plasma protein fraction
PRBCs: Packed red blood cells
SIRS: Systemic inflammatory response syndrome
SNS: Sympathetic nervous system
Svo_2: Mixed venous oxygen saturation
Vo_2: Oxygen consumption

REFERENCES
Ackerman M: The systemic inflammatory response, sepsis, and multiple organ dysfunction, *Crit Care Nurs Clin North Am* 6(2): 243-250, 1994.

American College of Chest Physicians/Society of Critical Care Medicine Consensus Conference Committee: Definitions for sepsis and organ failure and guidelines for the use of innovative therapies in sepsis, *Crit Care Med* 20(6): 864-874, 1992.

Aragon D, Parson R: Multiple organ dysfunction syndrome in the trauma patient, *Crit Care Nurs Clin North Am* 6(4): 873-881, 1994.

Hammond LC: When organs fail one by one, *RN* 57(10): 36-40, 1994.

Rauen CA: To old to live, too young to die: multiple organ dysfunction syndrome in the elderly, *Crit Care Nurs Clin North Am* 6(3): 535-542, 1994.

Shoemaker WC: Pathophysiology, monitoring, and therapy of acute circulatory problems, *Crit Care Nurs Clin North Am* 6(2): 295-307, 1994.

Author: **Janet Hicks Keen**

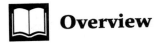 **Overview**

PATHOPHYSIOLOGY

Outcomes predicted according to object producing injury; type of energy released (kinetic, thermal, chemical); energy force (velocity of vehicle or missile); use of protective devices (seat belt, helmet).

Types of Injury

Blunt: Does not penetrate skin. Injury outcome related to compressibility, deformation of involved structures.

Penetrating: Enters tissue, causing direct damage. High-velocity missiles displace surrounding tissue, creating cavitation and massive destruction.

Do_2 and Vo_2: Profound fluid shifts and blood loss create severe fluid volume deficit. O_2 debt created by imbalance between O_2 supply and demand as cellular tissue inadequately perfused. When circulating fluid volume restored, a compensatory hyperdynamic circulatory state develops, improving survival. Inability to achieve hyperdynamic state associated with shock-related organ failure.

Neuroendocrine Stress Response: Release of catecholamines (epinephrine, norepinephrine) mobilizes glycogen stores, suppresses insulin secretion, and promotes peripheral use of glucose, resulting in net ↑ in blood glucose.

SIRS: Inflammatory response triggered by multiple foreign bodies and ↑ catecholamines, which stimulate release and production of WBCs.

MODS: Results from the overwhelming inflammation associated with SIRS or infection; can lead to death.

Other Complications: Hypovolemia, ARDs, ARF, coagulopathy, hypothermia.

INCIDENCE

- >150,000 deaths/yr in US
- Leading cause of death in US for all persons <44 yrs of age

HISTORY/RISK FACTORS

- Alcohol/other intoxicants
- Thrill-seeking behaviors, including high-risk sports
- Act of violence
- Failure to use safety device
- Preexisting medical conditions: COPD, cerebrovascular disorder, renal failure, and immune disorders produce physiologic alterations that impair adaptive responses to injury

INITIAL CLINICAL PRESENTATION

- Mild tenderness to severe pain that can be localized to site of injury, diffuse, or referred
- Dyspnea, agitation, restlessness, anxiety if tissue perfusion/oxygenation impaired

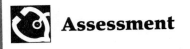 **Assessment**

PHYSICAL ASSESSMENT

Presence of alcohol, other intoxicants may confound CNS assessment and obscure pain, other diagnostic signs.

Inspection

Abrasions and ecchymoses: Suggest involvement of underlying structures. Absence does not preclude internal injury.

Protruding instruments: Do not remove; additional harm/renewed bleeding may occur.

Auscultation

- Breath sounds: ↓ or absent
- Bowel sounds: ↓ or absent

Palpation

- Cool, clammy skin
- Weak, thready pulse
- Swelling and point tenderness over injured area

Percussion

- Dullness over solid organs, large hematomas
- Tympany over lung fields if pneumothorax present

VITAL SIGNS/HEMODYNAMICS

RR: ↑

HR: ↑

BP: Nl, slightly ↑, or ↓ depending on degree of blood loss and circulating catecholamines. Young adults maintain nl BP until major blood loss occurs.

CVP/PAWP: ↓

CO: ↓; if hyperdynamic, ↑

SVR: ↑; if hyperdynamic, ↓

Other: Variable hemodynamic response r/t blood loss, fluid resuscitation, endogenous catecholamines (24 h), hyperdynamic state (48-72 h)

LABORATORY STUDIES

Hct/Hgb: Nl <1 h after injury; then ↓ according to degree of blood loss and dilutional anemia with resuscitation

WBC Count: ↑ initially; left shift with SIRS or infection

ABGs: Possible ↓ Pao_2; possible metabolic acidosis: pH <7.35, HCO_3^- <22

Type and Cross-Match: For transfusion

IMAGING

X-rays: Check for fractures, abnormal air/fluids, foreign objects, location of large organs; C-spine, chest, abdomen, pelvic, extremity x-rays usually necessary

CT Scan: Detects soft tissue injury, major organ hematomas, subtle fractures

▣ Collaborative Management

Oxygenation: Secure airway; intubation or cricothyroidotomy may be necessary. Stabilize C-spine. High-flow supplemental O_2; subsequent O_2 therapy titrated to ABG values, pulse oximetry.

Fluid Management: Underresuscitation contributes to shock, MODS, death. ≥ 2 large-bore (≥ 16 gauge), short catheters placed for rapid delivery of fluids and blood. Trauma/blood tubing, no stopcocks, use of external pressure, and dilution of PRBCs to ↓ viscosity promote rapid infusion of IV fluids. Warm all fluids to body temp to prevent hypothermia. Fluid needs derived from estimated blood loss and hemodynamic parameters.

Crystalloids: 0.9% NaCl or LR commonly used. Sustained use of NS can lead to hyperchloremic metabolic acidosis; therefore LR generally preferred. *Exception:* NS used when infused simultaneously through same IV line as blood products.

Colloids: Generally supplemental to crystalloid therapy. Albumin, dextran, hetastarch used.

PRBCs: If blood loss very rapid during initial resuscitation, immediate transfusion with O-negative blood may be required. Complications of multiple/massive transfusion include hypocalcemia, which may ↓ myocardial contractility. One ampule 10% $CaCl$ administered after every 4 U PRBCs. Abnormal hemostasis may occur as a result of deficient clotting factors in stored PRBCs.

PASG/MAST: To stabilize patients with hypovolemic shock. Inflatable trousers and optional inflatable abdominal compartment ↑ external pressure, resulting in ↑ SVR/MAP. Use is controversial. *Contraindications:* Uncontrolled thoracic bleeding, severe head injury, diaphragmatic rupture.

Gastric Intubation: To prevent vomiting, aspiration.

Urinary Drainage: For UA specimen and to monitor UO qh.

Pharmacotherapy

Broad-spectrum antibiotics: Used initially to prevent infections.

Opiate analgesia: Seldom used in early injury; used after full surgical evaluation and during immediate postop period. IV route preferred. Chronic opiate, alcohol users require larger amounts.

Tetanus prophylaxis: Td required if hx unknown, >10 yr since last immunization and wound clean/minor, or >5 yr and wound large/contaminated.

Parenteral Nutrition: Usually necessary because of ileus, injury to GI tract, ↑ metabolic needs.

Surgery: Need depends on injury type/extent. When multiple systems injured, surgical order coordinated carefully to preserve life and limit disability.

PATIENT-FAMILY TEACHING

- Medications: drug name, purpose, dosage, schedule, precautions, food-drug and drug-drug interactions, potential side effects
- Injury prevention education: instructions regarding seat belt application, firearm safety, injury prevention strategies suitable for persons involved
- Referral to trauma support groups
- Alcohol/substance abuse rehab program

Nursing Diagnoses/Interventions

Fluid volume deficit r/t active loss
Desired outcomes: Patient normovolemic within 12 h: MAP $\geq$70 mm Hg, HR 60-100 bpm, CVP 2-6 mm Hg, PAWP 6-12 mm Hg, CI $\geq$2.5 L/min/m^2, UO $\geq$0.5 ml/kg/h, warm extremities, brisk capillary refill, distal pulses $\geq$2+.

- Monitor BP q5-15min for $\downarrow$ or consistent downward trend.
- Monitor ECG for $\uparrow$ HR and myocardial ischemic changes caused by dilutional anemia.
- With volume depletion or active blood loss, administer pressurized fluids rapidly through several large-caliber catheters. Warm all fluids to prevent hypothermia. Use rapid warmer/infuser for blood products.
- Measure PA pressures q1-2h or more frequently. Measure CO/CI and calculate SVR and PVR q4-8h, or more often with instability. $\uparrow$ HR, $\downarrow$ PAWP, $\downarrow$ CO/CI, and $\uparrow$ SVR suggest inadequate fluid resuscitation. Be alert for pulmonary hypertension, which occurs with thoracic injury, smoke inhalation, ARDS.
- During hyperdynamic phase, anticipate $>$ nl CO/CI and $<$ nl SVR. Support status by administering fluids and supplemental O$_2$.
- Measure UO q1-2h. UO $<$0.5 ml/kg/h for 2 consecutive h suggests inadequate intravascular volume.
- Monitor for physical indicators of hypovolemia: cool extremities, capillary refill $>$2 sec, absent/$\downarrow$ amplitude of distal pulses.
- Estimate ongoing blood loss. Measure bloody or dark drainage from tubes/catheters. Estimate amount of blood loss *via* wound site.
- Administer O$_2$ to maximize delivery to tissues. Use continuous Spo$_2$ to check for adequacy.

Pain r/t physical injury
Desired outcomes: Within 2 h, patient's score on subjective evaluation of discomfort improves. Nonverbal indicators (eg, grimacing) absent.

- Use pain scale or devise communication methods for patients with ET tubes or other barriers. Preop pain is an anticipated and vital diagnostic aid.
- Administer opiates/other analgesics. Avoid preop opiates until thorough evaluation by trauma surgeon. Once prescribed, administer promptly *via* IV route before pain becomes severe.
- Substance abuse often involved in traumatic events; victims may be drug or alcohol users with $>$average tolerance to opiates and may develop symptoms of alcohol or opiate withdrawal that require treatment.
- Be aware that opiate analgesics can $\downarrow$ GI motility and may delay return to nl bowel functioning.

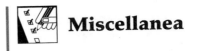 # Miscellanea

CONSULT MD FOR
- Abnormal VS: RR $>$20 breaths/min, HR $>$100 bpm, SBP $<$90 mm Hg
- Abnormal hemodynamics: CVP $<$2 mm Hg, PAWP $<$6 mm Hg, CI $<$2.5 L/min/m^2
- Spo$_2$ $<$90%
- UO $<$0.5 ml/kg/h $\times$ 2
- Altered mentation
- Occult blood in vomitus, blood-tinged stool/urine
- $\uparrow$ or uncontrolled pain
- Abnormal or purulent wound drainage

RELATED TOPICS
- Adult respiratory distress syndrome
- Anxiety
- Disseminated intravascular coagulation
- Hypothermia
- Mechanical ventilation
- Multiple organ dysfunction syndrome
- Nutritional support, enteral
- Systemic inflammatory response syndrome
- Wounds healing by primary intention
- Wounds healing by secondary intention

ABBREVIATIONS
Do$_2$: Oxygen delivery
FDP: Fibrin degradation product
MODS: Multiple organ dysfunction syndrome
PRBCs: Packed red blood cells
SIRS: Systemic inflammatory response syndrome
Td: Combined tetanus diphtheria toxoid
Vo$_2$: Oxygen consumption

Altered protection r/t clotting factor alterations or ↓ Hgb level
Desired outcomes: Patient exhibits no bleeding. Coagulation profiles nl by transfer from ICU.
- Obtain blood for PT, PTT, Hct, Hgb, fibrinogen levels, and FDPs. FDP >40 µg/ml = critical value; ≤10 = nl.
- Check for bleeding at venipuncture sites, mucous membranes, catheter insertion sites, incisions, GI tract. Test gastric drainage, vomitus, stool for occult blood.
- Give H_2-receptor antagonists, antacids, sucralfate to ↓ gastric acid, prevent mucosal erosion.
- Avoid IM injection/multiple venipunctures; use IV route instead.
- If invasive procedure necessary, press over insertion site for ≥3-5 min for venous; ≥10-15 min for arterial.

Risk for infection r/t inadequate primary/secondary defenses, tissue destruction, environmental exposure, multiple invasive procedures
Desired outcome: Patient infection free: core/rectal temp ≤37.8° C; HR ≤100 bpm; orientation × 3; no unusual redness, warmth, drainage at incisions/drain sites.
- Monitor VS for infection: ↑ temp, RR, HR. ↑ CO and ↓ SVR suggest sepsis.
- Evaluate LOC q2-4h. Altered mentation suggests sepsis.
- Keep all surgically placed tubes or drains patent by irrigating or attaching to low-pressure suction.
- Check incisions and wound sites for infection: redness, warmth, delayed healing, purulent or unusual drainage.
- Aid in removal of eschar by irrigation or wound packing, or prepare for surgical débridement.
- Culture drainage if foul smelling or abnormal.
- Give parenteral antibiotics in timely fashion. Reschedule if dosage delayed ≥1 h.
- Give tetanus immunoglobulin and tetanus toxoid as necessary.
- Change dressings q24h or more often if wet or soiled.

Posttrauma response r/t unanticipated serious physical injury or event
Desired outcome: By discharge, patient states impact of event has ↓; cooperates with treatment plan; does not exhibit severe stress reaction.
- Evaluate for severe stress reaction: display of affect inconsistent with statements or behavior, suicidal or homicidal statements or actions, extreme agitation or depression, failure to cooperate with care.
- Anticipate some reexperience of traumatic event. Reassure that this is common.
- Consult with specialist such as psychiatric nurse clinician for signs of severe stress reaction.
- Consider organic causes that may contribute to posttraumatic stress response (eg, severe pain, alcohol withdrawal, impaired cerebral perfusion).

REFERENCES
Bishop MH: Relationship between supranormal circulatory values, time delays, and outcome in severely traumatized patients, *Crit Care Med* 21(1): 56-63, 1993.
Cardona VC et al: *Trauma nursing: from resuscitation through rehabilitation,* ed 2, Philadelphia, 1994, WB Saunders.
Fontaine DK: The cutting edge in trauma, *Crit Care Nurse* (June Suppl): 14-21, 1993.
Lekander B, Cerra F: The syndrome of multiple organ failure, *Crit Care Nurs Clin North Am* 2(2): 331-342, 1990.
Reilly E, Yucha C: Multiple organ failure syndrome, *Crit Care Nurse* 14(2): 25-31, 1993.
Sommers MS: Alcohol and trauma: the critical link, *Crit Care Nurse* 14(2): 82-93, 1993.

Author: **Janet Hicks Keen**

Overview

PATHOPHYSIOLOGY

Chronic, progressive autoimmune disorder manifesting as weakness and abnormal fatigability of voluntary striated skeletal muscles. Abnormality occurs on postsynaptic membrane, where there is marked ↓ in AChRs. In ≈ 85%-90% of cases, an anti-AChR antibody is believed to cause structural damage to postsynaptic AChRs, inhibit receptor site synthesis, and cause receptor site blockade. Disease course depends on muscle groups involved and degree of involvement. Remissions and exacerbations can occur.

Myasthenic Crisis: Caused by medication tolerance or disease exacerbation from infection, trauma, surgery, temp extremes, stress, endocrine imbalance, or drugs with neuromuscular-blocking properties such as sedatives, tranquilizers, narcotics, certain antibiotics (eg, neomycin, gentamicin, tetracycline).

Cholinergic Crisis: Caused by anticholinesterase overdose; blocks AChR sites, causing neuromuscular depolarizing blockade.

HISTORY/RISK FACTORS

- Autoimmune disorders: RA, thyrotoxicosis, SLE, ulcerative colitis, pernicious anemia
- Women between 20-30 yrs; men >age 40
- Ratio of women to men: 3:2

CLINICAL PRESENTATION

Generalized Form: Weakness, abnormal fatigability of skeletal muscles that worsens as effort sustained and day progresses.

Ocular Form: Limited to eyes; can be mild. Responds poorly to drug therapy, but may remit spontaneously. Eye signs include ptosis, diplopia, inability to maintain upward gaze.

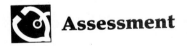

Assessment

PHYSICAL ASSESSMENT

Generalized Forms

Mild: Slow onset, usually begins with eye signs and spreads to bulbar nerves and skeletal muscles, sparing respiratory muscles. May remit; responds well to drug therapy.

  Eye signs: Ptosis, diplopia, inability to control extraocular muscles

  Bulbar signs: Difficulty chewing, dysphagia, dysarthria, inability to close mouth or raise chin off chest, nasal regurgitation of fluids, neck muscle weakness

  Limbs/girdle: Weakness

Moderate: Onset slow to moderate with early eye involvement. All muscle groups involved to varying degrees. Less responsive to drug therapy; remission possible.

Eye and bulbar signs: Similar to mild form; bulbar S&S may be severe

Skeletal muscle involvement: ↓ strength in all extremities; inability to maintain position without support

Resp muscle involvement: Diaphragmatic and intercostal weakness, dyspnea, ineffective cough, secretion accumulation, risk of respiratory arrest

Severe or acute fulminating: Rapid onset with severe bulbar and skeletal weakness. Early respiratory muscle involvement. Incidence of myasthenic or cholinergic crisis high; response to treatment poor. S&S similar to but more severe than moderate form.

Myasthenic Crisis: ↑ muscle weakness, anxiety, apprehension; severe ocular, bulbar weakness; rapid respiratory muscle weakness; respiratory arrest possible.

Cholinergic Crisis: ↑ muscle weakness, anxiety, apprehension; fasciculations (twitching) around eyes, mouth; diarrhea, cramping; sweating; pupillary constriction; excessive salivation; difficulty breathing, swallowing.

VITAL SIGNS/HEMODYNAMICS

MYASTHENIC CRISIS

RR: ↑; arrest possible

HR: ↑, ↓, or nl, depending on exacerbating factors or side effects of anticholinesterase

BP: ↑ or ↓, as with HR

Temp: Nl or ↑; if crisis caused by infection, ↑

CHOLINERGIC CRISIS

RR: ↑

HR: ↑ or ↓, depending on exacerbating factors or side effects of anticholinesterase

BP: ↑ or ↓, as with HR

Temp: Nl or ↑

Hemodynamics: Vary according to age, general health status

LABORATORY STUDIES

Tensilon Test: Short-acting anticholinesterase that delays breakdown of ACh, permitting ACh to act repeatedly over a longer period of time. With MG, symptoms improve within 30-60 sec of IV injection (2-10 mg). In myasthenic crisis, weakness improves with Tensilon; with cholinergic, symptoms worsen. Keep atropine sulfate at bedside to reverse Tensilon effects if cholinergic crisis occurs during test.

Serum Antibody Titer: ↑ against AChRs in 80%-90% of cases.

Thyroid Studies: Hyperthyroidism frequently present in young women with MG.

Others: CPK, ESR, and antinuclear antibody levels tested because of frequency of other immunologic disorders with MG.

IMAGING

CT Scan of Thymus Gland: To evaluate for thymic abnormality.

DIAGNOSTIC PROCEDURES

EMG: Amplitude of evoked muscle action potentials ↓ rapidly in MG.

Mediastinoscopy: Evaluates for thymic hyperplasia (80% of patients) and gross or microscopic thymomas (10%-15%).

Collaborative Management

Myasthenic or Cholinergic Crisis: Anticholinesterase withheld or ↓ temporarily. "Drug holiday" improves subsequent responsiveness to medication. In severe MG, plasmapheresis may hasten improvement in S&S.

Pharmacotherapy

Anticholinesterase agents: Pyridostigmine bromide (Mestinon), neostigmine bromide (Prostigmin Bromide), and ambenonium chloride (Mytelase) inhibit ACh breakdown. Pyridostigmine (drug of choice) is longer acting and has fewer side effects.

Corticosteroids (eg, ACTH, prednisone): Clinical improvement shown in 70%-100% of patients. Used for weakness uncontrolled by anticholinesterase drugs or surgery and patients who refuse surgery. Given alone or in combination with anticholinesterase drugs.

Immunosuppressive drugs: Cytotoxic drugs such as azathioprine (Imuran) and cyclophosphamide (Cytoxan) used alone or in combination with other therapies when response to steroids poor. Serious side effects: toxic hepatitis, thrombocytopenia, leukopenia, infections, nausea, vomiting, alopecia; leukemia and lymphoma possible.

Immune globulin: High doses may give rapid, brief symptom relief in some patients.

Thymectomy: May lead to clinical improvement, especially with thymic hyperplasia. Two approaches: transcervical or thoracotomy. Former may be less successful because of residual thymic tissue.

Plasmapheresis: Enables removal of abnormal circulating antibodies that interfere with AChRs. *Complications:* hypovolemia, impaired clotting, hypokalemia, hypocalcemia, myasthenic or cholinergic crisis.

Radiotherapy: For severe cases unresponsive to other therapies.

Resp Support: ET tube or tracheostomy with mechanical ventilation may be necessary.

Nutritional Support: Enteral or parenteral feedings may be needed for dysphagia.

PATIENT-FAMILY TEACHING

- S&S of myasthenic and cholinergic crises
- Need for resuscitator bag and suction apparatus at home
- Myasthenia Gravis Foundation: 222 South Riverside Plaza, Suite 1540, Chicago, IL 60606; 1-800-541-5454

Nursing Diagnoses/Interventions

Impaired gas exchange r/t altered O_2 supply associated with ↓ chest expansion and air movement secondary to weakness and abnormal fatigability of muscles of respiration
Desired outcomes: Within 12-24 h of treatment initiation, patient has adequate gas exchange: orientation × 3; RR ≤20 breaths/min with eupnea; Pao_2 ≥80 mm Hg; $Paco_2$ ≤45 mm Hg; and O_2 saturation ≥94%.

- Assess for indicators of altered respiratory function: restlessness, somnolence, ↓/adventitious breath sounds; changes in respiratory rate, rhythm, and depth; changes in skin color.
- Monitor ventilatory capability *via* pulmonary function tests. VC <75% of predicted value, tidal volume <1000 ml (or < nl/baseline volume), and RR >34 breaths/min signal need for assisted ventilation.
- Monitor ABG and pulse oximetry results. Falling Pao_2 (<60 mm Hg), rising $Paco_2$ (>50 mm Hg), and ↓ O_2 saturation, coupled with changes in VC, tidal volume, and increasing RR, indicate need for ET intubation or tracheostomy and mechanical ventilation.
- Provide pulmonary toilet q2h when patient awake and prn.

Ineffective airway clearance r/t ineffective cough; ↓ energy; and abnormal fatigability of diaphragmatic, intercostal, pharyngeal, and accessory muscles of respiration
Desired outcome: Within 24-48 h of intervention/treatment, patient's airway clear as evidenced by absence of adventitious breath sounds.

- Assess breath sounds, effectiveness of cough, and quality, amount, and color of sputum. Monitor for inability to raise secretions and secretions that are tenacious, thick, or voluminous. Send sputum for C&S if infection suspected.
- Suction as indicated, using hyperoxygenation before/after procedure. If patient has a tracheostomy, always suction trachea and mouth before deflating tracheostomy cuff. Especially important with MG because of ↑ saliva.
- Place in semi- to high-Fowler's position at all times to facilitate chest excursion and ↓ risk of aspiration. If patient has a tracheostomy, keep cuff inflated during feedings.
- ↑ activity as allowed and tolerated to minimize stasis of secretions and facilitate lung expansion.
- Keep another tracheostomy tube of the same size and an obturator at bedside in the event of inadvertent extubation.

Impaired swallowing r/t ↓ or absent gag reflex, ↓ strength or excursion of muscles involved in mastication, facial paralysis, or mechanical obstruction (tracheostomy tube)
Desired outcome: Patient demonstrates capability for safe and effective swallowing before oral foods and fluids given or reintroduced: presence of gag reflex and adequate strength and excursion of muscles involved in mastication.

- Assess for gag reflex, ability to swallow, and strength and excursion of muscles involved in mastication. As indicated, consult with speech therapist to determine patient's ability to swallow. If patient has an artificial airway, add a few drops of blue food coloring to tube feedings to facilitate assessment of aspiration.
- If patient cannot swallow, confer with physician regarding alternate method of nutritional support, such as enteral or parenteral nutrition.
- After return of gag reflex and ability to swallow, begin oral feedings cautiously.
  Start with a small quantity of ice chips, which may help stimulate swallowing reflex, and progress to semisolid foods and then to solid foods. If patient has a tracheostomy, inflate tracheostomy cuff for 30 min before/after feedings to prevent aspiration.
  Elevate HOB ≥70 degrees to facilitate gravity flow through pylorus.
  Provide small feedings at frequent intervals.
  Avoid cold foods and beverages, which cause bloating and upward pressure on diaphragm and may impede respiratory excursion.
  Keep suction equipment at bedside; suction excess secretions as necessary after each feeding. Inspect buccal surface pc for residual food particles. Provide materials for oral hygiene pc.
- If patient unable to communicate verbally, be alert to signs of respiratory distress, which can occur in response to aspiration: dyspnea, change in rate/depth of respirations, restlessness or agitation, pallor, adventitious breath sounds. If these signs occur, discontinue feeding immediately, ensure that HOB elevated, and provide O_2. If tracheostomy tube in place, suction through tube to remove food or secretions that may be obstructing airway.

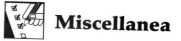 # Miscellanea

CONSULT MD FOR
- Advancement of myasthenic crisis
- Precipitation of cholinergic crisis
- Respiratory impairment: RR >24 breaths/min, Pao_2 <60 mm Hg, $Paco_2$ >50 mm Hg, Spo_2 <90%, inability to clear secretions
- Respiratory tract infection: change in sputum color, temp ≥37.8° C, ↑ WBCs

RELATED TOPICS
- Hypocalcemia
- Hypokalemia
- Mechanical ventilation
- Pneumonia, aspiration
- Psychosocial needs, patient
- Respiratory failure, acute

ABBREVIATIONS
ACh: Acetylcholine
AChR: Acetylcholine receptor
ACTH: Adrenocorticotropic hormone
ESR: Erythrocyte sedimentation rate
RA: Rheumatoid arthritis
SLE: Systemic lupus erythematosus
VC: Vital capacity

REFERENCES
Hardy EM, Rittenberry K: Myasthenia gravis: an overview, *Orthop Nurs* 13(6): 37-42, 1994.
Kernich CA, Kaminski HJ: Myasthenia gravis: pathophysiology, diagnosis, and collaborative care, *J Neurosci Nurs* 27(4): 207-218, 1995.
O'Donnel L: Caring for patients with myasthenia gravis. . . find out your role in assessing and managing this debilitating disorder, *Nursing* 25(3): 60-61, 1995.
Stowe AC: Myasthenia gravis. In Swearingen PL, Keen JH (eds): *Manual of critical care nursing,* ed 3, St Louis, 1995, Mosby.
Willig TN et al: Swallowing problems in neuromuscular disorders, *Arch Phys Med Rehabil* 75(11): 1175-1181, 1994.

Author: **Ann Coghlan Stowe**

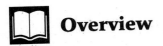 **Overview**

PATHOPHYSIOLOGY

Necrosis of myocardial tissue caused by lack of myocardial blood supply. Most AMIs caused by atherosclerosis, resulting in progressive narrowing of the coronary artery, thrombus formation, and, ultimately, occlusion of blood flow. Occlusion also caused by coronary artery spasm. Site of infarction determined by location of arterial occlusion.

HISTORY/RISK FACTORS

- Family hx of CAD
- Hyperlipidemia, hypercholesterolemia
- Hypertension, DM, obesity
- Age >65 yr
- Male; postmenopausal female
- Cigarette smoking
- ↑ stress
- Sedentary life-style

CLINICAL PRESENTATION

Classic: Substernal chest pain/pressure that radiates from jaw to epigastrium. Radiates to left arm, down inner aspect along ulnar nerve. Differs from angina in that it is constant and unrelieved by rest, position, or nitrates; duration ≥30 min. Denial of symptoms, severity is common.

Less Typical: Vague symptoms of GI upset or epigastric distress. May have no chest discomfort and only arm or shoulder blade pain. Approximately 25% of AMIs "silent," with vague symptoms not at all suggestive of AMI.

Assessment

PHYSICAL ASSESSMENT

Neuro: Anxiety, apprehension, weakness, fatigue

Resp: Dyspnea, orthopnea, cyanosis, crackles

CV: Tachycardia, bradycardia, dysrhythmias, S_4 gallop, pericardial friction rub, murmurs. If heart failure present, split S_1 and S_2, S_3 gallop

GI: Nausea, vomiting

Integ: Diaphoresis

VITAL SIGNS/HEMODYNAMICS

RR: ↑

HR: ↑ or ↓

BP: Nl or mild ↑; ↓ with ↓ CO

Temp: Nl or mild ↑ caused by inflammatory response

CVP: ↑ with RV infarct or advanced heart failure

PAWP: ↑ with LV infarct, heart failure

CO: ↓ with heart failure; or large area of akinetic ventricle

SVR: ↑

Other: Hemodynamics reflect response to ↑ sympathetic tone or impaired ventricular contractility

ECG: Mild tachycardia, bradycardia, AV block, ventricular dysrhythmias

LABORATORY STUDIES

Serum Enzymes: ↑ CK within 24 h of AMI. Isoenzyme levels more diagnostic of cardiac muscle damage. Generally, CK-MB level >10% of total CK signals myocardial muscle damage. If hx strongly suggestive of MI, and CK total and MB are wnl, testing for lactic dehydrogenase (LD) isoenzyme may be helpful. If total LD ↑ and LD_1 is the predominant isoenzyme, this is diagnostic of MI. Cardiac troponin I levels ≥3.1 ng/ml specific for myocardial injury.

Cholesterol: Level <200 mg/dl desirable.

Mg^{2+}, K^+: Often drop in AMI; low levels associated with ↑ incidence of dysrhythmias.

Leukocytes and ESR: ↑ as a result of inflammatory process.

IMAGING

Chest X-ray: May reveal cardiomegaly and signs of LV failure (interstitial pulmonary edema).

Technetium Pyrophosphate: May help to localize area of infarction. Necrotic tissue appears as darkened area or "hot spot" on scan up to 10 days after MI.

MUGA Scan: IV injection of isotope evaluates LV function and detects aneurysms, wall motion abnormalities, and intracardiac shunting.

Echocardiogram: Detects abnormalities of LV wall motion, measures EF, evaluates valve function, and estimates LVEDP. Normal EF >60%.

PET: Use of isotopes to assess metabolic activity of areas of infarct to determine if viable, but jeopardized, tissue present.

DIAGNOSTIC PROCEDURES

ECGs: Done immediately to direct therapy, then serially (24 h apart) or if condition changes. Changes in certain lead groups identify area, evolution of infarct.

ST-segment changes: Elevated in lead over or facing infarcted area. Reciprocal changes (ST-segment depressions) found in leads 180 degrees from area of infarction.

T-wave changes: Early, "giant" upright T waves seen in leads over infarct. Within several h to days, T wave becomes inverted. Gradually over time, ST-segment becomes isoelectric and T wave may remain inverted. T-wave changes may last for wks and return to nl or remain inverted for life.

Q waves: Indicative of MI; meet one of two criteria: wide (>.04 sec) or deep (>25% of total voltage of QRS).

Hemodynamic Monitoring: Used with complicated MI that results in failure with possible progression to cardiogenic shock.

Coronary Angiography: Identifies extent of CAD, location of lesions, and suitability for CABG, angioplasty, or atherectomy.

Collaborative Management

IV NTG: Titrated until relief of chest pain occurs while ensuring that SBP remains >90 mm Hg. Usually started at 10 μg/min and gradually $\uparrow$ q5−10min. Hypotension possible, especially if RV infarction present, since prompt vasodilatation results in $\downarrow$ venous return and reduction in preload.

IV Morphine Sulfate: Used with nitrates to relieve chest pain and $\downarrow$ anxiety, preload, sympathetic tone. Usual dosage 2-4 mg initially; given in 2-mg increments.

O$_2$: $\geq$2-4 L/min *via* nasal cannula; titrate to maintain Sao$_2$ $\geq$96%-98%.

Thrombolytic Therapy: With alteplase (Activase), anistreplase (APSAC, Eminase), streptokinase to lyse the clot in selected patients. May be given intracoronary in some instances.

Reduction of Cardiac Workload: Achieved with bed rest, β blockers, calcium channel blockers.

Prevention, Recognition, Treatment of Dysrhythmias: ACLS algorithms or agency protocol implemented.

Antiplatelet/Anticoagulant Therapy: For prevention of thrombus. Aspirin $\downarrow$ platelet aggregation; heparin prevents clot formation.

Management of Fluid Imbalance: To optimize preload. Oral and IV fluids given for dehydration; diuretics and vasodilators given for volume overload.

PTCA: May be performed emergently for residual stenosis after thrombolytic therapy.

IABP: For hemodynamic compromise refractory to NTG and other measures. Balloon inflation during diastole $\uparrow$ coronary perfusion; rapid deflation just before systole $\downarrow$ SVR (afterload) and LV workload.

CABG: Surgical indications include stable angina with 50% stenosis of left main coronary artery, stable angina with 3-vessel CAD, unstable angina with 3-vessel CAD or severe 2-vessel CAD, recent MI, ischemic heart failure with cardiogenic shock, and ischemia or impending MI after angiography.

PATIENT-FAMILY TEACHING

- Importance of activity limitation and its rationale: to minimize O$_2$ requirements and thus $\downarrow$ chest pain
- Necessity of reporting any further episodes of chest pain
- Measures that prevent complications of $\downarrow$ mobility, such as active ROM exercises
- Risk factor modification: diet low in cholesterol and saturated fat, smoking cessation, stress management
- Actions to take if chest pain unrelieved or $\uparrow$ in intensity:

  Stop and rest; sit or lie down.

  Take one NTG; wait 5 min. If pain not relieved, take second NTG; wait 5 min. If pain not relieved, take third NTG.

  Lie down if headache occurs, since vasodilatation effect of NTG causes $\downarrow$ in BP and transient headache.

  If pain not relieved after 3 NTGs taken over 15-min period, call physician or dial 911 or local emergency number.

- Post-MI activity progression, including guidelines for resuming post-MI sexual activity
- Phone number for American Heart Association: 1-800-242-8721; phone numbers for local and state Heart Associations

Nursing Diagnoses/Interventions

Pain (chest) r/t biophysiologic injury secondary to ↓ myocardial O_2 supply
Desired outcomes: Within 1 h of intervention, subjective evaluation of discomfort improves, as documented by pain scale.

- Assess and document character of chest pain: location, duration, quality, intensity, precipitating and alleviating factors, presence/absence of radiation, and associated symptoms. Have patient rate discomfort from 0 (no pain) to 10 (severe).
- Measure BP and HR with each episode. ↑ possible because of sympathetic stimulation as a result of pain. Alternately, if chest pain caused by ischemia, cardiac output may ↓, resulting in low BP.
- Obtain 12/18-lead ECG during chest pain. Ischemia is usually demonstrated by ST-segment depression and T-wave inversion.
- Administer O_2 per nasal cannula at 2-4 L/min.
- Position according to comfort level. Keep patients on IV NTG on complete bed rest until condition stabilizes. Profound orthostatic hypotension possible.
- Provide care in calm and efficient manner; reassure and support patient during chest pain episodes.
- Maintain quiet environment and group care activities to enable periods of uninterrupted rest.
- Administer nitrates, titrating IV NTG so that chest pain is relieved, yet SBP remains >90 mm Hg.
- If hypotension occurs (SBP 80-90 mm Hg), ↓ flow rate to ≤ ½ of infusing dose and administer small fluid challenge (eg, 250-500 ml) unless contraindicated by overt heart failure. If severe hypotension (SBP <80 mm Hg) occurs, stop infusion and contact physician, who may prescribe a low-dose positive inotropic agent (eg, dopamine, dobutamine).
- Monitor for NTG side effects: headache, hypotension, syncope, facial flushing, and nausea. If side effects occur, place in supine position and consult physician.
- Administer β blockers and calcium channel blockers, which relieve chest pain by diminishing coronary artery spasm, causing coronary and peripheral vasodilatation and ↓ myocardial contractility and O_2 demand. Monitor for side effects, including bradycardia and hypotension. Be alert to indicators of heart failure, eg, fatigue, SOB, weight gain, and edema, and heart block, eg, syncope and dizziness.
- Administer heparin and aspirin as prescribed. Monitor for excessive anticoagulation, including PTT value.

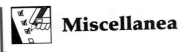 ## Miscellanea

CONSULT MD FOR
- Symptomatic or significant hypotension: SBP ≤80 mm Hg or associated with chest pain, dysrhythmias, SOB
- Serious or symptomatic dysrhythmias (eg, runs of VT, advancing heart block)
- Significant changes in 12-lead ECG: presence of Q waves, ST-segment elevation/depression
- Complications: cardiogenic shock, pulmonary edema

RELATED TOPICS
- Cardiac catheterization
- Cardiac surgery: CABG
- Coronary artery disease
- Coronary thrombolysis
- Hemodynamic monitoring
- Shock, cardiogenic

ABBREVIATIONS
EF: Ejection fraction
ESR: Erythrocyte sedimentation rate
IABP: Intraaortic balloon pump
ICS: Intercostal space
LVEDP: Left ventricular end-diastolic pressure
MCL: Midclavicular line

Decreased cardiac output r/t electrical factors (altered rate, rhythm, conduction) secondary to cardiac injury and infarcted tissue

Desired outcome: Within 24 h of treatment, patient in NSR; incidence of dysrhythmias ↓.

- Monitor continuously in modified chest lead V_I to detect ventricular ectopy vs aberrancy. Monitor on V_{II} if supraventricular dysrhythmias are present or if it is imperative to identify axis deviations. Keep alarms on at all times (eg, 50-100).
- Assess apical HR qh. Monitor for irregularities in rhythm.
- Auscultate for systolic murmur at fifth ICS, MCL; if present it could signal papillary muscle ischemia and mitral regurgitation.
- Document rhythm strip every shift and prn if dysrhythmias occur.
- Administer antidysrhythmics according to ACLS or agency guidelines.
- Monitor K^+ for levels >5.0 mEq/L or <3.5 mEq/L. Hypokalemia or hyperkalemia can cause dysrhythmias. Replace potassium as indicated.
- Deliver O_2 *via* nasal cannula at 2-4 L/min or as prescribed. O_2 may be beneficial for treating dysrhythmias caused by ischemia.

Decreased cardiac output r/t negative inotropic changes in the heart secondary to myocardial injury

Desired outcomes: Within 24 h of treatment, patient has adequate cardiac output: SBP ≥90 mm Hg, CO ≥4 L/min, CI ≥2.5 L/min/m^2, HR ≤100 bpm, warm and dry skin, UO ≥0.5 ml/kg/h, PAWP ≤18 mm Hg.

- Assess for the following as evidence of myocardial dysfunction: SBP <90 mm Hg, HR >100 bpm, RR >20 breaths/min, JVD, dependent edema, hepatomegaly, fatigue, weakness, ↓ activity level, and SOB with activity. Additional S&S include:
  Mental status: Restlessness, ↓ responsiveness
  Lung sounds: Crackles, rhonchi
  Heart sounds: S_3 gallop, murmur, ↑ HR
  Skin: Pallor, mottling, cyanosis, coolness, diaphoresis
- Record hemodynamic readings q1-2h and prn. Be alert to PAWP >18 mm Hg, CO <4 L/min, and CI <2.5 L/min/m^2.
- Keep accurate I&O records and weigh patient qd. Be alert to fluid volume excess.
- Help minimize cardiac workload by administering β blockers, placing in Fowler's or semi-Fowler's position as BP allows, and encouraging bed rest.
- Have patient perform active ROM and deep-breathing exercises. Encourage position changes from side to side q2h.
- Administer nitrates and afterload reducing agents, such as nitroprusside and preload reducing agents such as NTG, to maintain SVR within 900-1200 dynes/sec/cm^{-5} and PAWP ≤18 mm Hg; diuretics, such as furosemide and metolazone, to keep PAWP ≤18 mm Hg and UO ≥0.5 ml/kg/h; and inotropic agents, such as dopamine and dobutamine, to keep SBP >90 mm Hg.

REFERENCES

Adams J et al: Cardiac troponin I: a marker with high specificity for cardiac injury, *Circulation* 88(1): 101-106, 1993.

Engler MB, Engler MM: Assessment of the cardiovascular effects of stress, *J Cardiovasc Nurs* 10(1): 51-63, 1995.

Habib GB: Current status of thrombolysis in acute myocardial infarction, *Chest* 107(1): 225-232, 1995.

Paul S: The pathophysiologic process of ventricular remodeling: from infarct to failure, *Crit Care Nurs Q* 18(1): 7-21, 1995.

Reinhart SI: Uncomplicated acute myocardial infarction: a critical path, *Cardiovasc Nurs* 31(1): 1-7, 1995.

Stewart S, Kucia A, Poropat S: Early detection and management of right ventricular infarction: the role of the critical care nurse, *Dimens Crit Care Nurs* 14(6): 282-292, 1995.

Author: **Barbara Tueller Steuble**

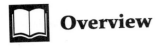 **Overview**

PATHOPHYSIOLOGY
Hypothyroidism results in ↓ circulating thyroid hormone, in which overall metabolic rate is significantly slowed. In severe cases in which hypothyroidism is untreated, a life-threatening condition known as myxedema coma can occur. Myxedema is a type of non-pitting edema that may be present in all patients with thyroid disease.

INCIDENCE/MORTALITY
Seen infrequently, but mortality rate >50%.

HISTORY/RISK FACTORS
- Hypothyroidism resulting from primary thyroid disease or anterior pituitary/hypothalamic disease
- Recent infection
- Severe emotional stress
- Adrenal insufficiency
- Rheumatologic or immunologic diseases
- Failure to take thyroid replacement medications

CLINICAL PRESENTATION
Extreme fatigue, unconsciousness with slow RR, bradycardia, hypoglycemia, hypothermia, hypotension, shock

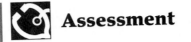 **Assessment**

PHYSICAL ASSESSMENT
Neuro: ↓ LOC, coma, seizures, hypothermia, cold intolerance
Resp: Slow, shallow respirations; possible basilar crackles
CV: Bradycardia, ↓ BP, activity intolerance, dysrhythmias or ECG findings reflective of ischemia.
Endo: Hypoglycemia, possible goiter
GI: Constipation, enlarged tongue
Integ: Dry, cracked, skin; coarse, brittle hair; myxedema in extremities

VITAL SIGNS/HEMODYNAMICS
RR: ↓
HR: ↓
BP: ↓
Temp: ↓
CVP/PAWP: Nl, ↑, or ↓
SVR: Nl, ↑, or ↓
CO: ↓
12/18-Lead ECG: May reveal changes r/t myocardial ischemia if hypotension ensues. Sinus bradycardia or AV heart block may be present. If myocardial perfusion altered, PACs or PVCs may be seen.

LABORATORY STUDIES
TSH: ↑ unless disease longstanding or severe
TRH Stimulation Test: ↑ basal
FTI and T_4 Levels: ↓
Antimicrosomal Antibodies: Positive test represents Hashimoto's thyroiditis.
Electrolytes: May reflect hyponatremia r/t associated adrenal insufficiency.

IMAGING
^{131}I Scan and Uptake: Will be <10% in a 24-h period. In secondary hypothyroidism, uptake ↑ with administration of exogenous TSH. With myxedema, treatment cannot await test results.

Collaborative Management

Goal of therapy: to ↑ metabolic rate sufficiently enough to normalize VS and organ function.
Supplemental O_2: To promote oxygenation to tissues. ET intubation/mechanical ventilation may be necessary.
Treatment of Hypotension: IV isotonic fluids (0.9% NS or RL). D_5W avoided. Vasopressors may not be effective because of ↓ metabolism.
Treatment of Hypoglycemia: D_{50} IV push
Treatment of Hyponatremia: Fluid restriction; 3% saline solution infusion may be necessary.
Identification of Cause/Stressor with Appropriate Treatment
Pharmacotherapy
IV thyroid supplements (rapid infusion): For hypothyroidism.
Concomitant IV hydrocortisone: May be given to avoid hyperadrenalism associated with aggressive thyroid replacement therapy.
Hypertonic (3%) saline: By continuous infusion for hyponatremia.

PATIENT-FAMILY TEACHING
- Importance of lifelong compliance with medications, especially thyroid replacement medications: purpose, dosage, schedule, precautions, drug-drug and food-drug interactions, and potential side effects
- Purpose, expected results, anticipated sensations of all nursing/medical interventions
- Expected changes that occur with hormone replacement: ↑ energy level, weight loss, ↓ peripheral edema; improvement of neuromuscular problems
- Importance of avoiding physical/emotional stress and ways to maximize coping mechanisms for handling stress
- S&S that signal need for prompt medical attention: fever, signs of infection, symptoms of hyperthyroidism (which may result from excess hormone replacement)

Nursing Diagnoses/Interventions

Altered protection r/t myxedema coma secondary to inadequate treatment of hypothyroidism or inadequate management of a stressor (infection, emotional stress) in a hypothyroid patient
Desired outcome: Within 24 h, patient has improved physiologic status: return of VS within 10% baseline *or* HR 60-100 bpm, SBP >90 mm Hg, RR 12-20 breaths/min, blood glucose >70 mg/dl, orientation × 3, and absence of seizures.
- Monitor VS at frequent intervals; be alert to bradycardia, ↓ BP, or ↓ RR.
- Monitor for signs of hypoxia: circumoral or peripheral cyanosis.
- Monitor serum electrolytes and glucose levels for ↓ sodium and glucose.
- Restrict fluids and/or administer hypertonic saline as prescribed to correct hyponatremia.
- Administer IV thyroid replacement hormones with IV hydrocortisone to support adrenals and IV glucose to treat hypoglycemia.
- Monitor for S&S of heart failure: JVD, crackles in lung bases, SOB, pitting edema of extremities, ↓ peripheral pulses, ↓ BP.
- Keep oral airway and manual resuscitator at bedside in event of seizure, coma, or need for additional ventilatory assistance.
- Monitor Spo₂ continuously.
- If mechanical ventilation implemented, monitor ABGs and assess for weaning potential as patient improves.
- Monitor I&O qh for ↓ UO.

Risk for infection r/t compromised immunologic status secondary to alterations in adrenal function caused by hypothyroidism
Desired outcome: Patient infection free: negative cultures of blood, secretions, and body fluids.
- Be alert to early indicators of infection: fever, erythema, swelling, discharge from wounds or IV sites, urinary frequency/urgency, dysuria, changes in sputum.
- Provide good skin care to ↓ possibility of wound and subsequent infections.
- Administer antibiotic/antifungal therapy as prescribed.

Miscellanea

CONSULT MD FOR
- ↓ RR, inability to arouse/awaken, loss of patent airway, Spo₂ <90%, hypotension, bradycardia, dysrhythmias, ↑ crackles in lung bases, ↑ JVD, hypoglycemia, hyponatremia
- Possible complications: extreme hypoventilation, respiratory arrest, heart failure, seizures, AV heart block, adrenal insufficiency, MI

RELATED TOPICS
- Antimicrobial therapy
- Heart block: AV conduction disturbance
- Hypoglycemia
- Hyponatremia
- Hypothyroidism
- Myocardial infarction, acute
- Respiratory failure, acute

ABBREVIATIONS
D₅₀: 50% dextrose
FTI: Free thyroxine index
T₄: Thyroxine
TRH: Thyrotropin-releasing hormone
TSH: Thyroid stimulating hormone

REFERENCES
Bromelow I: Transformed by thyroxine, *Nurs Times* 88(8): 40-42, 1992.
Epstein CD: Adrenocortical insufficiency in the critically ill patient, *AACN Clin Issues* 3(3): 705-713, 1992.
Rose BD: *Clinical physiology of acid-base and electrolyte disorders*, ed 4, New York, 1994, McGraw-Hill.
Sanford SJ: Endocrine crises and patient care. In Kinney M, Packa D, Dunbar S (eds): *ACN's clinical reference for critical care nursing*, ed 3, St Louis, 1993, Mosby.
Toto K: Endocrine physiology: a comprehensive review, *Crit Care Nurs Clin North Am* 6(4): 637-659, 1994.

Author: **Marianne Saunorus Baird**

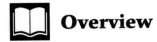 **Overview**

DESCRIPTION
During malnutrition the body initially uses its own skeletal muscle and adipose tissue. With severe stress (trauma, major surgery, sepsis), hypermetabolism, insulin resistance/hyperglycemia, and depletion of lean body mass occur. Because GI system remains active, enteral feedings *via* oral, nasogastric, intestinal routes are used to prevent bacteria from invading host, thus eliminating a major source of sepsis and possible organ failure while fostering wound healing and immunocompetence.

HISTORY/RISK FACTORS (for malnutrition)
- Weight: 80% below, 120% above standard
- Chewing or swallowing difficulties
- Nausea, vomiting, pain with eating
- Altered pattern of elimination
- Presence of chronic disease
- Chronic use of alcohol
- Medications: OTC/prescribed
- Recent trauma, major surgery, sepsis, burns
- NPO with IV fluid therapy >5 days

CLINICAL PRESENTATION (for malnutrition)
Brittle hair, pale and dry skin, poor skin turgor, fat and muscle wasting, redness/bleeding of mucous membranes, hepatomegaly

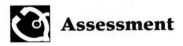 **Assessment**

PHYSICAL ASSESSMENT
Anthropometrics
Height: Used to determine BMI.
Weight: Compare to previous weight, standard weight charts, or use to calculate BMI. Changes may reflect fluid retention (edema, third spacing), diuresis, dehydration, surgical resections, traumatic amputations, weight of dressings or equipment.
BMI: Used to evaluate adult weight.

$$BMI = \frac{Weight(kg)}{Height(m) \times Height(m)}$$

BMI values of 20-25 optimal; values >25 indicate obesity; values <20 indicate underweight status.
TSF: Specially trained clinicians use calipers to measure skinfold. TSF <3mm signals severely depleted fat stores.

LABORATORY STUDIES
Protein Status: Evaluated *via* serum albumin (3.5-5.5 g/dl), transferrin (180-260 mg/dl), thyroxine-binding prealbumin (20-30 mg/dl), retinol binding protein (4-5 mg/dl). If hydration status nl and anemia absent, albumin and transferrin levels used as baseline indicators of adequacy of protein intake/synthesis. For evidence of response to therapy, values for short turnover proteins (thyroxine-binding prealbumin and retinol binding protein) are most useful.
Nitrogen Status: If more N taken in than excreted, N state is positive and an anabolic state exists. If more N excreted than taken in, N state is negative and a catabolic state exists. Accurate measurement of 24-h food intake and UO required to determine N state.
Creatinine-Height Index: Quantity of creatinine produced is directly r/t degree of skeletal muscle wasting.

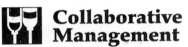 **Collaborative Management**

NUTRITIONAL SUPPORT MODES
Enteral Formulas
Standard: Include blended whole-food diets and commercial formulas
Modular: Single nutrient that may be combined with other modules (nutrients) for specific deficits
Nutritional Composition
Carbohydrates (50%)
Lactase: Aids in digestion of lactose; may be deficient in people with mucosal damage and especially in African-Americans, Asians, Native Americans, and Jews. Symptoms: watery diarrhea, abdominal cramps, flatulence, nausea.
Fiber: Included in many commercial preparations; may be helpful to control blood glucose, ↓ hyperlipidemia, control bowel disorders. Preparations highly viscous; require large-bore feeding tube (10F) or infusion pump.
Protein (15%)
Polymeric: Complete and original form; requires nl levels of pancreatic enzyme.
Hydrolyzed: Has been broken down into smaller forms; helpful in short-bowel syndrome or pancreatic insufficiency.
Elemental: Requires no further digestion; ready for absorption in hepatic and renal disorders.

Fat (35%)
Major source of essential fatty acids, fat-soluble vitamins, and calories.
Feeding Sites
Stomach: Reserved for alert patients with intact gag and cough reflexes.
Small bowel: Used for ↓ protective pharyngeal reflexes; small bowel less affected than stomach and colon by postop ileus. Tube placement more difficult. Continuous feedings approximate nl function and are better tolerated.
Types of Feeding Tubes
Small-bore: For long-term use; may have one port for feeding into jejunum and second port for stomach aspiration and decompression.
Large-bore: For short-term feeding of highly viscous fluids.
Gastrostomy: Soft tube inserted directly into stomach; temporary or permanent.
PEG: Soft tube inserted into stomach *via* esophagus; drawn through abdominal skin using stab incision.
Infusion Rates
Intermittent: 120 ml q2h: 30-60 ml initially, then ↑ by 60 ml q8h
Continuous: 40-50 ml/h initially, then ↑ by 25 ml q8h

MANAGEMENT OF COMPLICATIONS
Nausea and Vomiting
Cause: Fast rate of feeding, fat or lactose intolerance, hyperosmolality, delayed gastric emptying, product odor
Management: ↓ rate of feeding, ↓ fat, change to lactose-free formula, dilute feeding/mask odor with flavoring as indicated.
Blocked Tube
Cause: Viscous formula/medications; inadequate flushing
Management: Flush tube with 30 ml water after each administration/ aspiration; do not deliver crushed medications in small-bore tubes.

PATIENT-FAMILY TEACHING
- Purpose, expected results, anticipated duration of tube feeding
- Technique for home tube feeding as indicated

Nursing Diagnoses/Interventions

Altered nutrition: Less than body requirements r/t inability to ingest, digest, or absorb nutrients
Desired outcome: Within 7 days of initiating enteral nutrition, patient has adequate nutrition: stabilized weight at desired level/steady weight gain of 2-4 oz/day, improved protein stores, nitrogen balance, presence of wound granulation, absence of infection.
- Ensure nutritional assessment within 72 h of admission. Reassess weekly.
- Monitor electrolytes, BUN, glucose qd until stabilized; serum proteins, trace elements weekly.
- Weigh patient qd; record I&O carefully, tracking fluid balance trends.
- Administer formula within 10% of prescribed rate. Check volume infused and rate qh.
- Ensure that patient receives prescribed amount of calories.

Risk for aspiration r/t GI feeding, delayed gastric emptying, and site of feeding tube
Desired outcome: Patient free of aspiration: clear lung sounds, ABGs and arterial oximetry wnl for patient, and absence of respiratory distress.
- Check x-ray for tube position after placement. Insufflation with air/aspiration of stomach contents may not confirm placement of small-bore feeding tubes. Mark and secure tubing.
- Assess temp, respiratory rate/effort, and breath sounds q4h.
- Assess abdomen q8h. Consult physician if bowel sounds absent, abdomen distended, or nausea and vomiting occur.
- Elevate HOB $\geq$30 degrees during and for $\geq$1 h after feeding. If not possible or comfortable, turn patient to a slightly elevated right side-lying position.
- If residual feeding >50% of hourly feed, hold feeding for 1 h and recheck residual.
- Stop tube feeding ½-1 h before chest physical therapy, suctioning, placing patient supine.
- Consider placing feeding tube well beyond pylorus.
- Administer GI stimulants (eg, metoclopramide HCl [Reglan]).

Diarrhea (or risk of same) r/t bolus feeding, lactose intolerance, bacterial contamination, osmolality intolerance, medications, and low fiber content
Desired outcome: Patient has formed stools within 24-48 h of intervention.
- Assess GI status: bowel sounds, distention, bowel movements, cramping.
- Monitor hydration and I&O status carefully.
- If intermittent feeding: switch to continuous feeding method.
- If lactose intolerance: switch to lactose-free products.
- Prevent bacterial contamination: use clean technique, and discard feedings hanging >8 h; obtain stool sample for C&S.
- Most formulas are isotonic. If hypertonic, $\downarrow$ rate. If problem continues, dilute to ½ strength but maintain rate.
- Many medications are hypertonic, especially those containing sorbitol; consult pharmacist. Administer *Lactobacillus acidophilus* or diphenoxylate.
- Low fiber content: add psyllium or fiber.

Impaired tissue integrity (or risk of same) r/t mechanical irritant (presence of enteral tube)
Desired outcome: Tissue intact and similar in color/texture to surrounding area.
NASOGASTRIC/ENTERAL TUBE
- Assess nares for irritation or tenderness.
- Use small-bore tube.
- If long-term support needed, consider using gastrostomy/jejunostomy tube.
- Give ice chips, chewing gum, hard candies prn if permitted.
- Apply petrolatum ointment to lips q2h; brush teeth and tongue q4h.
- Alter tube's position qd. Use hypoallergenic tape to anchor tube.
GASTROSTOMY/JEJUNOSTOMY TUBE
- Assess site for erythema, drainage, tenderness, and odor q4h.
- Monitor tube placement q4h.
- Secure tube so there is no tension on tube and skin.
- Wash surrounding skin with soap and water qd; pat dry.

Risk for fluid volume deficit r/t failure of regulatory mechanisms, hyperglycemia
Desired outcome: Hydration status adequate: baseline VS, glucose <300 mg/dl, balanced I&O.
- Weigh patient qd.
- Monitor serum osmolality and electrolytes qd.
- Monitor for hyperglycemia. Perform finger stick q6h prn until blood glucose is stable. Administer sliding scale insulin to keep blood glucose levels <200 mg/dl.
- Assess rate/volume of nutritional support qh. Reset as indicated.
- Provide 1 ml water/kcal of enteral formula.

Miscellanea

CONSULT MD FOR
- Diarrhea
- Absent bowel sounds
- Residual >50% of hourly feed after 2 h
- Blood glucose >200 mg/dl
- Complications: eg, electrolyte imbalance, aspiration

RELATED TOPICS
- Hyperglycemia
- Hyperkalemia
- Hypernatremia
- Hypokalemia
- Hyponatremia
- Hypophosphatemia
- Nutritional support, parenteral
- Pneumonia, aspiration

ABBREVIATIONS
BMI: Body mass index
TSF: Triceps skinfold thickness

REFERENCES
Gianino S, St John RE: Nutritional assessment of the patient in the intensive care unit, *Crit Care Nurs Clin North Am* 5(1): 1-15, 1993.
Keithley JK, Eisenberg P: The significance of enteral nutrition in the intensive care unit patient, *Crit Care Nurs Clin North Am* 5(1): 23-29, 1993.
Metheny J: Minimizing respiratory complications of nasoenteric tube feedings: state of the science, *Heart Lung* 22(3): 213-223, 1993.
Webber K: Providing nutritional support. In Swearingen PL, Keen JH (eds): *Manual of critical care nursing*, ed 3, St Louis, 1995, Mosby.

Author: **Karen S. Webber**

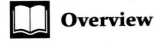 **Overview**

DESCRIPTION
Initiated *via* peripheral or central vein for partial or total inability to meet nutritional needs using GI tract. Necessary in protein-calorie malnutrition complicated by severe stress, since mortality/morbidity ↑, including compromised immunity, ↓ wound healing, and organ failure. PN often results in bowel mucosal atrophy and need for period of adjustment before bowel can fully resume digestion and absorption.

HISTORY/RISK FACTORS (for malnutrition)
- Weight: 80% below, 120% above standard
- Chewing or swallowing difficulties
- Nausea, vomiting, pain with eating
- Altered pattern of elimination
- Presence of chronic disease
- Chronic use of alcohol
- Medications: OTC/prescribed
- Recent trauma, major surgery, sepsis, burns
- NPO with IV fluid therapy >5 days

CLINICAL PRESENTATION (for malnutrition)
Brittle hair, pale and dry skin, poor skin turgor, fat and muscle wasting, redness/bleeding of mucous membranes, hepatomegaly

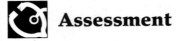 **Assessment**

PHYSICAL ASSESSMENT
Anthropometrics
Height: Used to determine BMI.
Weight: Compare to previous weight, standard weight charts, or use to calculate BMI. Changes may reflect fluid retention (edema, third spacing), diuresis, dehydration, surgical resections, traumatic amputations, weight of dressings or equipment.
BMI: Used to evaluate adult weight.

$$BMI = \frac{Weight(kg)}{Height(m) \times Height(m)}$$

BMI values of 20-25 optimal; values >25 indicate obesity; values <20 indicate underweight status.
TSF: Specially trained clinicians use calipers to measure skinfold. TSF <3mm signals severely depleted fat stores.

LABORATORY STUDIES
Protein Status: Evaluated *via* serum albumin (3.5-5.5 g/dl), transferrin (180-260 mg/dl), thyroxine-binding prealbumin (20-30 mg/dl), retinol binding protein (4-5 mg/dl). If hydration status nl and anemia absent, albumin and transferrin levels used as baseline indicators of adequacy of protein intake and synthesis. For evidence of response to nutritional therapy, values for short turnover proteins (thyroxine-binding prealbumin and retinol binding protein) are most useful.
Nitrogen Status: If more N taken in than excreted, N state is positive and an anabolic state exists. If more N excreted than taken in, N state is negative and a catabolic state exists. Accurate measurement of 24-h food intake and UO required to determine N state.
Creatinine-Height Index: Quantity of creatinine produced directly related to degree of skeletal muscle wasting.

Collaborative Management

PARENTERAL SOLUTIONS
Dextrose Solutions 5%-50%: To meet part of energy needs. When hypertonic solutions infused, insulin demand, CO_2 production, and O_2 consumption ↑, which may lead to respiratory distress and hypermetabolism.
Essential and Nonessential Amino Acid Solutions 3%-15%: Special amino acid formulations for specific disorders available.
Lipids 10%-20%: Provide essential fatty acids and a source of concentrated calories; infused with carbohydrates and protein. Infuse slowly to avoid adverse reaction: fever, chills, shivering, pain in chest and back.

FEEDING SITES
Central: Used for hypertonic infusions *via* large central vein.
Peripheral: Need for low osmolality of solutions can limit usefulness, but combining solutions of dextrose, amino acids, and lipids can ↓ osmolality. Used for short periods when CVC access unavailable.

TYPES OF CATHETERS
Single Lumen: If used for multiple tasks of specimen retrieval, feeding, and medication administration, can ↑ infection risk.
Multilumen: Dedicate one lumen for feeding, and use others for medications and laboratory specimens.
Right Atrial (eg, Hickman, Broviac): For long-term use.
Implantable (eg, Infuse-a-Port, Port-a-Cath): Designed for repeated access, making repeated venipuncture unnecessary.

INFUSION RATES
Using infusion pump, PN given at consistent rate according to nutritional and fluid volume status; gradual acceleration on initiation and deceleration on cessation prevents fluctuations in blood glucose. If infusion falls behind, do not attempt to "catch up."

PATIENT-FAMILY TEACHING
- Purpose, expected results, anticipated sensations of all nursing/medical interventions

Nursing Diagnoses/Interventions

Altered nutrition: Less than body requirements r/t inability to ingest, digest, or absorb nutrients
Desired outcome: Within 7 days of initiating PN, patient has adequate nutrition: stabilized weight at desired level/steady weight gain of 2-4 oz/day, improved protein stores, nitrogen balance, wound granulation, absence of infection.
- Ensure nutritional assessment within 72 h of admission. Reassess weekly.
- Monitor electrolytes, BUN, and blood glucose qd until stabilized.
- Monitor serum proteins and trace elements weekly.
- Weigh patient qd.
- Record I&O carefully, tracking fluid balance trends.
- Check volume infused and rate qh.
- Ensure that patient receives prescribed amount of calories.

Risk for infection r/t invasive procedures or malnutrition
Desired outcome: Patient infection free. Temp and VS wnl, total lymphocytes 25%-40%, WBCs 5000-11,000 µl, and absence of S&S of sepsis: erythema and swelling at catheter insertion site, glucose intolerance.
- Monitor temp, VS, total WBC count and differential for values outside nl per agency policy.
- Check blood glucose q6h for values outside nl.
- Examine catheter insertion site(s) q8h for erythema, swelling, or purulent drainage.
- Use sterile technique when changing central line dressing, containers, or lines.
- Dedicate one lumen to nutritional support only.
- Change all administration sets within time frame established by agency.
- Culture catheter tip and exit site prn.
- Take blood specimens if sepsis is suspected; administer antibiotics as prescribed.

Risk for fluid volume deficit r/t failure of regulatory mechanisms, hyperglycemia
Desired outcome: Patient's hydration status adequate: baseline VS, glucose <300 mg/dl, balanced I&O.
- Weigh patient qd.
- Monitor serum osmolality and electrolytes qd.
- Monitor for hyperglycemia. Perform finger stick q6h prn until blood glucose stable. Administer sliding scale insulin to keep blood glucose levels <200 mg/dl.
- Assess rate/volume of nutritional support qh. Reset as indicated.

Miscellanea

CONSULT MD FOR
- Catheter occlusion
- Suspected air embolus: dyspnea, chest pain, ↑ RR, ↑ HR, ↓ BP
- Blood glucose >200 mg/dl
- Complications: eg, electrolyte imbalance, septicemia

RELATED TOPICS
- Hyperglycemia
- Hyperkalemia
- Hyperosmolar hyperglycemic nonketotic syndrome
- Hypoglycemia
- Hypokalemia
- Hypophosphatemia
- Nutritional support, enteral
- Pneumothorax
- Pulmonary emboli, air

ABBREVIATIONS
BMI: Body mass index
CVC: Central nervous catheter
PN: Parenteral nutrition
TSF: Triceps skinfold thickness

REFERENCES
Gianino S, St John RE: Nutritional assessment of the patient in the intensive care unit, *Crit Care Nurs Clin North Am* 5(1): 1-15, 1993.

McMahon MM, Farnell MB, Murray MJ: Nutritional support of critically ill patients, *Mayo Clin Proc* 68: 911-920, 1993.

Payne-James JJ, Khawaja HT: First choice for total parenteral nutrition: the peripheral route, *J Parenter Enter Nutr* 17(5): 468-478, 1993.

Seshadri V, Meyer-Tettambel OM: Electrolyte and drug management in nutritional support, *Crit Care Nurs Clin North Am* 5(1): 31-36, 1993.

Webber K: Providing nutritional support. In Swearingen PL, Keen JH (eds): *Manual of critical care nursing,* ed 3, St Louis, 1995, Mosby.

Author: **Karen S. Webber**

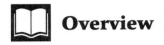 **Overview**

PATHOPHYSIOLOGY

Major problem of organ transplantation is graft rejection; if untreated, it results in complete organ destruction. When a foreign substance is detected, the body mounts a defense of nonspecific inflammation and phagocytosis. The next level of response involves the following:

Antibody-Mediated Immune Response: Related to B lymphocytes, which trigger production of antigen-specific immunoglobulins, or antibodies.

Cell-Mediated Immune Response: Involves T lymphocytes, which promote release of chemicals that kill foreign cells and facilitate phagocytosis and inflammatory response.

CLINICAL PRESENTATION

Signs of organ failure; depends on specific graft. General indicators include fever, malaise. Rejection may be classified as follows:

Hyperacute: Occurs immediately

Accelerated Acute: Occurs 3-5 days posttransplant

Acute: Occurs wks, mos, yrs posttransplant

Chronic: Develops slowly over mos to yrs

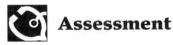 **Assessment**

PHYSICAL ASSESSMENT

Heart: Fever, lethargy, dyspnea, ↓ exercise tolerance, atrial or ventricular dysrhythmias, S_3/S_4 gallop, pericardial friction rub, JVD, crackles, hypotension, ↓ CO

Kidney: ↓ UO, tenderness over graft, hypertension, ↑ BUN/creatinine

Liver: Malaise; fever; abdominal discomfort; swollen, hard, tender graft; ↑ HR; RUQ or flank pain; ↓/cessation of bile flow; colorless bile; jaundice; ↑ PT, bilirubin, transaminase, ALP

Lung: ↓ lung ventilation and perfusion; respiratory insufficiency; ↑ PVR

Pancreas: Hyperglycemia, pancreatitis, pain over graft

VITAL SIGNS/HEMODYNAMICS

HEART

HR: ↑

Temp: ↑

CVP/PAWP: ↑

CO: ↓

ECG: Atrial and ventricular dysrhythmias; ↓ QRS voltage

KIDNEY

Temp: ↑

BP: ↑

CVP/PAWP: ↑ as a result of fluid overload

UO: ↓

LIVER

HR: ↑

Temp: ↑

CVP/PAWP: ↑ as a result of fluid retention

LUNG

HR: Sudden ↑

BP: Sudden ↑

Temp: ↑

CO: Sudden ↑

SVR: Sudden ↑

PANCREAS

HR: ↑

Temp: ↑

HEART

LABORATORY STUDIES

CBC: ↑ total lymphocytes

IMAGING

Chest X-ray: ↑ cardiac silhouette late in rejection

DIAGNOSTIC PROCEDURES

Biopsy: For definitive diagnosis; reveals presence, type, severity of rejection

KIDNEY

LABORATORY STUDIES

BUN/Creatinine: ↑

24-h Urine: ↓ creatinine clearance; ↑ protein excretion; ↓ sodium excretion.

IMAGING

Ultrasound with Doppler Flow: Change in Doppler wave forms

Renal Scan: ↓ RBF

DIAGNOSTIC PROCEDURES

Biopsy: Reveals presence, type, severity of rejection

LIVER

LABORATORY STUDIES

Serum Bilirubin Level: ↑ relative to baseline postop level

Transaminase Level: ↑ relative to baseline; ↑ early in rejection

ALP Level: ↑ from baseline

PT: Prolonged

CBC: ↓ platelets and ↑ total lymphocytes

DIAGNOSTIC PROCEDURES

Biopsy: Reveals presence, type, severity of rejection

LUNG

Transbronchial biopsy not helpful to detect rejection; morbidity risk ↑ with open biopsy.

LABORATORY STUDIES

Leukocyte and Absolute Lymphocytes: ↑ during rejection

ABGs: ↓ Pao_2, ↑ $Paco_2$ with rejection

PANCREAS

Open biopsy is the only way definitive diagnosis can be made.

LABORATORY STUDIES

Fasting and 2-h Postprandial Plasma Glucose: ↑ > nl

Serum Amylase: May ↑, signaling pancreatitis, a marker of rejection

C peptide (serum and urine): May ↓

IMAGING

Pancreas Radioisotope Flow Scan: Determines organ viability. ↓ flow may indicate rejection.

Collaborative Management

Goal of therapy: to achieve enough immunosuppression to prevent graft rejection but not so much as to leave patient defenseless.

PHARMACOTHERAPY

Azathioprine (Imuran): Affects rapidly replicating cells at early stage of lymphocyte activation; believed to block proliferation of helper T cells and cytotoxic T cells.

Corticosteroids: Suppress production of cytotoxic T lymphocytes from noncytotoxic precursor cells.

Antilymphocyte Sera (ALG or ATGAM): Antilymphocyte antibodies in the sera are useful in treating steroid-resistant rejection; potent suppressors of cell-mediated immunity.

Monoclonal Antibody (Orthoclone OKT3): Binds to T3 antigen on T cell surface, enhancing phagocytosis and entrapment of cells in spleen and liver. Lymphocytes removed from circulation by this process in ≈ 10-15 min.

Cyclosporine (Sandimmune): Inhibits production and release of lymphokines and generation of cytotoxic and plasma cells by blocking response of cytotoxic T lymphocytes to IL-2.

Tacrolimus (Prograf): Mechanism of action similar to cyclosporine: inhibits earliest steps of T-cell activation.

Mycophenolate Mofetil: Selective inhibitor of inosine monophosphate dehydrogenase, a pathway T and B lymphocytes depend on for proliferation.

PATIENT-FAMILY TEACHING

- Purpose, expected results of nursing/medical interventions, including immunosuppressive therapy
- S&S of organ rejection

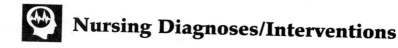

Nursing Diagnoses/Interventions

Anxiety/Fear r/t threat of change in health status secondary to potential loss of transplanted organ as a result of rejection

Desired outcomes: Patient expresses anxieties and fears regarding possibility of organ loss and verbalizes accurate information about S&S of organ rejection. Within 12 h of this diagnosis, fear and anxiety controlled: BP wnl for patient, HR ≤100 bpm, RR ≤20 breaths/min with eupnea.

- Encourage patient to discuss concerns and fears.
- Assess knowledge about rejection process and S&S that occur.
- Use short, simple sentences to explain current organ function and S&S of organ rejection.
- Reassure that appropriate medications are being given to prevent ongoing rejection. Review medication names, dosage, and action.
- Explain that rejection does not necessarily mean organ loss. Under most circumstances, rejection can be reversed.
- Reassure that retransplantation is a viable option if organ loss occurs.

Fluid volume excess (or risk for same) r/t compromised regulatory mechanism secondary to ↓ organ function associated with rejection episode

Desired outcome: Patient normovolemic: stable weight, UO ≥0.5 ml/kg/h, BP wnl for patient, HR 60-100 bpm, RR 12-20 breaths/min with eupnea, and absence of edema, crackles, and other S&S of fluid overload.

- Measure weight qd. Remember that a 1-kg weight gain can signal ≈ 1 L of fluid retention.
- Measure I&O q4h; note 24-h trends.
- Assess BP, HR, and RR q4h. Be alert to ↑ BP, tachycardia, and tachypnea, which indicate fluid overload.
- Auscultate for crackles and pericardial friction rub at least q8h.
- Assess and document peripheral, sacral, and periorbital edema on 0-4+ scale.

Powerlessness r/t actual or perceived helplessness with controlling organ rejection episodes

Desired outcome: Within 72 h of this diagnosis, patient relates that he or she can control aspects of daily care and assume responsibility for taking medications appropriately and obtaining follow-up care.

- Encourage patient to express feelings of frustration and powerlessness regarding organ rejection.
- Encourage participation in decisions about care routines. Help identify areas of the care plan patient can control, such as timing of morning care or initiation of rest periods.
- Reinforce that taking medications appropriately and keeping appointments for follow-up care *are* within patient's control and are significant in preventing rejection and organ destruction.
- Emphasize that rejection is a nl body response to foreign tissue.
- Solicit comments and opinions; honor opinions and preferences.

Risk for infection r/t inadequate secondary responses as a result of immunosuppression

Desired outcome: Patient infection free: normothermia; absence of erythema, swelling, and drainage at catheter and wound sites; absence of adventitious breath sounds and cloudy and foul-smelling urine; negative cultures; and WBCs 4500-11,000 μl.

- Assess and record temp q4h. Be alert to ↑ ≥37.8° C (100° F).
- Assess and document condition of indwelling IV/catheter sites and graft incision q8h. Be alert to swelling, erythema, tenderness, and drainage.
- Be alert to WBCs >11,000 μl or <4500 μl. Below-normal WBCs with ↑ differential (shift to left) may signal acute infection.
- Record urine volume, appearance, color, odor. Be alert to foul-smelling or cloudy urine, frequency and urgency of urination, and complaints of flank or labial pain, all of which signal renal-urinary infection.
- Auscultate lung fields q8h, noting presence of rhonchi, crackles, and ↓ breath sounds.
- Use meticulous sterile technique when dressing and caring for wounds and catheter sites.

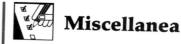

Miscellanea

CONSULT MD FOR
- S&S of fluid overload
- S&S of infection: fever ≥37.8° C; erythema, tenderness, drainage from surgical site, wound, or IV insertion site; WBCs ↑ or with ↑ band neutrophils (shift to left)

RELATED TOPICS
- Cardiac transplantation: postoperative
- Renal transplantation

ABBREVIATION
RBF: Renal blood flow

REFERENCES
Bass M: Pancreas transplantation: Detecting rejection and patient care, *ANNA J* 19(5): 476-482, 1992.

Bass PS, Bindon-Perler PA, Lewis RJ: Liver transplantation: the recovery phase, *Crit Care Nurs Q* 13(4): 51-61, 1991.

Nettles AT: Pancreas transplantation: a University of Minnesota perspective, *Diabetes Educator* 18(3): 232-238, 1992.

Vaska PL: OKT3 monoclonal antibody in cardiac transplant patients, *Dimens Crit Care Nurs* 10(3): 126-132, 1991.

Weiskittel PD: Organ rejection. In Swearingen PL, Keen JH (eds): *Manual of critical care nursing,* ed 3, St Louis, 1995, Mosby.

Author: **Patricia D. Weiskittel**

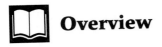 **Overview**

PATHOPHYSIOLOGY

Acute or chronic infection involving a bone. Although it often remains localized, it can spread through marrow, cortex, and periosteum. Acute hematogenic form most frequently caused by *Staphylococcus aureus* (90%-95%), but also can result from gram-negative rods (eg, *Escherichia coli*, *Pseudomonas* species, *Klebsiella*) or other organisms. Osteomyelitis often involves multiple infectious agents. TB of the musculoskeletal system is on the rise in the US and should be considered, especially with spinal symptoms.

Primary: Direct implantation of microorganisms into bone *via* compound fractures, penetrating wounds, diagnostic bone marrow aspiration, surgery.

Secondary or Acute Hematogenic: Infection of bone occurring through its own blood supply or by infection from contiguous soft tissues (especially ischemic, diabetic, neurotrophic ulcers), IV drug abuse, joints with septic arthritis.

HISTORY/RISK FACTORS

- Compound fracture, penetrating trauma
- Bone marrow aspiration, orthopaedic surgery
- IV drug abuse, malnutrition
- Disorders affecting blood supply/oxygenation: DM, sickle cell disease, COPD, vascular insufficiency
- Advanced age

CLINICAL PRESENTATION

Acute: Pain in involved area, fever, malaise, limited ROM.

Chronic: Bone infection persisting intermittently for yrs, usually flaring up after minor trauma to affected area or lowered systemic resistance. Edema and erythema over involved bone and generalized signs of sepsis can occur. With implant arthroplasty osteomyelitis, symptoms involve loosening and pain 3-5 months postop. TB of the spine (Pott's disease) presents with back pain and possible radiculopathy.

 Assessment

PHYSICAL ASSESSMENT

Weakness, pain, warmth, swelling, limited ROM in involved area; purulent drainage from sinus tract, surgical site

VITAL SIGNS/HEMODYNAMICS

RR: ↑
HR: ↑
BP: May be ↓ if septicemia present
Temp: ↑
Hemodynamics: May reflect systemic sepsis: ↓ CVP/PAP and initial ↓ SVR/↑ CO, with later ↑ SVR/↓CO as sepsis progresses.

LABORATORY STUDIES

CBC: Reveals leukocytosis and anemia.
ESR: ↑
Blood or Sequestrum Cultures: Identify causative organism *via* Gram's stain and C&S. Sequestrum is a piece of necrotic bone separated from surrounding bone because of osteomyelitis.
C-Reactive Protein: More quickly responsive to infection/inflammation than ESR; its relative values can be used to discern bone from joint infection.

IMAGING

X-rays: May reveal subtle areas of radiolucency (osteonecrosis) and new bone formation. Changes not evident until disease has been active ≥2-3 wks in adults.

Technetium Bone Scanning: May reveal areas of ↑ vascularity (called *hot spots*), which usually indicate osteomyelitis. False-positive results can occur with contiguous soft tissue infection. Negative results do not guarantee osteomyelitis is not present.

CT, MRI Scans: CT scans may demonstrate bone damage and soft tissue inflammation. MRI will not reveal bone changes, but is an excellent means for identifying pockets of purulence, especially intramedullary infections and osteitis and diskitis in Pott's disease.

DIAGNOSTIC PROCEDURES

Bone Biopsy: "Gold standard" for diagnosis of osteomyelitis. Considered positive when there is evidence of necrosis, acute or chronic inflammatory cells, and aggregates of lymphocytes and/or plasma cells. Also may provide infectious material for C&S studies. Especially important in establishing musculoskeletal TB.

Collaborative Management

IV Antimicrobial Therapy: When agent-specific antibiosis possible, may be given for 2 wks, followed by 2-4 wks of oral therapy. When infective agent not specifically identified, broad spectrum IV therapy may be required for 4-6 wks. In some cases long-term (3-6 mo) antibiotic therapy necessary. Powerful, potentially toxic agents may be required (eg, vancomycin, aminoglycosides, third-generation cephalosporins, clindamycin, fluoroquinolones, or combinations of these).

Immobilization of Affected Extremity: With splint, cast, or traction to relieve pain and ↓ potential for pathologic fracture.

Blood Transfusions: To correct any accompanying anemia.

Removal of Internal Fixation Device, Endoprosthesis: To help control infection. If total joint replacements are removed, a flail joint will result until prosthesis can be replaced.

Surgical Decompression of Infected Bone: May be followed by primary closure, myocutaneous flaps to cover denuded bone, or the area may be left open to drain and heal by secondary intention or with secondary closure. Radical débridement, bone grafting, and anti-TB chemotherapy used to prevent kyphotic deformity in Pott's disease.

Drains: May be inserted into affected bone to drain the site or act as ingress/egress tubes to funnel topical antibiotics directly into infected area.

Topical Antibiotics: May be used *via* continuous or intermittent infusion into the wound and continued until three successive drain cultures are negative. Alternatively, antibiotic impregnated polymethyl-methacylate (PMMA) beads may be packed into affected sites for 2-4 wks, after which the wound is reopened, beads are removed, and bone graft is packed in the deficit.

Hyperbaric O₂: Used to treat refractory osteomyelitis associated with adjacent pressure necrosis.

Amputation: May be required for extremities in which persistent infection/pain severely limits function.

PATIENT-FAMILY TEACHING

- Necessary care after hospital discharge (eg, analgesia, dressing changes, warm soaks, ROM exercises, activity limitations, use of ambulatory aids)
- When parenteral antibiotic therapy is to be given at home (usually *via* long-term VAD), the method of administering medications and care of device used
- Medications: drug name, route, dosage, purpose, schedule, precautions, drug-drug and food-drug interactions, and potential side effects
- Involving public health, visiting nurse, or similar home health care service professional to ensure adequate follow-up at home
- Indicators of potential complications, eg, recurring infection, pathologic fracture, joint contracture, pressure necrosis, medication reactions or toxic effects

Nursing Diagnoses/Interventions

Risk for infection *(for others)* r/t risk of cross-contamination; *(for patient)* r/t disease chronicity, suppression of nl flora during long-term antimicrobial therapy

Desired outcomes: At time of hospital discharge, patient, other patients, staff members are free of symptoms of infection: normothermia and WBCs ≤11,000/μl. Within 24 h of instruction, patient verbalizes potential of disease chronicity, importance of strict adherence to antibiotic therapy.

- As available, provide private rooms for patients with open, draining wounds. If this is not possible, avoid assigning roommates with recent surgery, open wounds, or those who are immunocompromised.
- Use Transmission-Based Precautions: Contact, for patients known to be or suspected of being infected or colonized with epidemiologically important microorganisms (eg, MRSA, VRE) that can be transmitted by direct contact.
- In addition to Standard Precautions, wear gloves when providing direct care or having hand contact with potentially contaminated surfaces or items in patient's environment.
- When possible, dedicate use of noncritical patient care equipment to single patient to avoid sharing between patients.
- Monitor for fever, ↑ pain, and laboratory data indicative of infection (eg, ↑ WBCs, ↑ ESR).
- Assess exposed wounds and dressings for erythema, ↑ wound drainage, purulent wound drainage, ↑ wound circumference, edema, warmth, localized tenderness.
- Assess neurovascular structures for deficit, which can signal infection or pressure from adjacent inflamed tissues.
- After primary closure or grafting of wound, continue to assess wound for S&S of infection.
- Observe for superimposed infections, especially fungal, by assessing for fever, black or furry tongue, sore mouth and tongue, nausea, diarrhea, oral monilial growth, or vaginal monilial growth. If VAD is used for antibiotic administration, monitor infusion site closely for irritation that does not respond to usual treatments with topical antibiotics. As indicated, obtain cultures of suspicious areas of inflammation.

Pain r/t joint changes and corrective therapy

Desired outcomes: Within 1-2 h of intervention, subjective perception of pain ↓, as documented by pain scale. Objective indicators, such as grimacing, are ↓/absent. Patient demonstrates ADL without complaints of discomfort.

- Explain and help patient use rating system to evaluate pain and analgesic relief on scale of 0 (no pain) to 10 (severe).
- Administer analgesics and antiinflammatory agents as prescribed (or 30 min before strenuous activity); document effectiveness, using pain scale. As appropriate, teach function of epidural anesthesia or PCA.
- Teach nonpharmacologic methods of pain control, including guided imagery, graduated breathing (as in Lamaze), enhanced relaxation, massage, biofeedback, cutaneous stimulation (*via* a counterirritant, such as oil of wintergreen), TENS device, warm or cool thermotherapy, music therapy, and tactile, auditory, visual, verbal distractions.
- Use traditional nursing interventions to counteract pain, including backrubs, repositioning, and encouraging verbalization of feelings.
- Incorporate rest, local warmth or cold, and elevation of affected joints, when possible, to help control discomfort.
- Advise coordinating time of peak effectiveness of antiinflammatory agent with periods of exercise or mandatory use of joints.
- Teach use of moist heat and hydrotherapy, which will help reduce long-term discomfort.

Impaired physical mobility r/t musculoskeletal impairment, bone pain

Desired outcome: Patient maintains appropriate body alignment; external fixation devices remain in place; traction remains intact. At time of hospital discharge, patient exhibits full or optimal ROM/function in limbs with affected bones.

- Position in proper body alignment, most commonly neutral position.
- Provide active/passive ROM of adjacent joints q8h as appropriate.
- Maintain traction by allowing weights to hang free. Do not remove weights even when repositioning.
- Use caution when turning and positioning to maintain body alignment. If patient has an unstable fracture that has not yet been reduced, consult orthopedist before moving patient.
- When external fixator is in place, support limb when turning; do not use fixator as a handle.
- As indicated, provide assistive device for ambulation. Demonstrate use and observe patient during return demonstration.

 # Miscellanea

CONSULT MD FOR

- S&S of new or ↑ infection: ↑ pain; ↑ WBCs; ↑ ESR; purulent wound drainage, ↑ erythema, tenderness, warmth over affected area; new-onset or joint instability
- S&S of superimposed fungal, other infections
- Potential complications: septicemia, endocarditis
- Adverse effects of antimicrobial therapy:
  Aminoglycosides: Ototoxicity/nephrotoxicity
  Penicillins: Anemia, hypersensitivity reactions, jaundice
  Cephalosporins: ↑ liver enzymes, nephrotoxicity
  Sulfonamides: Nephrotoxicity, agranulocytosis, thrombocytopenia, urinary calculi

RELATED TOPICS

- Antimicrobial therapy
- Endocarditis, infective
- Methicillin-resistant *Staphylococcus aureus*
- Shock, septic
- Vancomycin-resistant enterococci

ABBREVIATIONS

ESR: Erythocyte sedimentation rate
MRSA: Methicillin-resistant *Staphylococcus aureus*
VAD: Vascular access device
VRE: Vancomycin-resistant enterococci

REFERENCES

Deloach ED et al: The treatment of osteomyelitis underlying pressure ulcers, *Decubitus* 5(6): 32-41, 1992.

Gray MA: Local application of antibiotics in orthopaedic infections, *Orthop Nurs* 14(5): 69-70, 1995.

Laughlin RT et al: Osteomyelitis, *Curr Opin Rheumatol* 7: 315-321, 1995.

Ross DG: Osteomyelitis. In Swearingen PL (ed): *Manual of medical-surgical nursing*, ed 3, St Louis, 1994, Mosby.

Yandrich TJ: Preventing infection in total joint replacement surgery, *Orthop Nurs* 14(2): 15-19, 1995.

Author: **Dennis G. Ross**

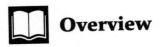 **Overview**

PATHOPHYSIOLOGY

Significant stressor for critically ill patients; contributes to such problems as confusion, inadequate ventilation, immobility, sleep deprivation, depression, and immunosuppression. Characteristic pain patterns develop according to area affected and underlying pathophysiologic process. Superficial structures, eg, subcutaneous tissue, ligaments, tendons, and parietal pleura, contain numerous small pain fibers. Pain affecting these areas usually is well localized and often described as pricking and burning. Pain associated with deeper visceral structures is often poorly localized and usually described as aching, although it may be sharp or burning. Pain associated with muscle injury is similar to visceral pain and is mediated through the same deep sensory systems. Acute ischemia causes burning or aching pain distal to area of vascular occlusion.

CONTRIBUTING FACTORS
Patient
- Fear, anxiety
- Barriers to communication
Caregiver
- Failure to assess pain intensity accurately
- Concern for respiratory depression or iatrogenic addiction

HISTORY/RISK FACTORS
- Pathologic conditions
- Tissue ischemia, injury
- Surgery, invasive procedures

CLINICAL PRESENTATION

Because pain is subjective, only patients can evaluate pain intensity accurately. Use one or more of several pain assessment tools to assist patient in rating pain. In addition, ask patient to describe nature of pain (eg, dull, sharp, pressure, cramping), location, and aggravating and relieving factors.

Numerical Rating Scale: Patient ranks pain numerically, usually from 1-5 or 1-10.

Visual Analog Scale: Patient marks 10-cm line to indicate pain intensity.

Adjective Rating Scale: Patient selects adjective that best describes pain intensity.

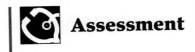 **Assessment**

PHYSICAL ASSESSMENT
Physiologic Findings (acute pain)
- Diaphoresis, pallor
- Vasoconstriction
- ↑ SBP and DBP
- ↑ pulse rate: >100 bpm
- Pupillary dilatation
- Change in RR: usually ↑ to >20 breaths/min
- ↑ muscle tension or spasm
- ↓ intestinal motility: nausea, vomiting, abdominal distention, ileus
- Endocrine imbalance: sodium and water retention, mild hyperglycemia

Nonverbal Indicators
- Skeletal muscle tension: facial grimace, tension; guarding or splinting of affected part; restlessness; ↑ or ↓ motor activity
- Psychic reactions: short attention span, irritability, anxiety, sleep disturbances, anger, crying, fearfulness, withdrawal

Collaborative Management

Opioid Agonists: Used to manage moderate to severe acute pain. Titrate in small increments to produce desired analgesia with minimal side effects. PCA pumps, continuous peripheral or epidural infusions, or small frequent IV bolus doses are effective methods. Physiologic or psychologic dependence and addiction are unusual when opioids are used in patients without hx of chemical dependency.

Precautions: Parenteral opioids may cause hypotension in patients with hypovolemia. Restore fluid volume before or concurrent with administration. Dose-related respiratory depression is a significant disadvantage, particularly with chronic hypoxia, debilitation, or advanced age. Keep naloxone (Narcan) immediately available to reverse respiratory depression.

Morphine: Most frequently used opioid. Vasodilatory effects beneficial for patients with LV failure, pulmonary hypertension, or pulmonary edema. Rapid IV injection may trigger histamine release with related ↓ in SVR and ↓ in CO/CI and MAP. Histamine-related bronchospasm may occur in patients with asthma.

Hydromorphone (Dilaudid): Highly effective opioid; substitute analgesic for patient with morphine allergy or intolerance.

Meperidine (Demerol): Indicated for brief courses (ie, <48 h) in patients with allergy or intolerance to other opiates. Its toxic metabolite, normeperidine, is a cerebral irritant and may cause seizures.

Fentanyl: Especially useful in critical care because of minimal CV effects, short duration of action, and rapid onset of action.

Opioid Agonist-Antagonists: Stimulate and antagonize opiate receptors to varying degrees, depending on agent and dose. May precipitate withdrawal in patients receiving opiates on a regular basis.

Pentazocine (Talwin): Predominant agonist effects but with weak antagonist activity. May cause ↑ MAP, LVEDP, and MPAP, and thus ↑ myocardial workload.

Butorphanol (Stadol): Adverse effects reported in patients with heart failure or AMI. May be useful to ↓ side effects associated with epidural morphine.

NSAIDs: Diminish effects of prostaglandins, rendering afferent receptors less sensitive to bradykinin, histamine, and serotonin, which in turn, ↓ pain receptor stimulation. Most NSAIDs given orally (eg, ibuprofen, aspirin), but injectable NSAIDs such as ketorolac (Toradol) are available. Prostaglandin inhibition ↓ platelet adhesiveness and may result in bleeding complications.

Other Pharmacologic Interventions: Sedatives and anxiolytics (eg, midazolam [Versed]) often used to ↓ anxiety associated with pain and promote amnesia when painful procedures are planned. Spinal analgesia with a local anesthetic agent may be used with epidural opiates. Intermittent or continuous local neural blockade, such as intercostal nerve block, is used for specific localized pain.

Nonpharmacologic Interventions: Used for mild pain and anxiety and as adjuncts to pharmacologic management of moderate to severe pain. Many of these techniques may be taught to and implemented by patient and significant others.

Physical therapies/modalities: Massage, ROM exercises, heat/cold applications, TENS

Emotional interventions: Prevention/control of anxiety, progressive relaxation, promotion of self-control

Cognitive interventions: Preparatory information, teaching of methods for preventing and reducing pain, distraction, humor, guided imagery, biofeedback

Nursing Diagnoses/Interventions

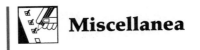 **Miscellanea**

Pain r/t biophysical injury secondary to pathology; surgical, diagnostic, or treatment interventions; trauma

Desired outcomes: Within 2 h of initiating therapy, patient's subjective evaluation of discomfort improves, as documented by pain scale. Patient does not exhibit nonverbal indicators of pain. Autonomic indicators ↓ or absent. Verbal responses, such as crying or moaning, absent.

- Develop a systematic approach to pain management for each patient. Primary nurse should collaborate with surgeon, anesthesiologist, and patient for optimal pain management. Consultation with pain management team recommended for prolonged or unusual pain.
- Monitor patient at frequent intervals for discomfort. Use a formal method of assessing pain.
- Evaluate patients with acute and chronic pain for nonverbal indicators of discomfort.
- Evaluate patients with acute pain for autonomic indicators of discomfort. Be aware that patients with chronic pain (> 6 mos duration) will not exhibit an autonomic response.
- Evaluate health hx for evidence of alcohol and drug (prescribed and nonprescribed) use. Individuals with hx of chemical dependence may require higher doses for effective analgesia. Persons with chronic or acute hepatic insufficiency require ↓ dose and careful selection of appropriate analgesics. Consult pain control team if available. All care providers must be consistent in setting limits while providing effective pain control through pharmacologic and nonpharmacologic methods. Psychiatric or mental health consultation may be necessary.
- Be aware that some opioid agonist-antagonist analgesics (eg, butorphanol, buprenorphine, pentazocine) have strong narcotic antagonist activity and may trigger withdrawal symptoms in individuals with opiate dependency.
- Administer opioid and other analgesics as prescribed. Monitor for side effects, such as respiratory depression, excessive sedation, nausea, vomiting, constipation. Be aware that meperidine may produce excitation, muscle twitching, and seizures, especially in conjunction with phenothiazines. Do not administer mixed agonist-antagonist analgesics concurrently with morphine or other pure agonist, because reversal of analgesic effects may occur.
- Administer nonnarcotic agents and NSAIDs as prescribed for relief of mild to moderate pain or on alternating schedule with opiate analgesics for moderate to severe pain. NSAIDs are especially effective when pain is associated with inflammation and soft tissue injury. Ketorolac (Toradol) may be given IM or IV when oral agents are contraindicated. Monitor for excessive bleeding, gastric irritation, and renal compromise in patients receiving NSAIDs.
- Administer prn analgesics before pain becomes severe. Prolonged stimulation of pain receptors results in ↑ sensitivity to painful stimuli and will ↑ amount of drug required to relieve pain.
- Administer intermittently scheduled or supplemental analgesics before painful procedures (suctioning, chest tube removal), ambulation, and at hs, so that their peak effect is achieved at inception of the activity or procedure.

CONSULT MD FOR
- Unrelieved pain or discomfort
- Complications: sustained respiratory depression, hypotension

RELATED TOPICS
- Agitation syndrome
- Anxiety
- Drug overdose: opioids
- Equianalgesic doses of opioid analgesics (see Appendix)
- Psychosocial needs, patient

ABBREVIATIONS
I/E: Inspiration to expiration
LVEDP: Left ventricular end-diastolic pressure
VC: Vital capacity

- Augment analgesic therapy with sedatives and tranquilizers to ↓ anxiety and promote relaxation. Avoid substituting sedatives and tranquilizers for analgesics.
- Wean patient from opioid analgesics by ↓ drug dosage or frequency. When changing route of administration or medication, be certain to employ equianalgesic doses of the new drug (see Appendix).
- Augment action of medication by employing nonpharmacologic methods of pain control. Many of these techniques may be taught to and implemented by patient and significant others.
- Maintain a quiet environment to promote rest. Plan nursing activities to enable long periods of uninterrupted rest at night.
- Evaluate for and correct nonoperative sources of discomfort (ie, position, full bladder, infiltrated IV site).
- Position patient comfortably, and reposition at frequent intervals to relieve discomfort caused by pressure.
- Sudden or unexpected changes in pain intensity can signal complications such as internal bleeding or leakage of visceral contents. Carefully evaluate patient and consult surgeon immediately.
- Document efficacy of analgesics and other pain control interventions, using pain scale or other formalized method.

Ineffective breathing pattern r/t neuromuscular impairment secondary to central respiratory depression

Desired outcome: Patient exhibits effective ventilation within 30 min of this diagnosis: relaxed breathing, RR 12-20 breaths/min with eupnea, clear breath sounds, nl color, Pao_2 ≥80 mm Hg, pH 7.35-7.45, $Paco_2$ 35-45 mm Hg, HCO_3^- 22-26 mEq/L, and Spo_2 ≥92%.

- Assess and document respiratory rate and depth qh. Note signs of respiratory compromise: RR <10 or >26; shallow or grunting respirations; use of accessory muscles of respiration; prolonged I/E ratio; pallor or cyanosis; ↓ VC; and ↑ residual volume.
- Monitor Spo_2 and ABGs. Be alert to ↓ Spo_2 (<90%-92%) or ↑ $Paco_2$ (>45 mm Hg).
- Assess and document LOC q1-2h.
- Use apnea monitor as indicated.
- Keep naloxone (Narcan) at bedside during and for 24 h after epidural or intrathecal administration.
- Maintain IV access for immediate administration of naloxone to reverse respiratory depression.
- Respiratory depression may persist for as long as 24 h after last dose of epidural morphine. Monitor for respiratory depression during and for 24 h after patient's receipt of epidural or intrathecal opioids.

Urinary retention r/t inhibition of reflex arc secondary to opioid action

Desired outcomes: Within 4 h of this diagnosis, complete bladder emptying achieved. Overflow incontinence absent.

- Monitor for symptoms of urinary retention: bladder distention, frequent voiding of small amounts of urine, sensation of bladder fullness, residual urine, dysuria, and overflow incontinence.
- Monitor I&O precisely.
- Catheterize bladder intermittently or insert indwelling catheter as prescribed.
- Administer IV naloxone as prescribed.

REFERENCES

Acute Pain Management Guideline Panel: *Acute pain management: operative and medical procedures and trauma, clinical practice guideline,* AHCPR Publication No 9200032, Rockville, Md, 1992, US Department of Health and Human Services.

Hauer M et al: Intravenous patient-controlled analgesia in critically ill postoperative/trauma patients: research-based practice recommendations, *Dimens Crit Care Nurs* 14(3): 144-152, 1995.

Jensen D, Justic M: An algorithm to distinguish the need for sedation, anxiolytic, and analgesic agents, *Dimens Crit Care Nurs* 14(2): 58-65, 1995.

Keen JH: Pain. In Swearingen PL, Keen JH (eds): *Manual of critical care nursing,* ed 3, St Louis, 1995, Mosby.

Pasero C, McCaffery M: Avoiding opioid-induced respiratory depression, *Am J Nurs* 94(4): 25-30, 1994.

Puntillo K: Dimensions of procedural pain and its analgesic management in critically ill patients, *Am J Crit Care* 3(2): 116-122, 1994.

Author: **Janet Hicks Keen**

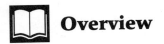 **Overview**

PATHOPHYSIOLOGY

Obstruction of pancreatic ductal flow resulting in injury to adjacent acinar cell where pancreatic enzymes are stored in their inactive form. Once acinar cell damage has occurred, enzymes are released and activated, resulting in autodigestion of the organ. Spillage of pancreatic enzymes causes chemical peritonitis and third spacing of vast amounts of fluid within peritoneum. Vascular damage and release of vasoactive amines, including bradykinin and kallikrein, contribute to capillary leakage and depress myocardial function. Net effect is hypovolemia and CV failure. Mortality high, especially with widespread necrosis and hemorrhage.

COMPLICATIONS

- Depletion of intravascular volume
- ↓ vascular tone and hyperdynamic circulatory state
- Life-threatening hemorrhage from rupture of necrotic pancreatic tissue
- Respiratory insufficiency r/t shunting and alveolocapillary leakage
- Intravascular coagulopathy
- Hypocalcemia
- Pancreatic pseudocysts or abscesses
- Sepsis

HISTORY/RISK FACTORS

- Mechanical blockage of pancreatic ducts: eg, biliary disease, structural abnormalities
- Alcohol consumption
- Infection: eg, hepatitis, mumps
- Pancreatic trauma: eg, abdominal injury, complications of ERCP
- Ischemia: eg, prolonged/severe shock, vasculitis

- Drugs: eg, NSAIDs, glucocorticoids, sulfonamides

CLINICAL PRESENTATION

- Sudden onset of mild to severe abdominal pain, often after excessive food or alcohol ingestion; may radiate to the back
- Possible nausea, vomiting, diarrhea, melena, and hematemesis
- Possible serious complications: dyspnea and cyanosis (signs of ARDS)

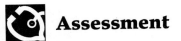 **Assessment**

PHYSICAL ASSESSMENT

- ↓/absent bowel sounds: reflect GI dysfunction and ileus
- Localized tenderness in RUQ or diffuse discomfort over upper abdomen
- Mild to moderate ascites
- ↓/absent breath sounds: suggest focal atelectasis or pleural effusion
- Crackles: reflect hypoventilation caused by pain, early ARDS, microemboli
- Delayed capillary refill, ↓ peripheral pulses: reflect hemorrhage or severe hypovolemia
- Chvostek's and Trousseau's signs: present if hypocalcemia severe

VITAL SIGNS/HEMODYNAMICS

RR: ↑
HR: ↑
BP: ↓
Temp: ↑
PAP: ↓
CO: ↓ caused by hypovolemia, myocardial depression; ↑ if SIRS present
PVR: ↑ caused by ↑ lung water/ARDS

SVR: ↓ if SIRS present
ECG: ST-segment depression, T-wave inversion may be seen with shock state, severe pain that causes coronary artery spasm, or effect of trypsin and bradykinins on the myocardium. Hypocalcemia results in widening of ST segment.

LABORATORY STUDIES

Hematology: ↑ WBCs reflective of inflammatory process. Hct and Hgb levels vary, depending on presence of hemorrhage (↓) or dehydration (↑).

Chemistry

Serum amylase: ↑ 3-5 × nl initially, but may become nl or ↓ as a result of urinary excretion (especially after fluid challenges/diuretics) or ↓ amylase secretion associated with severe necrosis.

Serum lipase: Parallels amylase level; more specific for pancreatitis.

Hypocalcemia, hypomagnesemia: Frequent findings.

Hyperglycemia: Consequence of glucagon release and damage to pancreatic β cells.

Liver enzymes: Persistent ↑ suggests hepatic inflammation attributable to alcohol or viral hepatitis.

Serum bicarbonate and potassium: ↑ HCO_3^- and ↓ K^+ reflect metabolic alkalosis, usually resulting from vomiting or gastric suctioning.

Coagulation Studies: ↓ platelets and fibrinogen. ↑ circulating levels of fibrin associated with microthrombi in pancreas and other tissues.

ABGs: ↓ Pao_2 may be present even without other symptoms of pulmonary insufficiency. Early hypoxia produces mild respiratory alkalosis. If ARDS ensues, respiratory failure present, with ↓ Pao$_2$, ↑ Paco$_2$, and respiratory acidosis.

IMAGING
Radiology
Abdominal x-ray: May show dilatation of bowel and ileus.

Chest x-ray: Findings helpful in distinguishing effusions from atelectasis and in diagnosing ARDS.

CT Scan: Estimates pancreatic size; identifies fluid collection, cystic lesions, abscesses, masses; visualizes biliary tract abnormalities; monitors inflammatory swelling of pancreas.

Endoscopic Pancreatography: To visualize opening to the pancreas directly and observe for swelling, ductal abnormalities, tumors, and stones.

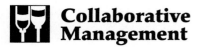 **Collaborative Management**

Efforts directed at pain relief and resting pancreas until autodigestion subsides.

Analgesia: Continuous or intermittent IV opiate analgesics to relieve severe pain. Morphine, fentanyl, meperidine (Demerol) may cause spasm of pancreatic ducts and impede ductal flow. Some authorities believe meperidine is less likely to cause ductal spasm and therefore recommend it for pancreatitis. Epidural blockade may be employed for severe pain.

Fluid/Electrolyte Management: Fluid sequestration and extensive intravascular volume loss, nausea, vomiting, gastric suctioning, and hemorrhage contribute to hypovolemic state. Colloids and crystalloids given to replace volume losses and minimize interstitial edema. Crystalloids alone may be used initially if serum protein levels adequate. Fluid sequestration in peritoneum and interstitium continues until acute phase arrested; therefore continual volume replacement essential. K$^+$ and Ca^{2+} replaced as needed. Because hypercalcemia has been implicated in the genesis of pancreatitis, calcium replacement is prescribed cautiously.

Suppression of Pancreatic Secretions: Accomplished by withholding oral feedings including water, aspirating gastric secretions *via* gastric suction, reducing gastric acidity *via* histamine H$_2$-receptor antagonists and other acid-suppression therapies, and ↓ physical activity.

Resp Support: Pulmonary congestion, pleural effusion, and atelectasis result in respiratory insufficiency. Abdominal distention and retroperitoneal fluid sequestration cause diaphragmatic elevation and ventilatory restriction. Frequent or continuous Spo$_2$ evaluated during first 2-3 days of therapy to detect early hypoxemia. O$_2$ initiated because of ↑ tissue needs and likelihood of impaired O$_2$ transport. If severe pulmonary insufficiency develops, ET intubation and positive pressure ventilation may be required. IV fluids monitored closely to prevent overload, ↑ lung water.

Nutritional Support: Initiation of parenteral feedings that provide nutrients necessary for tissue healing. High-glucose parenteral regimens compound hyperglycemia; therefore a higher percentage of calories as fats may be preferable. Oral feedings not indicated during acute episode because they cause pancreatic inflammation by stimulating glandular secretions.

Peritoneal Lavage: Removes toxic factors present in peritoneal exudate. Generally, 2 L of isotonic, balanced electrolyte solution infused into peritoneum over a 15-min period. Solution dwells in peritoneum for 20-30 min and then is drained. Common lavage additives include potassium, heparin, and a broad-spectrum antibiotic.

Surgical Management: In general, nonsurgical management most effective. Because acute pancreatitis is easily confused with acute abdominal emergencies that require urgent surgery, exploratory laparotomy necessary for some patients. More aggressive surgical procedures, such as early pancreatic drainage or débridement, remain controversial.

PATIENT/FAMILY TEACHING
- For patients whose pancreatitis is caused by excessive alcohol intake: the availability of alcohol rehabilitation programs
- Medications: drug name, dosage, purpose, schedule, precautions, drug-drug and food-drug interactions, and side effects
- Importance of adhering to a low-fat diet if prescribed
- S&S of actual or impending GI hemorrhage: nausea, vomiting of blood, dark stools, lightheadedness, passage of frank blood in stools
- S&S of infection: fever, unusual drainage from surgical incisions or peritoneal lavage site, warmth or erythema surrounding surgical sites, and abdominal pain
- Importance of seeking medical attention promptly if signs of recurrent pancreatitis (ie, pain, change in bowel habits, passing of blood in stools, or vomiting blood) or infection appear

Nursing Diagnoses/Interventions

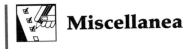 **Miscellanea**

Fluid volume deficit r/t active loss secondary to fluid sequestration within peritoneum and hemorrhage associated with tissue necrosis; and r/t insufficient oral intake

Desired outcome: Within 24 h of this diagnosis, patient normovolemic: MAP >70 mm Hg, HR 60-100 bpm, NSR on ECG, CVP 2-6 mm Hg, PAWP 6-12 mm Hg, CO ≥4 L/min, CI ≥2.5 L/min/m^2, SVR 900-1200 dynes/sec/cm^{-5}, PVR 60-100 dynes/sec/cm^{-5}, brisk capillary refill (<2 sec), peripheral pulses >2+ on 0-4+ scale, UO ≥0.5 ml/kg/h.

- Administer crystalloids, colloids, or combination of both as necessary according to serum albumin levels, electrolyte replacement needs.
- Monitor BP qh if losses caused by fluid sequestration, inadequate intake, or slow bleeding. Monitor BP q15min if patient has active blood loss or unstable VS.
- Monitor HR, ECG, and CV status. Be alert to ↑ HR, which suggests hypovolemia. ↑ HR also may result from fever or hypermetabolic state.
- Measure hemodynamic parameters. Be alert to low/↓ CVP, PAWP, and CO. ↑ HR, ↓ PAWP, ↓ CO (CI <3.0 L/min/m^2), and ↑ SVR suggest hypovolemia. As available, monitor Svo$_2$ to evaluate adequacy of tissue perfusion. Pulmonary hypertension anticipated in patients with ARDS. Monitor for signs of overaggressive fluid resuscitation: dyspnea, orthopnea, ↑ respiratory rate/effort, S$_3$ gallop, or crackles.
- Measure UO qh. Be alert to output <0.5 ml/kg/h for 2 consecutive h. Evaluate intravascular volume and CV function. ↑ fluids promptly if ↓ UO caused by hypovolemia, hypoperfusion.
- Monitor for physical indicators of hypovolemia, including cool extremities, delayed capillary refill (>2 sec), and ↓/absent distal pulses.
- Estimate ongoing fluid losses. Measure all drainage from tubes, catheters, and drains. Note frequency of dressing changes because of saturation with fluid or blood.
- Evaluate character of all fluid losses. Note color and odor. Be alert to particulate matter, fibrin, and clots. Test GI aspirate, drainage, and excretions (including stool) for occult blood.
- Administer inotropic agents as prescribed. Monitor hemodynamic parameters carefully and use lowest effective dose to minimize adverse effects of inotropic therapy (see Appendix).
- Provide frequent rest periods. Cluster procedures and treatments to enable long periods (at least 90 min) of uninterrupted rest.

Pain r/t chemical injury to peritoneum and surrounding tissue secondary to release of pancreatic enzymes

Desired outcomes: Within 2-4 h of this diagnosis, patient's subjective evaluation of discomfort improves, as documented by pain scale. Ventilation and hemodynamic status uncompromised: MAP 70-105 mm Hg, HR 60-100 bpm, and state of eupnea.

- As prescribed, administer IV opiate analgesia before pain becomes severe. Be aware that fentanyl, morphine, meperidine, and other narcotic analgesics have been linked with biliary spasm; their use may ↓ intestinal motility and delay return to nl bowel functioning.
- Pancreatitis can be very painful. Prepare significant others for personality changes and behavioral alterations associated with extreme pain and narcotic analgesia. Family members sometimes misinterpret patient's lethargy or unpleasant disposition and may even blame themselves. Reassure them that these are nl responses.
- Supplement analgesics with nonpharmacologic maneuvers to aid in pain reduction. Modify patient's body position to optimize comfort. Many patients with abdominal pain find dorsal recumbent or lateral decubitus bent-knee position most comfortable.
- Ensure consistency and promptness in delivering analgesia to relieve anticipation anxiety.
- Patients and family members are sometimes distressed at health team members' inability to relieve pain. Reassure continually that all possible measures are being implemented.
- Monitor respiratory pattern and LOC closely because both may be depressed by large amounts of opiate analgesics usually required to control pain.
- Monitor HR, BP, CVP, and PAWP. Be aware that opiates cause vasodilatation and can result in serious hypotension, especially with volume depletion.
- Evaluate effectiveness of medication; consult physician for dose and drug manipulation. If medications are not effective, prepare for splanchnic block, other pain-relieving procedure.

Impaired gas exchange r/t alveolocapillary membrane changes secondary to microatelectasis and pulmonary fluid accumulation

CONSULT MD FOR
- S&S of inadequate tissue perfusion: altered mental status, restlessness; ↓ BP, peripheral pulses; UO <0.5 ml/kg/h × 2 h; Svo$_2$ <60% or >80%; ↓/absent bowel sounds
- S&S of complications: DIC, SIRS, septic shock
- S&S of GI or other hemorrhage
- Inability to control pain with prescribed therapy
- New-onset absent bowel sounds or ↑ abdominal distention

Desired outcome: Within 4 h of this diagnosis, patient has adequate gas exchange: SaO_2 ≥92%, PaO_2 ≥80 mm Hg, $PaCO_2$ 35-45 mm Hg, RR 12-20 breaths/min with eupnea, patient oriented × 3, clear and audible breath sounds.

- Monitor and document RR. Note pattern, degree of excursion, use of accessory muscles.
- Monitor for crackles, rhonchi, wheezes, or ↓ breath sounds.
- Be alert to early signs of hypoxia, such as restlessness, agitation, altered mentation.
- Monitor SaO_2 *via* continuous pulse oximetry or ABGs frequently during first 48 h. Many patients with pancreatitis do not have obvious clinical symptoms of respiratory failure; ↓ SaO_2 may be the first sign of failure. Be alert for PaO_2 <60-70 mm Hg or O_2 saturation <92%.
- Administer O_2. Check O_2 delivery system at frequent intervals to ensure proper delivery and titrate to SpO_2.
- Maintain body position that optimizes ventilation and oxygenation. Elevate HOB ≥30 degrees, depending on comfort. If pleural effusion or other defect present on one side, position with unaffected lung dependent to maximize V/Q relationship.

Risk for infection r/t tissue destruction with resulting necrosis secondary to release of pancreatic enzymes

Desired outcome: Patient free of infection: core or rectal temp ≤37.8° C (≤100° F), negative culture results; HR 60-100 bpm, RR 12-20 breaths/min, BP wnl for patient, CI ≤4 $L/min/m^2$, SVR 900-1200 $dynes/sec/cm^{-5}$, and orientation × 3.

- Check for ↑ rectal or core temp q4h. Hypothermia may precede hyperthermia in some patients.
- If there is a sudden ↑ in temp, obtain specimens for culture of blood, sputum, urine, and appropriate sites as prescribed. Monitor culture reports; report positive findings promptly.
- Evaluate orientation and LOC q2-4h.
- Monitor BP, HR, RR, CO, and SVR. Be alert to ↑ HR and RR associated with temp ↑. ↑ CO and ↓ SVR suggest SIRS or sepsis.
- Administer parenteral antibiotics in a timely fashion. Reschedule if dose delayed for >1 h. Failure to give antibiotics on schedule can result in inadequate blood levels, treatment failure. Monitor peak and trough levels for patients receiving aminoglycoside antibiotics. Aminoglycosides used frequently; therefore monitor for hearing loss. Elders are especially susceptible to their ototoxic, nephrotoxic effects. Monitor BUN/creatinine and UO.

Impaired tissue integrity: GI tract, r/t release of chemical irritants into pancreatic parenchyma and surrounding tissue, including peritoneum

Desired outcomes: By time of hospital discharge, patient exhibits no further GI tissue destruction: ↓ pain; GI aspirate, stools, drainage, and vomitus negative for blood; and return of bowel sounds and bowel functioning. Gastric pH value remains >5.

- Withhold oral feedings to avoid stimulation of pancreatic enzymes.
- Ensure patency of gastric sump tube to provide continual drainage and prevent pancreatic stimulation. Do not occlude air vent of double-lumen tube because this may result in vacuum occlusion. Check placement of gastric tube at least q8h, and reposition as necessary.
- Administer antacids and histamine H_2-receptor antagonists as indicated to ↓ gastric and pancreatic secretions and reduce gastric pH. Monitor gastric pH, and administer antacids to maintain pH value >5.
- Because ↑ activity can stimulate gastric secretions, limit physical activity during acute phase.
- Test GI aspirate, drainage, and excretions for occult blood q12-24h.
- Initiate peritoneal lavage as prescribed to remove irritants from peritoneum.

Altered nutrition: Less than body requirements, r/t ↓ oral intake secondary to nausea, vomiting, and NPO status; and ↑ need secondary to tissue destruction or infection

Desired outcome: Patient maintains baseline body weight and demonstrates a state of nitrogen balance on nitrogen studies.

- Collaborate with physician, dietitian, pharmacist to estimate metabolic needs based on activity level, presence of infection or other stressor, nutritional status before hospitalization.
- Provide PN during acute phase. Monitor closely for hyperglycemia (eg, Kussmaul's respirations; rapid respirations; fruity acetone breath odor; flushed, dry skin; deteriorating LOC), which is commonly associated with pancreatitis. Consider use of long-chain fatty acids and supplements instead of high-glucose parenteral regimens. Administer insulin as necessary.
- Administer enteral feedings *via* feeding jejunostomy for patients with intestinal peristalsis.
- Monitor bowel sounds q4h. Document and report deviations from baseline. "Hold" oral or jejunostomy feedings if bowel sounds absent.
- Monitor blood or urine glucose levels q4-8h or as prescribed. Alter therapy if blood levels >200 mg/dl.
- Begin low-fat oral feedings when acute episode has subsided and bowel function has returned. This may take several wks in some patients.

RELATED TOPICS
- Adult respiratory distress syndrome
- Disseminated intravascular coagulation
- Hypocalcemia
- Hypokalemia
- Hypovolemia
- Shock, septic
- Systemic inflammatory response syndrome

ABBREVIATIONS
ARDS: Adult respiratory distress syndrome
ERCP: Endoscopic retrocholangiopancreatography
PN: Parenteral nutrition
SIRS: Systemic inflammatory response syndrome
SvO_2: Mixed venous oxygen saturation

REFERENCES
Ambrose MS, Dreher HM: Pancreatitis: managing a flare up, *Nursing* 26(4): 33-39, 1996.

Brown A: Acute pancreatitis: pathophysiology, nursing diagnoses, collaborative problems, *Focus Crit Care* 18(2): 121-130, 1991.

Krumberger JM: Acute pancreatitis, *Crit Care Nurs Clin North Am* 5(1): 169-185, 1993.

Smith A: When the pancreas self-destructs, *Am J Nurs* 91(9): 38-48, 1991.

Author: **Janet Hicks Keen**

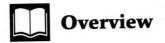 **Overview**

DESCRIPTION

NMBAs used when periods of complete paralysis are needed in intubated, mechanically ventilated patients. Generally used in the following situations: (1) to ↓ O_2 consumption when unable to maintain adequate O_2 saturation, (2) to alleviate specific medical conditions (see **HISTORY/RISK FACTORS**), (3) to immobilize patients for surgical and invasive procedures, (4) to manage ↑ ICP. If used in cases of extreme agitation, all possible causes of agitation (eg, pain, fear, suctioning, hypoxemia) must be investigated thoroughly before initiating NMBAs.

HISTORY/RISK FACTORS

- Status asthmaticus
- Tetanus
- Malignant hyperthermia
- Status epilepticus
- ARDS
- Severe, unrelieved agitation
- Hypoxemia unrelieved by mechanical ventilation

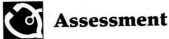 **Assessment**

PHYSICAL ASSESSMENT (during NMBA therapy)

Neuro: Fully aware and able to perceive pain and all stimuli but unable to respond because of paralysis

Resp: Apnea with respiratory muscle paralysis

CV: Tachycardia with some agents

GI: Possible constipation

VITAL SIGNS/HEMODYNAMICS (during NMBA therapy)

RR: Absent

HR: NI to ↑

BP: NI to ↑

Temp: NI

CVP/PAWP: NI to ↑

SVR: NI to ↑

CO: NI to ↑

12/18-Lead ECG: May reflect sinus tachycardia. If other dysrhythmias apparent, oxygenation and pain/anxiety management should be evaluated thoroughly.

LABORATORY STUDIES

ABGs: To evaluate for hypoxemia or pH imbalance. Acidosis ↑ effects of NMBAs, while alkalosis ↓ effects.

Serum Electrolytes: To identify abnormal value that may alter neuromuscular blockade. ↑ *Blockade:* Hypercalcemia, hypermagnesemia, hypocalcemia, hypokalemia, hyponatremia ↓ *Blockade:* Hyperkalemia, hypernatremia

Drug/Toxicology Screening: To r/o substance abuse/withdrawal with unmanageable anxiety.

IMAGING

Chest X-ray: May reflect "white out" characteristic of ARDS if NMBAs used to ↑ ventilation and ↓ O_2 consumption associated with respiratory failure.

DIAGNOSTIC PROCEDURE

Peripheral Nerve Stimulator: To quantify level/depth of neuromuscular blockade. Train-of-four technique most often used: four signals/"shocks" delivered down the nerve path in rapid succession. The muscle should move ≥1 × during four shocks. If no response, NMBA dosage may need to be ↓. If four twitches out of four shocks, dosage may need to be ↑, particularly if patient beginning to move around in bed.

4 twitches:	0%-50% blockade
3 twitches:	60%-70% blockade
2 twitches:	70%-80% blockade
1 twitch:	80%-90% blockade
no twitch:	>90% blockade

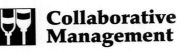 **Collaborative Management**

Depolarizing NMBAs: Succinylcholine (Anectine) is the only agent with widespread clinical use; provides rapid, brief paralysis. Long-term blockade impractical because of rapid tachyphylaxis and desensitization of receptors to blocking effects.

Nondepolarizing NMBAs: Used most often in critical illness for prolonged neuromuscular blockade. Most commonly used agents: pancuronium (Pavulon), vecuronium (Norcuron), atracurium (Tracrium), and rocuronium (Zemuron).

Medications that augment/↑ neuromuscular blockade: Aminoglycoside antibiotics (eg, gentamicin, tobramycin, neomycin), bretylium, calcium blockers, clindamycin, cyclosporine, lidocaine, procainamide, propranolol, quinidine, vancomycin

Medications that antagonize/↓ neuromuscular blockade: Anticholinesterase agents, azathioprine, carbamazepine, corticosteroids, phenytoin, ranitidine, theophylline

Mechanical Ventilation: For ventilation and blood oxygenation.

Spo_2 Monitoring: For continuous assessment of hemoglobin saturation/oxygenation.

ECG Monitoring: For continuous screening of dysrhythmias associated with hypoxemia or electrolyte imbalance.

Sedation: To ↓ LOC and thus anxiety associated with helplessness and inability to breathe without assistance while on NMBA therapy.

Anesthetics: Propofol

Antihistamines: Diphenhydramine, hydroxyzine

Antipsychotics: Haloperidol, chlorpromazine, thorazine

Barbiturates: Phenobarbital, pentobarbital

Benzodiazepines: Midazolam, diazepam, lorazepam, clonazepam

Analgesics: As appropriate for underlying conditions/procedures. Essential if pain expected, since patient will be unable to communicate pain.

Augmented Safety Measures: To ensure alarms are functional and remain on, particularly ventilator alarm, since patient unable to breathe if disconnected from ventilator or a mechanical problem ensues.

Alcohol Withdrawal Protocol: If patient ETOH user in withdrawal. Generally, benzodiazepines combined with thiamine and other vitamin therapy included in protocol.

PATIENT-FAMILY TEACHING

- Explanations that inability to move is not permanent and that patient is fully aware despite absence of response
- Encouragement for significant others to talk with patient
- Need for those who will touch patient to explain what they are about to do; patient is unable to open eyes to view environment
- Reminder to patient that recall of unpleasant procedures may be ↓ by sedatives administered
- Discharge medications: drug name, purpose, dosage, schedule, precautions, drug-drug and food-drug interactions, potential side effects

Nursing Diagnoses/Interventions

Impaired gas exchange (or risk for same) r/t ↓ ventilatory drive occurring with sedative use and CNS depression or ↓/absent chest wall movement with NMBA therapy
Desired outcome: Within 1 h of initiation of NMBA therapy, Pao_2 ≥80 mm Hg, $Paco_2$ 35-45 mm Hg, Spo_2 ≥90%.

- Assess depth of paralysis using peripheral nerve stimulator.
- Monitor lab values for electrolyte anomalies that ↑ or ↓ neuromuscular blockade.
- Monitor for hypotension if multiple agents for sedation used.
- Continuously monitor Spo_2 *via* pulse oximetry.
- Monitor chest wall movement *via* apnea monitor. Have appropriate antidote (pyridostigmine, atropine) for NMBAs at bedside. If patient ineffectively blockaded, chest wall will begin moving. If overly blockaded, ↓ NMBA dose as prescribed.
- When blockade has been terminated, continue to monitor respiratory status vigilantly; residual weakness from NMBAs may be present, as well as ↓ ventilatory drive from sedation.

Anxiety r/t actual or perceived threat of death and helplessness associated with NMBA-induced paralysis
Desired outcome: Within 4-6 h of therapy initiation, anxiety ↓: HR ≤100 bpm (unless NMBA used causes tachycardia), SBP ≤140 mm Hg, and cessation of extraneous motor movements.

- Administer medications for anxiety/sedation as prescribed.
- Consider giving pain medication based on underlying condition/procedure.
- Initiate nonpharmacologic measures to ↓ anxiety: guided imagery, biofeedback, therapeutic touch, verbal emotional support, explaining what you plan to do before performing activities that involve touching patient.

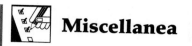

Miscellanea

CONSULT MD FOR

- Inability to manage patient's anxiety (evidenced by VS)
- Electrolyte imbalances or prescribed medications that may alter neuromuscular blockade
- Hypotension, hypertension
- Spo_2 <90%
- HR >150 bpm
- Possible complications: hypoxemia, prolonged weakness or paralysis following discontinuation of NMBA therapy, inability to wean from mechanical ventilation, inability to perform ADLs because of prolonged weakness

RELATED TOPICS

- Adult respiratory distress syndrome
- Agitation syndrome
- Alcohol intoxication, acute
- Anxiety
- Mechanical ventilation

ABBREVIATION

NMBAs: Neuromuscular blocking agents

REFERENCES

Davidson J: Neuromuscular blockade: indications, peripheral nerve stimulation, and other concurrent interventions, *New Horiz* 2(1): 75-84, 1994.

Puntillo K: Dimensions of procedural pain and its analgesic management in critically ill surgical patients, *Am J Crit Care Nurs* 3(2): 116-122, 1994.

Snider BS: Use of muscle relaxants in the ICU: nursing implications, *Crit Care Nurse* 13(6): 55-60, 1993.

Vender J: Sedation, analgesia, and neuromuscular blockade in critical care: an overview, *New Horiz* 2(1): 2-7, 1994.

Authors: **Marianne Saunorus Baird and Robert Aucker**

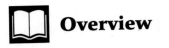 **Overview**

PATHOPHYSIOLOGY

Large force needed to fracture pelvis because these bones are stabilized by strong network of ligaments. The most serious complications are hemorrhage and exsanguination. Retroperitoneal space can hold as much as 4 L of blood before spontaneous tamponade occurs, thus acute blood loss difficult to identify until systemic symptoms, eg, hypotension, shock, appear. Damage to sciatic and sacral nerves may occur with sacral and sacroiliac disruption.

MORTALITY

Up to 50%

HISTORY/RISK FACTORS

- Motor vehicle or motorcycle collision, auto-pedestrian collision, fall, industrial accident, crush injury, sports-related injury
- Act of violence
- Intoxication, substance abuse
- Thrill-seeking behavior
- Failure to use safety device (eg, seat belt)
- Chronic illness
- Advanced age

CLINICAL PRESENTATION

- Suprapubic tenderness, pain over iliac spines
- Hemorrhagic shock: tachycardia, delayed capillary refill, pallor, hypotension
- Lacerations of perineum, groin, buttocks
- Urinary injuries: up to 15% of trauma victims with pelvic fracture have renal and LUT injuries

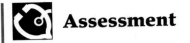 **Assessment**

PHYSICAL ASSESSMENT

- Groin, genitalia, suprapubic swelling or ecchymosis
- Pelvic instability
- Lower extremity involvement: shortening, abnormal rotation, "frog-leg" positioning, paresis
- Hematuria or urethral bleeding, blood in rectum
- Absent plantar flexion and ankle jerk reflexes

VITAL SIGNS/HEMODYNAMICS

RR: ↑
HR: ↑
BP: ↓
Temp: Nl; ↓ if hypothermic
CVP/PAWP: ↓
CO: ↓
SVR: ↑
Other: Hypovolemia likely because of significant blood loss. VS/hemodynamics reflect volume status.

LABORATORY STUDIES

Hct: Value that fails to stabilize, ↓, or fails to ↑ with transfusion is sign of ongoing bleeding. ↓ Hct is late sign of hemorrhage, occurring after significant blood loss.

IMAGING

Pelvic X-ray: Shows overall pelvic alignment and location of pelvic, sacral fractures.
CT Scan: Most reliable method for determining injury to posterior pelvis; identifies sacral and sacroiliac joint injury.
Angiogram: Identifies bleeding sites. Indicated for expanding pelvic retroperitoneal hematoma or suspected internal bleeding and pelvic injury.
Excretory Urogram (IVP), Cystography, Urography: Determine associated injuries.

Collaborative Management

Pelvic Stabilization

External immobilization: Device applied to immobilize pelvis externally or percutaneously through skin into bone. PASG sometimes used to immobilize bony injuries and provide tamponade effect, but is controversial. For abnormal shortening or rotation, lower extremities supported and stabilized in position in which they were found. Emergency external fixation devices, consisting of one pin in each iliac wing connected by a bar, can be inserted to provide pelvic stability. If emergency laparotomy needed, a more complex external fixation device may be applied.
Internal immobilization: Surgical open reduction and immobilization of unstable pelvic ring disruptions with plates, screws, or other devices that are surgically implanted internally. Permanent fixation requires close anatomic reduction because it will be final form of pelvic stabilization.
Surgical Exploration: Occurs along with ligation or vessel repair with hemorrhaging. Instead of surgical exploration, some patients undergo angiography and selective embolization of bleeding points with autologous blood clot or particulate gel foam.
Massive Fluid Resuscitation: With blood, colloids, or crystalloids. If >2 L blood required in 8 h after initial resuscitation, additional measures to manage bleeding indicated.

Pharmacotherapy

Antibiotics: For open fractures and positive cultures of wounds, blood, urine
Analgesics: IV morphine sulfate
Vasopressors: For hypotension only after sufficient volume replacement has occurred
Td Immunization: Booster given if hx unknown or booster needed

PATIENT-FAMILY TEACHING

- Medications: drug name, purpose, dosage, schedule, precautions, food-drug and drug-drug interactions, potential side effects
- Purpose, expected results, anticipated sensations of all nursing/medical interventions
- Need/technique used for pelvic immobilization
- Importance of reporting S&S of venous thrombosis, pulmonary embolus: calf tenderness, SOB, chest pain

Nursing Diagnoses/Interventions

Fluid volume deficit r/t active blood loss secondary to pelvic and pelvic sink injury
Desired outcomes: Within 12 h after injury, patient becomes normovolemic: regular HR ≤100 bpm, bilaterally strong/equal peripheral pulses, warm and dry extremities, brisk (<2 sec) capillary refill, SBP ≥90 mm Hg, UO ≥0.5 ml/kg/h. Patient awake, alert, and oriented × 3.
- Perform complete assessment of fluid balance qh until stable.
- Administer blood products, colloids, or crystalloids through large-bore peripheral IV catheter. Use pressure infusers and rapid-volume warmer/infusers for massive fluid/blood resuscitation. Be prepared to administer pressor agents only after fluid replacement in progress.
- Prepare to move patient to OR rapidly if necessary for repair of pelvic vasculature.
- Keep patient flat until fluid volume status stabilized if other injuries do not preclude position and if airway and breathing adequate in that position. Avoid Trendelenburg's position.
- If patient in PASG, wrap extremities in towels before application, maintain compartment pressures as prescribed, and check peripheral pulses and neurovascular status q2h. Deflate PASG slowly (eg, q6h in increments of 5 mm Hg) when prescribed. Deflate abdominal compartment before leg compartments.

Risk for infection r/t inadequate primary defenses secondary to open pelvic fractures, percutaneous external fixation devices, or surgical procedure
Desired outcome: Within 24 h after injury, soft tissues begin to heal without purulent drainage or erythema; WBCs <11,000 µl; cultures of blood and wounds negative; pin insertion site free of erythema, edema, purulent drainage; surgical wounds well approximated and without erythema, edema, or purulent drainage.
- For initial wound care, remove any gross contamination from wound and cover exposed soft tissue and bone with wet sterile dressings.
- Monitor all wounds, incisions, and pin insertion sites on external fixation devices q4h for erythema, drainage, edema.
- Perform pin care as prescribed. Pin care controversial and may include removing dried exudate to allow pin holes to drain freely. Unless contraindicated, wrap a loose, open gauze dressing around pin's insertion site.

Impaired physical mobility r/t pelvic immobilization secondary to pelvic ring instability
Desired outcomes: Immediately after pelvic immobilization, patient maintains appropriate body alignment; external fixation devices and traction remain in place. At time of hospital discharge, patient exhibits full ROM in uninjured extremities.
- Position in proper body alignment.
- Apply compression boots, if appropriate, to limit effects of venous stasis. Remove boots at least every shift to provide skin care.
- Provide active and passive ROM to uninjured extremities.
- Maintain traction by keeping it free hanging. Do not remove weights even when repositioning.
- Use caution when turning and positioning to maintain body alignment. For unstable fracture that has not yet been reduced, consult orthopedic surgeon before moving patient. Some patients can be turned from side to side until internal fixation accomplished. Keep HOB ↑ as indicated.
- Do not hold onto external fixation device when turning patient.

Impaired skin integrity r/t initial injury, physical immobility, and placement of external fixation or PASG secondary to pelvic injury
Desired outcomes: Within 12 h of injury and throughout hospitalization, patient has timely wound healing. Patient does not develop pressure ulcers nor experience tissue injury from external fixation device.
- Cover ends of all wires on external fixation device with cork or gauze to protect patient from injury.
- Apply padding to any traction slings.
- Use alternating air mattress or other specialty mattresses.
- If patient can be positioned laterally, pad external fixation device to prevent skin damage. Provide padding over bony prominences and any body area in contact with a rigid surface.
- Keep all skin areas clean and dry to minimize risk of pressure ulcers.

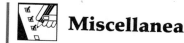 # Miscellanea

CONSULT MD FOR
- Signs of hemorrhage: altered mental status, hypotension, tachycardia, delayed capillary refill, pallor, ↓ UO
- Signs of infection: swelling, erythema, tenderness, ↑ or purulent drainage at pin sites or surgical incisions
- Signs of thrombotic or fat pulmonary emboli: sudden onset dyspnea, tachypnea, tachycardia, restlessness, crackles, ↑ temp, petechiae

RELATED TOPICS
- Multisystem injury
- Pulmonary emboli, fat and thrombotic
- Renal injury
- Shock, hemorrhagic
- Urinary tract injury, lower

ABBREVIATIONS
LUT: Lower urinary tract
Td: Combined tetanus diphtheria toxoid

REFERENCES
Berger JJ, Britt LD: Pelvic fracture hemorrhage, *Surg Annu* 27: 107-112, 1995.

Ghanayem AJ et al: Emergent treatment of pelvic fractures: comparison of methods for stabilization, *Clin Orthop* 318: 75-80, 1995.

Gokcen EC et al: Pelvic fracture mechanism of injury in vehicular trauma patients, *J Trauma* 36(6): 789-795, 1994.

Sommers MS: Pelvic fracture. In Swearingen PL, Keen JH (eds): *Manual of critical care nursing,* ed 3, St Louis, 1995, Mosby.

van Veen IH et al: Unstable pelvic fractures: a retrospective analysis, *Injury* 26(2): 81-85, 1995.

Ziglar MK, Parrish RS: An 18-year-old male patient with multiple trauma including an open pelvic fracture, *J Emerg Nurs* 20(4): 265-270, 1994.

Author: **Marilyn Sawyer Sommers**

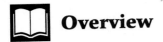 **Overview**

PATHOPHYSIOLOGY

Valvular heart disease involves obstruction to forward flow (stenosis) or valve insufficiency allowing backward flow (regurgitation). One or more valves may be affected by one or both process(es). Valve stenosis is usually caused by sclerosing, thickening, and calcification of valve leaflets. Stenotic valves obstruct blood flow, causing heart chamber hypertrophy and eventual failure. PBV involves use of a balloon-tipped catheter to dilate stenotic heart valves.

HISTORY/RISK FACTORS

- Advanced age
- Infective endocarditis
- Rheumatic fever
- Rheumatoid arthritis

CLINICAL PRESENTATION

Mitral Stenosis: Fatigue, debilitation, activity intolerance
Aortic Stenosis/LV Failure: Chest pain, dizziness, syncope, dyspnea, pulmonary edema

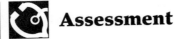 **Assessment**

PHYSICAL ASSESSMENT

Mitral Stenosis: Loud, long diastolic rumbling murmur at fifth ICS, MCL; may radiate to axilla; S_1 loud; opening snap with S_2; palpitations; crackles
Aortic Stenosis: Systolic, blowing murmur at second ICS, RSB; may radiate to neck; thrill, paradoxical splitting of S_2, slow carotid arterial uptake

VITAL SIGNS/HEMODYNAMICS

RR: ↑
HR: ↑
BP: *Aortic stenosis:* widened pulse pressure if nl DBP; if decompensated, narrow pulse pressure, ↓ MAP; *mitral stenosis:* nl or ↓
Temp: N/a
LVP: ↑ for aortic stenosis
PAEDP: ↑ for aortic stenosis
CO: ↓ for both aortic stenosis and mitral stenosis
MPAP: ↑ for mitral stenosis

LABORATORY STUDIES

Hgb/Hct: ↓ if blood loss
Electrolytes: To monitor for hypokalemia, other abnormalities.
Clotting Studies: Obtained before procedure to establish baseline and monitor need for anticoagulation.

DIAGNOSTIC PROCEDURES

Cardiac Catheterization: Ventriculogram may assist in visualizing blood flow. Measuring chamber pressures helps determine type of disorder present and degree of severity.
Echocardiography: To determine ventricular function, chamber size, and valve function.
Doppler flow studies: Continuous wave or pulsed wave frequencies to determine blood flow.
Color flow mapping studies: Uses colors to enhance image of blood flowing through the heart.
Transesophageal echocardiography: Uses endoscope that produces clear and undistorted image unimpeded by chest wall.

Collaborative Management

Procedure: Similar to PTCA technique. Femoral artery and vein cannulated; anticoagulation provided *via* heparin. For aortic valve dilatation, balloon valvuloplasty catheter passed into left ventricle *via* femoral artery. Balloon inflated × 3 over aortic valve for 12-30 sec at 12 atm pressure. To reach the mitral valve, balloon valvuloplasty catheter passed *via* femoral vein through atrial septum to mitral valve opening. Success evaluated by noting significant improvement in valve gradient and blood flow across valve.
Complications: Embolization to the brain, valve ring disruption, acute valve regurgitation, valvular restenosis, hemorrhage at catheter insertion site, LV perforation by guidewire, dysrhythmias.
Patient Selection: Typical candidates (1) are at high risk for surgery, (2) refuse surgery, (3) are elders (often >80 yrs), (4) are informed of treatment choices and choose this procedure over others.

PATIENT-FAMILY TEACHING

- Valve stenosis, purpose of valvuloplasty, expected results, anticipated sensations. Include the following:
  - Location of diseased valve, using drawing of heart
  - Use of local anesthesia and sedation during procedure
  - Insertion site of catheter: femoral artery and vein
  - Use of fluoroscopy during procedure, checking for hx contrast material sensitivity
  - Frequency of postprocedure observations
  - Importance of lying flat for prescribed time postprocedure to ↓ risk of bleeding

Nursing Diagnoses/Interventions

Decreased cardiac output (or risk for same) r/t altered preload and negative inotropic changes associated with valve regurgitation or hemorrhage secondary to PBV; or r/t altered rate, rhythm, or conduction associated with dysrhythmias secondary to PBV

Desired outcome: Throughout postop course, patient has adequate cardiac output: NSR on ECG, CO 4-7 L/min, CI $\geq$2.5 L/min/m², HR 60-100 bpm, RAP 4-6 mm Hg, PAWP 6-12 mm Hg, PAP 20-30/8-15 mm Hg, BP wnl, UO $\geq$0.5 ml/kg/h, peripheral pulses >2+ on 0-4+ scale, and orientation $\times$ 3.

- Monitor ECG for dysrhythmias; treat symptomatic or sustained dysrhythmias as indicated.
- Monitor CO/CI, HR, RAP, PAWP, and PAP qh. Note $\downarrow$ CO/CI, $\uparrow$ or $\downarrow$ in RAP, PAWP, or PAP.
- Monitor Hct and electrolytes. $\downarrow$ Hct suggests bleeding; a change in electrolyte levels (particularly of K$^+$) could precipitate dysrhythmias.
- Assess heart sounds immediately after procedure and q4h.
- Monitor for cardiac tamponade: hypotension, tachycardia, pulsus paradoxus, JVD, $\uparrow$ and plateau pressuring of PAWP and RAP.

Altered protection r/t risk of hemorrhage or hematoma formation secondary to heparinization with PBV

Desired outcomes: Minimal/absent bleeding or hematoma formation at catheter insertion site. PTT is within therapeutic range.

- Monitor insertion site for bleeding. Check for hematoma, and outline bleeding on the dressing for subsequent comparison.
- Keep catheterized leg straight. Check distal pulses frequently.
- Monitor heparin drip, which is usually maintained until 1-2 h before sheaths are removed.
- Monitor PTT for therapeutic range, usually 1½ $\times$ nl.
- When IVs or invasive lines (arterial or venous sheaths) are removed, apply firm pressure either manually or with a mechanical clamp for 30 min. Check for hematoma, bleeding, pulses after removal.

Miscellanea

CONSULT MD FOR
- New-onset A-fib, other dysrhythmias, or A-fib with rapid ventricular response
- CI <2.5 L/min/m2; PAWP >12-18 mm Hg
- UO <0.5 ml/kg/h $\times$ 2 consecutive h
- Altered mental status
- S&S of cardiac tamponade: $\uparrow$ HR, $\downarrow$ BP, paradoxical pulse, plateau pressuring of PAWP, RAP
- New onset murmur
- Hematoma, bleeding at catheter insertion site

RELATED TOPICS
- Aortic stenosis
- Cardiac tamponade
- Endocarditis, infective
- Heart failure, left ventricular
- Hemodynamic monitoring
- Mitral stenosis

ABBREVIATIONS
ICS: Intercostal space
MCL: Midclavicular line
RSB: Right sternal border

REFERENCES
Steuble BT: Valvular heart disease. In Swearingen PL, Keen JH (eds): *Manual of critical care nursing,* ed 3, St Louis, 1995, Mosby.

Vitello-Cicciu J, Lapsly D: Valvular heart disease. In Kinney M, Packa D, Dunbar S: *AACN's clinical reference for critical care nursing,* ed 3, St Louis, 1993, Mosby.

Author: **Cheryl L. Bittel**

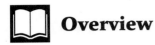 **Overview**

PATHOPHYSIOLOGY

Inflammatory process involving heart's epicardial surface and its protective covering, the pericardium. Occurs as result of MI, infection, or immunologic, chemical, or mechanical event. Initial findings include infiltration of polymorphonuclear leukocytes, ↑ vascularity, and fibrin deposit. Inflammation may spread from pericardium to epicardium or pleura. Eventually, the visceral layer develops exudates, and in some cases adhesions may occur. Excess fluid compresses the heart, impairs chamber filling, and retards ventricular ejection, resulting in ↓ CO.

HISTORY/RISK FACTORS

- Autoimmune cardiac injury: Dressler's syndrome, postcardiotomy syndrome
- Use of procainamide, hydralazine
- Infection, trauma, radiation injury
- MI, neoplasm, rheumatologic disease, uremia

CLINICAL PRESENTATION

Chief complaint is chest pain, usually aggravated by supine position, coughing, deep inspiration, and swallowing. Dyspnea develops because of shallow breathing to prevent pain.
Early Indicators: Fatigue, pallor, fever, anorexia
Late Indicators: ↑ dyspnea, joint pain, heart failure

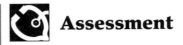 **Assessment**

PHYSICAL ASSESSMENT

Neuro: Fatigue, weakness
Resp: Crackles, tachypnea
CV: Intermittent friction rub composed of atrial systole, ventricular systole, or rapid ventricular filling; heard best with patient sitting and leaning forward and stethoscope diaphragm positioned at lower LSB.

VITAL SIGNS/HEMODYNAMICS

RR: ↑
HR: ↑
BP: Pulsus paradoxus of >10 mm Hg
Temp: ↑
CVP/PAWP: ↑
CO: ↓
ECG: During acute episodes, atrial dysrhythmias such as PAT, PACs, A-flutter, and A-fib. Late dysrhythmias include ventricular ectopy or bundle branch blocks (if there is ventricular involvement). Diffuse ST-segment elevation possible and often confused with that of AMI.

LABORATORY STUDIES

Cardiac Enzymes: May reveal ↑ CK-MB bands if epicardium inflamed.
Blood C&S: ASO titers ↑ when cause is immunologic. If caused by infection, will identify organism.

IMAGING

Echocardiogram: Essential for quantifying and evaluating trend of effusions; appears nl if pericarditis present without effusions. Transesophageal echocardiography may help identify some areas of effusion.
CT Scan: Differentiates restrictive pericarditis from constrictive myopathy *via* appearance of thickened pericardium, which occurs with pericarditis.
Cardiac Technetium Pyrophosphate Scan: May show diffuse regional uptake ("hot spot") in area of epicardial inflammation.

Collaborative Management

Bed Rest: Until pain and fever have disappeared. Activity limitations continue if effusions present.
Pharmacotherapy: In the presence of effusions, anticoagulants are contraindicated because of risk of cardiac tamponade.
NSAIDs: Preferred to ↓ inflammation, particularly after MI or cardiac surgery, since they do not delay healing as do corticosteroids.
Prednisone: Given if no response to NSAIDs.
Subxiphoid Pericardiocentesis: If effusions persist and cardiac status decompensates. Removes fluid compressing the heart. Echocardiography used to guide catheter tip and assess amount of effusion remaining. Catheter may be removed after fluid withdrawn or left in place for several days to enable gradual fluid removal. Catheter flushed with saline q4-6h after effusion withdrawal to prevent clotting. Sterile technique essential.
Pericardiectomy: To prevent cardiac compression or relieve the restriction.

PATIENT-FAMILY TEACHING

- Positions that may be helpful in relieving pain: side-lying, high-Fowler's, or sitting and leaning forward; avoidance of supine position
- Need for deep breathing, coughing at frequent intervals
- How to press arms against chest for added support with breathing, coughing
- Possibility of steroid myopathy with high-dose, long-term steroid therapy

Nursing Diagnoses/Interventions

Decreased cardiac output r/t ↓ preload secondary to ventricle compression by fluid in pericardial sac

Desired outcome: Within 2 days, patient has adequate cardiac output: RAP 4-6 mm Hg, mean PAWP 6-12 mm Hg, PAP 20-30/8-15 mm Hg, CO 4-7 L/min, SBP ≥90 mm Hg, HR 60-100 bpm, NSR on ECG, and absence of pulsus paradoxus.

- Evaluate heart sounds and neck veins frequently. Check for muffled heart sounds, new murmurs, new gallops, irregularities in rate/rhythm, and JVD, which may signal tamponade.
- Check for pulsus paradoxus, an abnormal ↓ in SBP during inspiration.
- Evaluate ECG for ST-segment changes. Maintain continuous cardiac monitoring.
- Have emergency equipment available for immediate PA catheterization, central line insertion, pericardiocentesis, or thoracotomy.

Ineffective breathing pattern r/t guarding resutling from chest pain

Desired outcome: Within 48 h of this diagnosis, patient demonstrates RR 12-20 breaths/min with eupnea and verbalizes that chest pain is controlled.

- Assess character and intensity of chest pain using 0-10 point scale. Provide pain medication as needed.
- Assess lung sounds q4h. If breath sounds ↓, encourage incentive spirometry, coughing, and deep-breathing exercises q2-4h.
- To facilitate coughing and deep breathing, support patient's chest by splinting with pillows.

Activity intolerance r/t bed rest, weakness, and fatigue secondary to impaired cardiac function, ineffective breathing pattern, or deconditioning

Desired outcome: Within 72 h of this diagnosis, patient exhibits cardiac tolerance to increasing levels of exercise: peak HR ≤20 bpm over resting HR, peak SBP ≤20 mm Hg over resting SBP, SBP during peak exercise ≤20 mm Hg under resting SBP, Svo_2 ≥60%, RR ≤24 breaths/min, NSR on ECG, warm and dry skin, and absence of crackles, murmurs, chest pain during/immediately after activity.

Note: High doses or long-term treatment with steroids may cause myopathy, especially in large proximal muscles. Patients experience difficulty in lifting objects and movement.

- Assess for evidence of muscle weakness; assist with activities as needed.
- Modify activity plan for patient with post-MI pericarditis who is receiving steroids. A lower activity level may help prevent ventricular wall thinning and ↓ risk of aneurysm or ventricular rupture.
- Teach patient to resume activities gradually, as prescribed, allowing for adequate periods of rest between activities.
- Assess RR, HR, BP, and clinical status before, during, and after activity. Encourage rest or slow activity progression if HR >20 bpm over resting HR, RR ↑ >24/breaths/min, or SBP ↑ or ↓ >20 mm Hg over resting SBP.

Miscellanea

CONSULT MD FOR
- New-onset murmurs, persistent or serious dysrhythmias
- Hemodynamic instability: CO <4 L/min, ↓ BP
- S&S of tamponade: JVD, muffled heart tones, ↓ pulse pressure
    Early: ↑ RAP with nl BP
    Late: ↑ PAP with ↓ BP

RELATED TOPICS
- Antimicrobial therapy
- Cardiac surgery: CABG
- Cardiac tamponade
- Immobility, prolonged
- Myocardial infarction, acute

ABBREVIATION
LSB: Left sternal border

REFERENCES

Baas LS, Steuble BT: Cardiovascular dysfunctions. In Swearingen PL, Keen JH (eds): *Manual of critical care nursing,* ed 3, St Louis, 1995, Mosby.

Dziadulewicz L, Shannon-Stone M: Postpericardiotomy syndrome: a complication of cardiac surgery, *AACN Clin Issues* 6(3): 464-470, 1995.

Kinney MR et al: *Comprehensive cardiac care,* ed 8, St Louis, 1996, Mosby.

Nikolic G: Myocardial infarction or inflammation? *Heart Lung* 24(2): 179-182, 1995.

Oliva PB, Hammill SC: The clinical distinction between regional postinfarction pericarditis and other causes of postinfarction chest pain, *Clin Cardiol* 17(9): 471-478, 1994.

Author: **Linda S. Baas**

Overview

DESCRIPTION
Form of RRT that employs patient's peritoneum as the semipermeable membrane. Indicated for volume excess, electrolyte disturbances, and metabolic acidosis caused by renal insufficiency. Special catheter is placed in the peritoneal cavity, and dialysate solution is instilled. Water, electrolytes, and waste products cross between peritoneal capillary bed and dialysate *via* osmosis and diffusion.

HISTORY/RISK FACTORS
- ATN
- Chronic renal failure
- Hepatorenal syndrome
- Hypertension

CLINICAL PRESENTATION
- Oliguria
- ↑ BUN/creatinine
- Edema: peripheral, periorbital, sacral
- Weakness, other evidence of electrolyte imbalance
- Bleeding tendencies

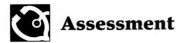 # Assessment

PHYSICAL ASSESSMENT
Neuro: Altered mental status, lethargy, disorientation
Resp: SOB, Kussmaul's respirations, crackles
CV: S_3 and S_4 gallop, pericardial friction rub, JVD, dysrhythmias, hypertension
GI: Nausea, vomiting, anorexia
GU: Oliguria, anuria
MS: Weakness, muscle tenderness, asterixis
Other: Uremic frost, pallor, ecchymosis, bleeding from puncture sites.

VITAL SIGNS/HEMODYNAMICS
RR: ↑
HR: ↑, irregular
BP: ↑
Temp: Nl, or slight ↑ with infection
Other: Hemodynamics usually reflect fluid volume excess with ↑ CVP/PAWP, ↑ SVR. CO may be ↓ if heart failure present.

ECG: Frequently shows dysrhythmias. May show hyperkalemic changes: peaked T waves, prolonged PR interval, ST depression, widened QRS.

LABORATORY STUDIES
Chemistries: BUN, creatinine, uric acid levels ↑ in renal failure, as may K^+, PO_4^{3-}, and possibly Mg^{2+}.
Creatinine Clearance: Most reliable estimation of GFR; usually <50 ml/min.
Urinalysis: Large amounts of protein and many RBC casts common. Sediment wnl when causes are prerenal.
Hematology: Hct may be low as result of renal failure; Hct and Hgb ↓ steadily if bleeding or hemodilution present. PT, PTT may be ↑ because of ↓ platelet adhesiveness.
ABGs: Metabolic acidosis (low $Paco_2$ and plasma pH).

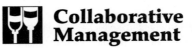 # Collaborative Management

System Components
Catheter: Two types commonly used.
  Trocar: Stiff Silastic catheter inserted at bedside to provide temporary access.
  Soft Silastic indwelling catheter (eg, Tenckhoff): Inserted in OR for permanent access.
Dialysate: Premixed sterile electrolyte solution with composition similar to nl plasma. Glucose concentrations variable inasmuch as hypertonic solutions are used to ↑ osmotic load for greater filtration. Potassium added according to need.

Methods
IPD: Usually 3-4 treatments/wk, lasting 8-10 h/session. Hospitalized patients with renal failure may undergo dialysis for 24 h qod.
CAPD: Extends amount of time fluid remains in abdomen (dwell time) to 4 h during day and 8 h during night, with 4-5 exchanges/day. Dialysis occurs 7 days/wk, 24 h/day. The most physiologic form of dialysis.

Complications
- Peritonitis: accounts for high incidence of failure with PD
- Hyperglycemic hyperosmolar nonketotic syndrome
- Hypernatremia, hypovolemia, metabolic alkalosis

Catheter-Related Problems
- Obstruction from clots, fibrin, or omentum
- Malposition
- Tunnel infection

Dietary Restrictions: Because more protein is lost through the peritoneal membrane, protein restriction liberalized to 1.2-1.5 g/kg/day to compensate for extra loss. If peritonitis develops, protein loss can ↑ from ≈10 g/day to 50 g/day. CAPD patients may need calorie restrictions as a result of added calories absorbed from glucose in the dialysate. Potassium may be less restricted in PD patients because the dialysate is potassium free. Sodium restricted to ≈80-100 mEq/day.
Fluid Restriction: Weight gain between treatments usually caused by fluid retention. Fluid intake may be limited to 1500-1800 ml in 24 h.
Phosphate Binders: To control hyperphosphatemia, which can occur because of inability to excrete excess dietary phosphates.
Vitamin D Analogs, Calcium Replacement: To prevent hypocalcemia and renal osteodystrophy. If hypocalcemia occurs, parathyroid glands release parathormone, which releases calcium from bone and may lead to bone demineralization and osteodystrophy.
Water-Soluble Vitamins and Folic Acid: Dialyzable, necessitating replacement after dialysis.

PATIENT-FAMILY TEACHING
- Importance of notifying staff members if S&S of infection occur.
- Dietary recommendations (eg, sodium, potassium restriction).
- For CAPD patients: begin teaching procedure and, as appropriate, have patient or significant others demonstrate technique to be used at home.

Nursing Diagnoses/Interventions

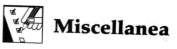 **Miscellanea**

Risk for infection r/t invasive procedure used to obtain peritoneal access for dialysis
Desired outcome: Patient infection free: normothermia, WBCs ≤11,000 μl, blood and dialysate free of infective organisms, and absence of erythema, purulent drainage, abdominal or access site pain, or cloudy dialysate.

- Assess condition of access site qd. Be alert to erythema, purulent drainage, tenderness.
- Use strict, aseptic technique when cleansing catheter site and connecting and disconnecting dialysate bags. Use antiseptic solution such as hydrogen peroxide or povidone-iodine to cleanse the access site. Maintain aseptic technique when cleansing and drying site. Cover site with dry, sterile dressing. Change dressing immediately if it becomes wet.
- Keep peritoneal catheters covered with dry, sterile dressing between treatments.
- Document appearance of PD effluent. If it becomes cloudy or contains flecks of material, send specimen for culture and obtain cell count to check for ↑ WBCs in the effluent.

Fluid volume excess (or risk for same) r/t dietary indiscretions of sodium and fluids and compromised regulatory mechanisms secondary to renal failure
Desired outcome: Within 24-48 h of admission, patient becomes normovolemic: balanced I&O; stable weight; HR ≤100 bpm; BP wnl for patient; RR 12-20 breaths/min; and absence of edema, crackles, and other S&S of hypervolemia.

- Monitor and record I&O q4h and weight qd. Be alert to weight gain >0.5-1 kg/24 h.
- Assess lung sounds, cardiac rate and rhythm, and for presence of peripheral, periorbital, and sacral edema. Be alert to crackles, tachycardia, pericardial friction rub, and pulsus paradoxus.
- Maintain prescribed fluid restrictions. Encourage participation in selection of fluids. Encourage ice chips, hard candy to relieve dry mouth.
- Elevate HOB during PD to relieve pressure of fluid against diaphragm.
- If outflow poor, change patient's position or irrigate catheter to determine patency.

Risk for fluid volume deficit r/t active loss secondary to excess fluid removal during dialysis
Desired outcomes: Patient remains normovolemic: balanced I&O, daily weight within 1-2 lbs of calculated dry weight (true body weight without any excess fluid), BP wnl for patient, CVP ≥2 mm Hg, and HR ≤100 bpm. Hct 20%-30% (acceptable range with renal failure).

- When using hypertonic dialysate, assess skin turgor, mucous membranes, CVP, BP, and HR for signs of dehydration, which can occur from excessive fluid loss: sudden ↓ in BP, tachycardia, poor skin turgor, dry mucous membranes, and change in mental status (eg, restlessness or unresponsiveness).
- When using hypertonic dialysate, check fingerstick glucose q4h.
- If hypotension occurs during PD, stop dialysis, consult physician, and encourage oral fluids up to 1000 ml (or per protocol).

Ineffective breathing pattern r/t ↓ lung expansion secondary to impaired respiratory mechanics occurring with dialysate in peritoneal cavity
Desired outcome: Patient becomes eupneic within 24 h of this diagnosis.

- Monitor respiratory rate, depth, and pattern, and assess breath sounds when dialysate is dwelling in the peritoneal cavity.
- Elevate HOB to ↓ pressure of fluid against the diaphragm and ↑ VC.
- Schedule deep-breathing exercises and incentive spirometry q2-4h.
- Get patient up in a chair 3-4 × day if possible.

CONSULT MD FOR

- Evidence of peritonitis/catheter-tunnel infection: erythema, purulent drainage, access site pain, abdominal pain/tenderness, cloudy dialysate, ↑ temp.
- Inability to drain peritoneal effluent after trying position changes or catheter irrigation to promote drainage.
- S&S of fluid volume excess: weight gain >0.5-1 kg/24 h, crackles, excessive edema.
- S&S of fluid volume deficit (when using hypertonic dialysate): ↓ BP, tachycardia, altered mental status, output >1500 over intake.
- Hyperglycemia (when using hypertonic dialysate): blood glucose >200 mg/dl.

RELATED TOPICS

- Acute tubular necrosis: oliguric
- Hyperkalemia
- Hypertensive crisis
- Metabolic acidosis, acute
- Metabolic alkalosis, acute
- Peritonitis
- Renal failure, acute and chronic

ABBREVIATIONS

CAPD: Continuous ambulatory peritoneal dialysis
GFR: Glomerular filtration rate
IPD: Intermittent peritoneal dialysis
RRT: Renal replacement therapy
VC: Vital capacity

REFERENCES

Brunier G: Peritonitis in patients on peritoneal dialysis: a review of pathophysiology and treatment, *ANNA J* 22(6): 575-584, 1995.

Currier H: Prevention, assessment, and treatment of peritonitis in PD patients, *ANNA J* 22(2): 129-130, 1995.

Prowant BF, Gallagher NM: Peritoneal dialysis. In Lancaster LE (ed): *Core curriculum for nephrology nursing*, ed 3, Pitman, NJ, 1995, AJ Janetti.

Stark JL: Dialysis options in the critically ill patient: hemodialysis, peritoneal dialysis, and continuous renal replacement therapy, *Crit Care Nurs Q* 14(4): 40-44, 1992.

Author: **Patricia D. Weiskittel**

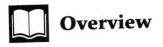 **Overview**

PATHOPHYSIOLOGY

Inflammation of all or part of peritoneal cavity caused by diffuse microbial proliferation or corrosion resulting from leakage of gastric/intestinal contents. Initial inflammation causes fluid shifts from intravascular to interstitial spaces because of ↑ vascular permeability. This transudated fluid contains high levels of fibrinogen and thromboplastin, which deposit around damaged area and form a barrier that harbors bacteria. As a result, multiple pockets of infection form, potentially leading to recurrent infection or septicemia. If prolonged or severe, can cause adhesions and bowel obstruction. Hypovolemic shock may ensue.

HISTORY/RISK FACTORS

- Disruption of GI tract integrity: perforated peptic ulcer; blunt or penetrating trauma, especially to hollow viscera
- Inflammatory bowel processes: diverticulitis, appendicitis, Crohn's disease
- Vascular events: ischemic colitis, mesenteric thrombosis, embolic phenomena
- Obstruction of small bowel and colon
- Severe hepatobiliary disease, CAPD
- General risk factors: advanced age, DM, vascular disease, advanced liver disease, malignancy, malnutrition, debilitation

CLINICAL PRESENTATION

- Moderate-to-severe pain, causing fetal position and resistance to movements that aggravate pain; onset sudden or insidious, with location varying according to underlying pathology
- Nausea, vomiting, anorexia, changes in bowel habits

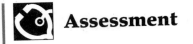 **Assessment**

PHYSICAL ASSESSMENT

Neuro: Restlessness, confusion resulting from impaired cerebral perfusion
Resp: Rapid RR, shallow ventilatory pattern caused by abdominal movement and pain
GI: ↓/absent bowel sounds (complete absence suggests ileus, a frequent complication); generalized or localized abdominal tenderness, rebound tenderness, guarding, involuntary rigidity, mild to moderate ascites

VITAL SIGNS/HEMODYNAMICS

RR: ↑
HR: ↑
BP: ↓
Temp: ↑
CVP/PAP: ↓
SVR: ↑ if hypovolemic; ↓ if SIRS present
CO: Usually ↓
Other: Endotoxemic vasodilatation manifested by low SVR, with initial ↑ in HR, CO. This state complicates initial hypovolemia and may result in dangerously low MAP, thus impairing renal, cardiac, cerebral perfusion.
ECG: Hypovolemia, fever stimulate sinus tachycardia. Hypokalemic changes may be present (ventricular ectopy, ST depression).

LABORATORY STUDIES

Hematology: WBCs usually >20,000 μl. Initially, Hgb and Hct ↑ because of hemoconcentration, but ↓ to baseline as nl intravascular volume restored.
Chemistries: Metabolic alkalosis expected as a result of nausea, vomiting, and gastric suction; reflected by high CO_2 and low Cl^-. Serum albumin often ↓, especially with bacterial peritonitis. Underlying disease process also affects chemistry, eg, ↑ amylase and lipase with pancreatitis.

IMAGING

Radiology: Abdominal x-ray usually reveals large and small bowel dilatation, with edema of small bowel wall. Free air in the abdomen suggests visceral perforation. With CT scanning, abscesses visualized and sometimes drained during procedure, thus avoiding surgery.

DIAGNOSTIC PROCEDURES

Abdominal Paracentesis: Involves catheter or trocar insertion to obtain specimens. Sterile saline infused, and return fluid analyzed for RBC, WBC, amylase, bacterial content. If ascites present, saline infusion may not be necessary because fluid can be removed directly for analysis.

Collaborative Management

Goal of therapy: to treat underlying disease process.
Antimicrobial Therapy: Both aerobic and anaerobic organisms found in abdomen, necessitating a combination of an aminoglycoside, such as gentamicin (Garamycin), and vancomycin (Vancocin) to provide full antimicrobial coverage.
Pain Management: Opiate analgesics used to ensure comfort but given cautiously to avoid abdominal and respiratory function compromise. Dose individually titrated. Initiation of analgesia delayed until full surgical evaluation, since important diagnostic clues can be masked.
Fluid, Electrolyte Management: Significant intravascular volume depletion may occur. In most cases crystalloids used initially. With evidence of ↓ intravascular proteins, colloids such as albumin indicated. Electrolyte replacement, typically potassium, implemented according to laboratory findings.
Nutritional Therapy: Motility minimal/absent. An enteric tube inserted to ↓/prevent distention. Patient on NPO status; PN may be necessary. When resumption of bowel sounds or passing of flatus signals return of GI motility, enteral nutrition begun.
Surgical Management: Often necessary, depending on cause of peritonitis. All intraabdominal foreign material removed, and nonviable tissue débrided. If present, bowel perforations and obstructions corrected, and abscesses drained.

PATIENT/FAMILY TEACHING

- Importance of seeking medical attention if indicators of infection or bowel obstruction occur (eg, fever, severe or unusual abdominal pain, nausea and vomiting, unusual drainage from wounds or incisions, change in bowel habits)

Nursing Diagnoses/Interventions

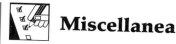 # Miscellanea

Fluid volume deficit r/t active loss secondary to fluid sequestration within peritoneum

Desired outcome: Within 8 h of this diagnosis, patient normovolemic: MAP 70-105 mm Hg, HR 60-100 bpm, NSR on ECG, CVP 2-6 mm Hg, PAWP 6-12 mm Hg, CI 2.5-4 L/min/m², UO ≥0.5 ml/kg/h, warm extremities, peripheral pulses >2+ on 0-4+ scale, brisk capillary refill (<2 sec), orientation × 3, stable weight.

- Monitor HR, BP, and ECG q1-4h or more often if VS unstable. Be alert to MAP ↓ ≥10 mm Hg from previous reading and to ↑ HR, which suggests hypovolemia. Usually ECG shows sinus tachycardia. If hypokalemia present as a result of prolonged vomiting or gastric suction, ventricular ectopy, prominent U wave, and ST-segment depression may be present.
- Measure CVP, PAWP, and CO q1-4h, depending on stability. Be alert to low/↓ CVP, PAWP, and CO. Calculate SVR q4-8h or more frequently in unstable patients. ↓ CVP and PAWP, ↓ CO (CI <2.5 L/min/m²), and ↑ SVR (>1200 dynes/sec/cm⁻⁵) suggest hypovolemia.
- Measure UO qh. Be alert to output <0.5 ml/kg/h for 2 consecutive h, which may signal intravascular volume depletion. Consider ↑ fluid intake promptly if ↓ UO caused by hypovolemia.
- Monitor for physical indicators of hypovolemia: cool extremities, capillary refill >2 sec, ↓ amplitude of peripheral pulses, and neurologic changes such as restlessness and confusion.
- Estimate ongoing fluid losses. Measure all drainage from tubes, catheters, drains. Note dressing change frequency because of saturation with fluid or blood. Weigh patient qd. Compare 24-h body fluid output with 24-h fluid intake.

Pain r/t biologic or chemical agents causing injury to peritoneum and intraperitoneal organs

Desired outcomes: Within 2 h of this diagnosis, patient's subjective evaluation of discomfort improves, as documented by pain scale. Nonverbal indicators of discomfort, such as grimacing, absent.

- Monitor for discomfort. Devise pain scale with patient, rating discomfort from 0 (no pain) to 10. Administer analgesics promptly, before pain becomes severe. Rate degree of pain relief by using pain scale. Be aware that opiate analgesics ↓ GI motility and may delay return of nl bowel functioning.
- Position patient to optimize comfort. Many patients find dorsal recumbent or lateral decubitus bent-knee position more comfortable than other positions.
- Monitor HR, BP, CVP, PAWP at least q4h. Be aware that IV opiates may cause vasodilatation and can result in serious hypotension, especially with volume depletion.
- Avoid giving analgesics to newly admitted patients until surgical evaluation has occurred.

Risk for infection r/t inadequate primary defenses (traumatized tissue, altered perfusion), tissue destruction, and environmental exposure to pathogens

Desired outcome: Septicemia does not develop: HR 60-100 bpm, RR 12-20 breaths/min, SVR 900-1200 dynes/sec/cm⁻⁵, CI 2.5-4 L/min/m², normothermia, negative culture results, and orientation × 3.

- Monitor VS and hemodynamics for signs of septicemia: ↑ HR, RR, CO and ↓ SVR. Check for ↑ rectal or core temp. Be aware that hypothermia may precede hyperthermia in some patients. Also note that elders and the immunocompromised may not exhibit fever, even with severe sepsis.
- If patient has a sudden temp ↑, obtain culture specimens of blood, sputum, urine, and appropriate sites as indicated. Monitor culture reports.
- Administer parenteral antibiotics in a timely fashion. Reschedule antibiotics if dose delayed >1 h. Recognize that failure to give antibiotics on schedule may result in inadequate drug blood levels and treatment failure. Aminoglycosides used frequently; therefore monitor for hearing loss. Check BUN/creatinine levels, and monitor UO to ensure patient has adequate renal function, since aminoglycosides are potentially nephrotoxic. Advanced age and hypovolemia ↑ risk of aminoglycoside toxicity.
- To minimize microbial growth, facilitate drainage of pus, GI secretions, old blood, necrotic tissue, foreign material such as feces, and other body fluids, from wounds. Ensure that gastric, intestinal, and other GI drainage tubes are functioning properly. Evaluate drainage character. Irrigate or reposition tubes as necessary.
- Evaluate wounds for evidence of infection: erythema, warmth, swelling, unusual drainage. Culture any unusual drainage.
- Evaluate orientation to time, place, and person and LOC. Document and report significant deviations from baseline.

CONSULT MD FOR
- Failure of prescribed analgesics to control pain
- UO <0.5 ml/kg/h × 2 h
- Loss of patency or other malfunction of drainage tubes
- Unusual characteristics or changes in wound drainage
- S&S of complications: hypokalemia, renal insufficiency, hypovolemic shock, septicemia

RELATED TOPICS
- Antimicrobial therapy
- Hypokalemia
- Hypovolemia
- Systemic inflammatory response syndrome

ABBREVIATIONS
CAPD: Continuous ambulatory peritoneal dialysis
SIRS: Systemic inflammatory response syndrome

REFERENCES
Keen JH: Peritonitis. In Swearingen PL, Keen JH (eds): *Manual of critical care nursing,* ed 3, St Louis, 1995, Mosby.
Krumberger J: Gastrointestinal disorders. In Kinney M, Packa D, Dunbar S (eds): *AACN's clinical reference for critical care nursing,* ed 3, St Louis, 1993, Mosby.

Author: **Janet Hicks Keen**

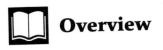 **Overview**

PATHOPHYSIOLOGY

Occurs as a result of aspiration of oral secretions or gastric contents. The more acidic or greater the volume of aspirate, the greater the pulmonary damage. Aspiration of inert or nontoxic substances (blood, barium, water, unchewed food) also can lead to inflammation. The aspirate flows to the dependent lung lobe(s), based on patient's position. Disrupted alveolar-capillary membrane and ↑ capillary permeability allow leakage of fluid across membrane resulting in noncardiac pulmonary edema, causing ↓ gas transport and hypoxemia. ↓ surfactant causes alveoli to collapse. These factors ↓ lung compliance and promote atelectasis. Bacterial pneumonia also possible because of susceptibility of injured lung to secondary infection.

HISTORY/RISK FACTORS

Delayed Gastric Emptying: Advanced age; obesity; shock; trauma; pain; Crohn's disease; diabetic autonomic neuropathy; use of anticholinergics (eg, atropine), ETOH, and opiates
↓ Swallowing Ability: Hypoxia, oropharyngeal local anesthesia, extubation following prolonged intubation, head and neck surgery, nasal CPAP, tracheostomy
Neuromuscular Disorders: MG, GBS, parkinsonism
Sedation, Therapeutic Paralysis
↓ LOC: Stroke, head trauma, ↑ ICP, metabolic disorders
Impaired Host Factors: ↑ oropharyngeal or gastric colony count, gingivitis, bowel obstruction, ↓ gastric acid (eg, acid suppression therapy leading to GI bacterial overgrowth), ↓ cough reflex, ↓ alveolar macrophage function, poor nutritional status, immobility, lung disease

CLINICAL PRESENTATION

Immediately After Aspiration: Period of apnea, followed by rapid-onset respiratory distress. Low-grade fever; scant amount of sputum
Later Signs: Large amount thin/frothy sputum, ↑ pulmonary congestion
Elders: May not exhibit initial signs; restlessness, weakness, anorexia, tachypnea likely; low-grade fever possible

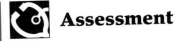 **Assessment**

PHYSICAL ASSESSMENT

Neuro: *Initially,* anxiety, restlessness; *later,* ↓ mentation as a result of hypoxemia
Resp: *Initially,* apnea followed by dyspnea, tachypnea, cough, small amount clear sputum, ↓ breath sounds over affected area, diffuse fine crackles, wheezing. *Later,* tachypnea; large amount thin, pink, frothy or thick purulent sputum; hemoptysis; hoarseness; fine or coarse crackles; wheezing
CV: Tachycardia, pulses weak if hypovolemic, ventricular dysrhythmias possible if hypoxemic
GI: Gurgling while eating, oral drooling, food left in mouth after swallowing, ↑ abdominal girth
Integ: *Initially,* cyanotic; *later,* warm and moist because of fever

VITAL SIGNS/HEMODYNAMICS

RR: ↑
HR: ↑
BP: ↑ at onset; then ↓ if hypovolemic
Temp: *Initially,* slight ↑; *later,* ↑ because of bacterial infection
CVP/PAWP/CO: ↓ if hypovolemic
PAP: Initially unchanged; ↑ with pulmonary congestion
ECG: Sinus tachycardia, hypoxia-related ventricular dysrhythmias

LABORATORY STUDIES

ABGs: *Initially,* hypoxemia with respiratory alkalosis; *later,* hypoxemia persists with respiratory acidosis
Sputum Culture: *Initially,* negative; *later,* evidence of one or more pathogens
WBCs: ↑ with bacterial pneumonia

IMAGING

Chest X-ray: Changes may not occur for 12-24 h after insult. *Large aspiration:* Initially, diffuse bilateral infiltrates; later, pulmonary edema. *Small localized aspiration:* Initially, atelectasis; later, large fluffy infiltrates.
Barium Swallow, UGI Series: To evaluate structural/functional abnormalities of esophagus.

DIAGNOSTIC PROCEDURES

Bronchoscopy: To remove aspirated particles or obtain uncontaminated sputum culture
Fine Needle Aspirate or Transtracheal Biopsy: To detect aspirated food particles or obtain uncontaminated sputum specimen
Intraesophageal pH Monitoring: To assess for gastric reflux

Collaborative Management

Airway: Bronchoscopy may remove material from pharynx and major airways. Small-volume lavage to clear the airway (controversial). Bronchodilators for bronchospasm.
Oxygenation: High Fio2 probable to maintain O2 saturation >90%. Mechanical ventilation and PEEP may be necessary to maintain satisfactory oxygenation. Prophylactic mechanical ventilation and PEEP controversial.
Fluid Management: Crystalloids to replace volume lost from pulmonary capillary leakage; colloids indicated in some instances. Use of either is controversial because both leak across the membrane.
Pharmacotherapy: Empirical antibiotics used prophylactically after aspiration or delayed until clinical, microbiologic, and radiographic evidence of bacterial pneumonia present.
Penicillin or clindamycin: For community-acquired aspiration
Cephalosporin, oxacillin, piperacillin with an aminoglycoside: For hospital-associated aspiration
Prophylactic parenteral corticosteroids: Frequently used; effectiveness not well established
Surgery: Closure or diversion of larynx may be done for intractable aspiration.

PATIENT-FAMILY TEACHING

- Purpose, expected results, anticipated sensations of all medical/nursing interventions
- Current level of pulmonary function and prognosis for recovery
- Risk factor modification to prevent recurrence: medications, diet, positioning, enteral tube feeding
- S&S of aspiration and steps to take if it occurs
- Necessity of completing full course of antibiotic therapy

Nursing Diagnoses/Interventions

Impaired gas exchange r/t fluid accumulation in the alveoli and ↓ surfactant secondary to alveolar-capillary membrane change
Desired outcome: Within 24 h of treatment initiation patient has adequate gas exchange: PaO_2 >60 mm Hg, $PaCO_2$ <45 mm Hg. Within 3 days, RR 12-20 breaths/min with eupnea; breath sounds clear bilaterally.

- If aspiration witnessed, position patient in slight Trendelenburg in right decubitus position to facilitate drainage of aspirate and ↓ risk of involving other lung. Suction oropharynx and trachea.
- Monitor ABGs and SpO_2. Hypoxemia is common and requires prompt treatment. Titrate supplemental O_2 to maintain SpO_2 >90%.
- ↓ PaO_2 levels despite high O_2 concentrations (up to 100%) require mechanical ventilation and use of PEEP. Be aware that PEEP will negatively impact CO, especially if patient hypovolemic.
- Administer bronchodilators, antibiotics.
- Monitor breath sounds q2h and prn. Suction as necessary to remove accumulated secretions.
- Monitor VS and hemodynamics qh. ↓ BP, PAWP, and CO, combined with ↑ RR, HR, and PAP, suggests ARDS.

Risk for infection r/t ↑ susceptibility of injured lung secondary to alveolar changes
Desired outcome: Patient infection free: normothermia, WBCs ≤11,000 μl, clear sputum, and no growth from sputum/blood cultures.

- Monitor temp q2h. Low-grade fever expected after aspiration. Temp >38.89° C (102° F) suggests infection.
- Monitor for ↑ WBCs. Nl or ↓ WBC, along with clinical signs of infection, may signal overwhelming infection and poor prognosis.
- Assess color, character, and amount of sputum. ↑ in amount and viscosity, change in color from clear to white, and foul odor signal infection.
- Monitor chest x-rays for progressive infiltrates. Bacterial pneumonia typically occurs 2-7 days after aspiration.
- Ensure frequent, thorough oral hygiene to ↓ colony count in the oropharynx and thus ↓ risk of infection caused by aspirated pathogens.

Risk for aspiration r/t ↓ swallowing ability, ↓ LOC, gastroesophageal reflex, or delayed gastric emptying
Desired outcome: Patient does not repeat aspiration incident during hospitalization as evidenced by absence of the following: S&S of aspiration, hypoxic episodes, new infiltrates on chest x-ray.

- Assess swallowing ability, cough, and gag reflex.
- Place unconscious patient on side in slight Trendelenburg position unless contraindicated.
- Assess bowel sounds and measure abdominal girth q8h. An ↑ in girth >8-10 cm reflects gastric retention.
- Suction oropharynx prn, even when artificial airway is in place. Aspiration frequently occurs despite appropriate airway cuff inflation.
- Administer medications that facilitate gastric emptying, eg, metoclopramide (Reglan).
- Implement safety procedures if patient receiving enteral tube feedings.
  Elevate HOB during feeding and for at least 30-60 min afterward.
  Monitor gastric residuals and withhold feeding accordingly.
  Check tube placement q4h and prn.
  Stop feeding 30-60 min before any procedure that requires patient to lie flat.
  Use glucose oxidase reagent strips to check tracheal secretions. Positive glucose signals aspiration of tube feeding.

Miscellanea

CONSULT MD FOR

- PaO_2 <50 mm Hg or ↓ despite high concentration of supplemental O_2 (suggests development of ARDS)
- Hypotension, ↓ PAWP and CO, especially if associated with ↑ PAP and ↑ pulmonary congestion
- Signs of pulmonary infection: ↑ WBCs, ↑ temp, sputum changes (foul odor, color changed from clear, ↑ viscosity)
- Tracheal secretions positive for glucose in patients with enteral feedings

RELATED TOPICS

- Adult respiratory distress syndrome
- Antimicrobial therapy
- Drowning, near
- Mechanical ventilation
- Nutritional support, enteral
- Pneumonia, community-acquired and hospital-associated

ABBREVIATIONS

GBS: Guillain-Barré syndrome
MG: Myasthenia gravis
UGI: Upper gastrointestinal

REFERENCES

Fox KA et al: Aspiration pneumonia following surgically placed feeding tubes, *Am J Surg* 170(6): 564-567, 1995.

Haines MM: AANA Journal course: update for nurse anesthetists: pulmonary aspiration revisited: changing attitudes toward preoperative fasting, *AANA J* 63(5): 389-396, 1995.

Mier L: Is penicillin G an adequate initial treatment for aspiration? *Intensive Care Med* 19(5): 270-284, 1993.

Nishino T: Swallowing as a protective reflex for the upper respiratory tract, *Anesthesiology* 70(3): 588-599, 1993.

Pratt JC, Tolbert CG: Tube feeding aspiration, *Am J Nurs* 96(5): 37, 1996.

Author: **Marguerite J. Murphy**

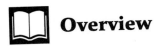 **Overview**

PATHOPHYSIOLOGY

Acute infection that inflames lung parenchyma (alveolar spaces and interstitial tissue). Involved lung tissue swells, and air spaces fill with fluid. Seldom requires hospitalization; seen in ICU only when an underlying medical condition such as COPD, cardiac disease, DM, or immunocompromised state causes respiratory decompensation.

Types

Pneumococcal: Causative organisms are *Pneumococcus pneumoniae, Streptococcus pneumoniae.* Often affects elders and the debilitated. Mortality rate ↑ if two or more lobes involved.

Legionnaire's: Causative organism is *Legionella pneumophila.* Typically affects smokers, elders, and the debilitated. Outbreaks associated with exposure to contaminated construction sites. Severe course possible with complications of ARF, shock, renal failure.

Viral influenza A: Pneumonia may occur 1 wk after onset of "flu" symptoms. Rapid deterioration may lead to respiratory failure, bacterial pneumonia.

HISTORY/RISK FACTORS

- COPD, DM, heart failure
- Alcoholism
- Immunosuppression
- Hypoventilation, hypoxia
- Chemical irritants, eg, smoke
- Advanced age

CLINICAL PRESENTATION

- Cough: productive or nonproductive
- Sputum: purulent or bloody
- Fever, chills
- Pleuritic chest pain, dyspnea
- Headache, myalgia

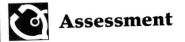 **Assessment**

PHYSICAL ASSESSMENT

Resp: Nasal flaring, use of accessory muscles, ↓ chest expansion, dullness on percussion, ↓/bronchial breath sounds, crackles

VITAL SIGNS/HEMODYNAMICS

RR: ↑
HR: ↑
BP: Nl or ↓
Temp: ↑
CVP: Nl; ↓ with dehydration
PAP/PAWP: Nl; ↑ with COPD, heart failure; ↓ with dehydration
SVR: Nl; ↑ with hypotension, dehydration

LABORATORY STUDIES

ABGs: ↓ Pao_2, ↓ $Paco_2$, respiratory alkalosis (pH >7.45) possible.
Spo2: Possible ↓ to <92%-94% in previously healthy individuals or <90%-92% with COPD.
WBCs: ↑ >11,000 μl with bacterial pneumonia; nl/↓ with viral pneumonia.
Sputum for C&S: Obtained before initiating antibiotic therapy. Identifies causative organism if bacterial; directs antibiotic therapy.
Serologic Studies: Acute and convalescent titers drawn to diagnose viral pneumonia.

IMAGING

Chest X-ray: To identify extent of disease.
  Lobar: Entire lobe involved.
  Segmental: Only parts of a lobe involved.
  Bronchopneumonia: Affects alveoli contiguous to involved bronchi.

Collaborative Management

O2: For hypoxemia. With chronic CO_2 retention, delivered in low concentrations while closely monitoring Spo_2. Titrate to maintain Spo_2 at 90%-92%.
Intubation and Mechanical Ventilation: If unable to maintain patent airway or maintain Pao_2 >60 mm Hg with supplemental O_2. High concentrations of O_2 with PEEP necessary in severe cases.

Pharmacotherapy

Antibiotics: PO erythromycin commonly used initially, but for critically ill, parenteral antibiotics used according to sensitivity of causative organism.

Antipyretics and analgesics: ↓ temp and provide relief for pleuritic pain. Opioid analgesia used cautiously because of risk of respiratory depression. Frequent monitoring of respiratory rate/depth and Spo_2 necessary.

Hydration: IV fluids to replace insensible loss.
Percussion/Postural Drainage: Promote mobilization of sputum.

PATIENT-FAMILY TEACHING

- Medications: drug name, purpose, dosage, schedule, precautions, drug-drug and food-drug interactions, and potential side effects
- Procedures for effective coughing, deep breathing
- Purpose, expected results, anticipated sensations for nursing/medical interventions

Nursing Diagnoses/Interventions

Ineffective airway clearance r/t ↑ tracheobronchial secretions and ↓ ability to expectorate secondary to fatigue

Desired outcome: Within 24-48 h of treatment initiation, airway free of excess secretions: presence of eupnea and absence of adventitious breath sounds and excessive coughing.

- Assess ability to clear secretions. Keep emergency suction equipment at bedside.
- Encourage oral fluid intake to help ↓ secretion viscosity.
- Encourage effective cough:
  Take several deep breaths.
  After last inhalation, cough 3-4 times on same exhalation until most of air expelled.
  Repeat several times until cough becomes productive.
- Ensure that patient receives chest physiotherapy as prescribed.
- Use humidified O_2 to liquefy secretions.

Impaired gas exchange r/t alveolar-capillary membrane changes secondary to fluid accumulation in lung or loss of surfactant

Desired outcome: Within 12 h of treatment, patient has adequate gas exchange: PaO_2 ≥60 mm Hg and $PaCO_2$ ≤45 mm Hg. Within 3 days, RR ≤20 breaths/min with eupnea, breath sounds clear, patient oriented × 3.

- Auscultate lung fields. Note adventitious breath sounds: crackles, rhonchi, friction rubs.
- Monitor SpO_2. Progressive hypoxemia may require ↑ concentrations of O_2.
- Assess for ↑ respiratory effort, SOB, tachypnea, use of accessory muscles, nasal flaring, grunting, restlessness, anxiety.
- Place in semi-Fowler's position to optimize lung expansion and ↓ WOB.
- Assess need for suctioning. Document color, consistency, amount of sputum.
- Provide rest periods between activities to ↓ O_2 demands.
- Explain all procedures, and provide emotional support to ↓ anxiety, which can contribute to O_2 consumption.

Risk for fluid volume deficit r/t ↑ insensible loss secondary to hyperventilation, fever, and use of supplemental O_2; and r/t ↓ fluid intake

Desired outcome: Patient normovolemic: UO ≥0.5 ml/kg/h, stable weight, BP wnl for patient, CVP 2-6 mm Hg, PAP 20-30/8-15 mm Hg, CO 4-7 L/min, MAP 70-105 mm Hg, HR 60-100 bpm, and SVR 900-1200 dynes/sec/cm^{-5}.

- Monitor I&O qh. Initially, intake should be > output.
- Monitor VS and hemodynamic pressures for hypovolemia. Be alert to ↓ BP, CVP, PAP, CO, and MAP, and to ↑ HR and SVR.
- Weigh qd.
- Administer PO and IV fluids. Document response to replacement therapy.
- Monitor for fluid overload or too rapid fluid administration: crackles, SOB, tachypnea, tachycardia, ↑ CVP, ↑ PAP, JVD, and edema.

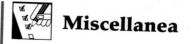 ## Miscellanea

CONSULT MD FOR

- Progressive decline in SpO_2, PaO_2 <60 mm Hg, $PaCO_2$ >45 mm Hg or >baseline
- UO <0.5 ml/kg/h × 2

RELATED TOPICS

- Antimicrobial therapy
- Mechanical ventilation
- Respiratory failure, acute

REFERENCES

Esler R et al: Patient-centered pneumonia care: a case management success story, *Am J Nurs* 94(11): 34-38, 1994.

Howard C: Respiratory dysfunctions. In Swearingen PL, Keen JH (eds): *Manual of critical care nursing,* ed 3, St Louis, 1995, Mosby.

Koziel H, Koziel MJ: Pulmonary complications of diabetes mellitus: pneumonia, *Infect Dis Clin North Am* 9(1): 65-96, 1995.

Moin P et al: Severe community acquired pneumonia: etiology, epidemiology, and prognosis factors, *Chest* 105(5): 1487-1495, 1994.

Author: **Cheri A. Goll**

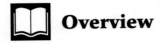 **Overview**

PATHOPHYSIOLOGY

Acute infection that inflames lung parenchyma (alveolar spaces and interstitial tissue) and fills air spaces with fluid. Can occur with altered resistance or impaired coughing mechanisms (eg, with thoracoabdominal surgery). Bacteria invade lower respiratory tract *via* three routes: aspiration of oropharyngeal organisms (most common), inhalation of aerosols that contain bacteria, or hematogenous spread to lung from another site of infection (rare). Any factor that alters lower airway integrity, thereby inhibiting ciliary action, ↑ likelihood of pneumonia.

TYPES

Gram-Negative Bacterial *(Klebsiella pneumoniae, Enterobacter, Serratia):* Characterized by copious purulent green or "currant jelly" sputum; 50% mortality rate. May result in lung abscess, necrotizing pneumonitis, ARF. Usually caused by aspiration of oropharyngeal flora.

Pseudomonas: Characterized by purulent sputum (green, foul-smelling). Rarely occurs in previously healthy adults; mortality rate high.

Staphylococcus aureus: Characterized by bloody sputum. Occurs in debilitating diseases, prior respiratory tract infection, or IV drug users. Slow response to antibiotics.

HISTORY/RISK FACTORS

- COPD, DM, cardiac disease
- Inhalation of smoke, other irritants
- Debilitation, alcoholism
- Immunosuppression
- Viral or influenzal respiratory tract infection
- Antibiotic therapy
- ET intubation
- General anesthesia, sedation
- Prolonged immobility

CLINICAL PRESENTATION

- Cough: productive or nonproductive
- Sputum: rust-colored, purulent, bloody, mucoid
- Pleuritic chest pain
- Headache, myalgia
- Elders may be confused, disoriented; may run low-grade fevers; initially may have few other S&S

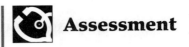 **Assessment**

PHYSICAL ASSESSMENT

Resp: Nasal flaring, expiratory grunt, use of accessory muscles, ↓ chest expansion, dullness on percussion over affected areas, ↓/bronchial breath sounds (absent if severe), high-pitched and inspiratory crackles (↑ by or heard only after coughing), low-pitched inspiratory crackles caused by airway secretions

CV: Tachycardia

Other: Fever, chills

VITAL SIGNS/HEMODYNAMICS

RR: ↑

HR: ↑

BP: Nl or ↓

Temp: ↑

CVP: Nl; ↓ with dehydration

PAP/PAWP: Nl; ↑ with COPD, heart failure; ↓ with dehydration

SVR: Nl; ↑ with hypotension, dehydration

LABORATORY STUDIES

ABGs: ↓ Pao_2 (<80 mm Hg), ↓ $Paco_2$ (<35 mm Hg), respiratory alkalosis (pH >7.45)

seen in absence of underlying pulmonary disease. In severe cases, $Paco_2$ can be >35 mm Hg because CO_2 elimination may be affected.

Spo_2: For continuous monitoring of O_2 saturation, response to therapy.

WBCs: $\uparrow >11,000$ μl with bacterial pneumonia.

Sputum for C&S: Obtained before initiating antibiotic therapy. Identifies causative organism, if bacterial, and directs antibiotic therapy.

IMAGING

Chest X-ray: To identify extent of disease.
Lobar: Entire lobe involved.
Segmental: Only parts of a lobe involved.
Bronchopneumonia: Affects alveoli contiguous to involved bronchi.

DIAGNOSTIC PROCEDURE

Bronchoscopy: To remove mucous plugs, define involved lung tissue, obtain specimen for biopsy.

Collaborative Management

O_2: For hypoxemia. With chronic CO_2 retention, O_2 delivered in low concentrations while closely monitoring Spo_2. Titrate to maintain Spo_2 of 90%-92%.

Intubation and Mechanical Ventilation: Necessary if unable to maintain patent airway or Pao_2 >60 mm Hg with supplemental O_2. High concentrations of O_2 with PEEP necessary in severe cases.

Pharmacotherapy

Antibiotics: Prescribed empirically based on clinical findings and chest x-ray until sputum or blood culture results available. Usually given parenterally and guided by sensitivity of causative organism. Many organisms responsible for nosocomial pneumonias (eg, MRSA, VRE) are resistant to multiple antibiotics. Identification of organism, determination of sensitivity, and attainment of therapeutic drug levels are critical for effective therapy.

Antipyretics and analgesics: To $\downarrow$ temp and provide relief for pleuritic pain, which may require opioid analgesia. Respiratory depression may occur. Frequent monitoring of respiratory rate/depth and Spo_2 necessary.

Hydration: IV fluids replace insensible loss.

Percussion/Postural Drainage: Promote mobilization of sputum.

PATIENT-FAMILY TEACHING

- Medications: drug name, purpose, dosage, schedule, precautions, drug-drug and food-drug interactions, and potential side effects.

- Before surgery, verbal and written instructions and demonstrations of turning, coughing, deep-breathing exercises to perform after surgery to prevent respiratory tract infection. Make sure patient not only verbalizes knowledge but *returns* demonstrations appropriately. Most patients can expand lungs effectively after surgery but will not do so unless encouraged.

- Purpose, expected results, anticipated sensations for medical/nursing interventions.

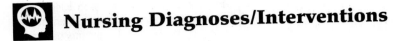

Nursing Diagnoses/Interventions

Risk for infection (nosocomial pneumonia) r/t inadequate primary defenses (↓ ciliary action), invasive procedure (intubation), chronic disease

Desired outcome: Patient infection free: normothermia, WBCs wnl, sputum clear to whitish in color.

- Perform good hand washing before/after contact with respiratory secretions and before/after contact with patient with tracheostomy or intubation. Inform visitors of precautions or pertinent isolation procedures.
- Identify candidate at ↑ risk for nosocomial pneumonia: >70 yrs, obese, hx of COPD or smoking, abnormal pulmonary function test results (especially ↓ forced expiratory flow rate), intubation for prolonged period, upper abdominal or thoracic surgery.

  Control pain, which interferes with lung expansion, by giving analgesics ½ h before deep-breathing exercises. Splint surgical wound with hands or pillows placed firmly across site of incision.

  For patients who cannot remove secretions effectively by coughing, perform gentle chest physiotherapy, including breathing exercises, postural drainage, percussion.

  If patient has ET or tracheostomy tube, provide a fast, deep breath with manual resuscitator to stimulate cough receptors.

- Identify patients at ↑ risk for aspiration: those with ↓ LOC, dysphagia, or gastric tube in place.

  For patient with ↓ LOC, determine feeding method with least risk of aspiration (eg, small-bore feeding tube with weighted tip that migrates to duodenum, TPN, gastrostomy).

  For patient with gastric tube, elevate HOB to at least 30 degrees during and for ≥1 h after feeding; turn onto right side rather than back; or deliver continuous rather than bolus feedings.

- Recognize risk factors for patients with tracheostomy or ET tube: underlying lung disease or other serious illness, ↑ colonization of oropharynx or trachea by aerobic gram-negative bacteria, greater access of bacteria to lower respiratory tract, cross-contamination caused by tube manipulation.

  Suction on as-needed rather than routine basis.

  Consider in-line suction system to ↓ risk of contamination.

Ineffective airway clearance r/t ↑ tracheobronchial secretions and ↓ ability to expectorate secondary to fatigue

Desired outcome: Within 24-48 h of treatment initiation, airway free of excess secretions: presence of eupnea; absence of adventitious breath sounds and excessive coughing.

- Assess ability to clear secretions. Keep emergency suction equipment at bedside.
- Encourage oral fluid intake to help ↓ secretion viscosity.
- Encourage effective cough:

  Take several deep breaths.

  After last inhalation, cough 3-4 times on same exhalation until most of air expelled.

  Repeat several times until cough becomes productive.

- Ensure that patient receives chest physiotherapy.
- Use humidified O_2 to liquefy secretions.

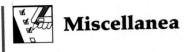

Miscellanea

CONSULT MD FOR

- Progressive decline in SpO_2, PaO_2 <60 mm Hg
- UO <0.5 ml/kg/h × 2

RELATED TOPICS

- Adult respiratory distress syndrome
- Antimicrobial therapy
- Mechanical ventilation
- Methicillin-resistant *Staphylococcus aureus*
- Pneumonia, immunocompromised
- Respiratory failure, acute
- Vancomycin-resistant enterococci

ABBREVIATIONS

MRSA: Methicillin-resistant *Staphylococcus aureus*

VRE: Vancomycin-resistant enterococci

Impaired gas exchange r/t alveolar-capillary membrane changes secondary to fluid accumulation in lung or loss of surfactant

Desired outcome: Within 12 h of treatment, patient has adequate gas exchange: $Pao_2 \geq 60$ mm Hg and $Paco_2 \leq 45$ mm Hg. Within 3 days, RR ≤ 20 breaths/min with eupnea, breath sounds clear, patient oriented $\times$ 3.

- Auscultate lung fields. Note adventitious breath sounds: crackles, rhonchi, friction rubs.
- Monitor Spo_2. Progressive hypoxemia may require $\uparrow$ concentrations O_2.
- Assess for $\uparrow$ respiratory effort: SOB, tachypnea, use of accessory muscles, nasal flaring, grunting, restlessness, anxiety.
- Place in semi-Fowler's position to optimize lung expansion and $\downarrow$ WOB.
- Assess need for suctioning. Document color, consistency, amount of sputum.
- Provide rest periods between activities to $\downarrow$ O_2 demands.
- Explain all procedures; provide emotional support to $\downarrow$ anxiety, which can contribute to O_2 consumption.

Risk for fluid volume deficit r/t $\uparrow$ insensible loss secondary to hyperventilation, fever, and use of supplemental O_2; and r/t $\downarrow$ fluid intake

Desired outcome: Patient normovolemic: UO ≥ 0.5 ml/kg/h, stable weight, BP wnl for patient, CVP 2-6 mm Hg, PAP 20-30/8-15 mm Hg, CO 4-7 L/min, MAP 70-105 mm Hg, HR 60-100 bpm, and SVR 900-1200 dynes/sec/cm^{-5}.

- Monitor I&O qh. Initially, intake should be $>$ output.
- Monitor VS and hemodynamic pressures for hypovolemia. Be alert to $\downarrow$ BP, CVP, PAP, CO, and MAP, and to $\uparrow$ HR and SVR.
- Weigh qd.
- Administer PO and IV fluids. Document response to replacement therapy.
- Monitor for fluid overload or too rapid fluid administration: crackles, SOB, tachypnea, tachycardia, $\uparrow$ CVP, $\uparrow$ PAP, JVD, edema.

REFERENCES

Centers for Disease Control: Guideline for prevention of nosocomial pneumonia, *Am J Infect Control* 22: 247-292, 1994.

Hanna D: Combating infection: using pulse oximeters safely, *Nursing* 25(7): 20-26, 1995.

Howard C: Respiratory dysfunctions. In Swearingen PL, Keen JH (eds): *Manual of critical care nursing,* ed 3, St Louis, 1995, Mosby.

Thompson CL: Critical care-acquired pneumonia, *Crit Care Nurs Clin North Am* 7(4): 695-702, 1995.

Author: **Cheri A. Goll**

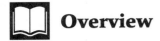 **Overview**

PATHOPHYSIOLOGY

Acute infection that inflames lung parenchyma (alveolar spaces and interstitial tissue) and fills air spaces with fluid. Underlying disease state a determining factor in susceptibility to specific pathogens. Usually patients with neutropenia from acute leukemia or cytotoxic agents have gram-negative bacilli as the source. Severely immunocompromised patients are affected not only by bacteria but also by fungi, viruses, and protozoa.

TYPES

Pseudomonas: Occurs with immunosuppression, neutropenia. Characterized by purulent sputum (green, foul-smelling); high mortality rate.

Staphylococcus aureus: Characterized by bloody sputum; slow response to antibiotics.

Pneumocystis carinii: Affects patients with AIDS or organ transplants. Characterized by night sweats; few auscultatory signs.

Aspergillosis (Aspergillus): Affects patients with AIDS, COPD, organ transplants. Characterized by high fever and nonproductive cough.

HISTORY/RISK FACTORS

- Neutropenia, immunosuppression, HIV infection
- Chemotherapy, cortisone therapy
- Organ, bone marrow transplant
- Antibiotic therapy
- ET intubation
- General anesthesia, sedation
- Prolonged immobility

CLINICAL PRESENTATION

- Cough: productive or nonproductive
- Sputum: rust-colored, purulent, bloody, mucoid
- Pleuritic chest pain
- Headache, myalgia
- Elders may be confused, disoriented; may run low-grade fevers; initially may have few other S&S

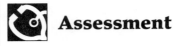 **Assessment**

PHYSICAL ASSESSMENT

Resp: Nasal flaring, expiratory grunt, use of accessory muscles, ↓ chest expansion, dullness on percussion over affected areas, ↓/bronchial breath sounds (absent if severe), high-pitched and inspiratory crackles (↑ by or heard only after coughing), low-pitched inspiratory crackles caused by airway secretions

CV: Tachycardia

Other: Fever, chills

VITAL SIGNS/HEMODYNAMICS

RR: ↑

HR: ↑

BP: Nl or ↓

Temp: ↑

CVP: Nl; ↓ with dehydration

PAP/PAWP: Nl; ↑ with COPD, heart failure; ↓ with dehydration

SVR: Nl; ↑ with hypotension, dehydration

LABORATORY STUDIES

ABGs: To check for ↓ Pao_2 (<80 mm Hg), ↓ $Paco_2$ (<35 mm Hg), respiratory alkalosis (pH >7.45) seen in absence of underlying pulmonary disease. In severe cases, $Paco_2$ can be >35 mm Hg because CO_2 elimination may be affected.

Spo$_2$: For continuous monitoring of O_2 saturation, response to therapy.

WBCs: ↑ >11,000 μl with bacterial pneumonia; nl/↓ with viral pneumonia.

Sputum for C&S: Obtained before initiation of antibiotic therapy. Identifies causative organism if bacterial and directs antibiotic therapy.

Serologic Studies: Acute and convalescent titers drawn to diagnose viral pneumonia.

IMAGING

Chest X-ray: To identify extent of disease.
  Lobar: Entire lobe involved.
  Segmental: Only parts of a lobe involved.
  Bronchopneumonia: Affects alveoli contiguous to involved bronchi.

DIAGNOSTIC PROCEDURE

Bronchoscopy: To remove mucous plugs, define involved lung tissue, obtain specimen for biopsy for definitive diagnosis of *Pneumocystis* or other pneumonia.

Collaborative Management

O$_2$: For hypoxemia. With chronic CO_2 retention, O_2 delivered in low concentrations while closely monitoring Spo$_2$. Titrate to maintain Spo$_2$ of 90%-92%.

Intubation and Mechanical Ventilation: Necessary if unable to maintain patent airway or Pao_2 >60 mm Hg with supplemental O_2. High concentrations of O_2 with PEEP necessary in severe cases.

Pharmacotherapy

Antibiotics: Prescribed empirically based on clinical findings and chest x-ray until sputum or blood culture results available. Usually given parenterally and guided by sensitivity of causative organism. Identification of organism, determination of sensitivity, and attainment of therapeutic drug levels critical for effective therapy.

Hydration: IV fluids to replace insensible loss.

Percussion/Postural Drainage: Promote mobilization of sputum.

PATIENT-FAMILY TEACHING

- Medications: drug name, purpose, dosage, schedule, precautions, drug-drug and food-drug interactions, and potential side effects
- Turning, coughing, and deep-breathing exercises
- Purpose, expected results, anticipated sensations for medical/nursing interventions

Nursing Diagnoses/Interventions

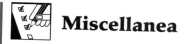 # Miscellanea

Risk for infection (pneumonia) r/t inadequate primary defenses (↓ ciliary action), invasive procedure (intubation), chronic disease

Desired outcome: Patient infection free: normothermia, WBCs wnl, sputum clear to whitish.

- Perform hand washing before/after contact with respiratory secretions and before/after contact with patient with tracheostomy or intubation. Inform visitors of precautions or pertinent isolation procedures.
- Control pain, which interferes with lung expansion, by giving analgesics ½ h before deep-breathing exercises. Splint surgical wound firmly across site of incision.
- For patients who cannot remove secretions effectively by coughing, perform gentle chest physiotherapy, including breathing exercises, postural drainage, and percussion.
- If patient has ET or tracheostomy tube, provide a fast, deep breath with a manual resuscitator to stimulate cough receptors.
- Identify patients at ↑ risk for aspiration: those with ↓ LOC, dysphagia, or gastric tube.
  For patient with ↓ LOC, determine feeding method with least risk of aspiration (eg, small-bore feeding tube with weighted tip that migrates to duodenum, TPN, gastrostomy).
  For patient with gastric tube, elevate HOB to ≥30 degrees during and for ≥1 h after feeding; turn to right side rather than back; or deliver continuous rather than bolus feedings.
- Recognize risk factors for patients with tracheostomy or ET tube: underlying lung disease or other serious illness, ↑ colonization of oropharynx or trachea by aerobic gram-negative bacteria, greater access of bacteria to lower respiratory tract, cross-contamination caused by tube manipulation. Suction on as-needed rather than routine basis; consider in-line suction system to ↓ risk of contamination.

Ineffective airway clearance r/t ↑ tracheobronchial secretions and ↓ ability to expectorate secondary to fatigue

Desired outcome: Within 24-48 h of treatment initiation, airway free of excess secretions: presence of eupnea and absence of adventitious breath sounds and excessive coughing.

- Assess ability to clear secretions. Keep emergency suction equipment at bedside.
- Encourage oral fluid intake to help ↓ secretion viscosity.
- Encourage effective cough: (1) take several deep breaths, (2) after last inhalation, cough 3-4 times on same exhalation until most of air expelled, (3) repeat several times until cough becomes productive.
- Ensure that patient receives chest physiotherapy.
- Use humidified O_2 to liquefy secretions.

Impaired gas exchange r/t alveolar-capillary membrane changes secondary to fluid accumulation in lung or loss of surfactant

Desired outcome: Within 12 h of treatment, patient has adequate gas exchange: PaO_2 ≥60 mm Hg and $PaCO_2$ ≤45 mm Hg. Within 3 days, RR ≤20 breaths/min with eupnea, breath sounds clear, patient oriented × 3.

- Auscultate lung fields. Note adventitious breath sounds: crackles, rhonchi, friction rubs.
- Monitor SpO_2. Progressive hypoxemia may require ↑ concentrations of O_2.
- Assess for ↑ respiratory effort: SOB, tachypnea, use of accessory muscles, nasal flaring, grunting, restlessness, anxiety.
- Place in semi-Fowler's position to optimize lung expansion and ↓ WOB.
- Assess need for suctioning. Document color, consistency, amount of sputum.
- Provide rest periods between activities to ↓ O_2 demands.
- Explain all procedures; provide emotional support to ↓ anxiety, which can contribute to O_2 consumption.

Risk for fluid volume deficit r/t ↑ insensible loss secondary to hyperventilation, fever, and use of supplemental O_2; and r/t ↓ fluid intake

Desired outcome: Patient normovolemic: UO ≥0.5 ml/kg/h, stable weight, BP wnl for patient, CVP 2-6 mm Hg, PAP 20-30/8-15 mm Hg, CO 4-7 L/min, MAP 70-105 mm Hg, HR 60-100 bpm, and SVR 900-1200 dynes/sec/cm^{-5}.

- Monitor I&O qh. Initially, intake should be > output.
- Monitor VS and hemodynamic pressures for hypovolemia. Be alert to ↓ BP, CVP, PAP, CO, and MAP, and to ↑ HR and SVR.
- Weigh patient qd.
- Administer PO and IV fluids. Document response to replacement therapy.
- Monitor for fluid overload or too rapid fluid administration: crackles, SOB, tachypnea, tachycardia, ↑ CVP, ↑ PAP, JVD, and edema.

CONSULT MD FOR
- Progressive decline in SpO_2, PaO_2 <60 mm Hg
- UO <0.5 ml/kg/h × 2

RELATED TOPICS
- Antimicrobial therapy
- Mechanical ventilation
- Organ rejection
- Respiratory failure, acute

REFERENCES
Howard C: Respiratory dysfunctions. In Swearingen PL, Keen JH (eds): *Manual of critical care nursing*, ed 3, St Louis, Mosby.

Timby BK: *Pneumocystis* in patients with acquired immunodeficiency syndrome, *Crit Care Nurse* 12(7): 64-73, 1992.

Walsh RD, Cunha BA: *Rhodococcus equi:* fatal pneumonia in a patient without AIDS, *Heart Lung* 23(6): 519-510, 1994.

Zurlo J: Respiratory infections and the acquired immunodeficiency syndrome. In Bone RC (ed): *Pulmonary and critical care medicine,* vol 2, St Louis, 1995, Mosby.

Author: **Cheri A. Goll**

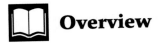 **Overview**

PATHOPHYSIOLOGY
Accumulation of air between parietal and visceral pleura. There are three types:

Spontaneous: Closed pneumothorax in which chest wall remains intact with no leak to atmosphere. It results from rupture of a bleb or bulla on pleural surface; may be life threatening.

Traumatic: Can be open or closed. Open occurs when air enters pleural space from atmosphere through an opening in the chest wall. Closed occurs when the visceral pleura is penetrated, but the chest wall remains intact.

Tension: Occurs when air enters pleural space through a pleural tear during inspiration. Air continues to accumulate but cannot escape during expiration. ↑ pressure causes a mediastinal shift toward the unaffected side, which further impairs ventilatory efforts. The ↑ pressure also compresses the vena cava, leading to ↓ CO and, ultimately, to circulatory collapse. Immediate intervention is critical.

HISTORY/RISK FACTORS
Spontaneous
Primary: Age 20-40, male, previously healthy, smoker
Secondary: COPD, cystic fibrosis, tuberculosis, malignant neoplasm

Traumatic
Open: Penetrating injury to thorax; invasive medical procedure (lung biopsy, thoracentesis, central line placement)
Closed: Blunt injury with rib fracture, CPR, positive-pressure ventilator
Tension: Spontaneous pneumothorax, trauma, infection, positive-pressure ventilator

CLINICAL PRESENTATION
Spontaneous/Traumatic: Sudden onset sharp, stabbing chest pain; may radiate to shoulder; moderate to severe dyspnea; anxiety

Tension: Severe dyspnea; chest pain; cool, clammy, mottled skin; anxiety and restlessness

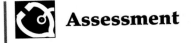 **Assessment**

PHYSICAL ASSESSMENT
Spontaneous/Traumatic
- Inspection: ↓ chest wall movement on affected side
- Palpation: tracheal shift toward unaffected side, subcutaneous emphysema (crepitus), tactile and vocal fremitus ↓/absent on affected side
- Percussion: hyperresonance on affected side
- Auscultation: absent/↓ breath sounds on affected side

Tension
- Inspection: ↓ chest wall movement on affected side, expansion of affected side throughout respiratory cycle, JVD
- Palpation: tracheal shift toward unaffected side, subcutaneous emphysema in neck and chest
- Percussion: hyperresonance on affected side
- Auscultation: absent/↓ breath sounds on affected side, distant heart sounds

VITAL SIGNS/HEMODYNAMICS
RR: ↑
HR: ↑
BP: Nl or ↓ if tension pneumothorax
Temp: Nl
ECG: Sinus tachycardia; may show ↓ QRS amplitude, precordial T-wave inversion, rightward shift of frontal QRS axis, and small precordial R voltage

LABORATORY STUDIES
ABGs: PaO_2 <80 mm Hg evident after moderate to large pneumothorax (≥15% of hemithorax). With resolution, arterial O_2 saturation returns to nl. ↓ pH (<7.35) and ↑ $PaCO_2$ (>45 mm Hg) possible.

IMAGING
Chest X-ray: Affected side shows air in pleural space, chest wall expansion, diaphragm lowering, partial to total lung collapse, and any tracheal shift.

Collaborative Management

O_2 Therapy: Administered when hypoxemia present, usually with a large pneumothorax.
Analgesia: Provides relief of pain of pneumothorax or its treatment.
Thoracentesis: Performed immediately in tension pneumothorax. Large-bore needle inserted in second ICS, MCL. A stylet introducer needle with a plastic sheath may be used. The needle is removed after penetration, and plastic catheter sheath left in place to allow decompression of chest cavity until chest tubes inserted.
Chest Tube Placement: Inserted in second or third ICS, MCL to remove air or in fifth or sixth lateral ICS to remove fluid. During insertion, patient in upright position so the lung falls away from chest wall. Usually connected to simple underwater-seal drainage for 6-24 h. Suction used if air leak or copious drainage present. One-way flutter valve may be used instead of underwater-seal drainage system if only air to be removed. After chest tube insertion and removal of air and fluid from the pleural space, the lung begins to re-expand. Chest tubes produce inflammation and, ultimately, pleural scarring, which may help prevent recurrent spontaneous pneumothoraces. Pleural inflammation may cause pleuritic pain, slight temp ↑, friction rub.
Thoracotomy: Often indicated because of risk of continuous recurrence if two or more spontaneous pneumothoraces on one side, or if pneumothorax resolution does not occur within 7 days. Mechanical/chemical abrasion of pleural surfaces may be performed to prevent recurrence.

PATIENT-FAMILY TEACHING
- Purpose, expected results, anticipated sensations of all nursing/medical interventions
- Information regarding chest tube placement and maintenance
- Medications: drug name, purpose, schedule, precautions, drug-drug and food-drug interactions, potential side effects
- Technique and need for frequent deep-breathing exercises
- How to splint affected side during coughing, moving, or repositioning
- Importance of maintaining active ROM on involved side to prevent development of a stiff shoulder from immobility

Nursing Diagnoses/Interventions

Impaired gas exchange r/t ↓ alveolar blood flow and ↓ O_2 supply secondary to ↑ pleural pressure

Desired outcome: Within 2-6 h of treatment initiation, patient exhibits adequate gas exchange: Pao_2 ≥60 mm Hg and $Paco_2$ ≤45 mm Hg (or values within 10% baseline values, which depend on underlying pathophysiology), RR ≤20 breaths/min with eupnea, and orientation × 3.

- Monitor serial ABGs for ↓ O_2 or ↑ CO_2. If unstable, monitor O_2 saturation *via* Spo_2 for continuous evaluation of oxygenation.
- Observe for early indicators of hypoxia: restlessness, anxiety, changes in mental status.
- Assess for ↑ respiratory distress: ↑ RR, ↓/absent movement of chest wall on affected side, ↑ dyspnea, cyanosis.
- Position to enable full expansion of unaffected lung. Semi-Fowler's position usually provides comfort and allows adequate expansion of chest wall. Or turn unaffected side down with HOB elevated to ensure better V/Q match.
- Change patient's position q2h to promote drainage.
- Encourage deep breaths; provide necessary analgesia to ↓ discomfort during deep-breathing exercises.
- Ensure delivery of prescribed concentrations of O_2.
- Assess and maintain closed chest-drainage system.

  Tape all connections and secure chest tube to thorax with tape.

  Avoid all kinks in tubing; ensure that bed and equipment not compressing any system component.

  Maintain fluid in underwater-seal chamber and suction chamber at appropriate levels.

  Suction amount is determined by water level in suction control chamber and not by suction apparatus. Minimal bubbling is optimal. Excessive bubbling causes rapid evaporative loss.

  Removing suction for short periods of time, such as for transporting, is not detrimental nor disruptive to the closed drainage system.

  Be aware that fluctuations in long tube of the underwater-seal chamber during inspiration indicate a patent chest tube. Fluctuations stop when either the lung has reexpanded or there is a kink or obstruction in the chest tube.

  Bubbling in underwater-seal chamber occurs on expiration and is a sign that air is leaving the pleural space.

  Continuous bubbling on both inspiration and expiration in the underwater-seal chamber is a signal that air is leaking into drainage system. Locate and seal system's air leak, if possible.

- Keep emergency supplies at bedside: (1) petrolatum gauze pad to apply over insertion site if the chest tube becomes dislodged and (2) sterile water for submerging chest tube if it becomes disconnected from the underwater-seal system. Never clamp a chest tube without a specific directive from physician, since clamping may lead to tension pneumothorax.
- Chest tube stripping controversial and can damage fragile lung tissue. Stripping may be indicated when bloody drainage or clots are visible in the tubing. Squeezing alternately hand-over-hand along drainage tube may generate sufficient pressure to move fluid along the tube.

Pain r/t biophysical injury as a result of chest tube placement and pleural irritation

Desired outcomes: Within 1-2 h of initiating analgesic therapy, patient's subjective evaluation of discomfort improves as documented by a pain scale. Nonverbal indicators of discomfort, eg, grimacing and splinting on inspiration, are absent.

- Rate discomfort on a scale of 0 (no pain) to 10 (worst pain). Medicate with analgesics, evaluating medication's effectiveness using the pain scale.
- Position on unaffected side to ↓ discomfort from chest tube site. Administer medication 30 min before initiating movement.
- Move patient as a unit to promote stability and comfort.
- Schedule activities to provide for periods of rest, which may ↑ patient's pain threshold.
- Stabilize chest tube to reduce pull or drag on latex connector tubing. Tape chest tube securely to thorax, and loop latex tubing on bed beside patient.

 # Miscellanea

CONSULT MD FOR
- New or persistent hypoxemia or hypercapnia
- Persistent large air leak in thoracic closed drainage system

RELATED TOPICS
- Bronchitis, chronic
- Chest trauma
- Emphysema
- Flail chest
- Mechanical ventilation
- Multisystem injury

ABBREVIATIONS
ICS: Intercostal space
MCL: Midclavicular line

REFERENCES
Hammond SG: Chest injuries in the trauma patient, *Nurs Clin North Am* 25(1): 35-43, 1990.

Howard C: Respiratory dysfunctions. In Swearingen PL, Keen JH (eds): *Manual of critical care nursing*, ed 3, St Louis, 1995, Mosby.

Rutter KM: Tension pneumothorax: how to restore normal breathing, *Nursing* 25(4): 33, 1995.

Wait MA, Dal Nogare AR: Treatment of AIDS-related spontaneous pneumothorax: a decade of experience, *Chest* 106(3): 693-696, 1994.

Young N, Gorzeman J: Managing pneumothorax and hemothorax, *Nursing* 21(4): 56-57, 1991.

Author: **Cheri A. Goll**

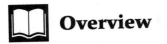 **Overview**

PATHOPHYSIOLOGY

Result from external pressure that exceeds capillary pressure, causing ischemia and eventually necrosis. Low pressure over a long period or high pressure over a brief period may produce ulcers. Friction and shear contribute because they damage vasculature and disrupt blood flow to area.

HISTORY/RISK FACTORS

- Obesity
- Advanced age
- Diabetes mellitus
- GI, digestive disorders
- Malignancy
- ↓ mobility
- Altered LOC
- Impaired sensation
- Debilitation, malnutrition
- Incontinence
- Sepsis/↑ temp

CLINICAL PRESENTATION

Optimal Healing: Initially, wound edges inflamed, indurated, tender. At first, granulation tissue on wound floor and walls is pink, progressing to deeper pink, then to beefy red; it should be moist. As healing occurs, wound edges become pink, angle between surrounding tissue and wound becomes less acute, and wound contraction occurs.

Impaired Healing: Exudate appears on wound floor and walls; does not abate as healing progresses. Undermining or tunneling develops. Skin surrounding wound may show damage: disruption, discoloration, ↑ pain.

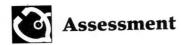 **Assessment**

PHYSICAL ASSESSMENT

High-risk individuals should be identified on admission and have assessments regularly with changes in condition.

Grade I: Nonblanchable erythema of intact skin. In dark-skinned individuals, heat may be the only indicator.

Grade II: Partial-thickness skin loss involving epidermis and/or dermis; seen as abrasion, blister, or shallow crater.

Grade III: Full-thickness skin loss involving subcutaneous tissue but does not extend through fascia.

Grade IV: Full-thickness injury that involves muscle, bone, or supporting structures.

VITAL SIGNS/HEMODYNAMICS

RR: Nl; ↑ with infection
HR: Nl; ↑ with infection

BP: Nl
Temp: Nl; ↑ with infection or inflammatory response
CVP/PAWP: Nl
CO: Nl; may ↑ with infection or inflammatory response
SVR: Nl; may ↓ with infection or inflammatory response

LABORATORY STUDIES

CBC with WBC Differential: To assess Hct and for infection. Watch for ↑ WBCs and shift to left, which indicates infection. Monitor lymphocyte count; ≤1800 μl is a sign of malnutrition. For optimal healing, Hct should be >20 g/dl.

Gram's Stain: If infection suspected, aids in selection of preliminary antibiotics.

C&S: Determines optimal antibiotic according to sensitivities of specific organism. Infection present when there are ≥10^5 organisms per gram of tissue or ≥4 organisms.

IMAGING

Ultrasound, Sonogram, or Sinogram: To determine wound size, especially when abscesses or tracts suspected.

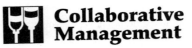 **Collaborative Management**

PHARMACOTHERAPY

Insulin: Controls glucose levels in individuals with DM, since ↑ blood glucose interferes with tissue healing.

Local or Systemic Antibiotics: Used prophylactically and when infection present.

Multivitamins, Especially C: Promote tissue healing.

Minerals, Especially Zinc and Iron: Prescribed, depending on serum levels, to promote healing.

Débriding Enzymes: Soften and remove necrotic tissue, eg, collagenase (Santyl).

DRESSINGS

Provide débridement, keep healthy wound tissue moist, enable application of antiinfective agents.

Moist Gauze With or Without Antiseptic: Insert and remove while moist. Provides means for topical antiinfective agent; good débridement; not painful; inexpensive. If excessively wet can cause tissue maceration.

Impregnated (Xeroform, Vaseline gauze): Provides topical antiseptic; keeps tissue hydrated; minimal pain with removal.

Transparent (eg, OpSite, Tegaderm, Bioclusive): Prevents wound fluid loss; protects from external contamination, friction, and fluid loss; minimal pain with removal. May withdraw excess exudate and reseal dressing;

presence of exudate may erroneously suggest infection.

Hydrocolloid (eg, Duoderm, Cutinova): Protects wound; provides autolytic débridement; easy to apply; minimizes pain.

Hydrogel (Hypergel, FLEXDERM): Protects wound; absorbent; autolytic; débrides; can administer topical drugs.

Foam (Lyofoam, NU-DERM, Allevyin): Insulates wound; provides padding; easy to apply.

Alginate (eg, Sorbsan, Kaltostat): Absorbs drainage; fills dead space; minimal pain; requires secondary dressing.

HYDROTHERAPY

Softens and removes debris mechanically.

WOUND IRRIGATION WITH OR WITHOUT ANTIINFECTIVE AGENTS

Dislodges and removes bacteria and loosens necrotic tissue, foreign bodies, and exudate.

DRAIN(S):

Remove excess tissue fluid or purulent drainage.

SURGICAL INTERVENTIONS

Débridement: Removes dead tissue and ↓ debris and fibrotic tissue.

Skin Graft: Provides wound coverage if necessary.

Tissue Flaps: Fill tissue defects and provide wound closure.

Cultured Keratinocytes: Sheet of skin cells grown from biopsy of patient's own skin to provide cover.

NUTRITION

Regular diet promotes positive nitrogen balance for optimal wound healing. Enteral supplements, tube feedings, PN may be necessary for malnourished patients or those with GI dysfunction.

GROWTH FACTORS

Stimulate new cell formation (eg, platelet-derived growth factor, insulin).

HYPERBARIC O$_2$

Supports oxidative processes in healing.

PRESSURE-RELIEVING DEVICE

↓ pressure to promote blood flow to "at risk" areas.

PATIENT-FAMILY TEACHING

- Need to maintain baseline activity level and change positions at frequent intervals
- Wound care procedure, expected results, anticipated sensations
- Signs of infection, impaired healing

Nursing Diagnoses/Interventions

Impaired tissue integrity (or risk of same) r/t excessive tissue pressure, shearing forces, or altered circulation

Desired outcomes: Patient's tissue remains intact. Following interventions/instructions, patient participates in preventive measures and verbalizes understanding of rationale for these interventions.

- Systematically assess skin over bony prominences qd.
- Establish and post a position-changing schedule.
- Assist patient with position changes. Heavier patients need to change position more frequently. Turn bed-bound patient q1-2h; have wheelchair-bound patient perform pushups in chair q15min to ensure periodic relief from pressure on buttocks. Use pillows or foam wedges to keep bony prominences from direct pressure. Patients with hx of previous tissue injury require pressure relief measures more frequently. Use low-Fowler's position, and alternate supine position with prone and 30-degree elevated side-lying positions.
- For immobile patients, totally relieve pressure on heels by raising them off bed surface with pillows inserted under length of lower leg.
- Minimize friction on tissue during activity. Lift rather than drag patient during position changes and transferring; use draw sheet to facilitate patient movement. Do not massage over bony prominences as this can result in tissue damage.
- Minimize skin exposure to moisture. Use moisture barriers and disposable briefs as needed.
- Use a mattress that reduces pressure, such as foam, alternating air, gel, or water.

Impaired tissue integrity: Presence of pressure ulcer, with ↑ risk for further breakdown r/t altered circulation and presence of contaminants or irritants

Desired outcomes: Stages I and II healed within 7-10 days; Stages III and IV may require mos to heal. Following intervention/instructions, patient verbalizes causes and preventive measures for pressure ulcers and successfully participates in plan of care to promote healing and prevent further breakdown.

- Maintain a moist physiologic environment to promote tissue repair and minimize contaminants. Change dressings as prescribed.
- Be sure patient's skin is kept clean with regular bathing; be especially conscientious about washing urine and feces from skin. Use soap and rinse it thoroughly from skin.
- If patient has excessive perspiration, ensure frequent bathing and change bedding as needed.
- To absorb moisture and prevent shearing when patient is moved, apply heel and elbow covers as needed.
- Use lamb's wool to keep areas between toes dry. Change wool periodically, depending on amount of moisture present.
- Do not use a heat lamp because it causes ↑ tissue metabolic rate.
- Provide wound care as prescribed.

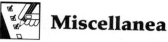 # Miscellanea

CONSULT MD FOR

- Signs of impaired wound healing: persistent or ↑ exudate, exudate with foul odor, presence of necrotic tissue, pale granulation tissue, no ↓ in wound size
- ↑ WBCs with left shift
- Positive wound C&S

RELATED TOPICS

- Alterations in consciousness
- Antimicrobial therapy
- Immobility, prolonged
- Methicillin-resistant *Staphylococcus aureus*
- Nutrition, enteral and parenteral
- Shock, septic
- Vancomycin-resistant enterococci

ABBREVIATION

PN: Parenteral nutrition

REFERENCES

Bennett MA: Report of the task force on the implications for darkly pigmented intact skin in the prediction and prevention of pressure ulcers, *Adv Wound Care* 8(6): 34-35, 1995.

Krasner D: The ABCs of wound care dressings, *Ostomy/Wound Management* 39(8): 66-72, 1993.

NPUAP position on reverse staging of pressure ulcers, *Adv Wound Care* 8(6): 32-33, 1995.

Stotts NA, Wipke-Tevis D: Co-factors in impaired wound healing, *Ostomy/Wound Management* 42(2): 44-56, 1996.

Stotts NA: Determination of bacterial burden in wounds, *Adv Wound Care* 8(4): 28-52, 1995.

Stotts NA: Wound and skin care. In Swearingen PL, Keen JH (eds): *Manual of critical care nursing*, ed 3, St Louis, 1995, Mosby.

Author: **Nancy Stotts**

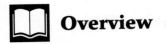 **Overview**

DESCRIPTION
Integral components of any care plan/care map are interventions that support psychosocial needs of patients' family/significant others. Important considerations are relationship to patient, mental status, self-concept and self-esteem, role relationships, age and developmental needs, sexuality, ethnocultural background, religious/spiritual needs, and family constellation and dynamics.

HISTORY/RISK FACTORS
- Family member/significant other who perceives that patient's life is threatened

CLINICAL PRESENTATION
Anxiety, fear, depression, or grief may be present.

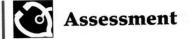 **Assessment**

PHYSICAL ASSESSMENT
Determine the following:
- Social, environmental, ethnic, and cultural factors
- Relationships
- Role patterns
- Developmental stage: be aware that other situational or maturational crises may be ongoing, eg, elderly parent or teenager with learning disability
- Previous adaptive behaviors: discuss observed conflicts and communication breakdown. ("I noticed that your brother would not visit your mother today. Has there been a problem we should be aware of? Knowing about it may help us better care for your mother.")

VITAL SIGNS
RR: Nl or slight ↑ with anxiety
Other: Release of endogenous catecholamines causes cardiopulmonary stimulation if individual anxious. HR, BP, temp usually not assessed in family/significant others.

Collaborative Management

Developmental Factors: Consider age and developmental stage when planning interventions. Assess impact of patient's disease process on meeting developmental goals.
Family Systems: Assess relationship of significant others to patient. Consider family constellation, relationships, roles, interactional dynamics, and support systems. Plan strategies to mobilize support if needed. Refer problems to appropriate psychiatric personnel.
Multicultural Factors: Consider characteristics and values of ethnocultural group and their influence on medical/nursing interventions.
Spiritual Needs: Refer to individuals who can assist in meeting religious or spiritual needs.
Consultation: Psychologist, psychiatric clinical nurse specialist, chaplain, OT, according to individual needs.

PATIENT-FAMILY TEACHING
- Referral to community or support groups (eg, ostomy support group, head injury rehabilitation group).
- Patient's current health status, therapies, and prognosis. Use individualized verbal, written, and audiovisual strategies to promote understanding.
- Evaluation at frequent intervals for understanding of provided information. Some individuals in crisis need repeated explanations before comprehension can be assured. Ask if needs for information are being met.
- Encouragement for family/significant others to relay correct information to patient. This reinforces comprehension for everyone.
- Assistance with using information received to guide health care decisions (eg, regarding patient's surgery, resuscitation, organ donation).

Nursing Diagnoses/Interventions

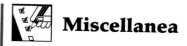 # Miscellanea

Altered family processes r/t situational crisis (patient's illness)
Desired outcome: Following intervention, family/significant others demonstrate effective adaptation to change/traumatic situation as evidenced by seeking external support when necessary and sharing concerns.
- Evaluate interactions with patient. Encourage reorganization of roles and priority setting as appropriate.
- Acknowledge involvement in patient care and promote strengths.
- Provide information and guidance related to patient. Discuss stresses of hospitalization and encourage discussions of feelings, eg, anger, guilt, hostility, depression, fear, sorrow.
- Encourage periods of rest, activity outside ICU and seeking of support when necessary.

Family coping: Potential for growth r/t use of support systems and referrals and choosing experiences that optimize wellness
Desired outcomes: At time of diagnosis, significant others express intent to use support systems and resources, identify alternative behaviors that promote communication and strengths, express realistic expectations, and do not demonstrate ineffective coping behaviors.
- Assess relationships, interactions, support systems, and individual coping behaviors. Permit movement through stages of adaptation.
- Acknowledge expressions of hope, future plans, and growth among significant others.
- Encourage development of open, honest communication. Provide opportunities in a private setting for interactions, discussions, and questions.
- Encourage exploration of outlets that foster positive feelings, eg, periods of time outside hospital area, meaningful communication with patient or support individuals, and relaxing activities.

Ineffective family coping: Compromised, r/t inadequate or incorrect information or misunderstanding, temporary family disorganization and role change, exhausted support systems, unrealistic expectations, fear, or anxiety
Desired outcomes: Following intervention, family/significant others verbalize feelings, identify ineffective coping patterns, identify strengths and positive coping behaviors, and seek information and support from the nurse or other support systems.
- Assist in identifying strengths, stressors, inappropriate behaviors, and personal needs.
- Assess for ineffective coping (eg, depression, substance abuse, violence, withdrawal) and identify factors that inhibit effective coping (eg, inadequate support system, grief, fear of disapproval by others, knowledge deficit).
- Provide information regarding patient's current health status and allow time for questions. Reassess understanding at frequent intervals.
- Provide opportunities in a private setting to talk and share concerns with nurses or other health care providers. If appropriate, refer to psychiatric clinical nurse specialist for therapy.
- Offer realistic hope. Help family/significant others develop realistic expectations for the future and identify support systems that will assist them with planning for the future.
- Reduce anxiety by promoting diversional activities, interaction with outside support system.

Fear r/t patient's life-threatening condition and/or knowledge deficit
Desired outcome: Family/significant others relate that fear has been lessened.
- Assess fears and understanding related to patient's clinical situation. Evaluate verbal and nonverbal responses.
- Acknowledge fears; provide opportunities for expressions of fears and concerns. Anger, denial, withdrawal, and demanding behavior may be adaptive coping responses during initial period of crisis.
- Assess hx of coping behavior. Determine resources, significant others available for support.
- Encourage positive coping behaviors by identifying fear(s), developing goals, identifying supportive resources, facilitating realistic perceptions, and promoting problem solving.
- Recognize anxiety and encourage family/significant others to describe their feelings.
- Be alert to maladaptive responses to fear: potential for violence, withdrawal, severe depression, hostility, and unrealistic expectations of staff or of patient's recovery. Provide referrals to psychiatric clinical nurse specialist or other as appropriate.
- Demonstrate a caring attitude. Offer *realistic* hope, even if it is the hope for the patient's peaceful death.
- Explore desires for spiritual, religious, or psychologic counseling.
- Assess your own feelings about patient's life-threatening illness. Acknowledge that your attitude and fear may be reflected to significant others.

RELATED TOPICS
- Agitation syndrome
- Anxiety
- Grieving
- Psychosocial needs, patient

REFERENCES
Demi AS, Miles MS: Bereavement, *Ann Rev Nurs Res* 4: 105-123, 1986.
Hall P: Critical care nursing: psychosocial aspects of care. In Burrell L (ed): *Adult nursing in hospital and community settings,* Norwalk, Conn, 1992, Appleton & Lange.
Hall P: Psychosocial support for the patient's family and significant others. In Swearingen PL, Keen JH (eds): *Manual of critical care nursing,* ed 3, St Louis, 1995, Mosby.
Kozier B et al: *Fundamentals of nursing: concepts, process, and practice,* ed 5, Redwood City, Calif, 1995, Addison-Wesley.

Author: **Patricia Hall**

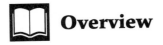 **Overview**

DESCRIPTION
Interventions that support psychosocial needs are founded on principles in which body, mind, and spirit operate in tandem to maintain homeostatic balance. Necessary considerations are mental status, self-concept and self-esteem, role relationships, age and developmental needs, sexuality, ethnocultural background, religious/spiritual needs, and family constellation/dynamics.

CLINICAL PRESENTATION
Varies according to patient's condition and circumstances. Thorough assessment of mental status and emotional state necessary in order to plan care. A Mini Mental Status Exam (see Appendix) is one important method of assessment. Scores <23 (out of total 25) signal cognitive dysfunction.

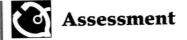 **Assessment**

VITAL SIGNS/HEMODYNAMICS
RR: NI or slight ↑ with anxiety
HR: NI or slight ↑ with anxiety
BP: NI or slight ↑ with anxiety
Temp: NI
Other: Release of endogenous catecholamines may cause CV stimulation if patient anxious.

Collaborative Management

Developmental Factors: Consider age and developmental stage when planning interventions. Assess impact of disease process on meeting developmental goals.
Family Systems: Assess family constellation, relationships, roles, interactional dynamics, and support systems. Plan strategies to mobilize support if needed; refer problems to appropriate psychiatric personnel.
Multicultural Factors: Consider ethnic or cultural group, ethnocultural characteristics and values, and influence on medical/nursing interventions.
Spiritual Needs: Refer to individuals who can assist in meeting religious/spiritual needs.
Sexuality: Assess sexual needs. Consider effects of specific disease process on sexual performance; provide counseling for dysfunctions.

PATIENT-FAMILY TEACHING
- Cognitive and emotional readiness to learn and current level of knowledge about health status.
- Barriers to learning, eg, ineffective communication, neurologic deficit, sensory alterations, fear, anxiety, or lack of motivation.
- Individualize verbal or written information, providing simple, direct instructions. Use audiovisual tools.
- Encourage family/significant others to reinforce correct information.
- Comprehension of information given. Ask patient to repeat what has been explained. Individuals in crisis or after general anesthesia often need repeated explanations.
- Informed consent: assist with using information received to make informed health care decisions.
- Process for executing advance directive for health care.

Nursing Diagnoses/Interventions

Ineffective individual coping r/t health crisis, sense of vulnerability, inadequate support systems

Desired outcomes: Within 24 h of this diagnosis, patient verbalizes feelings, identifies strengths, and begins using positive coping behaviors.

- Assess perceptions and ability to understand current health status.
- Establish honest communication. ("Please tell me what I can do to help you.") Assist with identifying strengths, stressors, inappropriate behaviors, personal needs.
- Support positive coping behaviors. ("I see that reading that book seems to help you relax.")
- Provide opportunities for expressions of concerns. Acknowledge feelings and assessment of current health status and environment.
- Identify factors that inhibit ability to cope (eg, unsatisfactory support system, knowledge deficit, grief, fear).
- Recognize maladaptive coping behaviors (eg, severe depression, drug or alcohol dependence, hostility, violence, suicidal ideation). Confront these behaviors. ("You seem to be requiring more pain medication. Are you experiencing more physical pain, or does it help to remove yourself from reality?")
- Help ↓ sensory overload by maintaining an organized, quiet environment.
- Encourage regular visits by significant others. Encourage them to engage in conversation to help ↓ patient's emotional and social isolation.
- Assess significant others' interactions with patient. Attempt to mobilize support systems by involving them in patient care whenever possible.
- As appropriate, explain to significant others that patient's ↑ dependency, anger, and denial may be adaptive coping behaviors in early stages of crisis until effective coping behaviors learned.

Spiritual distress r/t separation from spiritual/cultural support; challenged belief, value system

Desired outcomes: Within 24 h of this diagnosis, patient verbalizes spiritual or religious beliefs and expresses hope for the future, attainment of spiritual or religious support, and availability of the requisites for resolving conflicts.

- Assess spiritual or religious beliefs, values, and practices.
- Inform patient and family/significant others of availability of spiritual aids, such as a chapel or religious services.
- Be nonjudgmental toward religious or spiritual beliefs and values.
- Identify available support systems that may assist in meeting religious or spiritual needs.
- Be alert to comments r/t spiritual concerns, conflicts. ("Why is God doing this to me?")
- Use active listening and open-ended questioning to assist in resolving conflicts r/t spiritual issues. ("I understand that you want to be baptized. We can arrange to do that.")
- Provide privacy and opportunities for religious practices, such as prayer and meditation.
- If spiritual beliefs and therapeutic regimens are in conflict, provide honest, concrete information to encourage informed decision making.

Hopelessness r/t prolonged isolation or activity restriction, failing or deteriorating physiologic condition, long-term stress, or loss of faith in God or belief system

Desired outcomes: Before hospital discharge, patient verbalizes hopeful aspects of health status and relates that feelings of despair are absent/↓.

- Actively listen, provide empathetic understanding of fears and doubts, and promote an environment conducive to free expression.
- Assess understanding of health status and prognosis; clarify any misperceptions.
- Assess for indicators of hopelessness: unwillingness to accept help, pessimism, withdrawal, lack of interest, silence, loss of gratification in roles, hx of hopeless behavior, hypoactivity, inability to accomplish tasks, expressions of incompetence, closing eyes and turning away.
- Provide opportunities for patient to feel cared for, needed, and valued by others.
- Support significant others who seem to promote patient's feelings of hope.
- Recognize factors that promote sense of hope (ie, discussions about family members, reminiscing about better times).
- Promote anticipation of positive events (ie, mealtime, visits, bath time, extubation).
- Help patient recognize that although there may be no hope for returning to original lifestyle, there may be hope for a new, but different life.
- Avoid insisting that patient assume a positive attitude. Encourage hope for the future, even if it is the hope for a peaceful death.

Miscellanea

CONSULT MD FOR
- Severe or persistent depression
- Severe anxiety or panic
- As necessary, to clarify medical-surgical plan of care

RELATED TOPICS
- Agitation syndrome
- Alterations in consciousness
- Anxiety
- Delirium
- Grieving
- Psychosocial needs, family/significant others
- Sleep disturbances

REFERENCES

Carson VB: *Spiritual dimensions of nursing practice,* Philadelphia, 1989, Saunders.

Giger JN, Davidhizar R: Transcultural nursing assessment: a method for advancing nursing practice, *Int Nurs Rev* 37(1): 199-202, 1990.

Hall P: Psychosocial support. In Swearingen PL, Keen JH (eds): *Manual of critical care nursing,* ed 3, St Louis, 1995, Mosby.

Kozier B et al: *Fundamentals of nursing: concepts, process, and practice,* ed 5, Redwood City, Calif, 1995, Addison-Wesley.

Lazarus RS, Folkman S: *Stress: appraisal and coping,* New York, 1984, Springer.

Author: **Patricia Hall**

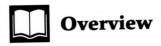 **Overview**

PATHOPHYSIOLOGY
When hydrostatic pressure in pulmonary vessels is > intravascular colloid osmotic pressure, fluid fills pulmonary interstitium and alveoli, impairing gas exchange. Physiologic shunting of blood through nonfunctional alveolar-capillary units results in profound hypoxemia. Common causes include ↑ hydrostatic pressure from LV failure or fluid volume excess or ↑ pulmonary capillary permeability and leakage of proteins into interstitial space (noncardiogenic pulmonary edema).

HISTORY/RISK FACTORS
Cardiac (Hydrostatic) Pulmonary Edema
- LV failure
- Cardiogenic shock
- Profound fluid volume overload

Noncardiac Pulmonary Edema
- All forms of shock
- Septicemia
- Near drowning
- Chemical, viral, other pneumonitis

CLINICAL PRESENTATION
Nocturnal dyspnea, dyspnea on exertion, orthopnea, cyanosis or pallor, palpitations, weakness, fatigue, anorexia, change in mentation

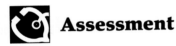 **Assessment**

PHYSICAL ASSESSMENT
Neuro: Somnolence, confusion, anxiety
Resp: Crackles, wheezing, moist cough, frothy sputum, dyspnea, tachypnea
CV: Tachycardia, S_3 or summation gallop, pulsus alternans, dysrhythmias, ↓ intensity of peripheral pulses, delayed capillary refill, peripheral edema
GU: Oliguria
Integ: Diaphoresis

VITAL SIGNS/HEMODYNAMICS
RR: ↑
HR: ↑

BP: ↓
Temp: N/a
CO/CI: ↓
PAP/PAWP: ↑
PVR: ↑
SVR: ↑
ECG: Dysrhythmias, ischemic changes possible (eg, ST-segment depression, T-wave inversion)

LABORATORY STUDIES
Chemistries: May reveal hyponatremia (dilutional), hyperkalemia if glomerular filtration ↓, or hypokalemia caused by diuretics. Also, ↑ bilirubin, ↑ liver enzymes caused by hepatic engorgement.
CBC: May reveal ↓ Hgb and Hct with anemia or dilution.
ABGs: Hypoxemia caused by ↓ gas exchange across fluid-filled alveoli; early respiratory alkalosis caused by ↑ RR; later, hypercarbia as respiratory failure ensues.
Digitalis Levels: Predisposition to digitalis toxicity caused by low CO state and ↓ renal excretion of the drug.

IMAGING
Chest X-ray: Pulmonary clouding, ↑ interstitial density, engorged pulmonary vasculature, cardiomegaly.

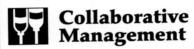 **Collaborative Management**

GENERAL
Treatment of Underlying Cause: Atherosclerotic heart disease, AMI, dysrhythmias, cardiomyopathy, fluid volume overload, systemic hypertension, cardiac valvular disorders and structural defects, cardiac tamponade, constrictive pericarditis. Goal: to remove fluid by improving myocardial function (optimize preload, afterload, contractility) and administering diuretics.
Sodium/Fluid Restriction: Extra salt and water are held in the circulatory system, causing ↑ volume. Limiting sodium will ↓ amount of fluid retained by the body. Total fluid intake may be limited to 1500 ml/day.
O_2: If mild, nasal cannula; if severe, nonrebreather mask or intubation with mechanical

ventilation may be necessary. Goal: to maintain SpO_2 ≥92%.
IABP: To ↓ afterload and improve coronary arterial perfusion if acute LV failure present.
Bed Rest: To ↓ cardiac workload and facilitate mobilization of fluid from extremities.
Stress Reduction: To ↓ endogenous catecholamine release and sympathetic tone.

PHARMACOTHERAPY
Initial Therapy
Morphine: To induce vasodilatation and ↓ venous return, preload, sympathetic tone, and anxiety and reduce myocardial O_2 consumption.
Diuretics: To ↓ blood volume and ↓ preload.
NTG: Given SL to improve coronary arterial blood flow, ↓ afterload.
Additional Therapy
Vasodilators: IV NTG to dilate venous or capacitant vessels, thereby ↓ preload and cardiac and pulmonary congestion. Nitroprusside and nifedipine dilate arterial or resistant vessels and ↓ afterload, thus ↑ forward flow.
Inotropic agents: Digitalis to strengthen contractions. For rapid inotropic response, use IV dobutamine, milrinone, and amrinone (see Appendix), and correct A-fib.
Bronchodilators: IV aminophylline at rate of 5 mg/kg may be indicated for wheezing.
Vasopressors: Dopamine used if SBP <100 mm Hg.

PATIENT-FAMILY TEACHING
- Physiologic process of LV failure; how fluid volume ↑ caused by poor heart functioning
- Importance of low-sodium diet and medications to help ↓ volume overload; how to read, evaluate food labels
- S&S of fluid volume excess that necessitate medical attention: irregular or slow pulse, ↑ SOB, orthopnea, ↓ exercise tolerance, and steady weight gain (≥1 kg/day for 2 successive days)
- If patient taking digitalis, technique for measuring HR; parameters for holding digitalis (usually HR <60/min) and notifying physician
- Warning signals to stop activity and rest: chest pain, SOB, dizziness or faintness, unusual weakness; use of prophylactic NTG

Nursing Diagnoses/Interventions

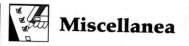 # Miscellanea

Impaired gas exchange r/t alveolar-capillary membrane changes secondary to fluid collection in alveoli and interstitial spaces

Desired outcome: Within 24 h of treatment initiation, patient has improved gas exchange: PaO_2 ≥80 mm Hg, RR 12-20 breaths/min with eupnea, and clear breath sounds.

- Monitor respiratory rate, rhythm, and character at frequent intervals. Be alert to RR >20 breaths/min, irregular rhythm, use of accessory muscles of respiration, cough, frothy sputum.
- Auscultate breath sounds, noting crackles, wheezes, and other adventitious sounds.
- Provide supplemental O_2 to maintain SpO_2 ≥92%. As indicated, prepare patient for aggressive O_2 delivery *via* nonrebreathing mask, mechanical ventilation.
- Assess ABGs; note changes in response to O_2 supplementation or treatment of altered hemodynamics. Be aware that O_2 administration may have minimal effect on hypoxemia because of physiologic shunting. Optimizing myocardial function *via* diuretic therapy, morphine, NTG, vasodilators, and positive inotropes will be more likely to improve condition.
- Suction secretions as needed. Consider intubation if patient has copious productive coughing with deteriorating SaO_2, PaO_2.
- If patient has bronchoconstriction/wheezing, consider IV aminophylline.
- Place in semi- or high-Fowler's position to maximize chest excursion.
- Maintain bed rest or activity restrictions to reduce tissue O_2 requirements.

Fluid volume excess r/t excessive fluid or sodium intake or r/t compromised regulatory mechanism secondary to ↓ cardiac output

Desired outcome: Within 24 h of treatment, patient normovolemic: clear lung sounds, UO ≥0.5 ml/kg/h, O > I + insensible losses, stable weight/weight loss, PAWP ≤18 mm Hg, SVR ≤1200 dynes/sec/cm^{-5}, and CO ≥4 L/min.

- Monitor I&O qh. Administer IV medications in smallest volume possible. Report positive fluid state or ↓ in UO to <0.5 mg/kg/h.
- Weigh qd; report significant ↑ in weight.
- Note changes from baseline to detect worsening of heart failure: ↑ crackles, rhonchi, ↑ pedal edema, JVD, S_3 heart sound or new murmur, and dysrhythmias.
- Monitor hemodynamic status q1-2h and prn. Note response to drug therapy as well as possible indicators for more aggressive therapy: ↑ PAWP and SVR and ↓ CO. Be aware that > nl PAWP (eg, 18-20 mm Hg) may be necessary to optimize CO with LV failure.
- Administer diuretics (furosemide), positive inotropes (dobutamine, milrinone), vasodilators (NTG, nitroprusside). Use concentrated solutions of inotropic, vasodilating agents. In general, use vasodilators if MAP >100 mm Hg or dopamine if MAP <100 mm Hg.
- Limit oral fluids; offer ice chips or frozen juice pops to ↓ thirst and discomfort of dry mouth.

CONSULT MD FOR
- Sustained hypoxemia: PaO_2 <80 mm Hg despite interventions
- Deteriorating cardiac performance: new-onset S_3 or summation gallop, murmur, dysrhythmias, frothy sputum, crackles, sustained hypotension
- Unacceptable hemodynamics: CO <4 L/min, PAWP >18 mm Hg, SVR >1200 dynes/sec/cm^{-5}, MAP <70 mm Hg
- UO <0.5 mg/kg/h × 2 consecutive h
- Complications: unrelieved chest pain, ECG evidence of ischemia, ARDS

RELATED TOPICS
- Adult respiratory distress syndrome
- Anaphylaxis
- Cardiomyopathy
- Heart failure, left ventricular
- Shock, cardiogenic
- Shock, septic
- Vasodilator therapy
- Vasopressor therapy

REFERENCES
Cross JA: Pharmacologic management of heart failure: positive inotropic agents, *Crit Care Nurs Clin North Am* 5(4): 589-597, 1993.

Dracup K, Dunbar SB, Baker DW: Rethinking heart failure, *Am J Nurs* 95(7): 22-28, 1995.

Robinson K: Reversing pulmonary edema, *Am J Nurs* 93(12): 45, 1993.

Steuble BT: Congestive heart failure/pulmonary edema. In Swearingen PL, Keen JH (eds): *Manual of critical care nursing,* ed 3, St Louis, 1995, Mosby.

Wright JM: Pharmacologic management of congestive heart failure, *Crit Care Nurs Q* 18(1): 32-44, 1995.

Author: **Janet Hicks Keen**

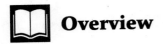 **Overview**

PATHOPHYSIOLOGY

Almost always an iatrogenic complication with multiple causes, including surgical procedures, insertion of PA and CV catheters, hemodialysis, endoscopy, and injection of contrast media. Small amounts of air may be completely asymptomatic because of rapid reabsorption. A larger bolus of air into the right ventricle may obstruct pulmonary blood flow completely, leading to cardiac arrest.

MORTALITY RATE

In severe cases, >50%. Rapid diagnosis and treatment essential.

RISK FACTORS

- Recent surgical procedure
- PA/CV catheter insertion
- Misuse of closed-wound suction unit
- Cardiopulmonary bypass
- Hemodialysis
- Endoscopy

CLINICAL PRESENTATION

Depends on severity of bolus. May result in sudden onset of agitation, confusion, cough, SOB, and chest pain.

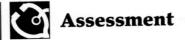 **Assessment**

PHYSICAL ASSESSMENT

Neuro: Confusion, delirium, coma
Resp: Tachypnea, dyspnea, wheezing
CV: Tachycardia, hypotension, mill wheel murmur

VITAL SIGNS/HEMODYNAMICS

RR: ↑
HR: ↑
BP: ↓
Temp: Nl
PAP: ↑ PVR results in sudden ↑ in PAS/PAD, while PAWP remains nl
CO: ↓
ECG: Sinus tachycardia, dysrhythmias possible because of hypoxemia

LABORATORY STUDIES

ABGs: PaO_2 <80 mm Hg, $PaCO_2$ >45 mm Hg, and respiratory acidosis (pH <7.35) generally present in severe cases.

IMAGING

Chest X-ray: Changes consistent with pulmonary edema or air fluid levels in the main PA system.

Collaborative Management

Prevention: Ensure that CV catheter is inserted with patient in Trendelenburg position. Luer-Lok all connections on IV tubing to prevent disconnection. Should venous air embolus occur despite precautions, the following are anticipated:
O_2: 100% FiO_2 initiated immediately.
Trendelenburg position with left decubitus tilt: To minimize further movement of air bolus through the heart and into the pulmonary vasculature and beyond.
Aspiration of air: If a CV catheter is in place near the right atrium, an attempt is made to aspirate the air.

PATIENT-FAMILY TEACHING

- Purpose, expected results, and anticipated sensations for nursing/medical interventions
- Necessity of remaining on left side in Trendelenburg position until stable

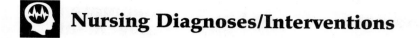 **Nursing Diagnoses/Interventions**

Impaired gas exchange r/t altered blood flow secondary to presence of air embolus
Desired outcome: Within 1 h of initiation of therapy, patient has adequate gas exchange: Pao_2 $\geq$60 mm Hg, $Paco_2$ 35-45 mm Hg, and pH 7.35-7.45.

- As soon as air embolus suspected, place in Trendelenburg position in a left decubitus tilt.
- Ensure delivery of 100% concentration O_2 *via* nonrebreathing mask or manual resuscitator if necessary.
- Attempt to aspirate air from right atrium *via* CV catheter.
- Monitor serial ABGs and O_2 saturation, assessing for adequate oxygenation and correction of respiratory alkalosis.
- Monitor for $\uparrow$ respiratory distress: $\uparrow$ RR, dyspnea, anxiety, cyanosis.

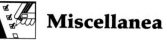 **Miscellanea**

CONSULT MD FOR
- Deteriorating ABGs: Pao_2 $\leq$60 mm Hg, $Paco_2$ >45 or <35 mm Hg, pH >7.45 or <7.35
- Respiratory distress: dyspnea, anxiety, cyanosis

RELATED TOPICS
- Adult respiratory distress syndrome
- Anxiety
- Hemodynamic monitoring
- Psychosocial needs, family/significant others
- Psychosocial needs, patient
- Respiratory failure, acute

REFERENCES

Currie DL: Pulmonary embolism: diagnosis and management, *Crit Care Nurs Q* 13(2): 41-49, 1990.

Henschke C, Mateescu I, Yankelevitz D: Changing practice patterns in the workup of pulmonary embolism, *Chest* 107(4): 940-945, 1995.

Howard C: Pulmonary dysfunctions. In Swearingen PL, Keen JH (eds): *Manual of critical care nursing,* ed 3, St Louis, 1995, Mosby.

Teplitz L: Responding to an air embolism, *Nursing* 22(7):33, 1992.

Author: **Cheri A. Goll**

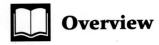 **Overview**

PATHOPHYSIOLOGY

Most common nonthrombotic cause of pulmonary perfusion disorders and result of two events: release of free fatty acids causing a toxic vasculitis, followed by thrombosis and obstruction of small pulmonary arteries by fat. V/Q mismatch occurs as nonperfused segments continue to be ventilated. There is profound pulmonary edema in ≈ 30% of patients. Thrombocytopenia and other clotting abnormalities are possible.

HISTORY/RISK FACTORS

- Osteomyelitis
- Sickle cell anemia
- Multiple long bone fractures, especially of femur and pelvis
- Trauma to adipose tissue or liver
- Burns
- Dehydration, other factors that could precipitate crisis in patients with sickle cell anemia

CLINICAL PRESENTATION

Typically, no S&S for 12-24 h after embolization; then sudden cardiopulmonary and neurologic deterioration

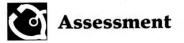 **Assessment**

PHYSICAL ASSESSMENT

Neuro: Restlessness, confusion, delirium, coma
Resp: Tachypnea, dyspnea, inspiratory crowing, expiratory wheezing, crackles
CV: Tachycardia, hypertension
Integ: Petechiae, especially of upper torso and axillae

VITAL SIGNS/HEMODYNAMICS

RR: ↑
HR: ↑
BP: ↑ initially; may ↓ with severe pulmonary hypertension, RV heart failure
Temp: ↑
CVP/PAP: ↑ caused by pulmonary hypertension
PAWP: Nl
PVR: ↑
CO: ↓ if pulmonary hypertension severe and RV heart failure present or if patient hypovolemic
ECG: Sinus tachycardia, possible dysrhythmias because of hypoxemia

LABORATORY STUDIES

ABGs: Pao_2 <80 mm Hg, $Paco_2$ >45 mm Hg, and respiratory acidosis (pH <7.35).
CBCs: To monitor for heparin-induced thrombocytopenia; ↓ Hgb and Hct present secondary to hemorrhage into the lung.

IMAGING

Chest X-ray: A pattern similar to ARDS is seen: diffuse, extensive bilateral interstitial and alveolar infiltrates.
Pulmonary V/Q Scan: To detect abnormalities of ventilation or perfusion. If there is V/Q mismatch (eg, nl ventilation with ↓ perfusion), vascular obstruction likely.

Collaborative Management

O₂: Based on clinical picture, ABGs, and prior respiratory status. Titrated to maintain Pao_2 >60 mm Hg, Spo_2 >90%. Intubation and mechanical ventilation may be required.
Steroids: Cortisone, 100 mg, or methylprednisolone, 30 mg/kg, used to ↓ local inflammation of pulmonary tissue and pulmonary edema.
Diuretics: Pulmonary edema may necessitate use of diuretics.

PATIENT-FAMILY TEACHING

- Purpose, expected results, anticipated sensations for nursing/medical interventions
- Medications: drug name, purpose, dosage, schedule, precautions, drug-drug and food-drug interactions, potential side effects

Nursing Diagnoses/Interventions

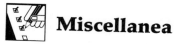 # Miscellanea

Impaired gas exchange r/t altered blood flow secondary to presence of PE

Desired outcome: Within 12 h of initiation of therapy, patient has adequate gas exchange: PaO_2 ≥60 mm Hg, $PaCO_2$ 35-45 mm Hg, and pH 7.35-7.45. Within 2-4 days of initiating therapy, RR 12-20 breaths/min with eupnea.

- Monitor serial ABGs and O_2 saturation, assessing for adequate oxygenation and correction of respiratory alkalosis.
- Monitor for ↑ respiratory distress:↑ RR, dyspnea, anxiety, cyanosis.
- Ensure delivery of prescribed concentrations of O_2.
- Position with unaffected side down; elevate HOB 30 degrees to optimize V/Q.
- Ensure deep-breathing exercises 3-5 × q2h.
- Assess temp q2-4h. As indicated, provide treatment to ↓ temp and thus O_2 demands.

Activity intolerance r/t imbalance between O_2 supply and demand secondary to ↓ alveolar O_2 supply and ↑ metabolic O_2 demands as a result of ↑ WOB

Desired outcome: Within 24-48 h of treatment initiation, patient verbalizes ↓ in fatigue and associated symptoms.

- Group procedures and activities to provide frequent rest periods (optimally, ≥90-120 min).
- ↓ metabolic demands for O_2 by limiting or pacing patient's activities and procedures.
- If patient is restless, which ↑ O_2 demand, ascertain cause of restlessness, eg, hypoxemia or anxiety.
- Schedule rest times after meals to avoid competition for O_2 supply during digestion.
- Monitor SpO_2 during activity to evaluate limits of activity.
- Assess temp q2-4h. As indicated, provide treatment to ↓ temp and thus O_2 demands.

CONSULT MD FOR

- Deteriorating ABGs: PaO_2 ≤60 mm Hg, $PaCO_2$ >45 or <35 mm Hg, pH >7.45 or <7.35
- Respiratory distress: dyspnea, anxiety, cyanosis

RELATED TOPICS

- Adult respiratory distress syndrome
- Heart failure, right ventricular
- Mechanical ventilation
- Pulmonary hypertension

REFERENCES

Currie DL: Pulmonary embolism: diagnosis and management, *Crit Care Nurs Q* 13(2): 41-49, 1990.

Henschke C, Mateescu I, Yankelevitz D: Changing practice patterns in the workup of pulmonary embolism, *Chest* 107(4): 940-945, 1995.

Howard C: Pulmonary dysfunctions. In Swearingen PL, Keen JH (eds): *Manual of critical care nursing,* ed 3, St Louis, 1995, Mosby.

Author: **Cheri A. Goll**

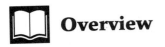 **Overview**

PATHOPHYSIOLOGY
Caused by a blood clot from the systemic circulation, typically deep veins of the legs or pelvis. The thrombus dislodges and travels to the pulmonary circulation, where it obstructs one or both branches of the PA or a subdivision. Total obstruction leading to pulmonary infarction is rare because the pulmonary circulation has multiple sources of blood. Although most thrombotic emboli resolve completely, chronic pulmonary hypertension may occur.

MORTALITY
Early diagnosis, appropriate treatment ↓ mortality to <10%.

HISTORY/RISK FACTORS
- Cardiac disorders: A-fib, heart failure, MI, rheumatic heart disease, low CO state
- Trauma: especially leg fracture, hip fracture in elders, burns, acute head injury, SCIs
- Carcinoma: particularly involving breast, lung, pancreas, GU/GI tracts
- Varicose veins or prior thromboembolic disease
- Prolonged immobilization: risk ↑ as length of immobilization ↑
- Surgical intervention: especially for pelvic, thoracic, and abdominal surgery and musculoskeletal injuries of hip or knee
- Obesity: ≥20% ↑ in ideal body weight
- Age: greatest risk between 55-65 yrs of age

CLINICAL PRESENTATION
Many patients do not exhibit S&S of DVT before experiencing PE.
- Sudden onset of dyspnea, tachypnea, restlessness, anxiety
- Nonproductive cough, palpitations, nausea, syncope
- With large embolus: oppressive substernal chest discomfort
- With pulmonary infarction: fever, pleuritic chest pain, hemoptysis

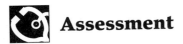 **Assessment**

PHYSICAL ASSESSMENT
Neuro: Restlessness, anxiety
Resp: Tachypnea, crackles, ↓ chest wall excursion, cyanosis; with pulmonary infarction, pleural friction rub
CV: Tachycardia, diaphoresis, edema, S_3/S_4 gallop

VITAL SIGNS/HEMODYNAMICS
RR: ↑
HR: ↑
BP: Nl/↓ with large emboli and RV heart failure
Temp: ↑ with pulmonary infarction
CVP/PAP: ↑ with RV heart failure
PAWP: Nl
CO: ↓
PVR: ↑
Other: PAP ↑ significantly (>20 mm Hg) if 30%-50% of pulmonary arterial tree affected. If massive PEs present and PAP ↑ to >40 mm Hg, RV failure can develop, leading to ↓ CO and BP.
ECG: Signs of acute pulmonary hypertension may be present: right-shift QRS axes, tall and peaked P waves, ST-segment changes, and T-wave inversion in leads V_1-V_4.

LABORATORY STUDIES
ABGs: Pao_2 <80 mm Hg, $Paco_2$ <35 mm Hg, and pH >7.45 usually present. Nl Pao_2 does not rule out presence of PE. Spo_2 used for continuous monitoring of O_2 saturation.

IMAGING
Chest X-ray: Initially nl, or elevated hemidiaphragm present. If large PE, abnormal blood vessel diameters and shapes. If pulmonary infarction present, infiltrates and pleural effusions may be seen within 12-36 h.
Pulmonary V/Q Scan: If there is V/Q mismatch (eg, nl ventilation with ↓ perfusion), vascular obstruction likely.
Pulmonary Angiography: Definitive study to visualize pulmonary vessels. Abrupt vessel "cut off" may be seen at embolization site.

DIAGNOSTIC PROCEDURES
P(A-a)o₂: Usually >10 mm Hg, depending on severity of perfusion disorder and degree of V/Q mismatch.
PAP: Acutely ↑ without ↑ of PAWP.

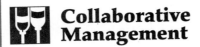 **Collaborative Management**

O₂: To maintain Pao_2 at >60 mm Hg.
Heparin: Started immediately in patients without bleeding or clotting disorders and in whom PE strongly suspected.
Initial dose: IV bolus of 5000-10,000 U
Maintenance dose: Continuous IV infusion of 1000 U/h or according to body weight (eg, 17 U/kg/h). Maintenance continues for 7-14 days, with patient confined to bed rest.
PTT: Maintain at 1.5-2.5 × nl by adjusting heparin. *Platelet counts* obtained q3d because thrombocytopenia and paradoxical arterial thrombosis can occur as a result of heparin therapy.

Protamine sulfate: Heparin antidote; keep readily available.
Oral Anticoagulants (warfarin sodium): Started 48-72 h after initiation of heparin therapy. The two given simultaneously for 6-7 days until warfarin inhibits vitamin K dependent clotting factors.
PT: Monitored qd, with goal of 1¼-1½ × nl. Once condition has stabilized, weekly monitoring of PT acceptable. INR should be 2:3.
Vitamin K: Reverses warfarin effects in 24-36 h. FFP may be required in cases of serious bleeding.
Thrombolytic Therapy (streptokinase, urokinase, tissue plasminogen activator): Given in first 24-72 h after PE to speed process of clot lysis, especially when severe cardiopulmonary compromise has occurred or there is >30% occlusion of pulmonary vasculature.
Thrombin time: Monitors effectiveness of thrombolytic therapy.
ϵ-Aminocaproic acid (eg, Amicar, unlabeled use): Primary dose of 4-5 g followed by continuous infusion of 1-1.25 g/h.
Surgical Interventions: Eg, inferior venal caval interruption, most often involving transvenous insertion of umbrella or filter that prevents passage of major emboli from DVTs in lower extremities.

PATIENT-FAMILY TEACHING
- Medications: drug name, purpose, dosage, schedule, precautions, drug-drug and food-drug interactions, potential side effects.
- Potential side effects and complications of anticoagulant therapy: easy bruising, prolonged bleeding from cuts, spontaneous nose bleeds, black and tarry stools, blood in urine and sputum.
- Importance of reporting promptly bleeding from any source.
- Necessity of using sponge-tipped applicators and mouthwash for oral care to minimize risk of gum bleeding during hospitalization when anticoagulant therapy most intensive. Instruct patient to shave with an electric rather than a straight razor.
- Rationale and application procedure for antiembolism hose.
- Importance of preventing impaired venous return from lower extremities by avoiding prolonged sitting, crossing legs, and constrictive clothing.
- Foods high in vitamin K (eg, fish, bananas, dark green vegetables, tomatoes, and cauliflower), which can interfere with anticoagulation.
- Purpose, expected results, and anticipated sensations of nursing/medical interventions.

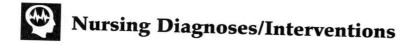

Nursing Diagnoses/Interventions

Impaired gas exchange r/t altered blood flow secondary to presence of PE

Desired outcome: Within 12 h of initiation of therapy, patient has adequate gas exchange: PaO_2 ≥60 mm Hg, $PaCO_2$ 35-45 mm Hg, and pH 7.35-7.45. Within 2-4 days of initiating therapy, RR 12-20 breaths/min with eupnea.

- Monitor serial ABGs and O_2 saturation, assessing for adequate oxygenation and correction of respiratory alkalosis.
- Monitor for ↑ respiratory distress:↑ RR, dyspnea, anxiety, cyanosis.
- Ensure delivery of prescribed concentrations of O_2.
- Position with unaffected side down; elevate HOB 30 degrees to optimize V/Q.
- Avoid positioning with knees bent (ie, "gatching" the bed) because this impedes venous return from legs and can ↑ risk of PE.
- Ensure deep-breathing exercises 3-5 × q2h.
- ↓ metabolic demands for O_2 by limiting or pacing patient's activities and procedures.
- Schedule rest times after meals to avoid competition for O_2 supply during digestion.
- Assess temp q2-4h. As indicated, provide treatment to ↓ temp and thus O_2 demands.

Altered protection r/t risk of clotting anomalies secondary to anticoagulation or thrombolytic therapy

Desired outcomes: Patient free of bleeding signs, or if bleeding occurs, it is not prolonged.

- Monitor serial PTT, PT, INR.
- Have antidotes readily available: protamine sulfate, vitamin K, ε-aminocaproic acid.
- Inspect the following for bleeding: entry site of invasive procedures, oral mucous membranes, wounds; inspect torso and extremities for petechiae or ecchymoses. Check stool, urine, sputum, and vomitus for occult blood. Be alert to complaints of back pain or other site-specific pain (eg, headache), which may signal occult bleeding.
- Apply pressure over puncture sites until bleeding stops, usually 5-10 min for vein and 10-20 min for artery. Apply pressure dressing over arterial puncture sites.
- Avoid giving IM injections.
- Monitor Hgb and Hct for ↓ in values or failure to see appropriate ↑ after transfusion.
- Numerous incompatibilities possible with heparin, and many drug-drug interactions possible with warfarin. Review of drug profile is recommended.
- Avoid use of any drug that contains aspirin or other nonsteroidal antiinflammatory drug; they are platelet aggregation inhibitors and can prolong bleeding.
- If patient is restless and combative, provide a safe environment: pad side rails, restrain as necessary to prevent falls, and use extreme care when moving to avoid bumping of extremities into side rails.

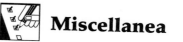

Miscellanea

CONSULT MD FOR

- Deteriorating ABGs: PaO_2 ≤60 mm Hg, $PaCO_2$ >45 or <35 mm Hg, pH >7.45 or <7.35
- Respiratory distress: dyspnea, anxiety, cyanosis
- PT, PTT, INR: values outside desired range

RELATED TOPICS

- Coronary thrombolysis
- Heart failure, right ventricular
- Pulmonary hypertension

ABBREVIATIONS

FFP: Fresh frozen plasma
INR: International normalized ratio
P(A-a)o2: Alveolar-arterial oxygen tension difference

REFERENCES

Apple S: New trends in thrombolytic therapy, *RN* 59(1): 30-35, 1996.

Currie DL: Pulmonary embolism: diagnosis and management, *Crit Care Nurs Q* 13(2): 41-49, 1990.

Henschke C, Mateescu I, Yankelevitz D: Changing practice patterns in the workup of pulmonary embolism, *Chest* 107(4): 940-945, 1995.

Howard C: Pulmonary dysfunctions. In Swearingen PL, Keen JH (eds): *Manual of critical care nursing*, ed 3, St Louis, 1995, Mosby.

Parenti C: Pulmonary embolism after coronary artery bypass surgery, *Crit Care Nurs Q* 17(3): 48-50, 1994.

Author: **Cheri A. Goll**

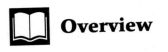 # Overview

PATHOPHYSIOLOGY

Defined as MPAP >20 mm Hg. No known cause for primary pulmonary hypertension, which is rare; but several causes identified for secondary pulmonary hypertension (see **HISTORY/RISK FACTORS,** below).

Rising PAP ↑ PVR, which causes standby vessels to open and capillaries to distend to accommodate ↑ blood flow. Although these responses ↓ PVR initially, the system eventually fails if ↑ pressure persists as a result of vasoconstriction that accompanies chronic alveolar hypoxia. The lower the pulmonary Pao_2, the more severe the vasoconstriction. Changes are reversible after resolution of hypoxia; however, with chronic hypoxia, pulmonary vasculature undergoes permanent thickening and narrowing. In addition, polycythemia develops, causing blood viscosity to ↑, which in turn causes ↑ PVR. RV dilatation and hypertrophy result in cor pulmonale or RV heart failure.

HISTORY/RISK FACTORS

- Obstruction to pulmonary venous outflow (congenital and acquired): eg, mitral valve disease, LV failure, stenosis of large pulmonary veins
- Chronic alveolar hypoxia: eg, COPD, sleep apnea, obesity
- Diffuse pulmonary fibrosis: eg, SLE, sarcoidosis
- Congenital heart disease with left-to-right shunt or ↓ pulmonary blood flow: eg, ventricular or atrial septal defect
- Systemic hypoxia: high-altitude hypoxia, V/Q disorders
- Local hypoxia: pulmonary embolism, thrombosis

CLINICAL PRESENTATION

Early: Hyperventilation, vague chest discomfort
Late: Tachypnea, dyspnea, orthopnea, chest congestion

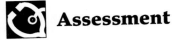 # Assessment

PHYSICAL ASSESSMENT

Resp: Cyanosis of lips, nail beds; distant breath sounds; basilar crackles
CV: Edema of hands and feet, anasarca (generalized, massive edema), JVD, RV heave (visible left parasternal systolic lift), accentuated pulmonary component of the second heart sound, RV diastolic gallop, pulmonary ejection click

VITAL SIGNS/HEMODYNAMICS

RR: ↑
HR: ↑
BP: Nl; ↓ if severe
Temp: Nl
PAP/MPAP: ↑ (>20 mm Hg with ↑ PVR)
CO: ↓
ECG: May show sinus tachycardia, right axis deviation, right bundle branch block, enlarged P waves

LABORATORY STUDIES

ABGs: Generally, Pao_2 <60 mm Hg; $Paco_2$ wnl (35-45 mm Hg). If cause is COPD, $Paco_2$ may be ↑.
RBC/Hct Values: ↑

IMAGING

Chest X-ray: May confirm RV dilatation or hypertrophy, enlarged PA.
Echocardiogram: May reveal enlarged right atrium and right ventricle, ↓ wall motion, pulmonic valve malfunction (midsystolic closure or delayed opening).
Pulmonary Angiography/Perfusion Scans: To r/o embolic event as underlying cause.

DIAGNOSTIC PROCEDURES

Pulmonary Function Tests: To diagnose, evaluate underlying pathologic condition.
Open Lung Biopsy: Avoided unless necessary to establish type of pulmonary vascular disease and extent of disease process.

Collaborative Management

O_2: Elimination of hypoxia to ↓ PVR and RV afterload.
Pharmacotherapy
Diuretics: ↓ circulating volume, PAP, and RV workload.
Digitalis: Generally used only with biventricular failure. Otherwise, inotropic effects can ↑ RV CO and PVR.
Bronchodilators (eg, aminophylline, isoproterenol, terbutaline): Act as afterload reducers by ↓ PVR and ↑ RV ejection fraction. May ↓ hypoxic vasoconstriction of pulmonary vascular bed.
Vasodilators (eg, nitrates, hydralazine, calcium channel blockers): Reverse pulmonary vasoconstriction, which ↓ RV afterload and enhances pulmonary blood flow.
Hemodynamic Monitoring: To differentiate or quantify contribution of LV or RV failure and measure response to pharmacotherapy.

PATIENT-FAMILY TEACHING

- Purpose, expected results, anticipated sensations for nursing/medical interventions
- Progressive muscle relaxation technique
- Relationship between activity, anxiety, and ↑ O_2 demands
- Medications: drug name, purpose, dosage, schedule, precautions, drug-drug and food-drug interactions, potential side effects

Nursing Diagnoses/Interventions

Impaired gas exchange r/t alveolar-capillary membrane changes secondary to fluid accumulation in lung

Desired outcome: Within 12 h of treatment, patient has adequate gas exchange: $Pao_2 \geq 60-80$ mm Hg and $Paco_2 \leq 45$ mm Hg. Within 3 days RR ≤ 20 breaths/min with eupnea, breath sounds clear/bilaterally equal, orientation $\times$ 3.

- Auscultate lung fields. Note type and extent of adventitious breath sounds.
- Monitor ABGs/Spo_2. Progressive hypoxemia may require $\uparrow$ concentrations O_2 or mechanical ventilation.
- Assess for SOB, tachypnea, use of accessory muscles, nasal flaring, grunting, restlessness, anxiety.
- Place in semi-Fowler's position to optimize lung expansion and $\downarrow$ WOB.
- With PEEP therapy, be aware that alveoli collapse when PEEP removed. O_2 levels achieved before suctioning will not be attained immediately after PEEP reinstituted because the effect PEEP exerts on alveoli is not instantaneous. To prevent dramatic $\downarrow$ in Pao_2 with suctioning, use PEEP adapter on manual resuscitator. In-line suction device may prevent hypoxia associated with suctioning.
- Provide rest periods between activities to $\downarrow$ O_2 demands.
- Explain all procedures; provide emotional support to $\downarrow$ anxiety, which can contribute to O_2 consumption.

Fluid volume excess r/t compromised regulatory mechanism secondary to $\downarrow$ cardiac output

Desired outcome: Within 24 h of treatment, patient becomes normovolemic: absence of adventitious lung sounds, $\downarrow$ peripheral edema, $\uparrow$ UO, weight loss, SVR ≤ 1200 dynes/sec/cm^{-5}, and CO ≥ 4 L/min.

- Auscultate lung fields for crackles and rhonchi or other adventitious sounds.
- Monitor I&O closely. Report positive fluid state or UO $\downarrow$ to <0.5 mg/kg/h.
- Weigh patient qd; report weight $\uparrow$ >1 kg/24 h.
- Assess for worsening heart failure: $\uparrow$ pedal edema, $\uparrow$ JVD, S_3 heart sound or new murmur, dysrhythmias.
- Monitor hemodynamic status q1-2h and prn. Note response to drug therapy and to indicators of need for more aggressive therapy, including $\uparrow$ MPAP and $\downarrow$ CO.
- Administer diuretics (furosemide) and vasodilators (nitroprusside) as prescribed.
- Limit oral fluids; offer ice chips or frozen juice pops to $\downarrow$ thirst and discomfort of dry mouth.
- Maintain bed rest restrictions to facilitate fluid movement from interstitial spaces in dependent extremities to intravascular spaces.

Activity intolerance r/t imbalance between O_2 supply and demand secondary to $\downarrow$ alveolar O_2 supply and $\uparrow$ metabolic O_2 demands as a result of $\downarrow$ WOB

Desired outcome: Within 24-48 h of treatment initiation, patient verbalizes $\downarrow$ in fatigue and associated symptoms.

- Group procedures and activities to provide frequent rest periods (optimally, $\geq 90-120$ min).
- $\downarrow$ metabolic demands for O_2 by limiting or pacing activities and procedures.
- Teach progressive muscle relaxation technique. Encourage significant others to coach patient in using this technique.
- If patient restless, which $\uparrow$ O_2 demand, ascertain cause of restlessness, eg, hypoxemia or anxiety.
- Explain procedures and offer support to $\downarrow$ fear and anxiety, which can $\uparrow$ O_2 demands.
- Schedule rest times after meals to avoid competition for O_2 supply during digestion.
- Monitor Spo_2 during activity to evaluate limits of activity and recommend optimal positions for oxygenation.
- Assess temp q2-4h. Provide treatment to $\downarrow$ temp and thus $\downarrow$ O_2 demands.

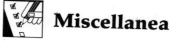

Miscellanea

CONSULT MD FOR

- Hypoxemia: $Spo_2 \leq 90\%$, $Pao_2 \leq 80$ mm Hg
- MPAP ≥ 20 mm Hg
- PVR ≥ 100 dynes/sec/cm^{-5}
- Intake > output or >1 kg weight gain/24 h

RELATED TOPICS

- Heart failure, right ventricular
- Hemodynamic monitoring
- Mechanical ventilation
- Psychosocial needs, patient
- Respiratory failure, acute

REFERENCES

Howard C: Respiratory dysfunctions. In Swearingen PL, Keen JH (eds): *Manual of critical care nursing*, ed 3, St Louis, 1995, Mosby.

Rubin LJ: Pulmonary hypertension and cor pulmonae. In Bone RC (ed): *Pulmonary and critical care medicine*, vol 2, St Louis, 1995, Mosby.

Thompson B, Hales C: Hypoxic pulmonary hypertension: acute and chronic, *Heart Lung* 15(5): 457-465, 1986.

Wollschlager C, Khan FA: Secondary pulmonary hypertension: clinical features, *Heart Lung* 15(4): 336-340, 1986.

Author: **Cheri A. Goll**

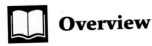 **Overview**

PATHOPHYSIOLOGY

Infection of renal parenchyma and pelvis; usually occurs secondary to UTI. Infecting organism may be a type of fecal flora (eg, *Escherichia* or *Klebsiella*) or nl flora from peri-urethral skin (eg, *Staphylococcus saprophyticus*). Recurrent infections common; CRF is a rare complication.

HISTORY/RISK FACTORS

- UTI or urinary obstruction
- Recent urologic procedure
- Pregnancy
- Female gender
- Advanced age

CLINICAL PRESENTATION

Fever, chills, flank pain, nausea, vomiting, malaise, frequency and urgency of urination, dysuria, cloudy and foul-smelling urine, nocturia

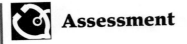 **Assessment**

PHYSICAL ASSESSMENT

Tender, enlarged kidneys; abdominal rigidity; CVA tenderness

VITAL SIGNS/HEMODYNAMICS

RR: ↑
HR: ↑
BP: Nl; ↓ if urosepsis present
Temp: ↑
Hemodynamics: May reflect early septic shock: ↑ CO, ↓ SVR. CVP/PAWP may be ↓ because of actual or relative hypovolemia.

LABORATORY STUDIES

Unless anatomic or preexisting renal disease present, renal function should remain nl.
Urine Culture: Should be positive for causative organism. Asymptomatic bacteriuria common in elders.
Urinalysis: Usually reveals WBCs, WBC casts, RBCs, bacteria.
Blood Culture: Positive for causative organism in hematogenous infection or when bacteremia develops. Obtained from patients who appear septic or are hypotensive.
CBC: Reveals ↑ WBCs.

IMAGING

IVP or Retrograde Pyelogram: Done with recurrent episodes or when obstruction suspected.

Collaborative Management

PHARMACOTHERAPY

Antibiotics: Initially parenteral, then oral. Low-dose antimicrobial prophylaxis may be indicated for women or children with recurrent UTI.
IV/Oral Fluids: To ensure adequate hydration and UO.
Acetaminophen: To control fever and treat discomfort.
Surgical Intervention: May be necessary for obstructive uropathy or infected stones.

PATIENT-FAMILY TEACHING

- Importance of taking medications for prescribed length of time, even if feeling "well"
- Necessity of reporting these S&S of UTI: urgency, frequency, dysuria, flank pain, cloudy or foul-smelling urine, fever
- Importance of perineal hygiene for female patients and necessity of wiping from front to back, wearing undergarments with cotton crotch, and voiding before and after intercourse
- Importance of emptying bladder at least q3-4h and once during the night to help prevent UTI caused by residual urine
- Necessity of maintaining fluid intake of ≥2-3 L/day and drinking fruit juices (cranberry, plum, prune) that leave an acid ash in urine
- Importance of continued medical follow-up because of high incidence of recurrence

Nursing Diagnoses/Interventions

Pain r/t dysuria secondary to infection

Desired outcomes: Within 1 h of intervention, subjective perception of discomfort ↓, as documented by pain scale. Objective indicators, such as grimacing, are ↓/absent.

- Monitor for CVA pain and tenderness, abdominal pain, dysuria. Devise pain scale with patient, rating pain from 0 (absent) to 10 (severe). Administer analgesics, and document their effectiveness, using pain scale.
- If not contraindicated, ↑ fluid intake to help relieve dysuria.
- As appropriate, assist with repositioning if it is effective in relieving discomfort.
- Use nonpharmacologic interventions when possible (eg, relaxation techniques, guided imagery, distraction).

Risk for infection (or its recurrence) r/t chronic disease process

Desired outcomes: Patient infection free: normothermia; urine clear and of nl odor; HR ≤100 bpm; BP ≥90/60 mm Hg (or wnl for patient); absence of flank, CVA, labial pain; absence of dysuria, urgency, frequency. Within 24-h period before hospital discharge, patient verbalizes knowledge about S&S of infection and importance of reporting them promptly if they occur.

- Monitor temp at least q4h. Be alert for temp >38° C (100° F). Monitor for flank, CVA, and labial pain; foul-smelling or cloudy urine; malaise; headache; and frequency and urgency of urination. Teach these S&S to patient and stress importance of reporting them promptly.
- Monitor BP and HR. Check for hypotension and tachycardia, which can signal sepsis and bacteremic shock.
- Monitor for ↓ SVR and ↑ CO, which can be indicators of early septic shock.
- Give antibiotics precisely as scheduled. Draw prescribed antibiotic serum levels at correct times to ensure reliable results. Most antibiotics are measured at peak (30-60 min after infusion) and trough (30-60 min before next dose) levels.
- Use urinary catheters only when mandatory. Use meticulous sterile technique when inserting, irrigating, or obtaining specimens. Provide perineal care qd. For indwelling catheters, maintain unobstructed flow, and keep urinary collection container below bladder level to prevent urine reflux. Tape catheter to thigh or abdomen to ↓ meatal irritation.
- Treat fever with prescribed antipyretics and tepid baths as needed.
- Stress importance of emptying bladder at least q3-4h and once during the night to help prevent UTI caused by residual urine.

Fluid volume deficit r/t ↓ intake secondary to anorexia or active loss secondary to vomiting and diaphoresis

Desired outcomes: Following treatment, patient normovolemic: balanced I&O, stable weight, UO ≥30-60 ml/h, and BP and HR wnl for patient. Within 24 h of admission, patient verbalizes knowledge about importance of fluid intake of ≥2-3 L/day.

- Maintain adequate fluid intake to avoid fluid volume deficit. Intake of ≥2-3 L/day is usually indicated; however, appropriate amount depends on output, which includes gastric, fecal, urinary, sensible, and insensible losses.
- Monitor I&O and daily weight as indicators of hydration status.
- Report indicators of volume deficit: poor skin turgor, thirst, dry mucous membranes, tachycardia, orthostatic hypotension.

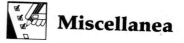

Miscellanea

CONSULT MD FOR

- Temp ≥38° C (100° F)
- S&S of possible urosepsis: ↓ BP, ↑ HR, ↓ SVR, ↑ CO
- Unrelieved or increasing flank pain

RELATED TOPICS

- Antimicrobial therapy
- Elder care
- Hypovolemia
- Shock, septic

ABBREVIATIONS

CVA: Costovertebral angle
UTI: Urinary tract infection

REFERENCES

Horne MM: Renal disorders and renal failure. In Swearingen PL: *Manual of medical-surgical nursing care,* ed 3, St Louis, 1994, Mosby.

Meares EM: Nonspecific infections of the genitourinary tract. In Tanagho EA, McAninch JW (eds): *Smith's general urology,* ed 14, Norwalk, Conn, 1995, Appleton & Lange.

Rose DB, Rennke HG: *Renal pathophysiology–the essentials,* Baltimore, 1994, Williams & Wilkins.

Author: **Mima M. Horne**

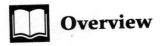 **Overview**

PATHOPHYSIOLOGY

Characterized by abrupt deterioration of renal function, resulting in accumulation of metabolic wastes, fluids, and electrolytes, usually accompanied by marked ↓ in UO. Generally, there are three identifiable phases.

First Phase: Characterized by oliguria, ↓ in 24-h UO to ≤400 ml; lasts ≈7-14 days.

Diuretic Phase: Evidenced initially by doubling of UO from previous 24-h total, producing as much as 3-5 L of urine in 24 h.

Recovery Phase: Marked by return to nl 24-h volume; may take 6 mo to 1 yr to return to baseline functional status.

Numerous fluid, electrolyte, and acid-base disorders occur with ARF, including hypervolemia, hyperkalemia, hyperphosphatemia, hypocalcemia, and metabolic acidosis.

HISTORY/RISK FACTORS

Prerenal (↓ renal perfusion)
- Hypovolemia
- Hepatorenal syndrome
- Edema-forming conditions
- Renal vascular disorders
- Hypertension

Intrarenal (parenchymal damage; ATN)
- Nephrotoxic agents
- Infection: gram-negative sepsis, pancreatitis, peritonitis
- Transfusion reaction
- Rhabdomyolysis with myoglobinuria
- Glomerular diseases
- Ischemic injury

Postrenal (obstructive)
- Calculi
- Tumor
- Benign prostatic hypertrophy
- Blood clots

CLINICAL PRESENTATION

Prerenal: Oliguria, ↑ specific gravity/osmolality, ↑ plasma BUN/creatinine ratio (20:1)

Intrarenal: Oliguric or nonoliguric, ↓ specific gravity/osmolality, presence of RBC casts and cellular debris in urine, ↓ plasma BUN/creatinine ratio (10:1)

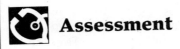 **Assessment**

PHYSICAL ASSESSMENT

Fluid Volume Excess: Peripheral edema, JVD, S_3 and S_4 gallops, crackles, hyperventilation, ↑ BP, oliguria

Fluid Volume Deficit: ↓ BP, poor skin turgor, flushed skin, dry mucous membranes, oliguria

Electrolyte Imbalances: Dysrhythmias, altered mental status, GI disturbances, neuromuscular dysfunction

Metabolic Acidosis: Weakness, disorientation, SOB, Kussmaul's respirations, CNS depression

Uremic Manifestations: Uremic frost (if severe); bleeding tendencies, purpura; fatigue and pallor; ↑ BP, heart failure, JVD, pericarditis; anorexia, nausea, vomiting, diarrhea; behavioral changes; ↓ wound healing; ↑ susceptibility to infection

VITAL SIGNS/HEMODYNAMICS

RR: ↑

HR: ↑

BP: ↑

Temp: Nl or ↑ with infection

CVP/PAWP: ↑ if oliguric; ↓ or nl if nonoliguric

SVR: ↑

CO: ↓ with heart failure or hypovolemia

ECG: If *hyperkalemic* (more likely at K^+ levels >6.5 mEq/L): tall, peaked T waves, loss of P waves, prolonged PR interval, widened QRS, cardiac arrest possible. If *hypokalemic* (more likely at K^+ <3 mEq/L): prolonged PR interval, flattened or inverted T waves, depressed ST segment, presence of U wave, ventricular dysrhythmias possible.

LABORATORY STUDIES

Chemistries: BUN, creatinine, and uric acid levels ↑ in ARF, as well as K^+, PO_4^{3-}, and possibly Mg^{2+}.

Creatinine Clearance: Most reliable estimation of GFR; usually <50 ml/min.

Urinalysis: Large amounts of protein and many RBC casts common: wnl when causes are prerenal.

Urinary Sodium: If prerenal, <10 mEq/L; if intrarenal, >20 mEq/L.

Hematology: Hct may be low as result of ARF; Hct and Hgb will fall steadily if bleeding or hemodilution present. PT, PTT may be ↑ because of ↓ platelet adhesiveness.

ABGs: Metabolic acidosis (low $Paco_2$ and plasma pH).

IMAGING

Ultrasonography: Identifies hydronephrosis, fluid collection, masses.

IVP: To diagnose partial or complete obstruction.

Renal Scan: Provides information about renal perfusion.

Renal Angiography and Venography: Detects presence/absence of thrombotic or stenotic lesions.

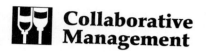
Collaborative Management

PRERENAL

Volume Replacement: Replacement solutions include free water plus electrolytes lost through urine, wounds, drainage tubes, diarrhea, vomiting. Losses replaced on volume-for-volume basis.

Diuretics: Furosemide (Lasix) and ethacrynic acid (Edecrin) may be used, after adequate hydration, to ↑ UO or prevent oliguria. Osmotic diuretics, such as mannitol, used to ↑ intravascular volume, promote RBF, and stimulate UO.

Dopamine: Low doses, usually ≤2 μg/kg/min, to stimulate dopaminergic receptors, encourage renal vasodilatation, and promote RBF.

INTRARENAL

Removal of Toxic Agent: Eg, aminoglycosides, dye load, chemicals.

Dialytic Therapy: Hemodialysis, PD, CAVH, CVVH.

Nutrition: Diet high in carbohydrates, low in sodium, low in potassium if retaining potassium, low in protein to minimize ↑ in azotemia.

Blood Transfusions: PRBCs given for anemia, which may be caused by ↓ erythropoietin, GI bleeding from mucosal ulceration, shortened life of RBCs.

Pharmacotherapy

Antihypertensives: Often necessary.

Phosphate binders: Aluminum hydroxide, calcium carbonate antacids control hyperphosphatemia; given with meals.

Sodium bicarbonate: Controls metabolic acidosis and promotes shift of K^+ back into cells.

Sodium polystyrene sulfonate (Kayexalate): Exchanges sodium for potassium in GI tract.

Water-soluble vitamin supplements: To replace vitamins removed during dialysis.

Drug dosage modification: Required for drugs excreted primarily by kidneys. Nephrotoxic drugs avoided.

POSTRENAL

Relief of Obstruction

Monitoring fluid and electrolyte balance: Postobstructive diuresis may result in hypovolemia, hyponatremia, hypokalemia, hypocalcemia, and hypomagnesemia.

PATIENT-FAMILY TEACHING

- S&S of biochemical alterations: weakness, paresthesias, HR <60 bpm, dry mucous membranes, confusion, abdominal cramps, diarrhea, vomiting.
- Lists of foods high in potassium, sodium, phosphorus, and magnesium, which are either added or avoided when planning meals. In addition, provide list of medications that contain magnesium, which should not be taken without physician approval.
- Importance of consuming only prescribed amount of protein and avoiding exposure to infection. Reinforce that patient should consume prescribed amount of carbohydrates and limit strenuous activity, which will spare protein and thus ↓ potassium release.
- Necessity of reporting ↑ in temp or other signs of infection.
- Importance of taking vitamins, mineral supplements, and medications exactly as prescribed.
- Relationship between calcium and phosphate levels. Emphasize that good control may help ↓ itching and prevent problems with bone disease.
- Importance of maintaining prescribed dialysis schedule and follow-up appointments.
- Use of lotions and oils to lubricate skin and relieve drying and cracking.

Nursing Diagnoses/Interventions

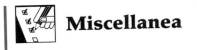 ## Miscellanea

Fluid volume excess r/t compromised regulatory mechanism secondary to ARF

Desired outcome: Within 24-48 h of onset, patient becomes normovolemic: balanced I&O, UO ≥0.5 ml/kg/h, body weight and BP wnl for patient, CVP 2-6 mm Hg, HR 60-100 bpm, and absence of S&S of fluid overload.

Note: Although patient is retaining sodium, sodium level may be wnl or ↓ because of dilutional effect of fluid overload.

- Document I&O qh. Replace output ml for ml at intervals of 4-8 h.
- Weigh patient qd.
- Assess for fluid volume overload: crackles, JVD, tachycardia, pericardial friction rub, gallop, ↑ BP, ↑ CVP/PAWP, or SOB.
- Assess for peripheral, sacral, or periorbital edema.
- Restrict total fluid intake to 1200-1500 ml/24 h, or as prescribed.
- If TPN delivered, total fluid intake may be >2000 ml/day. Ultrafiltration with dialysis or CAVH/CVVH may be necessary to maintain fluid balance.
- If patient retaining sodium, restrict sodium-containing foods; avoid sodium-containing IV diluents and medications, eg, sodium penicillin.

Fluid volume deficit r/t active loss secondary to diuresis, vomiting, diarrhea, and hemorrhage; or r/t failure of regulatory mechanism with fluid shift to interstitial compartments

Desired outcomes: Within 24 h of this diagnosis, patient becomes normovolemic: balanced I&O; UO ≥0.5 ml/kg/h with specific gravity of 1.010-1.020; CVP 2-6 mm Hg; HR 60-100 bpm; BP wnl for patient; and absence of S&S of hypovolemia. Weight stabilizes within 2-3 days.

- Weigh patient qd.
- Monitor I&O qh. 24-h intake should exceed output by 0.5-1 L.
- Be alert for excessive losses from vomiting, diarrhea, wound drainage, or diuresis.
- Observe for S&S of hypovolemia: poor skin turgor, dry and sticky mucous membranes, thirst, hypotension, tachycardia, and ↓ CVP.
- Encourage oral fluids if allowed. Frequently check IV fluid rates to ensure accurate administration.
- Monitor Hgb, Hct, and BUN levels. Expect baseline Hct in the range of 20%-30% because of the anemia that occurs with ARF. If GI bleeding present, BUN will ↑ without concomitant ↑ in serum creatinine.
- To minimize risk of bleeding, use small-gauge needles, minimize blood drawing, and use electric razors and soft-bristled toothbrushes. Limit invasive procedures as much as possible. If possible, avoid injections for 1 h after hemodialysis. Apply gentle pressure to injection sites for at least 2-3 min.
- Inspect gums, mouth, nose, skin, and perianal and vaginal areas q8h for bleeding. Inspect hemodialysis insertion and peritoneal access sites for bleeding.

Altered nutrition: Less than body requirements r/t catabolic state and excessive metabolic needs secondary to ARF; and r/t anorexia and psychologic aversion to dietary restrictions

Desired outcomes: Within 72 h, patient has adequate nutrition: caloric intake ranging from 35-45 cal/kg of nl body weight and protein intake consisting of 50%-75% of high-biologic-value proteins.

CONSULT MD FOR
- UO <0.5 ml/kg/h
- Weight gain/loss >0.5-1.5 kg/24 h
- Temp >38.22° C (100.8° F)
- S&S of infection: cloudy or blood-tinged peritoneal dialysate return, cloudy and foul-smelling urine, foul-smelling wound exudate, purulent drainage from any catheter site, foul-smelling and watery stools, foul-smelling vaginal discharge, purulent sputum, ↑ WBCs
- New-onset or worsening of electrolyte imbalances:

  Hyperkalemia (oliguric phase): Muscle weakness, irritability, paresthesias, peaked T waves, widened QRS

  Hypokalemia (diuretic phase): Lethargy; muscle softness, flabbiness; paresthesias; flattened or inverted T waves, presence of U wave

  Hypernatremia: Fatigue, restlessness, agitation, dry mucous membranes, hot and flushed skin

  Hyponatremia: Orthostasis, apprehension, personality changes, cold and clammy skin

  Hypocalcemia: Neuromuscular irritability, tonic muscle spasms, circumoral numbness

  Hypermagnesemia: Drowsiness, lethargy, diaphoresis, flushing, hypoventilation, ↓ HR, ↓ BP, ↓ DTRs

  Metabolic acidosis: Confusion, weakness, Kussmaul's respirations

  Uremia: Confusion, lethargy, itching, metallic taste, muscle twitching

- Assess and document nutrient intake every shift.
- Use cooling blanket or antipyretic agents to control fever, which ↑ metabolic needs.
- Encourage intake of high-biologic-value protein (eg, eggs, meat, fowl, milk, fish), which contains more essential amino acids necessary for cell building.
- Encourage high-caloric foods, which include honey, hard candy, gumdrops, sherbet.
- Restrict high-potassium foods. If oliguria present, sodium intake may be restricted. If diuresis present, sodium intake may be encouraged.
- Replace calcium orally (eg, with dairy products) or IV, and administer phosphate binders as prescribed.
- If patient anorexic or nauseated, provide small, frequent meals; eliminate any noxious odors. As indicated, administer antiemetic ½ h before meals.

Risk for infection r/t inadequate secondary defenses as a result of immunocompromised state associated with ARF; and r/t multiple invasive procedures

Desired outcome: At time of discharge from ICU, patient free of infection: normothermia, negative culture results of dialysate and body secretions, and WBCs ≤11,000/μl.

Note: After initial insult, infection is primary cause of death in ARF.

- Monitor temp q2-4h and q2h if it is >38° C (101° F). Because ARF may be accompanied by hypothermia, even slight ↑ in temp of 1°-2° may be significant.
- Uremia retards wound healing; therefore it is important that all wounds (including scratches resulting from pruritus) be assessed for infection. Send any suspicious fluid or drainage for C&S.
- Monitor WBCs for ↑.
- Be aware that catabolism of protein, which occurs with infection, causes release of K⁺ from the tissues. Monitor K⁺ levels.
- Avoid indwelling urinary catheter in patients with oliguria and anuria to ↓ risk of infection.
- Provide oral hygiene q2h.
- Reposition patient q2-4h. Provide skin care using non-alcohol-containing, mild lotions at least q8h.
- Encourage deep-breathing exercises and coughing q2-4h.

Altered protection r/t neurosensory changes secondary to electrolyte imbalance, metabolic acidosis, and uremia

Desired outcomes: Within 48-72 h of onset, patient verbalizes orientation × 3 and maintains nl mobility.

- Use simple and direct communication efforts because of ↓ attention level.
- To alleviate unpleasant metallic taste caused by uremia, provide frequent oral hygiene, using soft-bristled brushes. If appropriate, provide chewing gum or hard candy.
- Encourage isometric exercises and short walks to help maintain muscle strength and tone.
- ↓ environmental stimuli, and employ a calm, reassuring manner.
- Encourage establishment of sleep/rest patterns.

RELATED TOPICS
- Acute tubular necrosis: nonoliguric
- Acute tubular necrosis: oliguric
- Continuous arteriovenous hemofiltration/Continuous venovenous hemofiltration
- Hemodialysis
- Hyperkalemia
- Hyperphosphatemia
- Hypocalcemia
- Metabolic acidosis, acute
- Peritoneal dialysis

ABBREVIATIONS
CAVH: Continuous arteriovenous hemofiltration
CVVH: Continuous venovenous hemofiltration
DTR: Deep tendon reflex
GFR: Glomerular filtration rate
PD: Peritoneal dialysis
PRBCs: Packed red blood cells
RBF: Renal blood flow

REFERENCES
Baer CL, Lancaster LE: Acute renal failure, *Crit Care Nurs Q* 14(4): 1-21, 1992.

Stark JL: Acute renal failure in trauma: current perspectives, *Crit Care Nurs Q* 16(4): 49-60, 1994.

Fiehrer P: Nephrology nurse presents with acute cortical necrosis, *ANNA J* 21(6): 366-367, 1994.

Weiskittel PD: Renal-urinary dysfunctions. In Swearingen PL, Keen JH (eds): *Manual of critical care nursing*, ed 3, St Louis, 1995, Mosby.

Author: **Patricia D. Weiskittel**

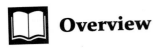 **Overview**

PATHOPHYSIOLOGY

Progressive, irreversible loss of kidney function that develops over days to yrs. Eventually can progress to ESRD, at which time renal replacement therapy (dialysis or transplantation) is required to sustain life. Retention of metabolic wastes and accompanying fluid and electrolyte imbalances adversely affect all body systems. Alterations in neuromuscular, CV, and GI function common. Renal osteodystrophy is an early and frequent complication. Collective manifestations of CRF are termed *uremia*.

HISTORY/RISK FACTORS

- Glomerulonephritis, polycystic kidney disease
- DM, hypertension
- SLE, chronic pyelonephritis
- Interstitial nephritis

CLINICAL PRESENTATION

All body systems adversely affected by uremia. S&S include weakness, malaise, anorexia, dry and discolored skin, peripheral neuropathy, irritability, clouded thinking, ammonia odor to breath.

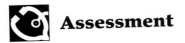 **Assessment**

PHYSICAL ASSESSMENT

Fluid Volume Abnormalities: Crackles, hypertension, edema, oliguria, anuria
Electrolyte Disturbances: Muscle weakness, dysrhythmias, pruritus, tetany
Metabolic Acidosis: Deep respirations, lethargy, headache
Anemia: Weakness, fatigue, SOB
Potential Acute Complications
Heart failure: Crackles, dyspnea, orthopnea
Pericarditis: Chest pain, SOB
Cardiac tamponade: Hypotension, distant heart sounds, pulsus paradoxus (exaggerated inspiratory drop in SBP)

VITAL SIGNS/HEMODYNAMICS

RR: ↑ rate and depth
HR: ↑ if fluid overload or anemia present
BP: ↑ because of fluid overload
Temp: Nl
CVP/PAP: ↑ because of fluid overload
SVR: Often ↑ because of hypertension associated with fluid overload, excessive renin secretion, arteriosclerosis

LABORATORY STUDIES

BUN/Serum Creatinine: Both ↑. Nonrenal problems, such as dehydration or GI bleeding, also can ↑ BUN, but with less effect on creatinine.
Creatinine Clearance: Measures kidneys' ability to clear the blood of creatinine and approximates the GFR. Creatinine clearance ↓ as renal function ↓. Dialysis usually begun when creatinine clearance <10 ml/min. Normally ↓ in elders.
Electrolytes: To determine presence of hyperkalemia, hypocalcemia, hypermagnesemia, hyperphosphatemia.

IMAGING

KUB X-ray: Documents presence of two kidneys, changes in size or shape, some forms of obstruction.
IVP, Renal Ultrasound, Renal Scan (using radionuclides), CT Scan: Additional tests for determining cause of renal insufficiency. Once ESRD occurs, these tests not performed.
Chest, Hand X-rays: To assess for development of heart failure, renal osteodystrophy.

DIAGNOSTIC PROCEDURES

Nerve Conduction Velocity Test: To assess for development/progression of uremic neuropathy.

Collaborative Management

Before ESRD, medical management aimed at slowing progression of CRF and avoiding complications. After ESRD, management aimed at alleviating uremic symptoms and providing dialysis or renal transplantation.
Diet: Carbohydrates ↑ in protein-restricted patients to ensure adequate caloric intake and prevent catabolism. Na limited to prevent thirst and fluid retention. K limited because of kidneys' inability to excrete excess K^+, and protein limited to minimize retention of nitrogenous wastes. Before ESRD, protein restriction may help slow CRF progression. Protein should be of high-biologic value only.
Fluid Restriction: For patients at risk for fluid volume excess. Fluid weight gain limited to 3%-4% of individual's "dry" weight.
Pharmacotherapy: Medications excreted primarily by the kidneys require modification of dosage or frequency. Dialyzable medications may need to be ↑ or held and given postdialysis.
Aluminum hydroxide, calcium carbonate, calcium acetate: To control hyperphosphatemia.

Antihypertensives: To control BP.
Multivitamins and folic acid: Given when dietary restrictions or dialysis in use (water-soluble vitamins are lost during dialysis).
Anabolic steroids, parenteral iron, ferrous sulfate, recombinant human erythropoietin (Epogen): To treat anemia.
Diphenhydramine: To treat pruritus, which is common in uremic patients, causing frequent and intense scratching.
Sodium bicarbonate: To treat metabolic acidosis.
Vitamin D preparations, calcium supplements: To treat hypocalcemia and prevent bone disease.
Deferoxamine: To treat iron or aluminum toxicity.
Packed Cells: To treat severe or symptomatic anemia. Anemia is usually proportional to the degree of azotemia. Hct can be ≤20%, but usually stabilizes at around 20%-25%. Typically transfusion does not occur unless Hct ≤20% or anemia is poorly tolerated.
Prevention of Complications: Volume depletion, hypotension, use of radiopaque contrast medium, nephrotoxic substances avoided.
Renal Transplantation or Dialysis: When above therapies inadequate to control uremia and prevent complications.

PATIENT-FAMILY TEACHING

- Importance of getting BP checked at frequent intervals and adhering to prescribed antihypertensive therapy, since control of hypertension may slow progression of chronic renal insufficiency
- Medications: drug name, purpose, dosage, schedule, precautions, drug-drug and food-drug interactions, and potential side effects
- Necessity of reading all OTC labels for potassium, sodium, phosphorus, or magnesium content
- Diet, including fact sheet listing foods to be restricted or limited
- Care and observation of dialysis access site if patient has one
- S&S that necessitate medical attention: irregular pulse, fever, unusual SOB or edema, sudden change in UO, unusual muscle weakness
- Need for continued medical follow-up; confirm date and time of next appointment
- Importance of avoiding infections and seeking treatment promptly should one develop; S&S of frequently encountered infections

Nursing Diagnoses/Interventions

Altered protection r/t neurosensory, MS, and CV changes secondary to electrolyte and acid-base imbalances

Desired outcomes: Following successful treatment, patient verbalizes orientation × 3 and remains free of injury caused by neurosensory, MS, and CV disturbances.

- Assess for and alert patient to indicators of the following:

  Hyperkalemia: Muscle cramps, dysrhythmias, muscle weakness, peaked T waves on ECG

  Hypocalcemia: Neuromuscular irritability and paresthesias

  Hyperphosphatemia: Soft tissue calcifications

  Uremia: Anorexia, nausea, metallic taste in the mouth, irritability, confusion, lethargy, restlessness, itching

  Metabolic acidosis: Rapid, deep respirations; confusion

- Depending on existing renal function, limit Na to prevent thirst and fluid retention.
- Avoid salt substitutes and "light" salts, which contain KCl, and K-containing medications.
- If multiple blood transfusions necessary, observe for indicators of hyperkalemia because old banked blood may contain as much as 30 mEq/L of K. Use fresh PRBCs when possible.
- Minimize tissue catabolism by controlling fevers, maintaining adequate nutritional intake (especially calories), and preventing infections. A high-carbohydrate diet helps to minimize production of nitrogenous wastes.
- Avoid magnesium-containing medications (eg, Maalox). Patients typically switched to aluminum hydroxide, calcium carbonate, or calcium acetate antacids.
- Administer antacids as prescribed to control hyperphosphatemia. Phosphate binders vary in aluminum or calcium content, however, and one may not be exchanged for another without first ensuring patient is receiving the same amount of elemental aluminum or calcium.
- Facilitate orientation through calendars, radios, familiar objects, and frequent reorientation.
- Ensure safety measures (eg, padded side rails, airway) for confused or severely hypocalcemic patients.

Activity intolerance r/t generalized weakness secondary to anemia and uremia

Desired outcome: Following treatment, patient RPE ≤3 on 0-10 scale and exhibits improving endurance to activity as evidenced by HR ≤20 bpm over resting HR, SBP ≤20 mm Hg over or under resting SBP, and RR ≤24 breaths/min with eupnea.

Note: Anemia is better tolerated in uremic than in nonuremic patients.

- Monitor patient during activity, and ask patient to RPE. Monitor for ↑ weakness, fatigue, dyspnea, chest pain, or further ↓ in Hct.
- Provide and encourage optimal nutrition.
- Administer epoetin alfa (Epogen) if prescribed.
- Administer anabolic steroids (eg, nandrolone) if prescribed. Prepare female patients for side effects, including facial hair, deepening voice, menstrual irregularities.
- Coordinate lab studies to minimize blood drawing.
- Monitor for occult blood and blood loss.
- Do not give ferrous sulfate at the same time as antacids. The two should be given at least 1 h apart to maximize absorption of ferrous sulfate.
- Assist with identifying activities that ↑ fatigue and adjusting those activities accordingly.
- Assist with ADL while encouraging maximal independence to patient's tolerance.
- Establish with patient realistic, progressive exercises and activity goals that are designed to ↑ endurance.

Impaired skin integrity r/t pruritus, dry skin secondary to uremia and edema

Desired outcome: Skin remains intact and free of erythema and abrasions.

- Pruritus often ↓ with reductions in BUN and improved phosphorus control. Encourage use of phosphate binders and ↓ in dietary phosphorus. Give phosphate binders with meals for maximal effects. If necessary, administer antihistamines as prescribed. Keep patient's fingernails short.
- Because uremia retards wound healing, instruct patient to monitor scratches for evidence of infection and seek early medical attention should S&S of infection appear.
- Uremic skin is often dry and scaly because of ↓ oil gland activity. Encourage use of skin emollients and bath oils and avoidance of hard soaps and excessive bathing.
- Clotting abnormalities and capillary fragility place uremic patients at ↑ risk for bruising. Protect patient during position changes and when moving.
- Provide scheduled skin care and position changes for persons with edema.

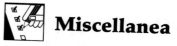

Miscellanea

CONSULT MD FOR

- Hct <20%-25%, occult bleeding, other significant blood loss.
- Chest pain at rest or with activity; dyspnea at rest
- Indicators of pulmonary edema: crackles, dyspnea, orthopnea

RELATED TOPICS

- Hemodialysis
- Hyperkalemia
- Hypernatremia
- Hyperphosphatemia
- Hypocalcemia
- Immobility, prolonged
- Metabolic acidosis, chronic

ABBREVIATIONS

ESRD: End-stage renal disease
GFR: Glomerular filtration rate
PRBCs: Packed red blood cells
RPE: Rate(d) perceived exertion
SLE: Systemic lupus erythematosus

REFERENCES

Horne MM: Renal disorders and renal failure. In Swearingen PL: *Manual of medical-surgical nursing care,* ed 3, St Louis, 1994, Mosby.

Price CA: Issues related to the care of critically ill patients with end stage renal failure, *AACN Clin Issues in Crit Care Nurs* 3(3): 585-596, 1992.

Rose DB, Rennke HG: *Renal Pathophysiology–the essentials,* Baltimore, 1994, Williams & Wilkins.

Author: **Mima M. Horne**

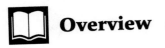

Overview

PATHOPHYSIOLOGY
Occurs infrequently but has potential for life-long complications or even death. Blunt injuries responsible for most renal trauma, but penetrating injuries also implicated.

INCIDENCE
Minor: 85%; bruising of renal parenchyma; superficial lacerations of renal cortex without rupture of renal capsule
Major: 10%-15%; major lacerations through cortex and medulla; continuation of laceration through renal capsule
Critical: <5%; renal vascular trauma in which kidney shattered and renal pedicle injured; fragmentation (renal fracture)

HISTORY/RISK FACTORS
- Vehicular collision
- Falls
- Sports-related injuries
- Assaults
- Stab/gunshot wounds

CLINICAL PRESENTATION
- Abdominal or flank pain, back tenderness, colicky pain with passage of blood clots
- Hemorrhage: pallor, diaphoresis, hypotension, tachycardia, restlessness, confusion
- Gross or microscopic hematuria; gross hematuria present in slightly > half of patients with renal trauma and considered unreliable diagnostic sign

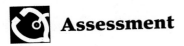

Assessment

PHYSICAL ASSESSMENT
Signs may be masked because of kidneys' protection by abdominal organs, back muscles, bony structures.
- Hematoma over flank of eleventh or twelfth ribs
- Obvious wounds, contusions, abrasions in flank or abdomen
- Abdominal distention
- Grey Turner's sign
- Pain at CVA
- Flank or abdominal mass

VITAL SIGNS/HEMODYNAMICS
RR: ↑ if hemorrhagic
HR: ↑ if hemorrhagic
BP: ↓ if hemorrhagic
Temp: Nl; ↓ if hypothermic, ↑ with infection
CVP/PAWP: ↓ if hemorrhagic
SVR: ↑ if hemorrhagic; ↑ or ↓ with infection

LABORATORY STUDIES
BUN Values: BUN level may ↑ because of renal dysfunction, body catabolism, or dehydration. Nl = 10-20 mg/dl.
Serum Creatinine: Creatinine excretion roughly proportional to GFR and a more accurate reflection of renal impairment than BUN. Nl = 0.7-1.5 mg/dl.
Clearance Tests: Evaluate extent of injury by assessing renal filtration, reabsorption, secretion, and RBF. Creatinine and urea usually tested.

IMAGING
KUB Radiography: Evaluates position, size, structure, and defects of kidney and LUT structures. Abnormal findings: retroperitoneal hematoma, fractured lower ribs or pelvis, foreign bodies, organ displacement, fluid accumulation.
Excretory Urogram/IVP: Contrast material given IV and filtered by kidneys before excretion through urinary tract. X-rays visualize nl or injured KUB structures. Check for hx of allergy to iodine or contrast material. Adequate hydration needed to rid body of contrast material after this test.
CT Scan: May reveal hematomas, renal lacerations, renal infarcts, or urine extravasation.
Renal Angiography: Arterial injection of contrast medium permits identification of renal pedicle injury, renal infarct, intrarenal hematoma, lacerations, and shattered kidney. Check for allergy to contrast medium; maintain adequate hydration during/after procedure.
Note: LUT injury often present with renal injury. The following may be performed to determine damage to LUT:
Retrograde urethrogram: To r/o urethral rupture.
Cystogram: If no urethral tear found on retrograde urethrogram, bladder filled with contrast material to determine if extravasation occurs, suggesting bladder tears/ruptures.

Collaborative Management

Antibiotics: For positive urine culture results, penetrating injuries, peritonitis.
Analgesics: IV morphine sulfate.
Diuretics: Osmotic diuretics (eg, mannitol) to promote RBF, ↑ GFR, and stimulate UO. Loop diuretics (eg, furosemide) ↓ filtrate reabsorption, promote water excretion. Used after adequate hydration to prevent oliguria.
Dopamine: Low doses of ≈ 2 μg/kg/min to promote renal vasodilatation and RBF.
Fluid Management: Restriction or hydration may be necessary, depending on presence of oliguric vs nonoliguric ARF.
Dietary Modifications: May be necessary with ARF. ↑ carbohydrates to prevent protein catabolism; ↓ Na^+, K^+ to correct electrolyte imbalances; protein restriction.
Renal Replacement Therapies: PD, CAVH, CVVH, or hemodialysis may be necessary to manage ARF.
Catheterization: If unable to void. Catheter passed only as far as it will progress without undue force. If resistance met, urethrogram indicated. If blood present at urethral meatus, catheterization contraindicated before urethrogram. Suprapubic catheter often used to manage severe urethral lacerations and urethral disruption.
Surgical Correction: For injuries accompanied by rapidly expanding, pulsating hematomas. Immediate surgical exploration indicated for critical renal trauma; rates of renal salvage low.

PATIENT-FAMILY TEACHING
- Medications: drug name, purpose, dosage, schedule, precautions, food-drug and drug-drug interactions, potential side effects
- Purpose, expected results, anticipated sensations of all nursing/medical interventions
- Need for ↑ fluid intake
- Necessity of reporting ↑ blood in urine; urge but inability to void

Nursing Diagnoses/Interventions

Altered pattern of urinary elimination r/t mechanical trauma secondary to injury to kidney and LUT structures

Desired outcome: Within 6 h after immediate trauma management, patient has UO of ≥0.5 ml/kg/h with no bladder distention.

- Ensure adequate urinary outflow. If patient unable to void, assess need for urinary catheterization or suprapubic drainage by palpating gently for full bladder. Monitor for these signs of kidney or LUT trauma:

  Urge but inability to void spontaneously

  Blood at urethral meatus

  Difficult or unsuccessful urinary catheterization

  Anuria after urinary catheterization

  Hematuria

- Do not catheterize if blood present at urethral meatus. Do not force catheter if resistance felt.
- Monitor serum BUN/creatinine. ↑ reflects renal impairment.
- Document I&O qh. Assess patency of urinary collection system qh to check for occlusion by clots. If indicated, gently irrigate catheter according to agency policy/prescription. Sudden cessation of urine flow through collection system may signal catheter obstruction. If irrigation does not resume urine drainage, consider changing urinary catheter.
- Ensure nephrostomy tube not occluded by patient's weight or external pressure. Irrigate nephrostomy tube *only* if prescribed, and with ≤5 ml fluid.
- Assess entrance site of nephrostomy tube for bleeding or urine leakage. Catheter blockage with clots or catheter dislodging can cause sudden ↓ in UO. Consult physician if blockage or displacement suspected.
- Assess urine for color and clots. Expect hematuria for first 24-48 h after nephrostomy tube insertion. Consult physician for gross bleeding.
- Ensure adequate hydration to promote clearing of contrast material after diagnostic testing.

Risk for infection r/t inadequate primary defenses and tissue destruction secondary to potential bacterial contamination of urinary tract system

Desired outcome: Patient infection free: normothermia, WBC count ≤11,000 μl, negative results of urine and wound drainage testing.

- Use aseptic technique when caring for urinary drainage systems. Maintain catheters and collection container at level lower than bladder; keep drainage tubing unkinked.
- Record color, odor, specific gravity of urine each shift. Culture urine specimen when infection suspected.
- Monitor WBC count qd and temp q4h for ↑.
- Assess for peritonitis each shift: abdominal pain, distention, rigidity; nausea, vomiting, fever, malaise, weakness.
- Assess catheter exit site for erythema, swelling, drainage.
- Assess surgical incision for approximation of suture line and evidence of wound healing. Culture purulent or foul-smelling drainage.
- Assess skin at all catheter entrance sites for irritation: erythema, drainage, swelling.
- Cleanse catheter insertion site q8h with antimicrobial solution. Change dressings q24h or as soon as wet. For erythema and swelling, consider use of pectin wafer skin barrier for extra protection.

Pain r/t physical injury associated with structural injury, procedures for urinary diversion, or surgical incisions

Desired outcomes: Within 2 h after giving analgesia, patient discomfort ↓, as documented by pain scale. Nonverbal indicators absent.

- Assess for pain using pain scale. Medicate promptly and document response to analgesia.
- Explain cause of pain.
- Assist into position of comfort. Often knee flexion helps reduce discomfort.
- Implement nonpharmacologic measures for coping with pain: diversion, touch, conversation.

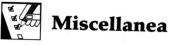 # Miscellanea

CONSULT MD FOR
- Blood at urethral meatus
- Inability to pass urinary drainage catheter
- UO <0.5 ml/kg/h
- New onset hematuria
- Blockage of nephrostomy or other urinary drainage tube
- Sudden cessation of urine flow
- ↑ BUN/creatinine

RELATED TOPICS
- Hemodialysis
- Continuous arteriovenous hemofiltration/ Continuous venovenous hemofiltration
- Multisystem injury
- Peritoneal dialysis
- Renal failure, acute
- Shock, hemorrhagic
- Shock, hypovolemic
- Urinary tract injury, lower

ABBREVIATIONS
CAVH: Continuous arteriovenous hemofiltration

CVA: Costovertebral angle

CVVH: Continuous venovenous hemofiltration

GFR: Glomerular filtration rate

LUT: Lower urinary tract

PD: Peritoneal dialysis

RBF: Renal blood flow

REFERENCES
Matthews LA, Spirnak JP: The nonoperative approach to major blunt renal trauma, *Semin Urol* 13(1): 77-82, 1995.

Miller KS, McAninch JW: Radiographic assessment of renal trauma: our 15-year experience, *J Urol* 154(2): 352-355, 1995.

Nash PA, Bruce JE, McAninch JW: Nephrectomy for traumatic renal injuries, *J Urol* 153(3 Pt 1): 609-611, 1995.

Nguyen HT, Carroll PR: Blunt renal trauma: renal preservation through careful staging and selective surgery, *Semin Urol* 13(1): 83-89, 1995.

Sommers MS: Renal and lower urinary tract trauma. In Swearingen PL, Keen JH (eds): *Manual of critical care nursing*, ed 3, St Louis, 1995, Mosby.

Author: **Marilyn Sawyer Sommers**

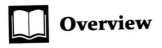

Overview

PATHOPHYSIOLOGY
Widely accepted mode of treatment for ESRD. Two types of transplant donors: living and cadaveric. 1-yr success rate with live donor transplantation: 90%-95%; with cadaveric transplantation since advent of cyclosporine: improved to 75%-85%. Majority placed on cadaveric waiting list, since demand far exceeds supply.

COMPLICATIONS
Rejection and infection. Rejection is immunologic response to transplanted kidney; can be categorized into four distinct types: hyperacute, accelerated acute, acute, and chronic.

HISTORY/RISK FACTORS
(pretransplantation)
- Chronic renal failure caused by glomerulonephritis: 30%-40%
- Pyelonephritis or other interstitial disease: 20%-30%
- Multisystem disease: 15%-20%
- Cystic kidney disease: 10%

CLINICAL PRESENTATION (with rejection)
Hyperacute: Occurs in OR; requires kidney removal.
Accelerated Acute: Occurs 48-72 h after transplant: ↓ UO, leukocytosis or leukopenia, tenderness over kidney, ↓ RBF on renal scan, profound thrombocytopenia. *Treatment:* Steroids, other immunosuppressives used for 3-4 days; poor prognosis for reversal.
Acute: Occurs 1-2 wks to several mos after transplant: fever, leukocytosis, enlarged/tender kidney, ↓ UO, weight gain, hypertension, ↑ BUN/creatinine. *Treatment:* Steroids, other immunosuppressives; good prognosis.
Chronic: Occurs mos to yrs after transplant: slow ↓ in renal function, hypertension, proteinuria. *Treatment:* None known; poor prognosis for long-term graft survival.

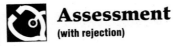

Assessment
(with rejection)

PHYSICAL ASSESSMENT
CV: Hypertension, peripheral edema
GU: Enlarged, firm kidney; graft tenderness; oliguria or anuria
Other: Weight gain

VITAL SIGNS/HEMODYNAMICS
RR: Nl or ↑
HR: ↑
BP: ↑ >10 mm Hg over baseline
Temp: ↑
Hemodynamics: Reflect volume status

LABORATORY STUDIES
BUN/Creatinine: ↑ from previous 24-h levels.
24-h Urine: Change in components, eg, ↓ creatinine clearance, total amount of creatinine excreted, urinary sodium excretion; ↑ protein excretion. In early postop period urinary protein concentration may be falsely ↑ because of presence of blood/blood proteins.

IMAGING
Renal Scan: Evaluates RBF and rate of excretion of substances into bladder.
Renal Ultrasound: To r/o possibility of obstruction.

DIAGNOSTIC PROCEDURE
Renal Biopsy: Determines presence, type, severity of rejection.

Collaborative Management

Pharmacotherapy
Corticosteroids: Megadoses of IV methylprednisolone (Solu-Medrol) to block production of interleukin-2 (IL-2), prevent transcription of IL-1. Also used for its antiinflammatory properties.
Azathioprine (eg, Imuran), cyclophosphamide (eg, Cytoxan): Block proliferation of immunocompetent lymphoid cells; affect rapidly dividing B and T cells.
Cyclosporine (eg, Sandimmune): To prevent IL-2 secretion, thus blocking activation of cytotoxic T lymphocytes.
Antilymphocyte sera (eg, ALG or ATGAM): Makes T cells susceptible to phagocytosis.
Monoclonal antibody (Orthoclone OKT3): Reacts with T_3 complex on surface of T cells, causing their removal from the circulation. Intensive monitoring necessary during first 2 doses because of high frequency of side effects, including bronchospasm and pulmonary edema.
Tacrolimus (eg, Prograf): Mechanism of action similar to cyclosporine: inhibits earliest steps of T-cell activation.
Mycophenolate mofetil (eg, Cellcept): Selective inhibitor of inosine monophosphate dehydrogenase, a pathway T and B lymphocytes depend on for proliferation.
Graft Irradiation: Destroys lymphocytes within graft. Irradiation performed with 150 rads for ≈ 3 successive days.

PATIENT-FAMILY TEACHING
- Verbal/written information about type of prescribed immunosuppressive agent. Discuss generic name, trade name, purpose, usual dosage, route, side effects, food-drug and drug-drug interactions, and precautions.
- Need for monthly urine cultures; S&S of UTI.
- Oral care: self-inspection of oral mucosa for exudate and lesions; use of soft-bristled toothbrush.
- Importance of daily skin care with water, nondrying soap, and lubricating lotion.

🧠 Nursing Diagnoses/Interventions

Fear and anxiety r/t threat to health status secondary to potential loss of kidney from rejection
Desired outcomes: Within 48 h posttransplant, patient verbalizes accurate information about S&S of rejection. Patient demonstrates ability to relax, discusses anxiety r/t rejection, and exhibits ↑ involvement in care activities.

- Provide opportunities for expressions of fears, concerns, and anxieties about kidney rejection.
- Ensure that patient/significant others verbalize knowledge of these S&S of rejection:
  Persistent, low-grade fever of 37.2°-37.8° C (99°-100° F)
  ↑ swelling of feet, ankles, hands, face
  Weight gain >1 kg/24 h
  Painful and swollen kidney
  ↑ BP
  ↓ 24-h UO
- Reassure that several medication regimens are available to treat rejection episodes.
- Reassure that rejection does not necessarily mean kidney loss. Under most circumstances, rejection can be reversed.
- Reassure that retransplantation is a viable option.

Risk for infection r/t inadequate secondary responses attributable to immunosuppression
Desired outcome: Patient infection free: normothermia; absence of erythema, swelling, and drainage at catheter and wound sites; absence of adventitious breath sounds and cloudy and foul-smelling urine; negative cultures; and WBCs 4500-11,000 μl.

- Assess and record temp q4h.
- Assess and document condition of indwelling IV/catheter sites and graft incision q8h. Be alert to swelling, erythema, tenderness, and drainage.
- Obtain blood, urine, and wound cultures when infection suspected.
- Be alert to WBCs >11,000 μl or <4500 μl. Below-nl WBCs with ↑ differential (shift to left) may signal acute infection.
- Record urine volume, appearance, color, and odor. Be alert to foul-smelling or cloudy urine, frequency and urgency of urination, and complaints of flank or labial pain, all of which are signs of renal-urinary infection.
- Auscultate lung fields q8h, noting presence of rhonchi, crackles, and ↓ breath sounds.
- Use meticulous sterile technique when dressing and caring for wounds and catheter sites.
- Obtain specimens for urine cultures 1 × wk during hospitalization.

Altered oral mucous membrane r/t treatment with immunosuppressive medication
Desired outcomes: Patient's oral mucosa, tongue, and lips are pink, intact, and free of exudate and lesions. Patient states swallowing occurs without difficulty within 24 h after treatment.

- Inspect mouth qd for signs of exudate and lesions.
- Assist in brushing with soft-bristled toothbrush and nonabrasive toothpaste after meals and snacks.
- Provide nystatin (Mycostatin) prophylactic mouthwash for "swish and swallow" pc and hs.

Impaired skin integrity (or risk for same): Herpetic lesions, skin fungal rashes, pruritus, and capillary fragility r/t treatment with immunosuppressive medications
Desired outcome: Patient's skin intact and free of open lesions or abrasions.

- Assess for/document the following qd: erythema, excoriation, rashes, bruises.
- Assess for/document herpetic lesions or other rashes in the perineal area.
- Inspect trunk area qd for flat, itchy fungal rashes.
- Use nonallergic tape only.
- Assist with changing position at least q2h; massage areas susceptible to breakdown.

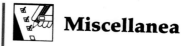

Miscellanea

CONSULT MD FOR
- Temp >37.8° C (100° F)
- S&S of infection: swelling, erythema, tenderness, drainage at surgical/catheter insertion sites
- UTI: foul-smelling, cloudy urine; ↑ frequency, urgency; graft or labial pain
- WBCs >11,000 or <4500 μl or with ↑ band neutrophils (shift to left)
- Exudate, lesions of oral mucosa
- S&S of rejection: ↓ UO, fever, leukocytosis, leukopenia, ↑ BUN/creatinine, enlarged and tender kidney, weight gain

RELATED TOPICS
- Anxiety
- Immobility, prolonged
- Nutritional support, enteral and parenteral
- Organ rejection
- Renal failure, acute

ABBREVIATIONS
ESRD: End-stage renal disease
RBF: Renal blood flow

REFERENCES
Fedric TN: Immunosuppressive therapy in renal transplantation, *Crit Care Nurs Clin North Am* 2(1): 123-131, 1990.

Holecheck MJ, Burrell-Diggs D, Navarro MO: Renal transplantation: an option for end-stage renal disease patients, *Crit Care Nurs Q* 13(4): 62-71, 1991.

Lancaster LE, Schanbaacher BA: Renal transplantation. In Lancaster LE (ed): *Core curriculum for nephrology nursing,* ed 3, Pitman, NJ, 1995, AJ Janetti.

Trusler LA: Management of acute renal transplant rejection, *J Urol Nurs* 9(4): 1012-1022, 1990.

Weiskittel PD: Renal-urinary dysfunctions. In Swearingen PL, Keen JH (eds): *Manual of critical care nursing,* ed 3, St Louis, 1995, Mosby.

Author: **Patricia D. Weiskittel**

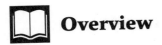 **Overview**

PATHOPHYSIOLOGY

Occurs secondary to alveolar hypoventilation and results in ↑ $Paco_2$. Degree to which ↑ $Paco_2$ alters pH depends on rapidity of onset and the body's ability to compensate. Although the blood buffer system acts immediately, it is usually insufficient to maintain nl pH. There is a delay of a few h to days before renal compensation is noted, so profound changes in pH can occur. Severe hypercapnia may cause cerebral vasodilatation, resulting in ↑ ICP.

HISTORY/RISK FACTORS

- Acute respiratory disorders: severe pneumonia, ARDS, pneumonia with COPD
- Chest wall trauma: flail chest, pneumothorax
- Respiratory center depression: drugs, CNS trauma/lesions
- Asphyxiation: mechanical obstruction, anaphylaxis
- Impaired respiratory muscles: hypokalemia, hyperkalemia, poliomyelitis, GBS
- Cardiac arrest
- Iatrogenic: inappropriate mechanical ventilation; high Fio_2 in the presence of chronic CO_2 retention

CLINICAL PRESENTATION

↑ respiratory effort, SOB, dyspnea, nausea, vomiting, headache. Restlessness and confusion, which are early signs, may be subtle but are important indicators.

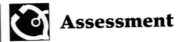 **Assessment**

PHYSICAL ASSESSMENT

Neuro: Fine tremors, asterixis, lethargy, coma, dilated conjunctival and facial blood vessels
Resp: Tachypnea, use of accessory muscles, cyanosis (late sign)
CV: Tachycardia, hypotension, diaphoresis, dysrhythmias

VITAL SIGNS/HEMODYNAMICS

RR: ↑
HR: ↑
BP: ↓
Temp: Nl; ↑ if bacterial pneumonia present
PAWP: ↑ with hypoxia caused by pulmonary vasoconstriction or if myocardial impairment present
PVR: ↑ in response to aveolar hypoxia
CO: ↓
ECG: Ventricular, other dysrhythmias

LABORATORY STUDIES

ABGs: $Paco_2$ >45 mm Hg and pH <7.35. If patient breathing room air, hypoxemia always present.
Serum Bicarbonate: Initially, values nl (22-26 mEq/L) unless a mixed disorder is present. Renal compensation does not occur for a few h to days.
Serum Electrolytes: Usually not altered; depend on cause of acidosis.
Drug Screen: Determines presence, quantity of drug if overdose suspected.

IMAGING

Chest X-ray: Determines presence of a respiratory disease.

Collaborative Management

Restoration of Effective Alveolar Ventilation: If $Paco_2$ >50-60 mm Hg, Pao_2 ≤50 mm Hg, and clinical signs of ventilatory failure present, intubation and mechanical ventilation usually required. Generally, use of bicarbonate avoided because of risk of alkalosis. Although life-threatening pH must be corrected to an acceptable level promptly, nl pH is not the immediate goal.
Treatment of Underlying Disorder: Eg, chest tube insertion for pneumothorax, naloxone (Narcan) for opiate overdose.

PATIENT-FAMILY TEACHING

- Reassurance that restlessness and confusion improve with treatment
- Importance for family to reorient patient to place, time, events and put familiar objects at bedside
- Explanations regarding all procedures and equipment, especially alarms and lights, rationale for their use

Nursing Diagnoses/Interventions

Impaired gas exchange r/t alveolar-capillary membrane changes secondary to pulmonary tissue disturbance/destruction

Desired outcome: Within 24 h of treatment initiation, patient has adequate gas exchange: $Paco_2$, pH, and Spo_2 wnl or within 10% of baseline.

- Monitor serial ABGs.
- Monitor O_2 saturation *via* pulse oximetry. Watch Spo_2 closely, especially when changing Fio_2 or evaluating response to treatment (eg, repositioning, chest physiotherapy).
- Assess and document respiratory status: respiratory rate and rhythm, exertional effort, and breath sounds. Compare pretreatment findings to posttreatment findings for evidence of improvement.
- Assess and document LOC. If $Paco_2$ ↑, be alert to subtle, progressive changes in mental status. Common progression: agitation → insomnia → somnolence → coma. Always evaluate "arousability" of patient with ↑ $Paco_2$ who appears to be sleeping.
- Ensure appropriate delivery of prescribed O_2 therapy. Assess respiratory status after every change in Fio_2.
- Assess for presence of bowel sounds and monitor for GI distention, which can impede diaphragm movement and restrict ventilation.

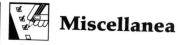 # Miscellanea

CONSULT MD FOR
- $Paco_2$ >50-60 mm Hg; Pao_2 ≤50 mm Hg
- Clinical S&S of ventilatory failure: confusion, lethargy, cyanosis (late sign)
- Hemodynamically significant dysrhythmias

RELATED TOPICS
- Chest trauma
- Guillain-Barré syndrome
- Increased intracranial pressure
- Mechanical ventilation
- Respiratory acidosis, chronic
- Respiratory failure, acute

ABBREVIATION
GBS: Guillain-Barré syndrome

REFERENCES
Heitz UE: Acid-base imbalances. In Swearingen PL, Keen JH (eds): *Manual of critical care nursing,* ed 3, St Louis, 1995, Mosby.

Horne MM, Heitz U, Swearingen PL: *Pocket guide to fluid, electrolytes, and acid-base balance,* ed 3, St Louis, 1997, Mosby.

Lovenstein J: *Acid and basics: a guide to understanding acid-base disorders,* New York, 1993, Oxford University Press.

Rose BD: *Clinical physiology of acid-base and electrolyte disorders,* ed 4, New York, 1994, McGraw-Hill.

Author: **Ursula Heitz**

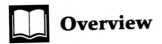 **Overview**

PATHOPHYSIOLOGY

Occurs in pulmonary diseases in which alveolar ventilation ↓ and V/Q mismatch present. Over time the amount of CO_2 eliminated is less than the amount generated, and thus $Paco_2$ levels ↑. In chronic lung disease, compensatory metabolic alkalosis (serum HCO_3^- >26 mEq/L) occurs and an acceptable acid-base environment is maintained despite $Paco_2$ as high as 60 mm Hg. If a superimposed disease state such as pneumonia is present, chronic compensatory mechanisms may be inadequate to meet sudden ↑ in $Paco_2$, and decompensation may occur.

HISTORY/RISK FACTORS

- COPD: emphysema, bronchitis; cystic fibrosis
- Restrictive disorders: extreme obesity (pickwickian syndrome), kyphoscoliosis
- Neuromuscular abnormality: ALS, muscular dystrophy
- Respiratory center depression: brain tumor, extreme obesity
- Exposure to pulmonary toxins: occupational risk; pollution

CLINICAL PRESENTATION

If $Paco_2$ does not exceed body's ability to compensate, no specific findings noted. If $Paco_2$ ↑ rapidly, the following may occur: dull headache, weakness, asterixis, dyspnea, agitation, and insomnia progressing to somnolence and coma.

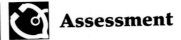 **Assessment**

PHYSICAL ASSESSMENT

Tachypnea, cyanosis. Severe hypercapnia ($Paco_2$ >70 mm Hg) may cause cerebral vasodilatation resulting in ↑ ICP, papilledema, and dilated conjunctival and facial blood vessels. If cor pulmonale present, RV failure may occur, causing peripheral edema, JVD, hepatomegaly.

VITAL SIGNS/HEMODYNAMICS

RR: ↑
HR: ↑
BP: Nl or ↓
Temp: ↑ if respiratory infection present
CVP: ↑ if RV failure present
PAP: ↑ because of hypoxemic-related pulmonary vasoconstriction and chronic pulmonary vascular changes
PVR: ↑ caused by ↑ PAP, compensatory polycythemia
ECG: Isoelectric P wave and isoelectric QRS complex in lead I in middle-aged or older adult suggest chronic bronchitis or emphysema. SVT or VT common during acute exacerbation.

LABORATORY STUDIES

ABGs: Determine diagnosis, severity of acidosis. $Paco_2$ will be ↑ and pH near nl, although on acidic (low) side, except in an acute pulmonary disorder (eg, pneumonia) superimposed on chronic hypercapnia. If $Paco_2$ ↑ abruptly from baseline, pH < nl may be seen.
Serum Electrolytes: Because of compensation, HCO_3^- expected to be ↑. If HCO_3^- nl or ↓, this could be diagnostic of a second pathologic process (eg, metabolic acidosis).
Sputum Culture: Determines presence of pathogens causing acute exacerbation of a chronic pulmonary disease (eg, pneumonia).

IMAGING

Chest X-ray: Determines extent of underlying pulmonary disease and identifies further pathologic changes that may be responsible for acute exacerbation (eg, pneumonia).

Collaborative Management

Oxygen Therapy: Used cautiously with chronic CO_2 retention when hypoxemia, rather than hypercapnia, stimulates ventilation. Continuous Spo_2 used to assess and maintain O_2 saturation of 90%-92%.
Pharmacotherapy: Bronchodilators and antibiotics, as indicated. Avoid narcotics and sedatives unless intubation and mechanical ventilation in place.
IV Fluids: To maintain adequate hydration.
Chest Physiotherapy and Postural Drainage: Aid in expectoration of sputum. Assess patient closely because it may be poorly tolerated.

PATIENT-FAMILY TEACHING

- Medications: drug name, dosage, route, schedule, precautions, drug-drug and food-drug interactions, and potential side effects, particularly of bronchodilators, antibiotics
- S&S that necessitate medical intervention: ↑ dyspnea unrelieved by medications, ↑ sputum production or change in color or consistency, fever and chills, ↑ cough, ↓ activity tolerance
- Pursed-lip breathing technique to promote air exchange:
  Sit upright with hands on thighs.
  Inhale normally through nose with mouth closed.
  Exhale slowly through mouth with lips pursed in a whistling position.
  Ensure that exhalation takes twice as long as inhalation, making a whistling sound while doing so.

Nursing Diagnoses/Interventions

Impaired gas exchange r/t alveolar-capillary membrane changes secondary to pulmonary tissue destruction

Desired outcome: Within 24 h of treatment initiation, patient has adequate gas exchange: $Paco_2$, pH, and Spo_2 wnl or within 10% of baseline.

- Monitor serial ABGs.
- Monitor O_2 saturation *via* pulse oximetry. Watch Spo_2 closely, especially when changing Fio_2 or evaluating response to treatment (eg, repositioning, chest physiotherapy).
- Assess and document respiratory status: respiratory rate and rhythm, exertional effort, and breath sounds. Compare pretreatment findings to posttreatment findings for evidence of improvement.
- Assess and document LOC. If $Paco_2$ ↑, be alert to subtle, progressive changes in mental status. Common progression: agitation → insomnia → somnolence → coma. Always evaluate "arousability" of patient with ↑ $Paco_2$ who appears to be sleeping.
- Ensure appropriate delivery of prescribed O_2 therapy. Assess respiratory status after every change in Fio_2.
- Patients with chronic CO_2 retention may be very sensitive to ↑ in Fio_2, resulting in depressed ventilatory drive. If patient requires mechanical ventilation, be aware of the importance of maintaining compensated acid-base status. If $Paco_2$ rapidly ↓ by excessive mechanical ventilation, severe metabolic alkalosis could develop. Sudden onset of metabolic alkalosis may lead to hypocalcemia, which can result in tetany or cardiac dysrhythmias.
- Assess for presence of bowel sounds and monitor for GI distention, which can impede diaphragm movement and restrict ventilation.
- In patient without intubation, encourage use of pursed-lip breathing (inhalation through nose, with slow exhalation through pursed lips), which helps airways to remain open and allows for better air excursion.

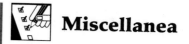 ## Miscellanea

CONSULT MD FOR
- ↑ $Paco_2$; ↓ pH, Pao_2
- Sao_2 ≤90%
- Hemodynamically significant dysrhythmias
- Deteriorating LOC, somnolence, difficult arousal from "sleep"
- Metabolic alkalosis resulting from excessive mechanical ventilation

RELATED TOPICS
- Increased intracranial pressure
- Mechanical ventilation
- Pneumonia, community-acquired
- Pneumonia, hospital-associated
- Pulmonary hypertension
- Respiratory acidosis, acute

ABBREVIATION
ALS: Amyotrophic lateral sclerosis

REFERENCES
Heitz UE: Acid-base imbalances. In Swearingen PL, Keen JH (eds): *Manual of critical care nursing,* ed 3, St Louis, 1995, Mosby.

Horne MM, Heitz U, Swearingen PL: *Pocket guide to fluid, electrolytes, and acid-base balance,* ed 3, St Louis, 1997, Mosby.

Lovenstein J: *Acid and basics: a guide to understanding acid-base disorders,* New York, 1993, Oxford University Press.

Rose BD: *Clinical physiology of acid-base and electrolyte disorders,* ed 4, New York, 1994, McGraw-Hill.

Author: **Ursula Heitz**

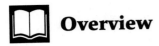 # Overview

PATHOPHYSIOLOGY

Defined as $Paco_2$ <35 mm Hg. Occurs as a result of alveolar hyperventilation, caused most frequently by anxiety but also by the initial stages of pneumonia, pulmonary edema, and pulmonary emboli. Hypocapnia results in ↑ pH, which is modified to a small degree by intracellular buffering. It is a subtle and early indicator of pathologic processes in the acutely ill and a poor prognostic sign in medical patients.

HISTORY/RISK FACTORS

- Anxiety, pain
- Pulmonary disorders: pneumonia, pulmonary edema, pulmonary thromboembolism
- Extremely high altitude: stimulates ventilatory effort causing respiratory alkalosis
- Hypermetabolic states: fever, sepsis
- Salicylate intoxication
- Excessive mechanical ventilation
- CNS injury: damage to respiratory center

CLINICAL PRESENTATION

Anxiety, dyspnea, lightheadedness, paresthesias, circumoral numbness, muscle cramps, hyperreflexia; *in extreme alkalosis:* confusion, syncope, seizures

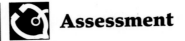 # Assessment

PHYSICAL ASSESSMENT

↑ rate and depth of respirations, confusion, tetany

VITAL SIGNS/HEMODYNAMICS

RR: ↑
HR: ↑
BP: ↑ if r/t pain or anxiety; ↓ if caused by sepsis
Temp: Nl unless infection present
Hemodynamics: Depend on underlying state
ECG: Dysrhythmias occur with even modest alkalosis in preexisting heart disease when inotropes are used. ST and T wave changes consistent with myocardial ischemia can occur when there is no known coronary disease. Supraventricular and ventricular dysrhythmias may be seen in the critically ill.

LABORATORY STUDIES

ABGs: $Paco_2$ <35 mm Hg, pH >7.45. ↓ Pao_2, along with the clinical picture (eg, pneumonia, pulmonary edema, pulmonary embolism), may help diagnose cause of respiratory alkalosis.

Serum Electrolytes
Bicarbonate: ↓ 2 mEq/L for each 10 mm Hg ↓ in $Paco_2$.
Sodium, potassium: May be ↓ slightly.
Calcium: May be ↓. Signs of hypocalcemia include muscle cramps, hyperactive reflexes, carpal spasm, tetany, convulsions.
Phosphorus: May ↓, especially with salicylate intoxication, sepsis.

Collaborative Management

Treatment of Underlying Disorder
Reassurance: If anxiety is the cause. If symptoms severe, may be necessary for patient to rebreathe exhaled air *via* paper bag.
Oxygen Therapy: If hypoxemia a cause.
Adjustments to Mechanical Ventilators: Respiratory rate and/or volume ↓ and dead space added.
Pharmacotherapy: Sedatives and tranquilizers for anxiety-induced respiratory alkalosis.

PATIENT-FAMILY TEACHING

- Explanation that S&S, such as paresthesias, lightheadedness, confusion, are reversible with correction of pH
- Pace breathing: explanation that patients are often unaware of their ↑ RR and should pace their breathing with yours or that of a family member who has been trained
- If alkalosis is r/t hypoxemia and supplemental O_2 is required, instruction in rationale for its use, importance of not removing delivery device, and safety precautions

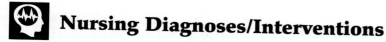 ## Nursing Diagnoses/Interventions

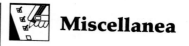 ## Miscellanea

Ineffective breathing pattern r/t anxiety

Desired outcome: Within 4 h of treatment initiation, patient's breathing pattern effective: state of eupnea, $Paco_2 \geq 35$ mm Hg, and pH ≤ 7.45.

- To help alleviate anxiety, reassure patient that a staff member will remain with him or her.
- Encourage slow breathing. Pace breathing pattern by having patient mimic your own breathing pattern.
- Monitor cardiac rhythm. With acute respiratory alkalosis, even modest alkalosis can precipitate dysrhythmias in patient with preexisting heart disease who is also taking inotropic drugs. In part, this is caused by hypokalemia, which occurs with alkalosis.
- Administer sedatives or tranquilizers as prescribed. Assess and document effectiveness.
- Have patient rebreathe into paper bag as indicated/prescribed.
- Ensure undisturbed rest after breathing pattern has stabilized. Hyperventilation can result in fatigue.
- Monitor for hypocalcemic tetany caused by ↑ binding of calcium. Be aware that tetany may occur despite nl calcium level.

CONSULT MD FOR

- Hemodynamically significant dysrhythmias
- Hypokalemic ECG changes
- Tetany, syncope, seizures

RELATED TOPICS

- Anxiety
- Hypocalcemia
- Mechanical ventilation
- Respiratory alkalosis, chronic

REFERENCES

Heitz UE: Acid-base imbalances. In Swearingen PL, Keen JH (eds): *Manual of critical care nursing,* ed 3, St Louis, 1995, Mosby.

Horne MM, Heitz U, Swearingen PL: *Pocket guide to fluid, electrolytes, and acid-base balance,* ed 3, St Louis, 1997, Mosby.

Lovenstein J: *Acid and basics: a guide to understanding acid-base disorders,* New York, 1993, Oxford University Press.

Rose BD: *Clinical physiology of acid-base and electrolyte disorders,* ed 4, New York, 1994, McGraw-Hill.

Author: **Ursula Heitz**

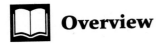

Overview

PATHOPHYSIOLOGY
State of chronic hypocapnia caused by respiratory center stimulation. ↓ $Paco_2$ stimulates the renal compensatory response and results in a proportionate ↓ in plasma bicarbonate. Maximal renal compensatory response requires several days to occur and can result in nl or near nl pH.

HISTORY/RISK FACTORS
- Cerebral disease: tumor, stroke
- Chronic hepatic insufficiency: terminal stages
- Restrictive lung diseases: interstitial pulmonary fibrosis; respiratory alkalosis throughout disease course except in terminal stages when $Paco_2$ ↑.
- Pregnancy
- Chronic hypoxia: high altitude, cyanotic heart disease

CLINICAL PRESENTATION
Patient usually symptom free

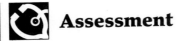

Assessment

PHYSICAL ASSESSMENT
↑ respiratory rate and depth

VITAL SIGNS/HEMODYNAMICS
RR: ↑
HR: ↑ if hypoxic
BP: Depends on underlying pathology
Temp: Nl unless concurrent infection present
PAP: ↑ possible if pulmonary fibrosis present

LABORATORY STUDIES
ABGs: $Paco_2$ <35 mm Hg, with nl or nearly nl pH; Pao_2 may be ↓ if hypoxemia a cause.
Serum Electrolytes: Probably nl, except for HCO_3^-, which ↓ as renal compensation occurs. Hypophosphatemia may be seen with severe hyperventilation. Alkalosis causes ↑ uptake of phosphate by the cells.

Collaborative Management

Treatment of Underlying Cause
Oxygen Therapy: If hypoxemia present and identified as causative factor.

PATIENT-FAMILY TEACHING
If alkalosis is r/t chronic hypoxia requiring supplemental O_2 use at home, provide rationale for use and safety precautions.

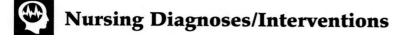 **Nursing Diagnoses/Interventions**

Nursing diagnoses/interventions are specific to the pathophysiologic process. Some patients may have the following:

Impaired gas exchange r/t alveolar-capillary membrane changes secondary to pulmonary tissue destruction

Desired outcome: Within 24 h of treatment initiation, patient has adequate gas exchange: $Paco_2$, pH, and Sao_2 wnl or within 10% of baseline.

- Monitor serial ABGs to assess response to therapy.
- Monitor O_2 saturation *via* pulse oximetry. Watch Spo_2 closely, especially when changing Fio_2 or evaluating response to treatment (eg, repositioning, chest physiotherapy).
- Assess and document respiratory status: respiratory rate and rhythm, exertional effort, and breath sounds. Compare pretreatment findings to posttreatment findings for evidence of improvement.
- Ensure appropriate delivery of prescribed O_2 therapy. Assess respiratory status after every change in Fio_2.

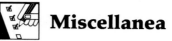 **Miscellanea**

CONSULT MD FOR
- Hypoxemia or hypophosphatemia

RELATED TOPICS
- Hypophosphatemia
- Respiratory alkalosis, acute
- Stroke: hemorrhagic
- Stroke: ischemic

REFERENCES

Heitz UE: Acid-base imbalances. In Swearingen PL, Keen JH (eds): *Manual of critical care nursing,* ed 3, St Louis, 1995, Mosby.

Horne MM, Heitz U, Swearingen PL: *Pocket guide to fluid, electrolytes, and acid-base balance,* ed 3, St Louis, 1997, Mosby.

Lovenstein J: *Acid and basics: a guide to understanding acid-base disorders,* New York, 1993, Oxford University Press.

Rose BD: *Clinical physiology of acid-base and electrolyte disorders,* ed 4, New York, 1994, Mc-Graw-Hill.

Author: **Ursula Heitz**

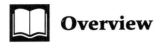 **Overview**

PATHOPHYSIOLOGY

Impairment of alveolar ventilation, pulmonary vascular perfusion, or both. ↑ WOB places demands on the cardiopulmonary system that exceed functional reserves. Clinically, ARF exists when Pao_2 <50 mm Hg with patient at rest and breathing room air, often accompanied by $Paco_2$ ≥50 mm Hg or pH <7.35. Three basic mechanisms involved.

Alveolar Hypoventilation: ↓ in alveolar minute ventilation. Indicators (cyanosis and somnolence) occur late, and condition may go unnoticed until hypoxia severe.

V/Q Mismatch: Most common cause of hypoxemia. Nl V/Q ratio is 0.8:1, eg, ventilation at 4 L/min with perfusion at 5 L/min. Interference with either side of the equation upsets the physiologic balance and can lead to respiratory failure.

Diffusion Disturbances: Processes that physically impair gas exchange across the alveolar-capillary membrane.

Right-to-left shunting (intrapulmonary shunt): Occurs when aforementioned processes untreated. Large amounts of blood pass from right side of the heart to left side and out into the general circulation without adequate ventilation. Hypoxemia secondary to right-to-left shunting does not improve with O_2 administration because additional Fio_2 is unable to cross the alveolar-capillary membrane.

HISTORY/RISK FACTORS

Impaired Alveolar Ventilation: COPD; restrictive pulmonary disease (interstitial fibrosis, pleural effusion, pneumothorax, obesity); neuromuscular defects (GBS, MG, MS); depression of respiratory control centers

V/Q Disturbances: Pulmonary emboli, atelectasis, pneumonia, emphysema, chronic bronchitis, ARDS

Diffusion Disturbances: Pulmonary/interstitial fibrosis, pulmonary edema, ARDS

CLINICAL PRESENTATION

Varies according to underlying disease process.
- Impaired LOC: common finding often erroneously attributed to heart failure, pneumonia, stroke
- Dyspnea, anxiety, headache, fatigue, ↑ BP, tachycardia, cardiac dysrhythmias

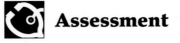 **Assessment**

PHYSICAL ASSESSMENT

Neuro: Restlessness, confusion, lethargy, coma if advanced

Resp: Dyspnea, tachypnea, crackles, wheezing, ↓ breath sounds; cyanosis and respiratory arrest if advanced

CV: Tachycardia, dysrhythmias, vasodilatation

Integ: Cool and dry at first, progressing to diaphoresis

VITAL SIGNS/HEMODYNAMICS

RR: ↑

HR: ↑

BP: ↑ at first; then ↓ because of vasodilatation

Temp: Nl unless infectious process present

CVP/PAWP: Depends on hydration, underlying disease process

PVR: ↑ in many cases, including pulmonary emboli, COPD, ARDS

SVR: initially ↑; then ↓ because of vasodilatation

CO: ↓ in late failure

ECG: Ventricular dysrhythmias, since hypoxemia ↑ ventricular irritability. A-fib/flutter with rapid ventricular response may be precipitated/exacerbated if COPD or heart failure also present. ECG evidence of ischemia (eg, ST-segment depression, T-wave elevation) possible if hypoxemia persistent or severe.

LABORATORY STUDIES

ABGs: Typical results are Pao_2 <60 mm Hg, $Paco_2$ ≥45 mm Hg, and pH <7.35. Pulse oximetry used for continuous monitoring of O_2 saturation.

Svo_2: Provides early indication of perfusion failure or ↑ tissue O_2 demands. Values <50% associated with impaired tissue oxygenation.

QS/QT: Ratio of shunt to cardiac output. Nl physiologic shunt 3%-4%; ↑ signals intrapulmonary shunting.

IMAGING

Serial Chest X-rays: Determine and monitor underlying pathophysiology and changes in patient's condition; often show diffuse infiltrates.

Collaborative Management

Correction of Hypoxemia: First treatment priority. O_2 therapy and inhaled or IV bronchodilators initiated *stat*. Goal: to maintain Pao_2 ≥90 mm Hg.

Correction of Abnormal pH Level: When pH <7.25, IV $NaHCO_3$ used conservatively and usually only when patient is mechanically ventilated. pH >7.45 managed by rebreathing mask or ↑ dead space on mechanical ventilator circuitry.

Intubation and Mechanical Ventilation: To restore alveolar ventilation, normalize pH, and ↓ WOB. Early intubation can prevent further airway collapse and tissue injury.

PEEP: Used with mechanical ventilation to promote better oxygenation with administration of lower levels of Fio_2. Also ↑ FRC by recruiting or maintaining open alveoli that otherwise are collapsed.

Pharmacotherapy

Bronchodilators (IV aminophylline, inhaled isoetharine [Bronkosol]): Dilate smooth muscles of the airways. Inhaled bronchodilators not effective with profound hypoventilation.

Corticosteroids: Short-term, high-dose corticosteroids (eg, methylprednisolone [Solu-Medrol]) may be useful in stabilizing the alveolar-capillary membrane to prevent further deterioration.

Antibiotics: Given if infectious pulmonary process suspected, as evidenced by fever, purulent sputum, or leukocytosis.

PATIENT-FAMILY TEACHING

- Explanation of need for frequent ABG analysis to patient and significant others
- Medications: drug name, purpose, dosage, schedule, precautions, drug-drug and food-drug interactions, potential side effects
- Purpose, expected results, and anticipated sensations of medical/nursing interventions
- Pursed-lip breathing technique, as indicated:
  Inhale through nose.
  Form lips in "O" shape as if whistling.
  Exhale slowly through pursed lips.

Nursing Diagnoses/Interventions

Impaired gas exchange r/t altered O_2 supply, alveolar-capillary membrane changes, or altered blood flow

Desired outcome: Within 12-24 h of therapy initiation, patient has adequate gas exchange: Pao_2 >60 mm Hg, $Paco_2$ <45 mm Hg, pH 7.35-7.45, RR 12-20 breaths/min with eupnea, and absence of adventitious breath sounds.

- Assess respiratory effort: rate, depth, rhythm, and use of accessory muscles and for respiratory distress: restlessness, anxiety, confusion, tachypnea.
- Administer O_2; monitor Fio_2 to ensure patient receiving prescribed concentrations.
- Auscultate breath sounds at frequent intervals. Monitor for ↓ or adventitious sounds (eg, wheezes, rhonchi).
- Monitor serial ABG/Spo_2. Be alert to ↓ Pao_2 and ↑ $Paco_2$ with ABG analysis or ↓ saturation levels with pulse oximetry, which are signals of respiratory failure.
- As applicable, encourage patient to slow rate of respirations by using pursed-lip breathing technique.
- Position patient to promote adequate gas exchange. Usually, semi- to high-Fowler's position is optimal. If the problem is unilateral, position patient to optimize ventilation and perfusion of unaffected lung.
- Keep oral airway and self-inflating manual ventilating bag at bedside for emergency use. Keep emergency intubation equipment nearby for use should condition deteriorate.

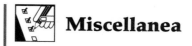

Miscellanea

CONSULT MD FOR
- Refractory hypoxemia: inability to maintain Pao_2 >60 mm Hg with Fio_2 ≤0.50
- Spo_2 <90%
- New-onset temp >38.33° C (101° F)
- Change in character of sputum (eg, clear, thin→yellow, thick)
- New-onset crackles, wheezes, rhonchi, especially if associated with ↓ Pao_2

RELATED TOPICS
- Adult respiratory distress syndrome
- Anxiety
- Bronchitis, chronic
- Chest trauma
- Emphysema
- Mechanical ventilation
- Multiple organ dysfunction syndrome
- Paralytic therapy
- Pneumonia, hospital-associated
- Pulmonary emboli, fat and thrombotic

ABBREVIATIONS
FRC: Functional residual capacity
GBS: Guillain-Barré syndrome
MG: Myasthenia gravis
MS: Multiple sclerosis
P(A-a)o$_2$: Alveolar-arterial oxygen tension difference
Svo$_2$: Mixed venous oxygen saturation

REFERENCES
Grossbach I: The COPD patient in acute respiratory failure, *Crit Care Nurse* 14(6): 32-40, 1994.

Howard C: Respiratory dysfunctions. In Swearingen PL, Keen JH (eds): *Manual of critical care nursing,* ed 3, St Louis, 1995, Mosby.

Kuhn MA: Multiple trauma with respiratory distress, *Crit Care Nurse* 14(2): 68-73, 77-80, 1994.

Tiernan PJ: Independent nursing interventions: relaxation and guided imagery in critical care, *Crit Care Nurse* 14(5): 47-51, 1994.

Author: **Cheri A. Goll**

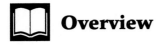 **Overview**

PATHOPHYSIOLOGY

Impaired cardiac function resulting in profound ↓ in peripheral blood flow incompatible with life. Usually caused by massive MI that renders ≥40% of the myocardium dysfunctional. With ↓ perfusion to heart, coronary flow ↓, further impairing cardiac function.
First Stage: Characterized by ↑ sympathetic discharge as the baroreceptors become stimulated by ↓ BP. Release of epinephrine and norepinephrine ↑ cardiac output by ↑ HR and contractility of uninjured myocardium, causing vasoconstriction.
Middle Stage: Characterized by ↓ perfusion to vital organs. Lactate and pyruvic acid accumulate in the tissues, and metabolic acidosis occurs. Blood is diverted from the skin, gut, and skeletal muscles to the vital organs.
Late Stage: Usually irreversible. Compensatory mechanisms ineffective and multiple organ failure occurs.

INCIDENCE

Occurs with 15%-20% of all MIs

MORTALITY

≥80%

HISTORY/RISK FACTORS

Massive MI, postcardiac surgery, massive pulmonary embolus, severe valvular dysfunction, end-stage cardiomyopathy, heart failure, cardiac tamponade

CLINICAL PRESENTATION

- S&S of biventricular failure: dyspnea, weakness, pallor, chest pain, diaphoresis
- With shock progression: ↓ mentation caused by ↓ cerebral perfusion. UO ↓ to <0.5 ml/kg/h as renal perfusion pressure ↓.

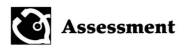 **Assessment**

PHYSICAL ASSESSMENT

Neuro: Agitation, restlessness, lethargy, confusion, unresponsiveness
Resp: Hyperventilation, dyspnea at rest, crackles
CV: Pulses weak/irregular, pulsus alternans, S_3/S_4
GU: Oliguria
Integ: Cold, clammy, mottled skin

VITAL SIGNS/HEMODYNAMICS

RR: ↑
HR: ↑
BP: ↓ with narrow pulse pressure
Temp: NI or ↓
RAP/PAP/PAWP: ↑
SVR: >1200/dynes/sec/cm^{-5}
CO: <4 L/min
CI: <1.5 L/min/m^2
Svo$_2$: <50%
ECG: Dysrhythmias may occur as a result of infarction or injury to areas of the conduction system or myocardium or as a result of electrolyte imbalance. ST-segment change may denote ischemia or injury patterns.

LABORATORY STUDIES

ABGs: Hypoxemia and metabolic acidosis result from impaired O_2 diffusion and tissue lactic acidosis.
Chemistries: May reveal hyperglycemia caused by epinephrine-induced glycogenolysis; ↑ lactate levels caused by anaerobic metabolism; hypernatremia, hypokalemia, or hyperkalemia with renal failure.
Urinalysis: To evaluate renal status.
Coagulation Profile: Often abnormal.

IMAGING

Chest X-ray: May show pulmonary congestion, possible cardiomegaly.

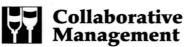 **Collaborative Management**

O$_2$ Therapy: To optimize tissue oxygenation. Intubation and mechanical ventilation may be necessary.
Morphine Sulfate: 2 mg IV push may assist in ↓ preload, pulmonary congestion and may relieve dyspnea.
Correction of Acidosis: IV sodium bicarbonate guided by serial ABGs.
Correction of Electrolyte Imbalance: Replacement of potassium and other electrolytes as indicated.

Diuretics: To ↓ preload. Furosemide or ethacrynic acid may be given. Nitrates such as NTG and IV nitroprusside (Nipride) may be used to ↓ filling pressures *via* venous dilatation. At times it may be necessary to ↑ preload if patient hypovolemic. In this situation, fluids are ↑ cautiously, the patient monitored carefully, and diuretics discontinued or avoided.
Positive Inotropes: To improve contractility. Dopamine at 2.0-20 μg/kg/min titrated to achieve desired effect. Higher doses ↑ myocardial workload. Dobutamine at 2.0-20 μg/kg/min to ↑ contractility and ↓ preload with less ↑ in HR. Amrinone, milrinone infusions provide similar inotropic effects but have mild vasodilator effects.
Vasopressors: To ↑ BP to adequate level (usually MAP ≥70 mm Hg). Accomplished by stimulating α-adrenergic receptors in the blood vessels. Dopamine, norepinephrine, epinephrine, phenylephrine, and methoxamine may be used.
IABP: Assists failing heart by ↓ afterload and ↑ coronary artery perfusion. Supports heart and circulation for ≤30 days; used as adjunct to medical therapy.
VAD: Mechanical device used to support the heart for massive LV and/or RV dysfunction. Provides conduit that diverts blood from ventricle to an artificial pump. Can maintain circulation and ↓ myocardial workload to promote ventricular recovery.
Emergency Cardiac Catheterization: To determine suitability for emergency PTCA, CABG, or arthrectomy.
Emergency CABG: To reperfuse areas with reversible injury patterns. Not as beneficial if tissue already necrotic as evidenced by Q waves on ECG.
Thrombolytic Therapy: For reperfusion of injured and noninfarcted myocardium.
Heart Transplantation: To replace failing heart with a suitably matched donor organ.

PATIENT-FAMILY TEACHING

- Purpose, expected results, anticipated sensations of all nursing/medical interventions
- Preparation of family for gravity of diagnosis, including possibility of death if shock is advanced

Nursing Diagnoses/Interventions

Decreased cardiac output r/t ↑ afterload, ↑ preload, or ↓ contractility
Desired outcome: Before weaning from assist device or pharmacologic agents is attempted, hemodynamic function is as near acceptable limits as possible: CO ≥4 L/min, BP ≥90/60 mm Hg, SVR ≤1200 dynes/sec/cm^{-5}, and PAWP ≤12 mm Hg.

- Monitor arterial BP, PAP, Svo$_2$, and heart rate and rhythm. Titrate vasoactive drugs to achieve CO between 4-7 L/min, arterial BP ≥90/60 mm Hg, and PAWP ≤12 mm Hg.
- Assess CO and SVR q1-4h and after every change in pharmacologic therapy. If SVR ↑ (>1200 dynes/sec/cm^{-5}), nitroprusside or similar medication may be needed.
- Auscultate lung sounds q1-2h and monitor UO. If crackles ↑ and UO ↓, additional diuretics may be necessary.
- To prevent further ↓ in BP, do not ↑ angle of HOB >30 degrees.
- Treat ventricular or other dysrhythmias according to ACLS guidelines.
- Be prepared to employ temporary transcutaneous or transvenous pacing if bradycardia or second- or third-degree heart block present.
- If preload is low, administer crystalloid IV fluids according to these fluid challenge guidelines:

Assessment	PAWP	Suggested fluids
CO low; PAWP low or nl	<6	200 ml over 10 min
	6-12	100 ml over 10 min
	≥12	50 ml over 10 min
PAWP ↑ during infusion	>6	Return to KVO rate
	≤3	Continue infusion
Assess PAWP after 10 min	If >3 or<6	Repeat challenge

- If medical management ineffective, prepare patient for insertion of IABP or left VAD.

Altered cerebral, renal, peripheral, and cardiopulmonary tissue perfusion r/t interrupted arterial blood flow to vital organs secondary to inadequate arterial pressure
Desired outcome: Within 96 h of this diagnosis, patient has adequate tissue perfusion: orientation × 3, equal and normoreactive pupils, nl reflexes, UO ≥0.5 ml/kg/h, warm and dry skin, peripheral pulses >2+ on 0-4+ scale, brisk capillary refill (<2 sec), and BP >90/60 mm Hg.

- Check neurologic status q1-2h to assess cerebral perfusion.
- Monitor I&O qh to assess renal perfusion. Assess extremities q1-2h, noting changes in skin color, temp, capillary refill, BP, and distal pulses.
- Titrate vasoactive drugs to maintain SBP >90 mm Hg.

Impaired gas exchange r/t alveolar-capillary membrane changes secondary to pulmonary congestion; and r/t altered O$_2$-carrying capacity of blood secondary to acidosis occurring with anaerobic metabolism
Desired outcome: Before weaning from supplemental O$_2$ or ventilatory assistance is attempted, patient has adequate gas exchange: Pao$_2$ ≥80 mm Hg, RR 12-20 breaths/min with eupnea, O$_2$ saturation ≥95%, and Svo$_2$ 60%-80%.

- At least qh, assess respiratory rate, depth, and effort for tachypnea or labored breaths. Also inspect skin and mucous membranes for pallor or cyanosis.
- Auscultate lung fields q1-2h for crackles, rhonchi, or wheezes.
- Monitor ABGs for hypoxemia (Pao$_2$ <80 mm Hg) or metabolic acidosis (pH <7.35 and HCO$_3^-$ <24 mEq/L).
- Deliver humidified O$_2$.
- Monitor transcutaneous O$_2$ saturation with pulse oximeter. Be alert to ↓ below 90%.
- Monitor Svo$_2$. When cardiac output drops, Svo$_2$ will ↓, indicating ↑ O$_2$ extraction.
- If condition continues to deteriorate, prepare for intubation and mechanical ventilation.

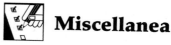

Miscellanea

CONSULT MD FOR

- SVR >1200 dynes/sec/cm^{-5}
- Svo$_2$ <50%
- CI <1.5 L/min/m^2
- New or ↑ crackles
- UO <0.5 ml/kg/h × 2
- Pao$_2$ <80 mm Hg, pH <7.35, Spo$_2$ <90%

RELATED TOPICS

- Cardiac surgery: CABG
- Cardiac transplantation: preoperative
- Hemodynamic monitoring
- Intraaortic balloon pump
- Mechanical ventilation
- Myocardial infarction, acute
- Ventricular assist device

ABBREVIATION

VAD: Ventricular assist device

REFERENCES

Baas LS, Steuble BT: Cardiovascular dysfunctions. In Swearingen PL, Keen JH (eds): _Manual of critical care nursing_, ed 3, St Louis, 1995, Mosby.

Chatterjee K et al: Gaining ground on cardiogenic shock, _Patient Care_ 28(15): 24-28, 1994.

Peppers M: Inotropes for heart failure, _Emergency_ 27(7): 18-25, 1995.

Rodgers KG: Cardiovascular shock, _Emerg Med Clin North Am_ 13(4): 793-810, 1995.

Shoemaker WC: Pathophysiology, monitoring, and therapy of acute circulatory problems, _Crit Care Nurs Clin North Am_ 6(2): 295-307, 1994.

Author: **Linda S. Baas**

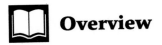 **Overview**

PATHOPHYSIOLOGY

A form of hypovolemic shock resulting from blood loss attributable to trauma, coagulopathy/bleeding disorder, GI tract bleeding, or any source that ↓ intravascular volume to the point that compensatory mechanisms are unable to maintain adequate tissue perfusion and nl cellular function. Altered cellular metabolism results in lactic acidosis, myocardial depression, intravascular coagulation, ↑ capillary permeability, and release of toxins.

HISTORY/RISK FACTORS

- GI bleeding, esophageal varices, liver disease, pancreatitis
- Recent surgery or other invasive procedure: eg, disruptions in vascular grafts or other vascular repairs
- Abdominal or thoracic aortic aneurysm
- Blood dyscrasia (von Willebrand's disease, hemophilia), DIC
- Heparinization/use of anticoagulants, thrombolytic therapy
- Major trauma, long bone fractures (femur), pelvic fracture
- Obstetric complications, cancer
- Alcohol or drug intoxication: leads to dangerous risk-taking behavior
- Chronic health conditions: impair physiologic response to injury or ↑ susceptibility to injury (hypertension, DM, COPD, CV disorders, renal failure, immunologic disorders)

CLINICAL PRESENTATION

Pallor, anxiety, restlessness, disorientation, cool and clammy skin. Unconsciousness, frank bleeding may be noted. Massive intraabdominal bleeding may present as distended, firm, tender abdomen, with or without ecchymosis.

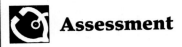 **Assessment**

PHYSICAL ASSESSMENT

Findings vary according to involved organs
Neuro: Restlessness, anxiety, confusion, unconsciousness
Resp: Rapid, shallow, ineffective respirations; in late shock, crackles signaling heart failure
CV: Heart tones nl to distant; rapid, thready pulses
GI: Possible ↓ in bowel sounds; ileus from ↓ mesenteric blood flow
GU: ↓ UO
Integ: Cool to cold temp with diaphoresis; pale to cyanotic color in face, extremities, and possibly, over entire body if blood loss profound

VITAL SIGNS/HEMODYNAMICS

Vary according to catecholamine response, volume status, drugs administered
RR: ↑ early; ↓ late
HR: ↑ early; ↓ very late
BP: Nl early; then ↓ SBP with orthostasis; later, SBP and DBP ↓
Temp: Nl; ↓ if shock severe or prolonged
CVP/PAWP: ↓
MAP: <70 mm Hg in late stages

CO: ↓
SVR: ↑
Svo₂: Usually low (<60%) reflecting high O₂ extraction from RBCs
12/18-Lead ECG: May reflect ST depression caused by myocardial ischemia, tachycardia. Ventricular irritability (PVCs, VT) may be present in later stages; PEA terminally.

LABORATORY STUDIES

CBC: Serial determination of Hgb/Hct reflects amount of blood lost. If drawn early, may be nl or slightly ↓. Platelets may ↑ in response to hemorrhage. WBCs may be ↑ or show shift to left, reflecting inflammatory response of SIRS.
Serum Lactate: May be >15 mg/dl, indicating lactic acidosis caused by hypoperfusion.
ABGs: If shock state severe, lactic acidosis occurs: arterial pH <7.25, HCO₃⁻ <22 mEq/L, Pao₂ <80 mm Hg. Anion gap may be ↑.
Coagulation Studies: Depending on preexisting disease, hypercoagulability may be present. ↑ in fibrinogen levels, FDPs, PT, and PTT may be seen.
Type and Crossmatch: Determines presence of antigens so that donor and recipient blood are compatible.

IMAGING

X-rays: To check for fractures, abnormal air or fluids, foreign objects, and to determine location of large organs.
CT Scan: Abdominal and thoracic scans detect soft tissue injuries, hematomas, subtle fractures, free air and fluid in abdomen (indicative of perforation) and large vascular tears or irregularities.

DIAGNOSTIC PROCEDURES

Angiography: To aid in visualization of bleeding site(s) if bleeding rapid and suspected of being arterial or from large vein. If GI bleeding clearly visible, therapeutic embolization may be attempted during angiography.

Hemodynamic Monitoring: PAP and invasive BP monitoring may be used to guide blood and fluid replacement and use of vasoactive drugs.

Peritoneal Lavage: Insertion of dialysis catheter into abdomen/peritoneum to check for intraabdominal bleeding.

Collaborative Management

Supplemental O$_2$: To fully saturate available Hgb.

Transfusion Therapy/Fluid Management: Two large-bore IV (16-18 gauge, short) catheters used for rapid delivery of blood/fluids. If blood loss rapid during initial phase, O-negative or type-specific blood may be needed until full crossmatch completed. One amp 10% CaCl given after every 4 U PRBCs, since blood calcium binds with citrate from banked blood.

Blood Products: Those appropriate for coagulopathies/bleeding disorders (eg, DIC, HIT, hemophilia) may be necessary if these disorders present.

Autotransfusion: Shed blood is filtered and reinfused into patient; used most often with thoracic cavity blood collected from draining chest tubes.

MAST/PASG: To ↑ external pressure on body/blood vessels, causing ↑ MAP and splinting of fractures. Considered controversial.

Gastric Intubation: To remove gastric contents, prevent vomiting and aspiration, and enable irrigation for gastric bleeding.

Indwelling Urinary Catheter: To monitor UO, which reflects organ perfusion.

Spo$_2$: To assess O$_2$ delivery; titrated to maintain Spo$_2$ >92%.

Nutritional Support: Short- and medium-chain fatty acids and branched-chain amino acids may stop protein catabolism caused by stress response.

Surgery: Specific to injury; may include abdominal exploration with repair of torn vessels or long bone/pelvic fractures associated with blood vessel injury or returning patient for reexploration of surgical site.

PHARMACOTHERAPY

Crystalloids: NS, LR to replace intravascular volume loss. Sustained use of NS can lead to hyperchloremic acidosis; therefore, LR preferred except with simultaneous blood administration.

Colloids (albumin, hetastarch, PPF): To restore intravascular volume, promote intravascular fluid retention.

Sodium Bicarbonate: To correct acidosis; guided by serial ABGs to assess effectiveness of treatment. Hyperventilation also may be used.

Replacements of K$^+$, Na$^+$, Cl$^-$, and Ca^{2+}: To correct electrolyte imbalances.

Vasopressors: Given IV to ↑ BP if unresponsive to fluid therapy alone (adequate MAP >70 mm Hg); includes catecholamines such as dopamine, norepinephrine, and epinephrine.

PATIENT-FAMILY TEACHING

- Need, purpose for all hemodynamic monitoring equipment and IV lines
- Need, purpose for blood products; associated risks
- Need, purpose for additional therapies, eg, mechanical ventilation; reassurance that this usually is only temporary
- Purpose, expected results, anticipated sensations of all nursing/medical interventions

Nursing Diagnoses/Interventions

Altered peripheral, cardiopulmonary, cerebral, renal, and gastrointestinal tissue perfusion r/t hypovolemia secondary to blood loss/hemorrhage

Desired outcome: Within 24 h of therapy initiation, patient has adequate perfusion: orientation $\times$ 3, peripheral pulses >2+ on 0-4+ scale, brisk capillary refill (<2 sec), UO $\geq$0.5 ml/kg/h, >5 bowel sounds/min, SBP >90 mm Hg, SVR 900-1200 dynes/sec/cm^{-5}, PAWP 6-12 mm Hg, CVP 2-6 mm Hg.

- Monitor hemodynamic pressures and adjust fluids, vasopressors, and O_2 accordingly. $\downarrow$ Svo_2 reflects high tissue extraction. Correct anemia, fluid status first; then consider inotropic therapy.
- Administer crystalloids or colloids for fluid replacement to maintain PAWP $\geq$6 mm Hg. Use NS, LR initially; use colloids as needed for significant third spacing or when serum albumin $\downarrow$.
- Monitor BP and peripheral pulses at least qh.
- Position patient supine with legs elevated to $\uparrow$ venous return and preload. This is effective only as a temporary measure until fluid volume is restored.
- Monitor for $\uparrow$ RR, $\uparrow$ HR, and cool and clammy skin at least q30min.
- Monitor neurologic status at least qh.
- Monitor ABGs for significant acidosis (pH <7.25) with hypercapnia ($Paco_2$ >45 mm Hg), signaling respiratory insufficiency with possible lactic acidosis. Administer sodium bicarbonate or hyperventilate as necessary.
- Auscultate bowel sounds at least q8h.

Impaired gas exchange r/t lack of RBCs to carry O_2 to vital organs and peripheral tissues

Desired outcomes: Within 24 h of treatment onset, patient has adequate gas exchange: HR and RR within 10% baseline or HR 60-100 bpm and RR 12-20 breaths/min; Hgb and Hct returned to baseline (Hgb 12 mg/dl and Hct >37%); O_2 saturation >90%; BP returned to within 10% baseline or SBP >90 mm Hg; and Svo_2 60%-80%.

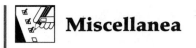 **Miscellanea**

CONSULT MD FOR

- Persistence of the following: Spo_2 <90%, Svo_2 <60%, temp >38.6° C (101.5° F), SBP <90 mm Hg while fluid and blood replacement or vasopressor therapy are active, HR >140 bpm, RR >30 breaths/min
- Potential complications: MODS, MI, stroke, renal failure, hypoxemia, bowel infarction

RELATED TOPICS

- Aortic aneurysm/dissection
- Bleeding, postoperative
- Cardiac surgery: CABG
- Cardiac surgery: valvular disorders
- Esophageal varices
- GI bleeding: upper and lower
- Multisystem injury
- Nutritional support, parenteral
- Pancreatitis, acute

ABBREVIATIONS

FDPs: Fibrin degradation products
HIT: Heparin-induced thrombocytopenia
MODS: Multiple organ dysfunction syndrome
PEA: Pulseless electrical activity
PPF: Plasma protein fraction
PRBCs: Packed red blood cells
SIRS: Systemic inflammatory response syndrome

- Administer supplemental O_2 as needed, using appropriate device. Advancement from nasal cannula to mask device to mechanical ventilation may be necessary in severe cases.
- Monitor O_2 saturation continuously.
- Maintain large-bore (16-18 gauge) IV catheter(s) in case additional transfusion/rapid volume expansion is necessary. Central lines may not be able to deliver volume as rapidly as needed to correct severe hypovolemia.
- Transfuse with PRBCs as prescribed to facilitate O_2 delivery and assist in volume expansion.
- Monitor breath sounds at least qh.
- Monitor Svo_2 for sustained/profound hypovolemic shock or if condition is complicated by LV failure. Standard PAP monitoring may not be adequate for assessment of perfusion/oxygenation with severe alterations in cellular metabolism.

Risk for infection r/t inadequate primary defenses secondary to presence of multiple invasive lines, movement restrictions, and stasis of body fluids

Desired outcome: Patient infection free: normothermia; WBCs <11,000 μl; negative culture results; and absence of erythema, swelling, warmth, tenderness, and purulent drainage.

- Monitor WBCs qd. Check for ↑ or left shifts.
- Assess all invasive sites for evidence of infection: redness, swelling, tenderness, drainage.
- Culture any suspicious drainage or secretions.
- Change IV tubing q72h (or per agency protocol).
- Administer prophylactic antibiotics if prescribed.
- Monitor temp q4h and prn. Recognize that even slight ↑ in temp may signal infection in these patients.

REFERENCES

Cone M: Cardiopulmonary support in the intensive care unit, *Am J Crit Care* 1(1): 98-108, 1992.

Edwards KP: Orthopedic trauma: pelvic fractures, *Today's OR Nurse* 15(1): 169-185, 1993.

Epstein CD, Henning RJ: Oxygen transport variables in the identification and treatment of tissue hypoxia, *Heart Lung* 22(4): 328-348, 1993.

Kerber K: The adult with bleeding esophageal varices, *Crit Care Nurs Clin North Am* 5(1): 153-162, 1993.

Krumberger JM: Acute pancreatitis, *Crit Care Clin North Am* 5(1): 169-185, 1993.

Lawrence DM: Gastrointestinal trauma, *Crit Care Clin North Am* 5(1): 127-140, 1993.

Neff JA, Kidd PS: *Trauma nursing: the art and science,* St Louis, 1993, Mosby.

Smith A, Fitzpatrick E: Penetrating cardiac trauma: surgical and nursing management, *J Cardiovasc Nurs* 7(2): 52-70, 1993.

Author: **Marianne Saunorus Baird**

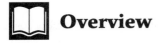 **Overview**

PATHOPHYSIOLOGY

A result of ECF depletion that ↓ intravascular volume to the point that compensatory mechanisms are unable to maintain adequate tissue perfusion and nl cellular function. Altered cellular metabolism results in lactic acidosis, myocardial depression, intravascular coagulation, ↑ capillary permeability, release of toxins, and, ultimately, death.

HISTORY/RISK FACTORS

- GI losses: vomiting, NG suctioning, diarrhea, intestinal drainage, enterocutaneous fistulas
- Skin losses: excessive diaphoresis from fever or exercise; burns
- Renal losses: diuretic therapy, DI, polyuric renal disease, adrenal insufficiency, osmotic diuresis (eg, hyperglycemia, postdye study), acute alcohol intoxication
- Third spacing or plasma-to-interstitial fluid shift: peritonitis, intestinal obstruction, burns, pancreatitis, hepatitis, cirrhosis
- Hemorrhage: major trauma, GI bleeding, obstetric complications
- Chronic health conditions: impair physiologic response to volume depletion (CV disease, DM, COPD, cerebrovascular disorders, hepatic or renal insufficiency, immunologic disorders)

CLINICAL PRESENTATION

Pallor, anxiety, restlessness, disorientation, cool and clammy skin, nausea, vomiting. Unconsciousness, frank bleeding may be noted.

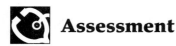 **Assessment**

PHYSICAL ASSESSMENT

Findings vary according to involved systems
Neuro: Restlessness, anxiety, confusion, unconsciousness
Resp: Rapid, shallow, ineffective respirations; in late shock, crackles signaling heart failure
CV: Rapid, thready pulses
GI: Possible ↓ in bowel sounds; ileus from ↓ mesenteric blood flow

GU: ↓ UO
Integ: Cool to cold temp with diaphoresis; pale to cyanotic color in face, extremities, and possibly over entire body if blood loss profound

VITAL SIGNS/HEMODYNAMICS

Vary according to catecholamine response, volume status, drugs administered
RR: ↑ early; ↓ late
HR: ↑ early; terminal ↓
BP: Nl early; then ↓ SBP with orthostasis; later, profound ↓ in MAP
Temp: Nl; ↓ if shock severe or prolonged
CVP/PAWP: ↓
MAP: <70 mm Hg in late stages
CO: ↓
SVR: ↑
12/18-Lead ECG: May reflect ST-segment depression caused by myocardial ischemia, tachycardia. Ventricular irritability (PVCs, VT) may be present in later stages; PEA terminally.

LABORATORY STUDIES

Hematology: Hct ↑ with dehydration; ↓ Hgb/Hct reflects amount of blood lost. WBCs may be ↑ or show shift to left, reflecting inflammatory response of SIRS.
Electrolytes: Variable according to type of fluid lost. GI, renal losses often cause hypokalemia. ↑ insensible loss, DI may cause hypernatremia.
Serum Lactate: May be >15 mg/dl, indicating lactic acidosis caused by hypoperfusion.
ABGs: If shock state severe, lactic acidosis occurs: arterial pH <7.25, HCO_3^- <22 mEq/L, Pao_2 <80 mm Hg. Anion gap may be ↑.
BUN: ↑ as a result of dehydration, ↓ RBF, or ↓ renal function. Plasma BUN/creatinine ratio >20:1 suggests hypovolemia.
Coagulation Studies: Depending on preexisting disease, hypercoagulability may be present. ↑ in fibrinogen levels, FDPs, PT, and PTT may be seen.
Type and Crossmatch: If shock caused by hemorrhage.

IMAGING

X-rays: To check for abnormal air or fluids. Possible findings include fluid in lungs and peritoneum; abnormal air/fluid in bowels because of obstruction.

CT Scan: Abdominal and thoracic scans detect soft tissue injuries, hematomas, subtle fractures, free air and fluid in abdomen (indicative of perforation), and large vascular tears or irregularities.

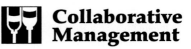 **Collaborative Management**

Treatment of Underlying Cause: Eg, surgery to correct GI bleeding or other hemorrhage, bowel obstruction; antibiotics for peritonitis.
Restoration of Tissue Perfusion
Crystalloids: For volume replacement; given rapidly as long as cardiac filling pressures and BP remain low. Overaggressive fluid resuscitation in uncontrolled hemorrhage avoided because of risk of secondary hemorrhage as intravascular hydrostatic pressure ↑.
Colloids: Eg, albumin, to prevent pulmonary edema; controversial.
Blood: Given only as necessary to maintain O_2-carrying capacity. Hct should not be ↑ >35%.
Vasopressors: To augment volume restoration if unresponsive to fluid resuscitation alone and/or SVR ↓. Given to maintain adequate MAP of >70 mm Hg. Includes catecholamines such as dopamine, norepinephrine, epinephrine.
Supplemental O_2: To ↑ O_2 available to the tissues.
Indwelling Urinary Catheter: To monitor UO, which reflects organ perfusion.
Gastric Intubation: To remove gastric contents, prevent vomiting and aspiration, and enable irrigation if there is gastric bleeding.

PATIENT-FAMILY TEACHING

- Need, purpose for all hemodynamic monitoring equipment and IV lines
- As applicable, need, purpose for blood products; associated risks
- Need for additional therapies, eg, mechanical ventilation; reassurance that this is usually only temporary
- Purpose, expected results, anticipated sensations of all nursing/medical interventions

Nursing Diagnoses/Interventions

Fluid volume deficit r/t abnormal loss of body fluids or ↓ intake
Desired outcome: Within 24 h of therapy initiation, patient normovolemic: peripheral pulses >2+ on 0-4+ scale, UO ≥0.5 ml/kg/h, SBP >90 mm Hg, SVR 900-1200 dynes/sec/cm^{-5}, PAWP 6-12 mm Hg, CVP 2-6 mm Hg.

- Position supine with legs elevated to ↑ venous return and preload. This is effective only as a temporary measure until volume is restored.
- Monitor hemodynamic pressures and adjust fluids, vasopressors, and O_2 accordingly. ↓ Svo$_2$ reflects high tissue extraction. Svo$_2$ monitoring especially helpful if hypovolemic shock is complicated by LV failure. Correct anemia, fluid status first; then consider inotropic therapy.
- Administer crystalloids or colloids for fluid replacement to maintain PAWP ≥6 mm Hg. Use LR, NS initially; use colloids as needed for significant third spacing or when serum albumin ↓.
- Document response to fluid therapy, and monitor for S&S of fluid overload or too rapid fluid administration: crackles, SOB, tachypnea, tachycardia, ↑CVP/PAP.
- Monitor BP and peripheral pulses at least qh.
- Monitor for ↑ RR and HR, and cool, clammy skin at least q30min.
- Monitor neurologic status at least qh.
- Monitor ABGs for significant acidosis (pH <7.25) with hypercapnia (Paco$_2$ >45 mm Hg), signaling respiratory insufficiency with possible lactic acidosis. Administer sodium bicarbonate or hyperventilate as necessary.
- Be aware that daily weight measurement is the single most important indicator of fluid status because acute weight changes usually signal fluid changes. Weigh at the same time of day on a balanced scale with patient wearing approximately the same clothing. A 10%-15% acute weight loss indicates severe ECF deficit; >15% may be fatal.

Altered cerebral, renal, and peripheral tissue perfusion r/t hypovolemia
Desired outcome: Within 12 h after therapy initiation, patient has adequate perfusion: alertness, warm and dry skin, BP wnl for patient, HR ≤100 bpm, UO ≥0.5 ml/kg/h, and capillary refill <2 sec.

- Monitor for ↓ cerebral perfusion: vertigo, syncope, confusion, restlessness, anxiety, agitation, excitability, weakness, nausea, and cool and clammy skin.
- Protect patients who are confused, dizzy, or weak. Keep side rails up and bed in lowest position with wheels locked. Raise to sitting or standing positions slowly. Assist with ambulation. Monitor for orthostatic hypotension: ↓ BP, ↑ HR, dizziness, and diaphoresis. If symptoms occur, return patient to supine position.
- To avoid unnecessary vasodilatation, treat fevers promptly. Cover with a light blanket to maintain body temp.
- Reassure patient and significant others that sensorium changes will improve with therapy.
- Palpate peripheral pulses bilaterally in arms and legs. Use a Doppler ultrasonic device if unable to palpate pulses.
- Monitor UO. Be alert to output <0.5 ml/kg/h for 2 consecutive h.

Risk for infection r/t inadequate primary defenses secondary to presence of multiple invasive lines, movement restrictions, and stasis of body fluids
Desired outcome: Patient infection free: normothermia; WBCs <11,000 μl; negative culture results; and absence of erythema, swelling, warmth, tenderness, and purulent drainage.

- Monitor WBCs qd. Check for ↑ or left shift.
- Assess all invasive sites for evidence of infection: redness, swelling, tenderness, drainage.
- Culture any suspicious drainage or secretions.
- Change IV tubing q72h (or per agency protocol).
- Administer prophylactic antibiotics if prescribed.
- Monitor temp q4h and prn. Recognize that even slight ↑ in temp may signal infection in these patients.

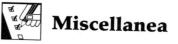

Miscellanea

CONSULT MD FOR

- Persistence of the following: Spo$_2$ <90%, Svo$_2$ <60%, temp >38.6° C (101.5° F), SBP <90 mm Hg while fluid and blood replacement or vasopressor therapy are active, HR >140 bpm, RR >30 breaths/min
- UO <0.5 ml/kg/h × 2 h
- Potential complications: MODS, MI, stroke, renal failure, hypoxemia, bowel infarction

RELATED TOPICS

- Bleeding, postoperative
- Burns
- Enterocutaneous fistulas
- Hypovolemia
- Multisystem injury
- Nutritional support, enteral and parenteral
- Pancreatitis, acute
- Shock, hemorrhagic

ABBREVIATIONS

ECF: Extracellular fluid
FDPs: Fibrin degradation products
MODS: Multiple organ dysfunction syndrome
PEA: Pulseless electrical activity
RBF: Renal blood flow
SIRS: Systemic inflammatory response syndrome

REFERENCES

Cone M: Cardiopulmonary support in the intensive care unit, *Am J Crit Care* 1(1): 98-108, 1992.

Cullen L: Interventions related to fluid and electrolyte balance, *Nurs Clin North Am* 27(2): 569-597, 1992.

Horne M, Heitz UE, Swearingen PL: *Pocket guide to fluid, electrolyte, acid-base balance,* ed 3, St Louis, Mosby, 1996.

Imm A, Carlson RW: Fluid resuscitation in circulatory shock, *Crit Care Clin* 9(2): 313-333, 1993.

Reilly E, Yucha C: Multiple organ failure syndrome, *Crit Care Nurse* 14(2): 25-31, 1993.

Author: **Janet Hicks Keen**

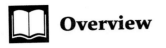 **Overview**

PATHOPHYSIOLOGY

Form of vasogenic shock in which trauma or surgery of spinal cord or brain (more rarely) causes massive vasodilatation, leading to "false hypovolemia" and hypotension. Bradycardia possible as a result of interruption of descending SNS pathways if injury to C- or upper T-spine present. Loss of sympathetic innervation causes venous pooling in extremities and splanchnic vasculature, resulting in ↓ venous return to the heart. Low CO and low tissue perfusion pressure cause bradycardia and add to hypotension. With SCIs lower than midthorax, effects are less severe.

HISTORY/RISK FACTORS

- Injury to C-spine, upper T-spine, or brain
- Spinal anesthesia
- Epidural catheter for pain control placed at or above T6
- Motor vehicle accident (especially if unrestrained); diving accident
- Alcohol or drug intoxication (leads to dangerous risk-taking behavior)
- Chronic health conditions that lead to impaired physiologic response to injury or ↑ susceptibility

CLINICAL PRESENTATION

- Pallor, anxiety, restlessness, disorientation
- Warm and clammy skin as a result of vasodilatation
- With severe SCI or head injury: weakness/paralysis of extremities and torso, impaired reflexes, hypotension

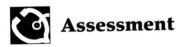 **Assessment**

PHYSICAL ASSESSMENT

Varies with injury cause/location
Neuro: Restlessness, anxiety, confusion → unconsciousness; *with SCI and head injury:* paralysis, paresis, altered reflexes, headache
Resp: Tachypnea, hyperpnea if ↑ ICP present; deep sighs, yawning, Cheyne-Stokes or irregular breathing pattern
CV: Bradycardia, hypotension
GI: ↓ bowel sounds; *with SCI:* possible fecal impaction or paralytic ileus
GU: ↓ UO; *with SCI:* bladder dysfunction, urinary retention, incontinence
Integ: Usually warm, diaphoretic skin

VITAL SIGNS/HEMODYNAMICS

RR: ↑
HR: ↓
BP: ↓

Temp: Nl; ↑ with head injury; or poikilothermic with SCI
CVP/PAWP: ↓
CO: ↓
SVR: ↓
12/18-Lead ECG: May reflect sinus bradycardia with possible ST-segment depression, indicating myocardial ischemia if SBP <90 mm Hg. ECG change seen with ↑ ICP for head injury: prominent U waves, notched T waves, prolongation of QT interval. SVT and ventricular dysrhythmias also may be present.

LABORATORY STUDIES

ABGs: To assess effectiveness of respirations and detect need for O_2/mechanical ventilation. ↓ Pao_2 or ↑ $Paco_2$ possible with pulmonary injury or ↓ LOC.
CBC with Differential: To identify complications of infection or other bleeding associated with injury.
Serum Osmolality: To assess for DI and SIADH in head-injured patients.
Urine Osmolality/Specific Gravity: To assess for DI.
Blood Alcohol Level/Toxicology Screen: To assess for substance abuse.
Venous Lactate Level: To assess for tissue hypoperfusion and anaerobic metabolism.

IMAGING

X-rays: Skull, cervical, lumbar spine films to detect structural injuries, including skull fractures and spinal injuries.
CT Scan: To diagnose cerebral hemorrhage, infarction, hydrocephalus, cerebral edema, structural shifts.
CSF Analysis: To check for infection.
MRI: To detect structural anomalies of head or spinal column. Defines structures, detects tissue changes, and evaluates flow patterns and blood vessels.

DIAGNOSTIC PROCEDURES

Evoked Responses: Evaluates brain's electrical potentials to external stimulus (visual, auditory, somatosensory) to help diagnose lesions of the cortex or ascending pathways of the spinal cord, brainstem, or thalamus.
Pulmonary Fluoroscopy: To evaluate degree of diaphragmatic movement with high cervical injury.
Angiography: To study cerebral vasculature if CT scan unavailable or inadequate to visualize vessels.

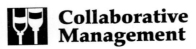 **Collaborative Management**

Maintenance of BP Within Acceptable Range: Hypotension may result in ↓ O_2 delivery to all cells, resulting in anaerobic metabo-

lism, which ↓ pH as a result of lactate production. May consider hemodynamic monitoring to guide management.
Management of ICP Dynamics: For head injury, *via* ICP monitoring. CPP should be maintained at 60-80 mm Hg.
Maintenance of Body Temp: With every 1° C ↑ in temp, a 10%-13% ↑ in metabolic rate occurs, which ↑ tissue O_2 demands. With head injury, central fever is caused by hypothalamic injury, resulting in plateaulike temp ↑, usually ≤41° C (105.8° F), with no tachycardia, sweating, or diurnal variation. Body temp variations managed with external cooling.
Supplemental O_2: To ↑ O_2 delivery to injured CNS tissues and provide ↑ O_2 to meet ↑ tissue needs.
Hyperventilation Therapy: Mechanical ventilation ↓ CO_2 levels and thus promotes cerebral vasoconstriction with resulting ↓ ICP.
Immobilization of Injured Site: Skeletal traction used to immobilize spinal fractures/dislocations.
Surgery: To evacuate mass lesions (intracranial hematoma), place ICP monitoring devices, elevate skull fractures, and stabilize T-spine and L-spine injuries. Surgery for acute C-spine injury controversial.

PHARMACOTHERAPY

Fluid Resuscitation: Blood volume nl, but vascular space enlarges because of vasodilatation. Fluid repletion, usually with crystalloids (0.9% NaCl, LR) used. Hypotonic glucose-containing solutions (D_5W) may ↑ cerebral edema and should be avoided.
Vasopressors: Epinephrine, norepinephrine, high-dose dopamine may be used to manage vasodilatation. BP that does not respond to vasopressor therapy is possible, as vasomotor control is lost below level of spinal cord lesion, leading to massive refractory vasodilatation.
Corticosteroids: Used in SCI and head injury to protect neuromembranes from further destruction.

PATIENT-FAMILY TEACHING

- Need/purpose for hemodynamics, IV fluid/medication administration devices, ECG/other equipment
- For SCI, need/purpose for specialty bed and other devices, including traction; after acute period, explanation of AD and methods to identify and manage the disorder for lesions at T6 and above
- With SCI and head injury, explanation regarding cognitive and sensorimotor deficits; after acute phase, need for rehabilitation
- If event r/t spinal anesthesia, explanation that shock should resolve within 24 h

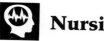 # Nursing Diagnoses/Interventions

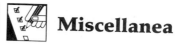 # Miscellanea

Impaired gas exchange r/t ↓ cellular O_2 supply secondary to low perfusion pressure during vasodilated state

Desired outcomes: Within 24 h of treatment onset, patient has adequate gas exchange: orientation × 3, Pao_2 >80 mm Hg, RR 12-20 breaths/min with eupnea. $Paco_2$ <30 mm Hg during acute phase if head-injured, then 35-45 mm Hg at discharge.

- Assess patient for hypoxia: confusion, agitation, restlessness, irritability.
- Ensure patent airway *via* proper neck positioning and frequent assessment of need for suctioning.
- Monitor ABGs, paying special attention to pH and $Paco_2$ values. Low pH may signal lactic acidosis unless $Paco_2$ ↑, indicating respiratory failure.
- Administer appropriate O_2 therapy as needed, including mechanical ventilation. Mechanical ventilation augments oxygenation and ↓ $Paco_2$.

Decreased cardiac output r/t relative hypovolemia secondary to enlarged vascular compartment as a consequence of neurogenic shock

Desired outcome: Within 24 h of this diagnosis, cardiac output adequate: SBP >90 mm Hg (or within 10% nl for patient), HR 60-100 bpm, CVP 4-6 mm Hg, PAP 20-30/8-15 mm Hg, SVR 900-1200 dynes/sec/cm^{-5}, peripheral pulses >2+ on 0-4+ scale, UO ≥0.5 ml/kg/h, and NSR on ECG.

- Monitor for indicators of low CO: SBP <90 mm Hg or a 10-20 mm Hg drop within 1 h, HR >100 bpm, possible irregular rhythm and ↓ amplitude of peripheral pulses, flushed skin, fainting, confusion, dizziness, UO <0.5 ml/kg/h for 2 consecutive h.
- Implement hemodynamic monitoring as prescribed. Anticipate ↓ CVP, PAP, PAWP, and SVR. Observe response to fluids and vasopressors/inotropes.
- Monitor continuous ECG for rate and rhythm.
- Administer IV fluids. If hypotension remains despite volume resuscitation, use vasopressors as prescribed.
- Change position slowly to minimize risk of severe hypotension.
- Perform ROM exercises q2h to help correct venous pooling.

Decreased adaptive capacity: Intracranial and autonomic, r/t to spinal cord or intracranial injury with resultant ↓ perfusion pressure during vasodilated state

Desired outcome: Within 12-24 h of treatment initiation, patient has adequate intracranial adaptive capacity: RR 12-20 breaths/min with eupnea; HR 60-100 bpm; ICP 0-15 mm Hg; CPP 60-80 mm Hg; absence of headache, vomiting, and other clinical indicators of altered ICP.

- Assess neurologic status at least qh, including pupils, LOC, motor and sensory function.
- Monitor VS at least qh, noting changes in respiratory pattern, fluctuations in BP and pulse, ↓ HR, and widening pulse pressure (for head injury).
- Monitor hemodynamic status to maintain CPP at 60-80 mm Hg. Be alert to ↓ SBP.

Dysreflexia (or risk for same) r/t abnormal response of SNS to a stimulus after spinal injury

Desired outcome: Patient has no symptoms of AD: dry skin above level of injury, BP wnl for patient, HR >60 bpm, and absence of headache and other indicators of AD.

- Assess for classic triad of AD. *Above level of injury:* throbbing headache, cutaneous vasodilatation, sweating; *below level of injury:* gooseflesh, pallor, chills, vasoconstriction.
- Be alert for other indicators of AD: marked ↑ in BP (250-300/140-170 mm Hg), bradycardia, nasal stuffiness, blurred vision, nausea.
- Maintain continuous cardiac monitoring. Observe for dysrhythmias (bradycardia) during first 2 wks after injury.
- Implement measures to prevent these factors that may precipitate AD: bladder (distention, infection, calculi, cystoscopy), bowel (fecal impaction, rectal examination, suppository insertion), skin (pressure from tight clothing or sheets, temp extremes, sores, areas of broken skin).
- If indicators of AD are present, place patient in sitting position or elevate HOB 60 degrees, monitor BP and HR q3-5min until stable, determine and remove AD stimulus.

CONSULT MD FOR

- Persistence of the following: hypotension despite fluid replacement or vasopressor therapy, O_2 saturation <90 mm Hg, swing in BP to profound hypertension (SBP >200 mm Hg), temp >38° C (101° F) that is unresponsive to antipyretic agents (especially in head injury), deterioration in LOC, papillary changes
- Potential complications: acute renal failure, bowel infarction, MI, stroke, MODS, AD (in T6 and higher with SCI)

RELATED TOPICS

- Autonomic dysreflexia
- Diabetes insipidus
- Head injury
- Multisystem injury
- Nutritional support, enteral and parenteral
- Spinal cord injury, cervical and thoracic
- Vasopressor therapy

ABBREVIATIONS

AD: Autonomic dysreflexia
CPP: Cerebral perfusion pressure
MODS: Multiple organ dysfunction syndrome
SIADH: Syndrome of inappropriate antidiuretic hormone
SNS: Sympathetic nervous system
SVT: Supraventricular tachycardia

REFERENCES

Ahrens T, Rutherford K: *Essentials of oxygenation: implications for clinical practice,* Boston, 1993, Jones & Bartlett.

Battle FJ, Northrup BE: Pathophysiology of acute spinal cord injury, *Trauma Q* 9(2): 29-37, 1993.

Cammermyer M, Appledorn C: *Core curriculum for neuroscience nursing,* Chicago, 1993, American Association of Neuroscience Nurses.

Cardona VC et al: *Trauma nursing: from resuscitation through rehabilitation,* ed 3, Baltimore, 1994, Williams & Wilkins.

Imm A, Carlson RW: Fluid resuscitation in circulatory shock, *Crit Care Clin* 9(2): 313-333, 1993.

Kinney M, Packa D, Dunbar S: *AACN's clinical reference for critical care nursing,* ed 3, St Louis, 1993, Mosby.

Vos H: Making headway with intracranial hypertension, *Am J Nurs* 93(2): 28-39, 1993.

Author: **Marianne Saunorus Baird**

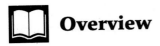 **Overview**

PATHOPHYSIOLOGY
Sepsis involves systemic inflammatory, immune, and hormonal responses to infection. Septic shock ensues as hypotension and inadequate tissue perfusion lead to lactic acidosis, oliguria, and acute alterations in mental status. It is believed that bacterial endotoxins released during sepsis trigger release of vasoactive kinins, which results in vasodilatation and ↑ capillary permeability. Later, progression to vasoconstriction and ↓ CO is stimulated by powerful catecholamines and prostaglandins released from ischemic tissues.

COMPLICATIONS
High risk for MODS, including DIC and ARDS

HISTORY/RISK FACTORS
- Infection: often caused by gram-negative bacteria, *Streptococcus pneumoniae*, *Staphylococcus aureus*, viruses, fungi
- Malnutrition, immunosuppression
- Chronic health problems: eg, CV, hepatic, renal disease
- Recent traumatic injury or major surgery
- Advanced age

CLINICAL PRESENTATION
Early Hyperdynamic (Warm) Stage: Fever, chills, flushed and warm skin, hyperventilation, fluid retention

Late (Cold) Stage: Pallor, cool skin, peripheral cyanosis, hypoventilation, profound hypotension

For Elders: Altered LOC, weakness, anorexia, normo/hypothermia, hyper/hypoglycemia

 Assessment

PHYSICAL ASSESSMENT
EARLY
Neuro: ↓ LOC, confusion, drowsiness
Resp: Tachypnea, crackles, dyspnea
CV: Tachycardia, hypotension, vasodilatation, strong and bounding peripheral pulses
GU: ↓ UO, ↑ specific gravity
LATE
Neuro: Stupor, coma
Resp: ↓ respiratory rate/depth, crackles, rhonchi, wheezes
CV: Extreme tachycardia, S_3 gallop, profound hypotension, ↓ peripheral pulses
GU: Oliguria, anuria

Other: Oozing from previous venipuncture sites; respiratory and metabolic acidosis

VITAL SIGNS/HEMODYNAMICS
EARLY
RR: ↑
HR: ↑
BP: ↓
Temp: ↑ >38.3° C; sometimes nl or ↓, especially with elders
PAWP: <6 mm Hg
SVR: <900 dynes/sec/cm^{-5}
CO: >7 L/min
CI: >4 L/min/m^2
Svo$_2$: >80% (reflects ↓ use of O_2 by cells)
LATE
RR: ↓
HR: ↑
BP: ↓
Temp: ↓
PAWP: >12 mm Hg
SVR: >1200 dynes/sec/cm^{-5}
CO: <4 L/min
CI: <2.5 L/min/m^2
Svo$_2$: ≤60% (reflects ↓ O_2 binding to Hgb caused by profound acidosis)

LABORATORY STUDIES
WBCs: ↑; may be ↓ because of binding with endotoxins that are removed from the circulation. Later after immune system activates, leukocytosis may occur with ↑ immature (band) forms.
Serum Glucose: Usually ↑ because of catecholamine-induced hepatic gluconeogenesis and glycogenolysis.
C&S: Identifies causative organism(s) in bloodstream as well as suspected infection sites (eg, urine, sputum, blood, vascular catheters, incisions).
ABGs: Reflect metabolic acidosis (low HCO_3^-). Early in sepsis, low $Paco_2$ may reflect hyperventilation. As shock progresses, respiratory acidosis (retention of CO_2) occurs and hypoxemia is present as a result of respiratory failure and metabolic derangements that impair O_2 transport/utilization.
BUN/Creatinine: ↑ reflects ↓ renal perfusion.
Clotting Studies: ↑ PT, PTT, bleeding time, FSPs; thrombocytopenia, reflecting activation of clotting cascade; may signal development of DIC.
Liver Studies: ↑ AST (SGOT), ALT (SGPT), LDH resulting from hepatic ischemia.

IMAGING
X-rays: Help determine causes such as pneumonia or perforated viscus. Serial chest x-rays monitor respiratory status, since ARDS is a potential complication.

Collaborative Management

Fluid Administration: Early IV volume expansion essential to maintain tissue perfusion yet avoid pulmonary edema. LR, NS, PPF (Plasmanate), albumin, and FFP used.
Oxygenation: Supplemental O_2, mechanical ventilation, and PEEP if S&S of ARDS present.
Hemodynamic/Flow Monitoring: To maximize Do_2, Vo_2, and CI. Goal: to maintain supradynamic values by adjusting fluids, inotropes, and vasopressors and ensuring adequacy of O_2-carrying capacity *via* optimal Hct and O_2 administration.
Pharmacotherapy
Antimicrobial therapy: Begun immediately after culture specimens obtained. Empirical treatment with broad-spectrum antibiotic. Specific agent prescribed after sensitivities available.
Positive inotropic drugs (eg, dopamine, dobutamine): To augment cardiac contractility and CO. If SVR ↑, may be given along with vasodilators, such as nitroprusside and NTG. See Appendix for "Inotropic and Vasoactive Agents."
Vasopressors (eg, dopamine, norepinephrine): For refractory hypotension. See Appendix for "Inotropic and Vasoactive Agents."
Immunomodulation: Recently developed monoclonal antibodies against endotoxins may be given to alter body's response to endotoxin release during gram-negative sepsis. Other monoclonal antibodies in development.
Other: Antipyretics; cooling blanket; ibuprofen for anti-inflammatory effects. Corticosteroids, used in the past, now considered of no benefit unless patient is on long-term corticosteroid therapy.
Nutritional Support: Enteral nutrition is optimal but often not possible. Short- and medium-chain fatty acids (absorbed more readily and metabolized more easily than long-chain fatty acids) given parenterally. Branched-chain amino acids, metabolized by muscle rather than the liver, may be used if there is evidence of hepatic failure.

PATIENT-FAMILY TEACHING
As appropriate, measures that prevent further infection: eg, for patients with long-term vascular access, valvular heart disease, immune suppression

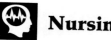 **Nursing Diagnoses/Interventions**

Fluid volume deficit r/t active loss from vascular compartment secondary to ↑ capillary permeability and shift of intravascular volume into interstitial spaces
Desired outcomes: Within 8 h of therapy initiation, patient normovolemic: peripheral pulses >2+ on 0-4+ scale, stable body weight, UO ≥0.5 ml/kg/h, SBP ≥90 mm Hg or wnl for patient, and absence of edema and adventitious lung sounds. PAWP 6-12 mm Hg, CO 4-7 L/min, and SVR 900-1200 dynes/sec/cm^{-5}.

- Assess fluid volume by monitoring BP, HR, and peripheral perfusion qh or more often.
- During acute hypotension, position patient supine with legs elevated to optimize preload.
- Administer crystalloids and colloids to maintain PAWP of 6-12 mm Hg or ≤18 mm Hg with LV failure. Assess PAWP and lung sounds frequently during fluid replacement to detect fluid overload: crackles, ↑ PAWP. As indicated, give PRBCs to ↑ O_2-carrying capacity of blood.
- Monitor hemodynamic pressures and Svo$_2$ as available.
    Anticipate ↓ BP, PAWP, and SVR and ↑ CO/CI in early stages. Support with fluids and inotropes as necessary.
    Anticipate ↓ BP, ↑ PAWP, ↑ SVR, and ↓ CO/CI in later stages.
    In general, use vasodilators if MAP >100 mm Hg or vasopressors if MAP <70 mm Hg.
    In late stage, fluids, inotropes, vasopressors, and vasodilators all may be necessary because of MODS and desensitization to endogenous catecholamines. Titrate carefully to optimize CI and maintain Svo$_2$ of 60%-80%.
- Weigh qd; monitor I&O every shift and UO qh, noting 24-h trends. Weight may ↑ despite actual fluid volume deficit because of shift of intravascular volume into interstitial spaces.
- Assess for interstitial edema as evidenced by pretibial, sacral, ankle, and hand edema, as well as lung crackles. Take measures to protect skin integrity.

Altered cerebral, renal, and GI tissue perfusion r/t hypovolemia secondary to vasodilatation (early stage) or interruption of arterial and venous blood flow secondary to microcirculatory sludging of blood (late stage)
Desired outcomes: Within 24 h of initiating therapy, patient has adequate perfusion: orientation × 3, peripheral pulses >2+ on 0-4+ scale, brisk capillary refill (<2 sec), UO ≥0.5 ml/kg/h, and ≥5 bowel sounds/min. BP 110-120/70-80 mm Hg (or wnl for patient), Svo$_2$ 60%-80%, SVR 900-1200 dynes/sec/$^{-5}$, CO 4-7 L/min, and CI 2.5-4 L/min/m^2.

- Assess for ↓ cerebral perfusion: ↓ LOC, restlessness.
- Assess for ↓ renal perfusion: UO <0.5 ml/kg and ↑ BUN/creatinine and serum K$^+$ levels.
- Monitor BP continuously. Be alert to ↓ SBP, nl/↑ DBP, ↓ pulse pressures that occur with ↓ perfusion.
- Assess for hypoperfusion: ↓ pulse amplitude, cool extremities, pallor or mottling, and delayed capillary refill.
- Monitor cellular O_2 consumption (Svo$_2$). With sepsis, cellular O_2 delivery ↓ because of precapillary vasoconstriction and thus cellular O_2 use ↓. This may result in abnormally high Svo$_2$.
- Treat underlying infection with appropriate antimicrobial therapy, being certain to administer precisely as scheduled to optimize bloodstream levels.
- Administer fluids, inotropes, and/or vasodilators or vasopressors to optimize SVR and CO/CI. Be aware that ↑ filling pressures may be necessary for optimal CO.
- Assess for ↓ splanchnic (visceral) circulation, including ↓/absent bowel sounds, ↑ amylase, ↑ liver enzymes, and ↓ platelet count.

Impaired gas exchange r/t alveolar-capillary membrane changes secondary to interstitial edema, alveolar destruction, and endotoxin release with activation of histamine and kinins
Desired outcome: Within 4 h of therapy initiation, patient's Pao$_2$ ≥80 mm Hg; Paco$_2$ ≤45 mm Hg; pH 7.35-7.45; and lungs clear.

- Administer supplemental O_2 to maximize O_2 available to tissues.
- If patient exhibits inadequate gas exchange (eg, Pao$_2$ <60 mm Hg on 100% oxygen *via* non-rebreathing mask), prepare for probability of endotracheal intubation.
- Assess for and maintain patent airway by assisting with coughing or suctioning as necessary.
- Assess ABGs. Be alert to ↓ Pao$_2$, ↑ Paco$_2$, acidosis. Monitor for dyspnea, SOB, crackles, restlessness. Adjust supplemental O_2, ventilator settings as indicated.
- Closely monitor PAWP and keep as low as possible to avoid contributing to excess lung water. A narrow range of optimal PAWP exists because of complex pathophysiology, including intravascular fluid volume deficit, ↑ capillary permeability, and possible LV failure.
- If patient is mechanically ventilated, monitor for ARDS: ↑ peak inspiratory pressures, Fio$_2$ >0.50, ↑ PEEP necessary to maintain adequate Pao$_2$, diffuse bilateral pulmonary infiltrates on chest x-ray.
- Turn q2h to maintain optimal V/Q ratios and prevent atelectasis.

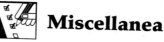 **Miscellanea**

CONSULT MD FOR
- S&S of inadequate tissue perfusion: altered mental status, restlessness; ↓ BP, peripheral pulses; UO <0.5 ml/kg/h × 2 h; Svo$_2$ <60% or >80%; ↓/absent bowel sounds
- S&S of complications: MODS, ARDS, ATN, DIC, mesenteric infarction

RELATED TOPICS
- Adult respiratory distress syndrome
- Antimicrobial therapy
- Disseminated intravascular coagulation
- Hemodynamic monitoring
- Mechanical ventilation
- Multiple organ dysfunction syndrome
- Renal failure, acute

ABBREVIATIONS
ATN: Acute tubular necrosis
Do$_2$: Oxygen delivery
FFP: Fresh frozen plasma
FSPs: Fibrin split products
MODS: Multiple organ dysfunction syndrome
PPF: Plasma protein fraction
PRBCs: Packed red blood cells
Vo$_2$: Oxygen consumption

REFERENCES
Beam TR: Antiinfective drugs in the prevention and treatment of sepsis syndrome, *Crit Care Nurs Clin North Am* 6(2): 275-293, 1994.
Brown K: Septic shock: stopping the deadly cascade, *Am J Nurs* 94(9): 20-26, 1994.
Brown K: Critical interventions in septic shock, *Am J Nurs* 94(10): 20-25, 1994.
Hazinski MF: Mediator-specific therapies for the systemic inflammatory response syndrome, sepsis, severe sepsis, and septic shock, *Crit Care Nurs Clin North Am* 6(2): 309-319, 1994.
Lawler DA: Hormonal response in sepsis, *Crit Care Nurs Clin North Am* 6(2): 265-274, 1994.
Stengle J, Dries D: Sepsis in the elderly, *Crit Care Nurs Clin North Am* 6(2): 421-427, 1994.

Author: **Janet Hicks Keen**

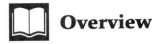 **Overview**

PATHOPHYSIOLOGY
The most common sleep disorder in the hospital setting is sleep deprivation as a result of noises and frequent interruptions for patient care. Patients who are ill have ↑ need for sleep; sleep deprivation will adversely affect recovery from illness.

HISTORY/RISK FACTORS
- Severe or prolonged illness
- Respiratory disorders, sleep apnea
- Depression, stress, anxiety
- Use of alcohol, CNS stimulants (eg, cocaine), other medications
- Dietary changes
- Life-style changes, including change in work habits, environment
- Excessive environmental stimuli (eg, noise, lights)
- Interrupted rest/sleep, daytime naps
- Caffeine ingestion
- Unrelieved pain

CLINICAL PRESENTATION
Inability to sleep at night, nighttime anxiety, agitation or confusion, restlessness, irritability, fatigue, ↓ concentration, emotional lability, physical discomfort

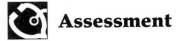 **Assessment**

PHYSICAL ASSESSMENT
Variable, depending on underlying disease process
Neuro: Anxiety, agitation, purposeless motor movement, hallucinations, depression
GU: Change in urinary habits
GI: Change in bowel habits, nausea

VITAL SIGNS/HEMODYNAMICS
RR: Possible ↑ as a result of stress, anxiety, underlying respiratory disorder (eg, sleep apnea, pickwickian syndrome)
HR: Possible ↑ resulting from stress, anxiety
BP: Possible ↑ resulting from stress, anxiety
Temp: Nl
Other: Endogenous catecholamines released during stress/anxiety may affect cardiopulmonary status, especially with chronic or debilitating disease

LABORATORY STUDIES
Hgb/Hct: Checks for ↓, which could impair tissue oxygenation and interfere with relaxation, sleep.
Blood Alcohol/Toxicology Screen: If intoxicant suspected as contributing factor.
ABGs/Spo$_2$: Checks for hypoxemia. Continuous Spo$_2$ monitoring may help detect ↓ O$_2$ with sleep apnea.

Collaborative Management

O$_2$ Therapy: Used continuously or prn during sleep if sleep apnea or hypoxemia contributes to sleep disturbance.
Apnea Monitor: When sleep apnea suspected or is an established component of sleep disturbance.
Pharmacotherapy: Never used as sole therapy. Must be initiated along with nonpharmacologic interventions.
Analgesics: Opiates or nonopiates given continuously or on regularly scheduled basis to control pain.
Sedatives/hypnotics: Used only after other treatable causes have been managed (eg, hypoxia, discomfort, pain). Examples include short-duration benzodiazepines, eg, Restoril, ProSom.
Nonpharmacologic Measures to Promote Sleep
Mask or eliminate environmental stimuli: Eg, *via* eyeshields, earplugs, soothing music, dimmed lights at bedtime.
Promote muscle relaxation: Ambulation as tolerated throughout day. Teach and encourage in-bed exercises and position changes. Perform back massage at bedtime. If not contraindicated, use heating pad.
Reduce anxiety: Ensure adequate pain control. Keep patient informed of progress and treatment measures. Avoid overstimulation by visitors or other activities immediately before bedtime. Avoid stimulant drugs (eg, caffeine).
Promote comfort: Encourage patient to use own pillows, bedclothes if not contraindicated. Adjust bed; rearrange linens. Regulate room temp.
Promote usual presleep routine: Oral hygiene at bedtime; reading or other quiet activity.
Minimize sleep disruption: Eg, maintain quiet environment throughout night via earplugs or ↓ alarm levels; use "white noise" (eg, low-pitched, monotonous sounds; electric fan; soft music); enable periods of at least 90 min of undisturbed sleep; limit visiting during these periods. Dim lights when checking patient during night
Consultation: PT to provide ROM exercises, appropriate activity. Some agencies employ massage therapists, who provide therapeutic massage at bedtime.

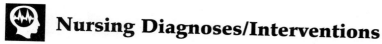 ## Nursing Diagnoses/Interventions

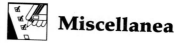 ## Miscellanea

Sleep pattern disturbance r/t environmental changes, illness, therapeutic regimen, pain, immobility, or psychologic stress

Desired outcomes: After discussion, patient identifies factors that promote sleep. Within 8 h of intervention, patient attains 90-min periods of uninterrupted sleep and verbalizes satisfaction with ability to rest.

- Assess usual sleeping patterns (eg, bedtime routine, number of h sleep per night, sleeping position, use of pillows and blankets, daytime napping, nocturia).
- Explore relaxation techniques that promote rest/sleep: imagining relaxing scenes, soothing music or taped stories, muscle relaxation exercises.
- Identify causes/activities that contribute to insomnia, adversely affect sleep patterns, or awaken patient: pain, anxiety, depression, hallucinations, medications, underlying illness, sleep apnea, respiratory disorder, caffeine, fear, medical/nursing interventions.
- If appropriate, limit daytime sleeping. Attempt to establish regularly scheduled daytime activity (eg, ambulation, sitting in chair, active ROM), which may promote nighttime sleep.

CONSULT MD FOR
- Persistent hypoxemia
- Prolonged periods of sleep apnea
- Ineffective pain relief

RELATED TOPICS
- Agitation syndrome
- Anxiety
- Delirium
- Pain
- Psychosocial needs, patient
- Respiratory failure, acute

REFERENCES
Adam K, Oswald I: Sleep is for tissue regeneration, *J Royal College of Physicians* 11: 376-388, 1977.

Kozier B et al: *Fundamentals of nursing: concepts, process, and practice,* ed 5, Redwood City, Calif, 1995, Addison-Wesley.

Webster RA, Thompson DR: Sleep in hospitals, *J Adv Nurs* 11: 447-457, 1986.

Author: **Patricia Hall**

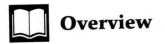 **Overview**

PATHOPHYSIOLOGY

Results from concussion, contusion, laceration, hemorrhage, or impaired blood supply to cervical area of spinal cord. With survival of initial injury, morbidity/mortality most often result from infection. Pulmonary and renal complications account for 30%-40% of all deaths. Higher incidence of left lower lobe pneumonia and atelectasis, possibly caused by changes in respiratory patterns, ineffective cough, positioning problems, and anatomy of left mainstem bronchus.

Classifications

By mechanism: Flexion (eg, diving into a swimming pool) or extension (eg, whiplash)

If injury complete: Absence of all voluntary motor, sensory, and vasomotor function below injury level

If injury incomplete: Some voluntary motor or sensory function below injury level

INCIDENCE

Cervical area involved in ⅔ of all SCIs

HISTORY/RISK FACTORS

- Vehicular collision, fall, sports-related injury
- Act of violence
- Intoxication
- Thrill-seeking behavior
- Failure to use safety device (helmet, seat belt, air bag)
- Chronic illness
- Advanced age

CLINICAL PRESENTATION

Flaccid paralysis, inability to maintain sitting position, ↓ LOC with concurrent head injury

(common), ↓ cerebral perfusion as a result of neurogenic shock

Spinal Shock: Experienced immediately after SCI. Loss of all reflex activity below level of injury, lasting min or prolonged over days and wks. During recovery phase of spinal shock, reflex emptying of bowel and bladder, extensor or flexor rigidity, hyperreflexic DTRs, and reflex priapism may occur.

Neurogenic Shock: CV instability as a result of interrupted descending sympathetic pathways, causing venous pooling in extremities, ↓ venous return to heart, ↓ cardiac output, bradycardia, and usually hypotension.

AD: Life-threatening response of ANS to a stimulus (eg, bladder distention, fecal impaction). If not identified promptly, treated, and reversed, consequences may include seizures, SAH, fatal stroke.

S&S: Severe and throbbing headache, hypertension, nasal congestion, bradycardia; cutaneous vasodilatation, flushed skin, and sweating above level of injury; gooseflesh, cool skin, and vasoconstriction below injury level.

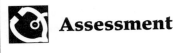 **Assessment**

PHYSICAL ASSESSMENT
Levels of Injury

C4 and above: Loss of all muscle function, including muscles of respiration. With complete cord transection death occurs unless immediate ventilation initiated.

C4-5: Same as preceding but with possible sparing of phrenic nerve; assisted ventilation probable. Patient will be tetraplegic/quadriplegic.

C6-8: Quadriplegia occurs, but with some function of diaphragm and accessory muscles of respiration and some movement of neck, shoulders, chest, upper arms.

Cord Syndromes

Central cord: Seen with hyperextension injuries or interrupted blood supply to cervical spinal cord. Motor and sensory deficits less severe in lower than in upper extremities because of central arrangement of cervical fibers in spinal cord.

Horner's: Seen after partial transection (incomplete injury) of cervical cord. Affects either preganglionic sympathetic trunk or postganglionic sympathetic neurons. S&S: ipsilateral miosis, enophthalmos (backward displacement of eye in its socket), ptosis, and absence of sweating.

Spinal Shock: Flaccid paralysis of all skeletal muscles; urinary and fecal retention. Absence of DTRs; cutaneous, visceral, somatic sensation; position sense; penile reflex; sweating.

Neurogenic Shock: Vasodilatation, profound bradycardia, hypotension.

VITAL SIGNS/HEMODYNAMICS

RR: ↓, irregular; absent with complete transection C4 or above

HR: ↓ with neurogenic shock

BP: ↓ with neurogenic shock; ↑ with AD

Temp: Nl; ↓ with hypothermia

CVP/PAWP: ↓ with neurogenic shock

CO: ↓ with neurogenic shock

LABORATORY STUDIES

ABG and Pulmonary Function Studies: Assess effectiveness of respirations and detect need for O₂, tracheostomy, mechanical ventilation.

Sputum/Urine Cultures: Detect onset of infection; determine appropriate antibiotic therapy.

IMAGING

Spinal X-rays: A-P/lateral films detect fractures or dislocations of vertebral bodies, narrowing of spinal canal, and hematomas. Additional views (odontoid, bilateral oblique, flexion-extension) may be necessary, particularly in the obese and heavily muscled.

CT Scan: Reveals soft tissue injury or subtle fractures.

MRI: Defines internal organ structures, detects tissue changes such as edema or infarction, and evaluates vascular integrity.

Pulmonary Fluoroscopy: Evaluates degree of diaphragmatic movement with a high cervical injury. Helps determine need for assisted ventilation.

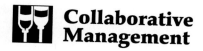 **Collaborative Management**

Skeletal Traction: To immobilize and reduce fracture or dislocation. May be achieved *via* Vinke, Gardner-Wells, Cone, or Crutchfield tongs, which are inserted through skull's outer table. Tongs attached to ropes and pulleys with weights to achieve bony reduction and proper alignment.

Special Frame or Bed: Eg, Roto Rest kinetic treatment table.

Halo Device with Plaster or Fiberglass Jacket: For skeletal fixation of head and neck and to enable earlier mobilization and rehabilitation.

Respiratory Management: Need for assisted ventilation based on level of injury, ABGs, and results of pulmonary function tests, pulmonary fluoroscopy, and physical assessment. Mechanical ventilation likely with injuries at C4 and above, patients >40 yrs of age, smokers, associated chest trauma, and immersion injuries. High cervical injury may require permanent tracheostomy with mechanical ventilation.

Aggressive Pulmonary Care: To prevent, detect, and treat atelectasis, pulmonary infection, and respiratory failure. Chest physiotherapy, intubation, and ventilation instituted as indicated.

Fluid Management: In neurogenic shock, blood volume nl but vascular space enlarged. Careful fluid replacement, usually with crystalloids, indicated. Pressor therapy initiated for unresponsiveness to fluid replacement.

Gastric Tube Placement: To decompress stomach, prevent aspiration, and ↓ risk of paralytic ileus.

Urinary Catheterization: Indwelling or intermittent to decompress atonic bladder in immediate postinjury phase. With return of reflex arc after spinal shock subsides, a reflex neurogenic bladder that fills and empties automatically is usual.

Pharmacotherapy

Methylprednisolone: Giving this adrenal steroid within 8 h of injury protects neuromembrane from further destruction and improves blood flow to injured site.

Osmotic diuretics (eg, mannitol, urea): ↓ edema at site of injury.

Acid suppression therapy (eg, antacids, histamine H_2-receptor antagonists): To suppress/neutralize gastric acid; ↓ risk of gastric ulceration.

Stool softeners/laxatives: Prevent fecal impaction, which could stimulate AD.

Analgesics: ↓ pain associated with injury or surgery. Titrated carefully to prevent respiratory depression.

Antihypertensives: Treat severe hypertension that occurs with AD.

Vasopressors (eg, dopamine): Treat hypotension caused by neurogenic shock. *Caution:* Orthostatic hypotension may become a permanent problem. Move patient slowly to avoid ↓ BP. Abdominal binders and Ace bandages or thigh-high antiembolic stockings also used.

Anticoagulants (heparin): Prevent thrombophlebitis, DVT, PE. Patients not candidates for anticoagulation may have inferior vena cava umbrella or filter inserted to trap emboli traveling from lower extremities to lungs.

Urinary antiseptic (eg, methenamine mandelate): Treats/prevents UTI.

Urinary acidifier (eg, vitamin E): Maintains urine pH ≈ 5.5.

Surgical Intervention: Controversial during immediate postinjury phase. May be performed if neurologic deficit progressing, compound fractures present, injury involves penetrating spine wound, bone fragments in spinal canal, or acute anterior spinal cord trauma present. Surgeries may include decompression laminectomy, closed or open fracture reduction, or spinal fusion for stabilization.

PATIENT-FAMILY TEACHING

- AD: causes, S&S, methods of treatment
- Medications: drug name, purpose, dosage, schedule, precautions, food-drug and drug-drug interactions, potential side effects
- Purpose, expected results, anticipated sensations of all nursing/medical interventions
- Address and phone numbers of National Spinal Cord Injury Association: 545 Concord Ave., Cambridge, MA 02138; 617-441-8500, 800-962-9629

Nursing Diagnoses/Interventions

Impaired gas exchange r/t altered O_2 supply associated with hypoventilation secondary to paralysis of muscles of respiration

Desired outcomes: Within 24 h of this diagnosis and throughout remaining hospitalization, patient has adequate gas exchange: orientation $\times$ 3, $Pao_2 \geq 80$ mm Hg; $Paco_2 \leq 45$ mm Hg, RR 12-20 breaths/min with eupnea, VC ≥ 1 L.

- Assess for respiratory dysfunction: shallow, slow, or rapid respirations; VC <1 L; changes in sensorium; anxiety; restlessness; tachycardia; pallor; inability to move secretions. Special vigilance required for nonintubated patients with low C-spine injuries because hemorrhage and edema can result in higher level of dysfunction and change in respiratory status that requires assisted ventilation.
- Monitor ABGs. Be particularly alert to Pao_2 <60 mm Hg and $Paco_2$ >50 mm Hg. These findings signal need for assisted ventilation.
- Monitor VC at least q8h. If <1 L, Pao_2/PAo_2 ratio ≤ 0.75, or copious secretions present, intubation recommended.
- Monitor for ascending cord edema: $\uparrow$ difficulty with swallowing or coughing, respiratory stridor with retraction of accessory muscles, bradycardia, fluctuating BP, and $\uparrow$ motor and sensory loss at level higher than initial findings.
- Do not hyperextend neck for resuscitation; instead, intubate using manual C-spine immobilization. Cricothyroidotomy also may be performed.
- If cranial tongs or halo traction in place, monitor respiratory status q1-2h for first 24-48 h and then q4h if condition stable. Ensure that plaster or fiberglass vest does not restrict diaphragmatic movement.

Ineffective airway clearance (or risk for same) r/t $\downarrow$/absent cough reflex secondary to C-spine injury

Desired outcome: Within 24-48 h of this diagnosis, patient has clear airway as evidenced by absence of adventitious breath sounds.

- Monitor respiratory status; be alert to indicators of ineffective airway clearance: crackles or rhonchi, $\downarrow$/absent breath sounds, $\uparrow$ HR (>100 bpm), $\uparrow$ BP (>10 mm Hg over nl for patient), $\downarrow$ tidal volume (<75%-85% of predicted value), $\downarrow$ VC (<1 L), shallow or rapid respirations (>20 breaths/min), pallor, cyanosis, $\uparrow$ restlessness, and anxiety.
- Suction as needed. Hyperoxygenate and hyperventilate before/after suctioning. Be alert for bradycardia associated with tracheal suctioning. Atropine may be necessary before suctioning.
- Implement following measures to improve airway clearance:
    Place in semi-Fowler's position unless contraindicated (eg, patient in cervical tongs with traction).
    Turn from side to side at least q2h to help mobilize secretions.
    Keep room humidified to help loosen secretions.
    Unless contraindicated, hydrate with at least 2-3 L/day of fluid.
    If patient has respiratory muscle control, teach coughing and deep-breathing exercises, which should be performed at least q2h.
    If patient's cough ineffective, implement "quad coughing": place palm of hand under diaphragm and push up on abdominal muscles as patient exhales.

Dysreflexia (or risk for same) r/t abnormal response of ANS to a stimulus

Desired outcomes: Patient has no symptoms of AD: dry skin above injury level, BP wnl for patient, HR ≥ 60 bpm, NSR on ECG, and absence of headache.

- Assess for S&S of AD: severe and throbbing headache, $\uparrow$ BP (eg, ≥ 250-300/150 mm Hg), nasal stuffiness, blurred vision, nausea, bradycardia. Assess for S&S of AD above level of injury: cutaneous vasodilatation, sweating, flushed skin. Also be alert to S&S of AD that occur below injury level: gooseflesh, pallor, chills, vasoconstriction.
- Assess for cardiac dysrhythmias *via* cardiac monitor during initial postinjury stage (2 wks).
- Avoid stimuli that cause AD: *bladder stimuli* (distention, infection); *bowel stimuli* (fecal impaction, suppository insertion); *skin stimuli* (pressure from tight clothing or sheets, temp extremes, areas of broken skin).
- If AD occurs, implement the following:
    Elevate HOB to induce postural hypotension.
    Monitor BP and HR q3-5min until stable.
    Remove offending stimulus.

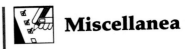 **Miscellanea**

CONSULT MD FOR
- Neurogenic shock: $\downarrow$ BP, $\downarrow$ HR, $\downarrow$ CO, $\downarrow$ SVR
- AD: throbbing headache, flushed skin and sweating above level of injury, $\uparrow$ BP
- Thrombophlebitis/DVT: calf pain with dorsiflexion, $\uparrow$ calf circumference, heat and erythema of calf
- Infection: URI, UTI, surgical site

Catheterize distended bladder using lubricant containing local anesthetic.

Check for urinary catheter obstruction.

Check for fecal impaction, using ointment containing local anesthetic (eg, Nupercainal).

Check for sensory stimuli, and loosen clothing, bed covers, other constricting fabric.

- Consult physician for severe hypertension or symptoms that do not abate.
- Administer antihypertensive agent.

Decreased cardiac output r/t relative hypovolemia secondary to enlarged vascular space occurring with neurogenic shock

Desired outcome: Within 24 h of this diagnosis, patient has adequate cardiac output: orientation $\times$ 3; SBP $\geq$90 mm Hg; HR 60-100 bpm; RAP 4-6 mm Hg; PAP 20-30/8-15 mm Hg; PAWP 6-12 mm Hg; SVR 900-1200 dynes/sec/cm^{-5}; nl amplitude of peripheral pulses (>2+ on 0-4+ scale); UO $\geq$0.5 ml/kg/h.

- Monitor for $\downarrow$ cardiac output: drop in SBP >20 mm Hg, SBP <90 mm Hg, HR >100 bpm, confusion, flushed skin, $\downarrow$ peripheral pulses, UO <0.5 ml/kg/h for 2 consecutive h. In the presence of neurogenic shock, anticipate $\downarrow$ RAP, PAP, PAWP, and SVR.
- Cardiac monitor indicated for 48-72 h or until stable; report changes in rate and rhythm.
- Implement measures to prevent orthostatic hypotension:

  Change patient's position slowly.

  Perform ROM exercises q2h to prevent venous pooling.

  Apply elastic antiembolic hose as prescribed to promote venous return.

  Avoid placing legs in dependent position.

  Collaborate with physical therapy in using tilt table.
- Administer fluids to control mild hypotension.
- Administer vasopressors for hypotension that fails to respond to volume repletion.

Altered peripheral and cardiopulmonary tissue perfusion (or risk for same) r/t interrupted blood flow associated with thrombophlebitis, DVT, and PE secondary to venous stasis, vascular intimal injury, and hypercoagulability occurring with $\downarrow$ vasomotor tone and immobility

Desired outcome: Patient free of symptoms of thrombophlebitis, DVT, and PE within 48 h of initiation of therapy: absence of heat, swelling, discomfort, and erythema in calves and thighs; HR $\leq$100 bpm; RR $\leq$20 breaths/min with eupnea; BP wnl for patient; Pao$_2$ $\geq$80 mm Hg; and absence of chest, shoulder pain.

- Assess for thrombophlebitis and DVT: heat and erythema of calf or thigh, $\uparrow$ circumference of calf or thigh, tenderness or pain in extremity (depending on whether injury complete or incomplete), pain in calf area with dorsiflexion.
- Assess for PE: sudden chest or shoulder pain, tachycardia, dyspnea, tachypnea, hypotension, pallor, cyanosis, cough with hemoptysis, restlessness, $\uparrow$ anxiety, $\downarrow$ Pao$_2$/Spo$_2$.
- Implement measures to prevent thrombophlebitis, DVT, and PE:

  Change position q2h.

  Perform ROM exercises.

  Avoid use of knee gatch or pillows under knees.

  Do not allow legs to be dependent for >½ -1 h.

  Apply sequential compression devices.

  Maintain adequate hydration of at least 2-3 L/day of fluid.

  Administer prophylactic heparin as prescribed.
- If signs of thrombophlebitis or DVT present, implement the following:

  Maintain bed rest.

  Keep affected extremity in neutral or elevated position.

  Administer anticoagulants and antiplatelet aggregating agents as prescribed.

Risk for impaired skin integrity r/t prolonged immobility secondary to immobilization device or paralysis

Desired outcome: Patient's skin remains intact during hospital course.

- Perform a complete skin assessment at least q8h. Pay close attention to skin that is particularly susceptible (ie, over bony prominences, around halo vest edges).
- Turn and reposition patient after spinal cord has been stabilized. Massage susceptible skin at least q2h. If turning allowed before immobilization with tongs, halo, or surgery, use logrolling technique.
- Keep skin clean and dry.
- Provide pressure-relief mattress most appropriate for patient's injury.

Altered nutrition (or risk for same): Less than body requirements, r/t $\downarrow$ oral intake secondary to inability to feed self because of paralysis of upper extremities; $\downarrow$ GI motility secondary to ANS dysfunction; fear of choking and aspiration

RELATED TOPICS
- Autonomic dysreflexia
- Immobility, prolonged
- Mechanical ventilation
- Multisystem injury
- Pulmonary embolus, thrombotic
- Shock, neurogenic
- Vasodilator therapy
- Vasopressor therapy

Desired outcome: Within 24-72 h of this diagnosis, patient has adequate nutrition: balanced nitrogen state, serum albumin 3.5-5.5 g/dl, thyroxine-binding prealbumin 20-30 mg/dl, and retinol binding protein 4-5 mg/dl.

- Perform baseline assessment of nutritional status.
- Assess readiness for oral intake: presence of bowel sounds, passing of flatus, or bowel movement. Paralytic ileus common within 72 h of injury.
- When patient begins oral diet, progress slowly from liquids to solids as tolerated.
- ↓ external stimuli to help patient concentrate on chewing and swallowing and thus ↓ aspiration risk.
- Provide small, frequent feedings.
- If patient in a Stryker wedge frame or Foster bed, feed in prone position to ↓ risk of aspiration. If in a halo device or already stabilized, feed in high-Fowler's position.
- Feed slowly, providing small, bite-size pieces.

Urinary retention r/t inhibition of spinal reflex arc secondary to spinal shock after SCI

Desired outcome: Within 24 h of this diagnosis, patient has UO of ≥0.5 ml/kg/h with output comparable to intake.

- Be aware that urinary retention with stretching of bladder muscle may trigger AD.
- Assess for urinary retention: suprapubic distention and intake > output.
- Expect an indwelling catheter for first 48-96 h after injury, followed by intermittent catheterization to retrain bladder.
- If AD triggered by a distended bladder, obstructed catheter, kinked tubing, or UTI, implement the following:
    Notify physician.
    Catheterize using anesthetic jelly.
    If catheter obstructed, gently instill ≤30 ml NS in attempt to open catheter.
    If catheter remains obstructed, remove it and insert another, using anesthetic lubricating agent.
    If UTI is the suspected trigger, obtain urine specimen for C&S testing.

Ineffective thermoregulation r/t inability of body to adapt to environmental temp changes secondary to poikilothermic reaction occurring with SCI

Desired outcome: Within 2-4 h of this diagnosis patient becomes normothermic.

- Monitor temp at least q4h, and assess for signs of ineffective thermoregulation: complaints of being too warm, excessive diaphoresis, warmth of skin above injury level, complaints of being too cold, gooseflesh, or cool skin above injury level.
- Implement measures to attain normothermia:
    Regulate room temp.
    Provide extra blankets to prevent chills.
    Protect from drafts.

ABBREVIATIONS
AD: Autonomic dysreflexia
ANS: Autonomic nervous system
DTR: Deep tendon reflex
SAH: Subarachnoid hemorrhage
URI: Upper respiratory infection
VC: Vital capacity

Provide warm food and drink if patient chilled; provide cool drinks if patient warm.

Use fans or air conditioners to prevent overheating.

Remove excess bedding to facilitate heat loss.

Provide tepid bath or cooling blanket to facilitate cooling.

Risk for injury r/t potential for paralytic ileus with concomitant risk of AD secondary to SCI

Desired outcome: Patient remains free of symptoms of paralytic ileus: nl bowel sounds present, no signs of AD.

- Assess for paralytic ileus, which occurs most often within first 72 h after injury: ↓ or absent bowel sounds, abdominal distention, anorexia, vomiting, and altered respirations as a result of pressure on diaphragm.
- Observe closely for signs of AD, which can be triggered by abdominal distention.
- If paralytic ileus occurs, implement the following:

  Restrict oral or enteral intake.

  Insert gastric tube to decompress stomach; attach to suction.

  Insert rectal tube, if prescribed, using local anesthetic lubricant.

Constipation or fecal impaction r/t neuromuscular impairment secondary to spinal shock

Desired outcome: Within 24-48 h of this diagnosis and subsequently q2-3 days (or within patient's preinjury pattern), patient has bowel elimination of soft and formed stools.

- Monitor for constipation (nausea, abdominal distention, malaise) and fecal impaction (nausea, vomiting, ↑ abdominal distention, palpable colonic mass, or presence of hard fecal mass on digital examination).
- Until bowel sounds present and paralytic ileus has resolved, maintain NPO status; continue gastric suction.
- Before return of rectal reflex arc, it may be necessary to remove feces from rectum manually. If fecal impaction present in atonic bowel, small-volume enema may be necessary. Use generous amounts of anesthetic lubricant when performing rectal examination or administering enema.

Risk for infection r/t inadequate primary defenses (broken skin) secondary to presence of invasive immobilization devices

Desired outcome: Patient infection free at insertion site for tongs or halo device: normothermia; negative culture results; and absence of erythema, swelling, warmth, purulent drainage, or tenderness at insertion site.

- Assess insertion sites q8h for infection: erythema, swelling, warmth, purulent drainage, and tenderness.
- Perform pin care as prescribed. Cleanse according to individual prescription using aseptic technique. Apply sterile dressings around pins, or leave area open to air according to physician or agency policy.

REFERENCES

Boss BJ et al: Self-care competence among persons with spinal cord injury, *SCI Nurs* 12(2): 48-53, 1995.

Campbell LS: Commentary on acute SCI: how to minimize the damage, *ENAS Nurs Scan Emerg Care* 4(3): 10-11, 1994.

Dalton JR: Urologic management of the patient with spinal cord injury, *Trauma Q* 9(2): 72-81, 1993.

Lemke DM: Defining assessment parameters in dual injuries: spinal cord injury and traumatic brain injury, *SCI Nurs* 12(2): 40-47, 1995.

Thomas E, Paulson SS: Protocol for weaning the SCI patient, *SCI Nurs* 11(2): 42-45, 1994.

Author: **Ann Coghlan Stowe**

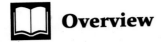 **Overview**

PATHOPHYSIOLOGY

Results from concussion, contusion, laceration, hemorrhage, or impaired blood supply to spinal cord. SCI may be secondarily ↑ by ischemia and subsequent edema. Although life expectancy is good after injury, morbidity/mortality most often result from infection. Pulmonary and renal complications account for 30%-40% of all deaths.

Classifications

By stability: Integrity of supporting structures (eg, ligaments or bony facets)

If injury complete: Absence of all voluntary motor, sensory, and vasomotor function below injury level

If injury incomplete: Some voluntary motor or sensory function below injury level

HISTORY/RISK FACTORS

- Vehicular collision, fall, sports-related injury
- Act of violence
- Intoxication
- Thrill-seeking behavior
- Failure to use safety device (seat belt, air bag)
- Chronic illness
- Advanced age

CLINICAL PRESENTATION

Weakness, possible flaccid paralysis of lower extremities; full function of upper extremities, chest, trunk muscles

Fractures Involving Vertebral Bodies: With "burst" fracture (fragmentation of a vertebral body with penetration of spinal cord) there is almost always paralysis. Penetration of spinal cord with bony fragments may cause hemorrhage, infection, and leakage of CSF.

Spinal Shock: Experienced immediately after SCI. Loss of all reflex activity below level of injury, lasting min or prolonged over days and wks. Generally, the more quickly signs of return to function appear, the better the prognosis.

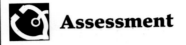 **Assessment**

PHYSICAL ASSESSMENT
Levels of Injury

T11-L2: Use of upper extremities, neck, and shoulders. Chest and trunk muscles provide stability; there is some muscle function of upper thigh. At this level there may be loss of voluntary bowel and bladder control, but there is reflex bowel emptying. Men may experience difficulty achieving and maintaining erections.

L3-S1: Muscle function of all muscle groups in upper body and most muscle function in lower extremities. Loss of voluntary bowel and bladder function, with reflex emptying. Men may experience ↓/lack of ability to have erections.

S2-4: Function of all muscle groups but some lower extremity weakness. May have flaccidity of bowel and bladder as well as loss of ability to have reflex erection.

Cord Syndromes

Anterior cord: Involves injury to anterior portion of spinal cord supplied by anterior spinal artery and may be associated with acute traumatic herniation of an intervertebral disk. Varying degrees of paralysis occur below injury level, along with diminution of pain and temp sensations.

Lateral cord (Brown-Séquard): Results from horizontal hemisection of spinal cord, eg, from a gunshot or stab wound. Patients usually have bilateral motor and sensory impairment, with a relative difference in function from one side to the other. While there are bilateral motor and sensory deficits, motor activity is better on one side and sensory activity better on the other.

Spinal Shock: Flaccid paralysis of skeletal muscles; urinary and fecal retention. Absence of DTRs; cutaneous, visceral, somatic sensation; position sense; penile reflex; sweating. As spinal shock subsides, patient may experience flexor spasms evoked by cutaneous stimulation, reflex emptying of bowel and bladder, extensor or flexor rigidity, hyperreflexic DTRs, and reflex priapism in males.

VITAL SIGNS/HEMODYNAMICS

RR: ↑ possible with pain
HR: ↑ possible with pain
BP: slight ↑ with pain
Temp: NI
CVP/PAWP: NI
CO: NI

SVR: NI
Other: Hemodynamic monitoring usually not necessary

LABORATORY STUDIES
Sputum/Urine Cultures: Detect onset of infection and determine appropriate antibiotic therapy.

IMAGING
Spinal X-rays: A-P/lateral films detect fractures or dislocations of vertebral bodies, narrowing of spinal canal, and hematomas.
CT Scan: Reveals soft tissue injury or subtle fractures.
MRI: Defines internal organ structures, detects tissue changes such as edema or infarction, and evaluates vascular integrity.
Myelography: Identifies site of spinal canal blockage, which can occur as a result of fractures, dislocations, or herniation or protrusion of an intervertebral disk.

Collaborative Management

Immobilization of Injured Site: With or without surgical intervention. Surgical stabilization with laminectomy and spinal fusion may be necessary. If injury stable, it may be treated with closed reduction. Some L-spine injuries may be immobilized with halo device with femoral distraction, which may be connected to traction with weights for reduction and stabilization before surgery.
Fluid Management: Neurogenic shock unlikely. Requirements for IV fluids depend on oral intake and existence of other injuries.
Urinary Catheterization: Indwelling or intermittent to decompress atonic bladder in immediate postinjury phase (spinal shock). Lesions at or below T12 generally result in atonic, areflexic neurogenic bladder that overfills, distending bladder and causing overflow incontinence. Intermittent catheterization instituted as soon as possible.
Pharmacotherapy
Methylprednisolone: Giving this adrenal steroid within 8 h of injury protects neuromembrane from further destruction and improves blood flow to injured site.
Osmotic diuretics (eg, mannitol, urea): ↓ edema at site of injury.
Acid suppression therapy (eg, antacids, histamine H$_2$-receptor antagonists): To suppress/neutralize gastric acid; ↓ risk of gastric ulceration.
Stool softeners/laxatives: Prevent fecal impaction.
Analgesics: To ↓ pain associated with injury or surgery.
Anticoagulants (heparin): Prevent thrombophlebitis, DVT, PE. Noncandidates for anticoagulation may have inferior vena cava umbrella or filter inserted to trap emboli traveling from lower extremities to lungs.
Urinary antiseptics (eg, methenamine mandelate): Prevents/treats UTI.
Urinary acidifiers: Maintain urine pH ≈ 5.5.

PATIENT-FAMILY TEACHING
- Purpose, expected results, anticipated sensations of all nursing/medical interventions
- Procedure for intermittent catheterization: proper hand washing and cleansing of urinary meatus before catheterization
- Indicators of UTI: incontinence, malaise, anorexia, fever, cloudy or foul-smelling urine; importance of adequate fluid intake and regular urine cultures
- Bladder-emptying techniques such as straining or Credé's method: even with these techniques, dribbling of urine may occur, necessitating catheterization or incontinence undergarments
- Bowel-emptying techniques: digital rectal stimulation, insertion of suppository, and abdominal massage to facilitate bowel movement
- Referral to sex therapist or other knowledgeable rehabilitation professional on resolution of critical stages of SCI
- Medications: drug name, purpose, dosage, schedule, precautions, food-drug and drug-drug interactions, potential side effects
- Address and phone numbers of National Spinal Cord Injury Association: 545 Concord Ave., Cambridge, MA 02138; 617-441-8500, 800-962-9629

Nursing Diagnoses/Interventions

Altered peripheral and cardiopulmonary tissue perfusion (or risk for same) r/t interrupted blood flow associated with thrombophlebitis, DVT, and PE secondary to venous stasis, vascular intimal injury, and hypercoagulability occurring with ↓ vasomotor tone and immobility
Desired outcome: Patient free of symptoms of thrombophlebitis, DVT, and PE within 48 h of initiation of therapy: absence of heat, swelling, discomfort, and erythema in calves and thighs; HR ≤100 bpm; RR ≤20 breaths/min with eupnea; BP wnl for patient; PaO_2 ≥80 mm Hg; and absence of chest or shoulder pain.

- Assess for thrombophlebitis and DVT: heat and erythema of calf or thigh, ↑ circumference of calf or thigh, tenderness or pain in extremity (depending on whether injury complete or incomplete), pain in calf area with dorsiflexion.
- Assess for PE: sudden chest or shoulder pain, tachycardia, dyspnea, tachypnea, hypotension, pallor, cyanosis, cough with hemoptysis, restlessness, ↑ anxiety, ↓ PaO_2/SpO_2.
- Implement measures to prevent thrombophlebitis, DVT, and PE:
  Change position q2h.
  Perform ROM exercises.
  Avoid use of knee gatch or pillows under knees.
  Do not allow legs to be dependent for >½-1 h.
  Apply sequential compression devices.
  Maintain adequate hydration of at least 2-3 L/day of fluid.
  Administer prophylactic heparin as prescribed.
- If signs of thrombophlebitis or DVT present, implement the following:
  Maintain bed rest.
  Keep affected extremity in neutral or elevated position.
  Administer anticoagulants and antiplatelet aggregating agents as prescribed.

Risk for impaired skin integrity r/t prolonged immobility secondary to immobilization device or paralysis
Desired outcome: Patient's skin remains intact during hospital course.

- Perform a complete skin assessment at least q8h. Pay close attention to skin particularly susceptible (ie, over bony prominences).

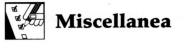 **Miscellanea**

CONSULT MD FOR
- Thrombophlebitis/DVT: calf pain with dorsiflexion, ↑ calf circumference, heat and erythema of calf
- Infection: URI, UTI, surgical site

RELATED TOPICS
- Immobility, prolonged
- Multisystem injury
- Pulmonary embolus, thrombotic

ABBREVIATIONS
DTRs: Deep tendon reflexes
URI: Upper respiratory infection

- Turn and reposition patient after spinal cord has been stabilized. Massage susceptible skin at least q2h. If turning allowed before surgical immobilization, use logrolling technique.
- Keep skin clean and dry.
- Provide pressure-relief mattress most appropriate for patient's injury.

Urinary retention (with overflow incontinence) r/t loss of reflex activity for micturition and bladder flaccidity secondary to cord lesion at or below T12

Desired outcome: Patient has UO without incontinence.

- As prescribed, either insert indwelling urinary catheter or catheterize patient intermittently on a regularly scheduled basis.
- If intermittent catheterization used and episodes of urinary incontinence occur, catheterize more frequently. If >400 ml of urine obtained, catheterize more often and reduce fluid intake.
- Measure amount of residual urine, and attempt to ↑ length of time between catheterizations, as indicated by ↓ amounts (ie, <50-100 ml) urine.
- Monitor and record I&O. Distribute fluids evenly throughout the day to prevent overdistention.
- ↓ fluid intake before bedtime to prevent nighttime incontinence. Discourage intake of caffeine-containing beverages and foods.

Sexual dysfunction or altered sexuality pattern r/t trauma associated with SCI

Desired outcome: Patient verbalizes sexual concerns before discharge from ICU.

- Assess level of sexual function or loss from a neurologic and psychologic perspective. General rule for men is that the higher the lesion, the greater the chance of having an erection, but there is less chance for ejaculation. For women, ovulation may stop for several mos as a result of postinjury stress. Ovulation usually returns, and nl pregnancy possible.
- If you are uncomfortable discussing this subject, arrange for knowledgeable staff member to speak with patient about his or her concerns.
- Reflex erection on resolution of spinal shock is nl for men. Reassure that there is nothing to be embarrassed about.
- Expect acting-out behavior related to patient's sexuality. This is a nl response to concerns regarding sexual prognosis.
- Provide accurate information regarding expected sexual function in an open, interested manner, based on your assessment of patient's readiness for information.
- Facilitate communication between patient and his or her partner.

REFERENCES

Boss BJ et al: Self-care competence among persons with spinal cord injury, *SCI Nurs* 12(2): 48-53, 1995.

Campbell LS: Commentary on acute SCI: how to minimize the damage, *ENAS Nurs Scan Emerg Care* 4(3): 10-11, 1994.

Dalton JR: Urologic management of the patient with spinal cord injury, *Trauma Q* 9(2): 72-81, 1993.

Lemke DM: Defining assessment parameters in dual injuries: spinal cord injury and traumatic brain injury, *SCI Nurs* 12(2): 40-47, 1995.

Stowe AC: Spinal cord injury. In Swearingen PL, Keen JH (eds): *Manual of critical care nursing,* ed 3, St Louis, 1995, Mosby.

Thomas E, Paulson SS: Protocol for weaning the SCI patient, *SCI Nurs* 11(2): 42-45, 1994.

Author: **Ann Coghlan Stowe**

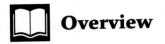 **Overview**

PATHOPHYSIOLOGY

Results from concussion, contusion, laceration, hemorrhage, or impaired blood supply to thoracic area of spinal cord. Although life expectancy is good after injury, morbidity/mortality most often result from infection. Pulmonary and renal complications account for 30%-40% of all deaths.

Classifications

By mechanism: Eg, flexion or extension
By stability: Integrity of supporting structures (eg, ligaments or bony facets)
If injury complete: Absence of all voluntary motor, sensory, and vasomotor function below injury level
If injury incomplete: Some voluntary motor or sensory function below injury level

HISTORY/RISK FACTORS

- Vehicular collision, fall, sports-related injury
- Act of violence
- Intoxication
- Thrill-seeking behavior
- Failure to use safety device (seat belt, air bag)
- Chronic illness
- Advanced age

CLINICAL PRESENTATION

Flaccid paralysis of lower extremities; may have difficulty maintaining sitting position; altered LOC with concurrent head injury (common); ↓ cerebral perfusion attributable to neurogenic shock

Spinal Shock: Experienced immediately after SCI. Loss of all reflex activity below level of injury, lasting min or prolonged over days and wks. Generally, the more quickly signs of return to function appear, the better the prognosis.

Neurogenic Shock: Injuries to upper thoracic and cervical regions may result in CV instability as a result of interrupted descending sympathetic pathways, causing venous pooling in extremities, ↓ venous return to heart, ↓ cardiac output, bradycardia, and usually hypotension.

AD: Life-threatening response of ANS to a stimulus (eg, bladder distention, fecal impaction). If not identified promptly, treated, and reversed, consequences may include seizures, SAH, fatal stroke. 80% of persons with lesions at or above T6 (tetraplegics/quadriplegics/high paraplegics) experience AD.

S&S: Severe and throbbing headache, hypertension, nasal congestion, bradycardia; cutaneous vasodilatation, flushed skin, and sweating above level of injury; gooseflesh, cool skin, and vasoconstriction below injury level.

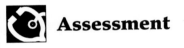 **Assessment**

PHYSICAL ASSESSMENT

Levels of Injury

T1-3: Neck, shoulder, chest, arm, hand, and respiratory function; difficulty maintaining sitting position.
T4-10: Same as preceding but with more stability of trunk muscles. The lower the lesion, the greater the independence. Will be paraplegic.

T11-L2: Use of upper extremities, neck, and shoulders. Chest and trunk muscles provide stability; some muscle function of upper thigh. At this level there may be loss of voluntary bowel and bladder control, but there is reflex emptying of the bowel.

Cord Syndromes

Anterior cord: Involves injury to anterior portion of spinal cord supplied by anterior spinal artery and may be associated with acute traumatic herniation of an intervertebral disk. Surgical decompression necessary. Varying degrees of paralysis occur below injury level, along with diminution of pain and temp sensations.

Lateral cord (Brown-Séquard): Results from horizontal hemisection of spinal cord, eg, from a gunshot or stab wound. Patients usually have bilateral motor and sensory impairment, with a relative difference in function from one side to the other. Motor activity better on one side and sensory activity better on the other.

Spinal Shock: Flaccid paralysis of all skeletal muscles; urinary and fecal retention. Absence of DTRs; cutaneous, visceral, somatic sensation; position sense; penile reflex; sweating.

Neurogenic Shock: Vasodilatation, profound bradycardia, hypotension. A phase of neurogenic shock experienced with SCIs lower than midthorax, with loss of sympathetic innervation to vasculature below injury level; effects of that loss may be limited. Susceptibility to bradycardia and hypotension in relation to position changes, but not likely to be a serious problem.

VITAL SIGNS/HEMODYNAMICS

RR: ↓, irregular
HR: ↓ with neurogenic shock
BP: ↓ with neurogenic shock; ↑ with AD

Temp: Nl; ↓ with hypothermia
CVP/PAWP: ↓ with neurogenic shock
CO: ↓ with neurogenic shock

LABORATORY STUDIES

ABG and Pulmonary Function Studies: Assess effectiveness of respirations and detect need for O_2, tracheostomy, mechanical ventilation.
Sputum/Urine Cultures: Detect onset of infection and determine appropriate antibiotic therapy.

IMAGING

Spinal X-rays: A-P/lateral films detect fractures or dislocations of vertebral bodies, narrowing of spinal canal, and hematomas.
CT Scan: Reveals soft tissue injury or subtle fractures.
MRI: Defines internal organ structures, detects tissue changes such as edema or infarction, and evaluates vascular integrity.
Myelography: Identifies site of spinal canal blockage, which can occur as a result of fractures, dislocations, or herniation or protrusion of an intervertebral disk.

Collaborative Management

Immobilization of Injured Site: With or without surgical intervention. May require surgery: laminectomy with or without fusion and insertion of Harrington rods for stabilization.
Respiratory Management: Need for assisted ventilation based on injury level, ABGs, and results of pulmonary function tests and physical assessment. Need for ventilatory assistance more likely with patients >40 yrs, smokers, associated chest trauma, and immersion injuries.

Aggressive Pulmonary Care: To prevent, detect, and treat atelectasis, pulmonary infection, and respiratory failure. Chest physiotherapy, intubation, and ventilation instituted as indicated.
Fluid Management: In neurogenic shock, blood volume nl but vascular space enlarged. Careful fluid replacement, usually with crystalloids, indicated. Pressor therapy initiated for unresponsiveness to fluid replacement.
Gastric Tube Placement: To decompress stomach, prevent aspiration, and ↓ risk of paralytic ileus.
Urinary Catheterization: Indwelling or intermittent to decompress atonic bladder in immediate postinjury phase. With return of reflex arc after spinal shock subsides, a reflex neurogenic bladder that fills and empties automatically is usual.
Pharmacotherapy
Methylprednisolone: Giving this adrenal steroid within 8 h of injury protects neuromembrane from further destruction and improves blood flow to injured site.
Osmotic diuretics (eg, mannitol, urea): ↓ edema at site of injury.
Acid suppression therapy (eg, antacids, histamine H_2-receptor antagonists): To suppress/neutralize gastric acid; ↓ risk of gastric ulceration.
Stool softeners/laxatives: Prevent fecal impaction, which could stimulate AD.
Analgesics: To ↓ pain associated with injury or surgery. Selected/titrated carefully to prevent respiratory depression.
Antihypertensives: Treat severe hypertension that occurs with AD.
Vasopressors (eg, dopamine): Treat hypotension attributable to neurogenic shock. *Caution:* Orthostatic hypotension may become a permanent problem. Move patient slowly to avoid ↓ BP. Abdominal binders and

Ace bandages or thigh-high antiembolic stockings also used.
Anticoagulants (heparin): Prevent thrombophlebitis, DVT, PE. Noncandidates for anticoagulation may have inferior vena cava umbrella or filter inserted to trap emboli traveling from lower extremities to lungs.
Urinary antiseptics (eg, methenamine mandelate): Treats/prevents UTI.
Urinary acidifiers (eg, vitamin E): Maintain urine pH ≈ 5.5.

PATIENT-FAMILY TEACHING

- AD: causes, S&S, methods of treatment
- Medications: drug name, purpose, dosage, schedule, precautions, food-drug and drug-drug interactions, potential side effects
- Purpose, expected results, anticipated sensations of all nursing/medical interventions
- Procedure for intermittent catheterization: proper hand washing and cleansing of urinary meatus before catheterization; possibility that with lesion above T12 and bladder indicating neurogenic reflex, bladder may eventually empty automatically and may not require catheterization
- Indicators of UTI: incontinence, malaise, anorexia, fever, cloudy or foul-smelling urine; importance of adequate fluid intake and regular urine cultures
- Individualized bowel program, including data regarding bulk-forming agents (eg, psyllium), high-roughage diet, ↑ fluid intake to 2-3 L/day, stool softeners, glycerine suppositories, intermittent use of bisacodyl, occasional use of enemas
- Address and phone numbers of National Spinal Cord Injury Association: 545 Concord Ave., Cambridge, MA 02138; 617-441-8500, 800-962-9629

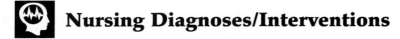 **Nursing Diagnoses/Interventions**

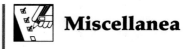 **Miscellanea**

Impaired gas exchange r/t altered O_2 supply associated with hypoventilation secondary to paralysis of muscles of respiration
Desired outcomes: Within 24 h of this diagnosis and throughout remaining hospitalization, patient has adequate gas exchange: orientation $\times$ 3, Pao_2 $\geq$80 mm Hg, $Paco_2$ $\leq$45 mm Hg, RR 12-20 breaths/min with eupnea, VC $\geq$1 L.
- Assess for respiratory dysfunction: shallow, slow, or rapid respirations; VC <1 L; changes in sensorium; anxiety; restlessness; tachycardia; pallor; and inability to move secretions. Special vigilance required for nonintubated patients with high thoracic lesions because hemorrhage and edema can result in higher level of dysfunction and change in respiratory status that requires assisted ventilation.
- Monitor ABGs. Be particularly alert to Pao_2 <60 mm Hg and $Paco_2$ >50 mm Hg. These findings signal need for assisted ventilation.
- Monitor VC at least q8h. If <1 L, Pao_2/PAo_2 ratio $\leq$0.75, or copious secretions present, intubation recommended.
- Monitor for ascending cord edema: $\uparrow$ difficulty with swallowing or coughing, respiratory stridor with retraction of accessory muscles, bradycardia, fluctuating BP, and motor and sensory deficits at level higher than initial findings.

Ineffective airway clearance (or risk for same) r/t $\downarrow$/absent cough or $\downarrow$ respiratory effort secondary to involvement of intercostal (T1 to T6) or abdominal muscles (T6 to T12)
Desired outcome: Within 24-48 h of this diagnosis, patient has clear airway as evidenced by absence of adventitious breath sounds.
- Monitor respiratory status; be alert to indicators of ineffective airway clearance: crackles or rhonchi, $\downarrow$ or absent breath sounds, $\uparrow$ HR (>100 bpm), $\uparrow$ BP (>10 mm Hg over nl for patient), $\downarrow$ tidal volume (<75%-85% of predicted value), $\downarrow$ VC (<1 L), shallow or rapid respirations (>20 breaths/min), pallor, cyanosis, $\uparrow$ restlessness, and anxiety.
- Suction secretions as needed. Hyperoxygenate and hyperventilate before/after suctioning. Be alert for bradycardia associated with tracheal suctioning. Atropine may be necessary before suctioning.
- Implement the following measures to improve airway clearance:
  Place in semi-Fowler's position unless contraindicated (eg, patient in cervical tongs with traction).
  Turn from side to side at least q2h to help mobilize secretions.
  Keep room humidified to help loosen secretions.
  Unless contraindicated, hydrate with at least 2-3 L/day of fluid.
  If patient has respiratory muscle control, teach coughing and deep-breathing exercises, which should be performed at least q2h.
  If patient's cough ineffective, implement "quad coughing": place palm of hand under diaphragm and push up on abdominal muscles as patient exhales.

Dysreflexia (or risk for same) r/t abnormal response of ANS to a stimulus
Desired outcomes: Patient has no symptoms of AD: dry skin above injury level, BP wnl for patient, HR $\geq$60 bpm, and absence of headache. ECG shows NSR.
- Assess for classic triad of AD: throbbing headache, cutaneous vasodilatation, and sweating above injury level. Also assess for $\uparrow$ BP (eg, $\geq$250-300/150 mm Hg), nasal stuffiness, flushed skin (above injury level), blurred vision, nausea, and bradycardia. Be alert to signs of AD that occur below injury level: gooseflesh, pallor, chills, vasoconstriction.
- Assess for cardiac dysrhythmias *via* cardiac monitor during initial postinjury stage (2 wks).
- Avoid stimuli that cause AD: *bladder stimuli* (distention, infection); *bowel stimuli* (fecal impaction, suppository insertion); *skin stimuli* (pressure from tight clothing or sheets, temp extremes, areas of broken skin).
- If AD occurs, implement the following:
  Elevate HOB to promote cerebral venous return.
  Monitor BP and HR q3-5min until stable.
  Remove offending stimulus.
  Catheterize distended bladder using lubricant containing local anesthetic.
  Check for urinary catheter obstruction.
  Check for fecal impaction, using ointment containing local anesthetic (eg, Nupercainal).
  Check for sensory stimuli, and loosen clothing, bed covers, other constricting fabric.

CONSULT MD FOR
- Neurogenic shock: $\downarrow$ BP, $\downarrow$ HR, $\downarrow$ CO, $\downarrow$ SVR
- AD: throbbing headache, flushed skin and sweating above level of injury, $\uparrow$ BP
- Thrombophlebitis/DVT: calf pain with dorsiflexion, $\uparrow$ calf circumference, heat and erythema of calf
- Infection: URI, UTI, surgical site

- Consult physician for severe hypertension or symptoms that do not abate.
- Administer antihypertensive agent.

Decreased cardiac output r/t relative hypovolemia secondary to enlarged vascular space occurring with neurogenic shock

Desired outcome: Within 24 h of this diagnosis, patient has adequate cardiac output: orientation × 3; SBP ≥90 mm Hg; HR 60-100 bpm; RAP 4-6 mm Hg; PAP 20-30/8-15 mm Hg; PAWP 6-12 mm Hg; SVR 900-1200 dynes/sec/cm^{-5}; nl amplitude of peripheral pulses (>2+ on 0-4+ scale); UO ≥0.5 ml/kg/h.

- Monitor for ↓ cardiac output: drop in SBP >20 mm Hg, SBP <90 mm Hg, HR >100 bpm, confusion, flushed skin, ↓ peripheral pulses, UO <0.5 ml/kg/h for 2 consecutive h. In the presence of neurogenic shock, anticipate ↓ RAP, PAP, PAWP, and SVR.
- Cardiac monitor indicated for 48-72 h or until stable; report changes in rate and rhythm.
- Implement measures to prevent orthostatic hypotension:
    Change patient's position slowly.
    Perform ROM exercises q2h to prevent venous pooling.
    Apply elastic antiembolic hose as prescribed to promote venous return.
    Avoid placing legs in dependent position.
    Collaborate with physical therapy in using tilt table.
- Administer fluids to control mild hypotension.
- Administer vasopressors for hypotension that fails to respond to volume repletion.

Altered peripheral and cardiopulmonary tissue perfusion (or risk for same) r/t interrupted blood flow associated with thrombophlebitis, DVT, and PE secondary to venous stasis, vascular intimal injury, and hypercoagulability occurring with ↓ vasomotor tone and immobility

Desired outcome: Patient free of symptoms of thrombophlebitis, DVT, and PE within 48 h of initiation of therapy: absence of heat, swelling, discomfort, and erythema in calves and thighs; HR ≤100 bpm; RR ≤20 breaths/min with eupnea; BP wnl for patient; Pao$_2$ ≥80 mm Hg; absence of chest, shoulder pain.

- Assess for thrombophlebitis and DVT: heat and erythema of calf or thigh, ↑ circumference of calf or thigh, tenderness or pain in extremity (depending on whether injury complete or incomplete), pain in calf area with dorsiflexion.
- Assess for PE: sudden chest or shoulder pain, tachycardia, dyspnea, tachypnea, hypotension, pallor, cyanosis, cough with hemoptysis, restlessness, ↑ anxiety, ↓ Pao$_2$/Spo$_2$.
- Implement measures to prevent thrombophlebitis, DVT, and PE:
    Change position q2h.
    Perform ROM exercises.
    Avoid use of knee gatch or pillows under knees.
    Do not allow legs to be dependent for >½-1 h.
    Apply sequential compression devices.
    Maintain adequate hydration of at least 2-3 L/day of fluid.
    Administer prophylactic heparin as prescribed.
- If signs of thrombophlebitis or DVT present, implement the following:
    Maintain bed rest.
    Keep affected extremity in neutral or elevated position.
    Administer anticoagulants and antiplatelet aggregating agents as prescribed.

Risk for impaired skin integrity r/t prolonged immobility secondary to immobilization device or paralysis

Desired outcome: Patient's skin remains intact during hospital course.

- Perform a complete skin assessment at least q8h. Pay close attention to skin that is particularly susceptible (ie, over bony prominences, around halo vest edges).
- Turn and reposition patient after spinal cord has been stabilized. Massage susceptible skin at least q2h. If turning allowed before surgical immobilization, use logrolling technique.
- Keep skin clean and dry.
- Provide pressure-relief mattress most appropriate for patient's injury.

Urinary retention r/t inhibition of spinal reflex arc secondary to spinal shock after SCI

Desired outcome: Within 24 h of this diagnosis, patient has UO of ≥0.5 ml/kg/h with output comparable to intake.

- Be aware that urinary retention with stretching of bladder muscle may trigger AD.
- Assess for urinary retention: suprapubic distention and intake > output.
- Expect an indwelling catheter for first 48-96 h after injury, followed by intermittent catheterization to retrain bladder.
- If AD triggered by a distended bladder, obstructed catheter, kinked tubing, or UTI, implement the following:
    Notify physician.

RELATED TOPICS

- Autonomic dysreflexia
- Immobility, prolonged
- Mechanical ventilation
- Multisystem injury
- Pulmonary embolus, thrombotic
- Shock, neurogenic
- Vasodilator therapy
- Vasopressor therapy

Catheterize using anesthetic jelly.

If catheter obstructed, gently instill ≤30 ml NS in attempt to open catheter.

If catheter remains obstructed, remove it and insert another, using anesthetic lubricating agent.

If UTI is the suspected trigger, obtain urine specimen for C&S testing.

Reflex incontinence r/t uninhibited activity of spinal reflex arc secondary to recovery phase from spinal shock in patients with cord lesions above T12

Desired outcomes: Patient does not experience urinary incontinence.

- As prescribed, catheterize patient on a regularly scheduled basis.
- If episodes of urinary incontinence occur, catheterize more frequently. If >400 ml of urine obtained, catheterize more often and reduce fluid intake.
- Measure amount of residual urine, and attempt to ↑ length of time between catheterizations as indicated by ↓ amounts (eg, <50-100 ml) urine.
- Monitor and record I&O. Encourage consistent intake of fluids, evenly distributed throughout the day, to prevent overdistention, which can cause incontinence and ↑ risk for AD.
- ↓ fluid intake before bedtime to prevent nighttime incontinence.
- Discourage intake of caffeine-containing beverages and foods.

Constipation r/t lack of voluntary control of anal sphincter and lack of sensation of fecal mass after return of reflex arc associated with neuromuscular impairment

ABBREVIATIONS
AD: Autonomic dysreflexia
ANS: Autonomic nervous system
DTR: Deep tendon reflex
SAH: Subarachnoid hemorrhage
URI: Upper respiratory infection
VC: Vital capacity

Desired outcome: Within 24-48 h of this diagnosis and subsequently q2-3 days (or within patient's preinjury pattern), patient has bowel elimination of soft and formed stools.

- Obtain hx of preinjury bowel elimination pattern.
- Assist with selection of high-fiber menu items.
- Unless contraindicated, maintain a minimum daily fluid intake of 2-3 L/day.
- Administer stool softeners (eg, docusate sodium) qd.
- If possible, avoid enemas for long-term bowel management, since patient with SCI cannot retain enema solution. If, however, impaction occurs, a gentle small-volume cleansing enema, followed by manual removal of fecal material, may be necessary.
- Assess readiness for bowel retraining program, including neurologic status and current bowel patterns, noting frequency, amount, and consistency. Usually bowel retraining initiated when patient neurologically stable and can resume sitting position.
- Because use of bedpan may impair ability to evacuate bowel, provide bedside commode, if allowed.

  Provide ample time each day for bowel elimination. Take advantage of gastrocolic reflex occurring ½ h after mealtime.

  Ensure privacy.

  Stimulate rectal sphincter with digital stimulation or insert suppository (eg, bisacodyl) to initiate reflex peristalsis with reflex evacuation. Bowel overdistention or anal sphincter stimulation caused by impaction, rectal examination, or enema may precipitate AD. Use generous amounts of anesthetic lubricant when performing rectal examination or administering enema.

  If patient has upper extremity function, teach how to perform digital rectal stimulation, insertion of suppository, and abdominal massage to facilitate bowel movement.

REFERENCES

Boss BJ et al: Self-care competence among persons with spinal cord injury, *SCI Nurs* 12(2): 48-53, 1995.

Campbell LS: Commentary on acute SCI: how to minimize the damage, *ENAS Nurs Scan Emerg Care* 4(3): 10-11, 1994.

Dalton JR: Urologic management of the patient with spinal cord injury, *Trauma Q* 9(2): 72-81, 1993.

Lemke DM: Defining assessment parameters in dual injuries: spinal cord injury and traumatic brain injury, *SCI Nurs* 12(2): 40-47, 1995.

Stowe AC: Spinal cord injury. In Swearingen PL, Keen JH (eds): *Manual of critical care nursing*, ed 3, St Louis, 1995, Mosby.

Thomas E, Paulson SS: Protocol for weaning the SCI patient, *SCI Nurs* 11(2): 42-45, 1994.

Author: **Ann Coghlan Stowe**

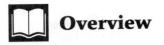 **Overview**

PATHOPHYSIOLOGY

State of recurring or continuous seizures of at least 30-min duration in which return to full consciousness from postictal state not attained before another seizure occurs. Metabolic demands of brain and heart ↑ greatly during seizure activity; thus adequate perfusion essential for organ function.
Convulsive: Generalized tonic-clonic seizures
Nonconvulsive: Includes simple partial status (focal motor), complex partial status (temporal or nontemporal seizures), and absence status (petit mal seizures)

COMPLICATIONS

Cardiac dysrhythmias, hyperthermia, aspiration, hypertension, hypotension, anoxia, hyperglycemia, hypoglycemia, dehydration, myoglobinuria, oral or musculoskeletal injuries

MORTALITY RATE

10%-12%

HISTORY/RISK FACTORS

- Epilepsy, especially with medication noncompliance, alcohol use, infection
- Acute metabolic disturbances: hypoglycemia, hyponatremia, hypocalcemia, hepatic encephalopathy
- CNS infection, trauma, tumors
- Stroke

CLINICAL PRESENTATION

Convulsive status, most common form, characterized by generalized tonic-clonic seizures

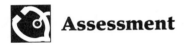 **Assessment**

PHYSICAL ASSESSMENT

Convulsive: Generalized tonic-clonic seizures without return to full consciousness. Respiratory depression or arrest, hypotension, dysrhythmias possible. Life-threatening medical emergency.

Nonconvulsive

Simple partial: Commonly manifested as focal motor status. Usually consciousness intact and motor activity localized to areas such as face and hand. May last a few h or days.
Complex partial: Prolonged confusional state. Automatisms (lip smacking, chewing, swallowing) and speech difficulty possible.
Absence: Some alterations in consciousness. Automatisms or mild clonic movements, such as eyelid fluttering, possible. Difficult to differentiate from complex partial status.

VITAL SIGNS/HEMODYNAMICS

RR: ↓, irregular, or absent
HR: ↑
BP: ↑ as a result of catecholamine excess; ↓ with anticonvulsant therapy
Temp: ↑
Other: CVP, PAP monitoring usually not necessary unless in prolonged or medically induced coma, in which event CVP assists with fluid management.
ECG: Dysrhythmias possible, especially with phenytoin administration.

LABORATORY STUDIES

Drug Screen: To r/o drug, alcohol intoxication
Chemistries: To r/o electrolyte imbalance or metabolic disturbance
CBC: ↑ WBCs suggest infection
Antiepilepsy Serum Drug Level
ABGs: To determine state of oxygenation

IMAGING

CT Scan: To check for brain lesion

DIAGNOSTIC PROCEDURE

EEG: Performed during seizure; can differentiate between absence or complex partial status.

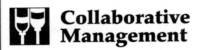 **Collaborative Management**

Maintenance of Alveolar Ventilation: Oral airway, O_2, and, if necessary, intubation and respiratory support initiated.
Prevention of Wernicke-Korsakoff Syndrome: 100 mg IV thiamine and 50 ml 50% glucose administered if chronic alcohol ingestion or hypoglycemia suspected.

Pharmacotherapy
Fast-acting anticonvulsant

Diazepam (Valium): 0.15-0.25 mg/kg IV to achieve high serum and brain concentrations. Not used as long-acting anticonvulsant. To avoid respiratory depression, do not administer faster than 5 mg/min.
IV lorazepam (Ativan): Similar to diazepam but has shorter half-life. Given 0.1 mg/kg up to 8 mg. To avoid respiratory depression, do not administer faster than 2 mg/min.

Long-acting anticonvulsant

IV phenytoin (Dilantin): Usual loading dose: 18-20 mg/kg. Do not infuse faster than 50 mg/min, since hypotension or dysrhythmias can develop. Flush line with NS only. If status persists after 20 mg/kg dose, additional 5 mg/kg up to maximum total dose of 30 mg/kg may be given.
IV phenobarbital: If allergic to phenytoin. *Usual dose:* 20 mg/kg. Respiratory depression and hypotension can occur, possibly necessitating ventilatory support.
Pentobarbital coma: If other therapies ineffective. *Loading dose:* 5 mg/kg. *Maintenance dose:* 0.5-3 mg/kg/h to stop seizure activity or maintain burst suppression on EEG. Monitor respiratory and CV activity continuously. Mechanical ventilation and vasopressors usually required.
Lidocaine, midazolam, neuromuscular blockade: Alternative therapies to stop seizure activity. Neuromuscular blockade stops movement but not electrical activity.

PATIENT-FAMILY TEACHING

- Disease, its cause, pathophysiology, and seizure classification
- Medications: drug name, purpose, dosage, schedule, precautions, drug-drug and food-drug interactions, potential side effects; importance of maintaining constant blood level of antiepilepsy agent by taking qd as prescribed
- Explanation of aura or warning occurring at beginning of seizure and importance of patient's lying down or getting into a safe position to prevent injury when it occurs
- Explanation that sleep deprivation can precipitate SE
- Referral to regional epilepsy support groups and Epilepsy Foundation of America (EFA)

Nursing Diagnoses/Interventions

Risk for trauma (oral and musculoskeletal) r/t seizure activity
Desired outcome: Patient's oral cavity and musculoskeletal system do not exhibit evidence of trauma after the seizure.

- As indicated, pad side rails, keep side rails up at all times, maintain bed in its lowest position, and keep an oral airway at bedside.
- Perform protective measures during seizures.
  - Turn to the side to enable tongue to fall forward to open the airway and drain secretions.
  - Avoid forcing airway into patient's mouth.
  - Avoid use of tongue blade, which could splinter.
  - Remove sharp or potentially dangerous objects.
  - Loosen any tight clothing.
  - Avoid restraining patient.
  - Stay with patient; assess and record seizure type and duration. Record any automatisms, motor activity, incontinence, tongue biting, postictal state.
- After seizure, reorient and reassure patient.

Impaired gas exchange r/t altered O_2 supply associated with hypoventilation and bradypnea secondary to depressant effect of seizures on respiratory center
Desired outcome: Within 1 h of treatment/intervention, patient has adequate gas exchange: $Pao_2 \geq 80$ mm Hg, $Paco_2$ 35-45 mm Hg, pH 7.35-7.45, and RR 12-20 breaths/min with eupnea.

- Assess respiratory status, including rate, depth, rhythm, and color. Be alert to use of accessory muscles, rapid or labored respirations, and cyanosis.
- Position an oral airway to help maintain open airway.
- Keep patient turned to the side to enable secretions to drain; suction as necessary.
- Monitor ABGs/Spo_2. Be alert to hypoxemia and respiratory acidosis. Administer O_2 as indicated.
- Keep intubation and suction equipment readily available for airway and ventilation assistance.
- Administer antiepilepsy medications carefully to avoid further depression of respiratory center.

Altered cerebral and cardiopulmonary tissue perfusion r/t interrupted blood flow secondary to continuous seizure activity or vasodilatory effects of some antiepilepsy medications
Desired outcome: Within 1 h of treatment/intervention, patient has adequate cerebral and cardiopulmonary perfusion: orientation × 3; NSR on ECG; BP wnl for patient; RR 12-20 breaths/min with eupnea; and absence of headache, papilledema, and other clinical indicators of ↑ ICP.

- Maintain airway and ventilation; provide supplemental O_2.
- Monitor VS q2-4 min. Respiratory depression, ↓ BP, and dysrhythmias can occur with rapid infusion of diazepam and phenytoin. Monitor closely and maintain BP to preserve cerebral perfusion.
- Monitor cardiac status *via* cardiac monitor. Be alert to dysrhythmias.
- Perform baseline and serial neurologic assessments to determine presence of focal findings that suggest an expanding lesion.

Ineffective individual coping r/t frustration secondary to unpredictable nature of the disease
Desired outcome: Within 24-48 h of this diagnosis, patient verbalizes feelings, identifies strengths and ineffective coping behaviors, and demonstrates a responsible role in his or her own care.

- Encourage patient to express feelings of frustration so that areas of major concern can be evaluated.
- Involve patient in decisions regarding care so that he or she has more of a sense of control over the disease.
- Help set realistic goals for employment and living arrangements.
- To involve patient in self-care, encourage him or her to educate others in what to do should a seizure occur.
- Encourage involvement in support groups.

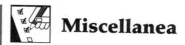

Miscellanea

CONSULT MD FOR

- Hypoventilation, respiratory depression, hypoxia, hypercapnia, $Spo_2 \leq 90\%$
- Phenytoin level <10 or >25 µg/ml.
- S&S of ↑ ICP
- Complications: dysrhythmias, suspected aspiration, ↑ or ↓ BP, hypoxemia, hyperglycemia, hypoglycemia, dehydration, oral or musculoskeletal injury

RELATED TOPICS

- Head injury
- Hypoglycemia
- Hyponatremia
- Increased intracranial pressure
- Pneumonia, aspiration

REFERENCES

Callanan M: Status epilepticus. In Swearingen PL, Keen JH (eds): *Manual of critical care nursing,* ed 3, St Louis, 1995, Mosby.

Hauser WA: Status epilepticus: epidemiologic considerations, *Neurology* 40(Suppl 2): 9-13, 1990.

Sierzant TL: Prolonged seizures (status epilepticus) or serial seizures. In Santilli N (ed): *A handbook for health care professionals,* Philadelphia, 1996, Lippincott-Raven.

Simon RP: Physiologic consequences of status epilepticus, *Epilepsia* 26(Suppl 1): S58-S66, 1985.

Working Group on Status Epilepticus: Treatment of convulsive status epilepticus: recommendations of the Working Group on Status Epilepticus, *JAMA* 270(7): 854-859, 1993.

Author: **Mimi Callanan**

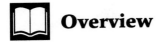

Overview

PATHOPHYSIOLOGY
Most common cause is hypertension, usually resulting in rupture of a small penetrating artery in the basal ganglia. Damage occurs as blood destroys and displaces brain tissue. Ischemia develops in area surrounding the already injured brain tissue, resulting in even greater damage. Intracerebral blood sometimes ruptures into the lateral ventricle, causing ↑ risk for communicating hydrocephalus.

HISTORY/RISK FACTORS
- Age >55
- Systemic arterial hypertension
- Cerebral aneurysm, cerebral vascular malformation
- Vasculitis
- Hematologic disorders
- Stimulant abuse
- Cerebral neoplasms

CLINICAL PRESENTATION
Severe hypertension; ↓ LOC, which ensues within a few h if stroke causes mass effects as a result of swelling or involves brainstem or thalamic regions bilaterally; mild to moderate headache.
Brainstem ICH: Quadriplegia, coma possible.

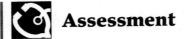

Assessment

PHYSICAL ASSESSMENT
NIH Stroke Scale: Quick and easy to use for evaluating cognitive, language, and motor deficits unique to stroke (see Appendix)
Deficits with Putamen Hemorrhage: Contralateral hemiplegia, hemisensory loss, hemianopia, slurred speech
Deficits with Thalamic Hemorrhage: Contralateral hemiplegia, hemisensory loss, small and poorly reactive pupils, ↓ LOC
Deficits with Pontine Hemorrhage: Locked-in syndrome (aware, unable to communicate verbally, quadriplegia), coma
Deficits with Cerebellar Hemorrhage: Occipital headache, ataxia, dizziness, headache, nausea, vomiting
Deficits with Lobar Hemorrhage: Mimics cerebral infarct (eg, contralateral motor and sensory signs); minimal deficit because of site
CNS: S&S of ↑ ICP, seizures
Resp: Hyperventilation, tachypnea, irregular pattern if ↑ ICP present
CV: Dysrhythmias, hypertension

VITAL SIGNS/HEMODYNAMICS (for large ICH)
RR: ↑, irregular, or ↓
HR: ↑, possible dysrhythmias
BP: ↑
Temp: ↑ if seizures, pneumonia, or ↑ ICP present
ICP: ↑ resulting from size of hematoma and edema associated with cerebral infarct, hydrocephalus, or seizure activity
CPP: ↓
ECG: QT prolongation, ST-segment depression, T-wave inversion, presence of U waves, ventricular ectopy; ↑ incidence of AMI after stroke

LABORATORY STUDIES
Hematology, Chemistry, Coagulation Profiles, Syphilis Tests, Sedimentation Rate: To assess for infection or vasculitis.
Drug Screen (eg, cocaine, amphetamine)
LP: To measure CSF pressures and obtain CSF specimen when infection such as meningitis or neurosyphilis suspected.

IMAGING
CT Scan: Performed immediately to differentiate ischemic from hemorrhagic stroke.
Xenon CT: Radioisotope used to calculate cerebral blood flow of ischemic brain tissue and assist in management.

MRI and Magnetic Resonance Arteriogram (MRA): Provide detailed information regarding area of injury or its vascular supply.

Transcranial Doppler Studies: To evaluate intracranial vessels. Also used for evaluating vasospasm, determining brain death *via* detection of cerebral circulatory arrest, and locating emboli.

Cerebral Angiography: Helps determine cause of stroke by identifying involved blood vessel.

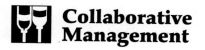

Collaborative Management

Early detection *via* accurate neurologic examination and immediate medical or surgical intervention help prevent stroke extension, ↑ brain edema, and hydrocephalus.

Prevention of Stroke Extension: ↓ potential infarct size depends on adequate perfusion to the penumbra, the ischemic brain tissue surrounding the hematoma. Controlling arterial BP essential and necessitates individual consideration.

ICP Monitoring: Necessary for large infarcts, ↑ edema, and hydrocephalus. CPP should be >60 mm Hg at all times. Raise HOB to 30 degrees to promote venous return and ↑ cerebral perfusion.

Optimizing Regulatory Function: Dysrhythmias corrected and fluid status optimized to improve CO and promote cerebral perfusion. Other considerations: maintenance of adequate nutrition, prevention of aspiration, acid suppression therapy, bowel and bladder retraining, ROM, sequential compression stockings, maintenance of skin integrity.

Pharmacotherapy: Neuroprotective agents hold great promise but remain experimental.

Antihypertensives: In acute phase, SBP often ↑ and requires careful management. Nicardipine (Cardene), which may have cerebral protection properties in addition to antihypertensive effects, or labetalol (Normodyne) often used. However, overaggressive therapy may result in relative hypotension and compromised cerebral perfusion. If BP suboptimal, dopamine or dobutamine titrated to keep MAP high enough to maintain CPP >60 mm Hg.

Anticonvulsant therapy: Phenytoin (Dilantin), lorazepam (Ativan), or diazepam (Valium) may be used for seizures.

Sedation: May be necessary to ↓ anxiety/agitation, which can contribute to ↑ ICP. Drugs used include midazolam (Versed), fentanyl (Sublimaze), or propofol (Diprivan).

Craniotomy: For evacuation of hematoma or aneurysmal clipping.

PATIENT-FAMILY TEACHING
- Definition/description of patient's stroke
- Risk factors and prevention measures
- Warning signs of stroke and need to report these to health care provider and call 911 or EMS
- National Stroke Association phone number: 1-800-STROKES
- Referrals to American Heart Association, local support groups

Nursing Diagnoses/Interventions

Decreased adaptive capacity: Intracranial, r/t interrupted blood flow secondary to ICH
Desired outcome: Within 72 h of this diagnosis (or optimally ongoing), patient has adequate cerebral tissue perfusion: no ↓ in LOC per NIH Stroke Scale; no deterioration in motor function on affected side; and no new or further deterioration of language, cognition, or visual field.

- Assess for neurologic changes qh in the acute phase. Use NIH Stroke Scale to record and monitor neurologic changes following stroke.
- Maintain ICP <15 mm Hg and CPP >60 mm Hg. CPP = MAP − ICP.
- Position to maintain adequate cerebral perfusion; avoid extreme hip flexion. When positioning, monitor tolerance to position change. Keep HOB raised at 30 degrees as tolerated.
- Maintain oxygenation by turning as tolerated and suctioning as needed. Assess breath sounds frequently. Avoid activities or conditions that can ↑ ICP, including excessive coughing, hypercapnia, and hypoxia.
- Maintain adequate SBP. Use vasodilators or vasopressors as necessary to optimize BP and maintain CPP >60 mm Hg.
- Medicate for sedation as prescribed. Monitor response, including effects of sedation and resulting changes in ICP.

Impaired physical mobility r/t ↓ motor function of upper and/or lower extremities and trunk following stroke
Desired outcome: At time of discharge from ICU, patient exhibits no evidence of complications of immobility such as skin breakdown, contracture formation, pneumonia, or constipation.

- Turn and position frequently as tolerated; transfer toward unaffected side.
- Teach methods for turning and moving using stronger extremity to move weaker extremity.
- Position weaker extremities when turning to avoid contracture formation, frozen shoulder, or foot drop.
- Begin passive ROM within first 24 h of admission. Monitor response and modify exercises if BP or ICP ↑.
- Obtain PT and OT referrals as soon as possible to establish appropriate therapy.
- Have patient cough and breathe deep at scheduled intervals. Provide percussion and postural drainage for patients for whom coughing and deep breathing ineffective for mobilizing secretions.

Impaired verbal communication r/t aphasia secondary to cerebrovascular insult
Desired outcome: At a minimum of 24-h period before discharge from ICU, patient demonstrates improved self-expression and relates ↓ in frustration with communication.

- Be aware that aphasia is the partial or complete inability to use or comprehend language and symbols and may occur with dominant (left) hemisphere damage.
  Receptive aphasia (eg, Wernicke's, sensory) characterized by inability to comprehend spoken words. Patient may respond to nonverbal cues.
  Expressive aphasia (eg, Broca's, motor) characterized by difficulty expressing words or naming objects. Gestures, groans, swearing, or nonsense words may be used. Use of a picture or word board may be helpful.

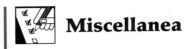 # Miscellanea

CONSULT MD FOR
- Significant BP changes that result in changes in neurologic examination
- ICP >15 mm Hg or CPP <60 mm Hg
- PaO_2 <80 mm Hg, SpO_2 <90%, $PaCO_2$ >40 mm Hg (or >30 mm Hg if on hyperventilation therapy)
- Deteriorating neurologic status or S&S of ↑ ICP
- Complications: ventricular dysrhythmias, AMI, pneumonia, sepsis, DVT, pulmonary emboli, seizures

RELATED TOPICS
- Agitation syndrome
- Atrial fibrillation
- Hypertensive crisis
- Immobility, prolonged
- Increased intracranial pressure
- Myocardial infarction, acute
- Pneumonia, aspiration
- Pulmonary emboli: thrombotic and embolic
- Status epilepticus
- Stroke: ischemic

ABBREVIATIONS
CPP: Cerebral perfusion pressure
ICH: Intracranial hematoma

- Evaluate nature and severity of the aphasia. Assess ability to point to specific object, follow simple directions, understand yes/no and complex questions, repeat simple and complex words, repeat sentences, name objects, relate purpose or action of the object, fulfill written requests, write requests, and read.
- Assess for dysarthria, which signals risk for aspiration resulting from ineffective swallowing and gag reflexes. Consult with speech therapist to plan measures to promote independence and facilitate swallowing.
- ↓ environmental distractions, such as television or others' conversations. Fatigue affects ability to communicate; plan adequate sleep/rest.
- Communicate with patient as much as possible. General principles include facing patient and establishing eye contact, speaking slowly and clearly, giving patient time to process communication and give answer, keeping messages short and simple, staying with one clearly defined subject, avoiding questions with multiple choices and instead phrasing questions so that they can be answered "yes" or "no," and using same words each time when repeating a statement or question. If patient does not understand after repetition, try different words. Use gestures, facial expressions, and pantomime to supplement and reinforce message.
- When helping patients regain use of symbolic language, start with nouns first, and progress to more complex statements. For continuity, keep a record at the bedside of words to be used (eg, "pill" rather than "medication").
- Treat patient as an adult. It is not necessary to raise the volume of your voice unless patient is hard of hearing. Be respectful.
- When patients have difficulty expressing words or naming objects, encourage them to repeat words after you for practice in verbal expression. Be prepared for labile emotions because these patients become frustrated and emotional when faced with their impaired speech.
- Patients who have lost the ability to monitor their verbal output may not produce sensible language but may think they are making sense. Avoid labeling patient "belligerent" or "confused" when the problem is aphasia and frustration.
- Patients with nondominant (right) hemisphere damage often have no difficulty speaking; however, they may use excessive detail, give irrelevant information, and get off on a tangent. Bring patient back to the subject by saying "Let's go back to what we were talking about."
- Provide supportive and relaxed environment for patients unable to form words or sentences or speak clearly or appropriately. If patient makes an error, avoid criticism and use encouragement, eg, "That was a good try." Acknowledge frustration. To validate patient's message, repeat or rephrase it aloud.
- Ensure that call light is available and patient knows how to use it. If patient is unable to use call light, check frequently and anticipate needs to ensure safety and trust.

REFERENCES

Barch C: Stroke. In Swearingen PL, Keen JH (eds): *Manual of critical care nursing,* ed 3, St Louis, 1995, Mosby.

Shepard T, Fox S: Assessment and management of hypertension in the acute stroke patient, *J Neurosci Nurs* 28(1): 5-12, 1996.

US Department of Health and Human Services: Post-stroke rehabilitation, *Clin Pract Guidel* 16, May 1995.

Author: **Carol Barch**

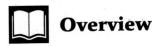 **Overview**

PATHOPHYSIOLOGY

Caused by event that interrupts blood flow to brain, resulting in ischemia, which leads to infarction. *Thrombi* usually form in arterial branches with low flow and plaque formation. Cerebral *emboli* usually form in heart and travel to brain. *Lacunar* infarcts occur as a result of blockages in small vessels deep in brain. The ischemic event compromises the Na^+/K^+ pump, causing massive flux of ions and water, resulting in brain cell edema. High concentrations of intracellular Ca^{2+} and lactic acid cause cellular metabolic alterations that ultimately lead to death. Lactic acidosis stimulates vasomotor center, causing marked ↑ in arterial pressure known as CNS ischemic response.

INCIDENCE

Comprises 75%-80% of all strokes

HISTORY/RISK FACTORS

- Strongest risk factors: hypertension, smoking, aging (>55 yrs), previous hx of TIA/stroke
- CV disease: A-fib, AMI, hypercholesterolemia, dilated cardiomyopathy, valvular heart disease
- Other: male gender, African-American ethnicity, family hx of stroke or AMI, sedentary lifestyle

CLINICAL PRESENTATION

Hemiparesis, visual field cut, aphasia, headache. Altered LOC if stroke causes mass effects because of swelling or involves brainstem or thalamic regions bilaterally.

Thrombotic: Likely to evolve over several h and may fluctuate over several h or days
Embolic: Usually maximal at onset; often occurs during activity
Lacunar: Pure motor or pure sensory deficit

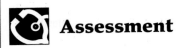 **Assessment**

PHYSICAL ASSESSMENT

NIH Stroke Scale: Quick and easy to use for evaluating cognitive, language, and motor deficits unique to stroke (see Appendix)
Deficits with ICA Stroke: Contralateral motor or sensory deficit, aphasia with dominant hemisphere, neglect with nondominant hemisphere, contralateral visual field deficit (hemianopia), contralateral eye deviation
Deficits with MCA Stroke: Contralateral hemiplegia (arm and face > leg), sensory involvement, aphasia of dominant hemisphere, neglect of nondominant hemisphere (denial of weakness), homonymous hemianopia
CNS: S&S of ↑ ICP, seizures
Resp: Hyperventilation, tachypnea, irregular pattern if ↑ ICP present
CV: Dysrhythmias, hypertension

VITAL SIGNS/HEMODYNAMICS

RR: Irregular
HR: ↑, dysrhythmias
BP: ↑, especially with large hemispheric stroke
Temp: ↑ if seizures, pneumonia, or ↑ ICP present
ICP: ↑ as a result of edema associated with cerebral infarct, hydrocephalus, or seizure activity
CPP: MAP − ICP = >60 mm Hg

ECG: QT prolongation, ST-segment depression, T-wave inversion, presence of U waves, ventricular ectopy; ↑ incidence of AMI after stroke

LABORATORY STUDIES

Hematology, Chemistry, Coagulation Profiles, Syphilis Tests, Sedimentation Rate: To assess for infection or vasculitis.
Drug Screen (eg, cocaine, amphetamine) Hypercoagulable Profile: To evaluate levels of proteins C and S, which may be deficient in young (<45 yrs) stroke patient who may have no other risk factors for stroke.
LP: To measure CSF pressures and obtain CSF specimen when infection such as meningitis or neurosyphilis suspected.

IMAGING

CT scan: To differentiate ischemic from hemorrhagic stroke. Often nl with ACI during first 24 h.
MRI and Magnetic Resonance Arteriogram (MRA): Provide detailed data regarding area of injury or its vascular supply.
Xenon CT: Radioisotope used to calculate cerebral blood flow of ischemic brain tissue and assist in management.
Doppler Studies: Include echocardiogram (transthoracic or transesophageal) to evaluate heart structure and function; carotid Doppler or duplex to evaluate blood flow in extracranial carotid arteries; and transcranial Doppler to evaluate intracranial vessels. The latter also used for evaluating vasospasm, determining brain death *via* detection of cerebral circulatory arrest, and locating emboli.
Cerebral Angiography: Helps determine cause of stroke by identifying involved blood vessel. In clinical trials, thrombolytic agents injected directly into clot *via* microcatheter to restore blood flow to brain.

Collaborative Management

Early detection *via* accurate neurologic examination and immediate medical or surgical intervention help prevent stroke extension, ↑ brain edema, and hydrocephalus.

Prevention of Stroke Extension: ↓ potential infarct size depends on adequate perfusion to the penumbra, the ischemic brain tissue surrounding the core infarct. Controlling arterial BP essential. "Normal" BP may be too low, causing further ischemia and infarct by ↓ cerebral perfusion. Arterial BP should not be lowered abruptly.

ICP Monitoring: Necessary for patients (especially those in 20s and 30s) with large infarcts, ↑ edema, and hydrocephalus. CPP should be >60 mm Hg at all times and HOB kept flat to ↑ cerebral perfusion.

Optimizing Regulatory Function: Dysrhythmias corrected and fluid status optimized to improve CO and promote cerebral perfusion. Additional considerations include maintenance of adequate nutrition, prevention of aspiration, acid suppression therapy, bowel and bladder retraining, ROM, sequential compression stockings, and maintenance of skin integrity.

Rehabilitation: Consults to physiatrist, PT, OT, and speech therapist should be made within first 24 h.

Pharmacotherapy: Neuroprotective agents hold great promise, but use is limited to clinical trials.

Thrombolytics: Alteplase (Activase) recently approved for use in acute ischemic stroke: given within first 3 h of symptom onset.

Anticoagulation: IV heparin indicated for progressing stroke, TIAs, and cardioembolic stroke.

Antiplatelet therapy: To ↓ risk of stroke and ↓ frequency of TIAs. Aspirin and ticlopidine (Ticlid) are agents in current use.

Antihypertensives: In acute phase, SBP often ↑ and requires careful management. Nicardipine (Cardene), which may have cerebral protection properties in addition to antihypertensive effects, or labetalol (Normodyne) often used. However, overaggressive therapy may result in relative hypotension and compromised cerebral perfusion. If BP suboptimal, dopamine or dobutamine titrated to keep MAP high enough to maintain CPP >60 mm Hg.

Anticonvulsant therapy: Phenytoin (Dilantin), lorazepam (Ativan), or diazepam (Valium) may be used for seizures.

Sedation: May be necessary to ↓ anxiety/agitation, which can contribute to ↑ ICP. Drugs used include midazolam (Versed), fentanyl (Sublimaze), or propofol (Diprivan).

Carotid Endarterectomy: Surgical removal of plaque in obstructed carotid artery considered choice treatment for >70% carotid stenosis.

Craniotomy: Dural incision or temporal lobectomy considered for young patient who has uncontrollable ↑ in ICP as a result of massive edema.

PATIENT-FAMILY TEACHING
- Definition/description of specific type of stroke (eg, thrombotic, embolic, lacunar)
- Risk factors and prevention measures
- Warning signs of stroke and need to report these to health care provider and call 911 or EMS
- National Stroke Association phone number: 1-800-STROKES

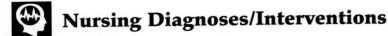 # Nursing Diagnoses/Interventions

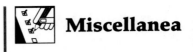 ## Miscellanea

Decreased adaptive capacity: Intracranial, r/t interrupted blood flow secondary to thrombus or embolus

Desired outcome: Within 72 h of this diagnosis (or optimally on an ongoing basis), patient has adequate cerebral tissue perfusion: no ↓ in LOC; no evidence of deterioration in motor function on affected side; and no evidence of new or further deterioration of language, cognition, or visual field per NIH Stroke Scale.

- Assess for neurologic changes qh in the acute phase. Use NIH Stroke Scale to record and monitor neurologic changes following stroke.
- Maintain ICP <15 mm Hg and CPP >60 mm Hg. CPP = MAP − ICP.
- Position patient to maintain adequate cerebral perfusion; avoid extreme hip flexion. When positioning, monitor tolerance to position change. Keep HOB flat as tolerated.
- Maintain oxygenation by turning as tolerated and suctioning as needed. Assess breath sounds frequently. Avoid activities or conditions that can ↑ ICP, including excessive coughing, hypercapnia, and hypoxia.
- Maintain adequate SBP. Higher pressures (typically 140-180 mm Hg) necessary to perfuse area of brain at risk of infarction. Use vasodilators or vasopressors as necessary to optimize BP and maintain CPP >60 mm Hg.
- Medicate for sedation as prescribed. Monitor response, including effects of sedation and resulting changes in ICP.

Impaired physical mobility r/t ↓ motor function of upper and/or lower extremities and trunk following stroke

Desired outcome: At time of discharge from ICU, patient exhibits no evidence of complications of immobility such as skin breakdown, contracture formation, pneumonia, or constipation.

- Turn and position frequently, as tolerated.
- Transfer toward unaffected side.
- Teach methods for turning and moving using stronger extremity to move weaker extremity.
- Position weaker extremities when turning to avoid contracture formation, frozen shoulder, or foot drop.
- Begin passive ROM within first 24 h of admission. Monitor response and modify exercises if BP or ICP ↑.
- Obtain PT and OT referral as soon as possible to establish appropriate therapy.
- Have patient cough and breathe deeply at scheduled intervals. Provide percussion and postural drainage for patients for whom coughing and deep breathing ineffective for mobilizing secretions.

Impaired verbal communication r/t aphasia secondary to cerebrovascular insult

Desired outcome: At a minimum of 24-h period before discharge from ICU, patient demonstrates improved self-expression and relates ↓ in frustration with communication.

- Be aware that aphasia is the partial or complete inability to use or comprehend language and symbols and may occur with dominant (left) hemisphere damage.
  Receptive aphasia (eg, Wernicke's, sensory) characterized by inability to comprehend spoken words. Patient may respond to nonverbal cues.
  Expressive aphasia (eg, Broca's, motor) characterized by difficulty expressing words or naming objects. Gestures, groans, swearing, or nonsense words may be used. Use of a picture or word board may be helpful.

CONSULT MD FOR

- SBP <140 or >180 mm Hg or other preestablished range
- ICP >15 mm Hg or CPP <60 mm Hg
- Pao_2 <80 mm Hg, Spo_2 <90%, $Paco_2$ >40 mm Hg (or >30 mm Hg if on hyperventilation therapy)
- Deteriorating neurologic status or S&S of ↑ ICP
- Complications: ventricular dysrhythmias, AMI, pneumonia, sepsis, DVT, pulmonary emboli, seizures

RELATED TOPICS

- Agitation syndrome
- Atrial fibrillation
- Hypertensive crisis
- Immobility, prolonged
- Increased intracranial pressure
- Myocardial infarction, acute
- Pneumonia, aspiration
- Pulmonary emboli: thrombotic, embolic
- Status epilepticus
- Stroke: hemorrhagic

ABBREVIATIONS

CPP: Cerebral perfusion pressure
ICA: Internal carotid artery
MCA: Middle cerebral artery

- Evaluate nature and severity of the aphasia. Assess ability to point to specific object, follow simple directions, understand yes/no and complex questions, repeat simple and complex words, repeat sentences, name objects, relate purpose or action of the object, fulfill written requests, write requests, and read.
- Assess for dysarthria, which signals risk for aspiration resulting from ineffective swallowing and gag reflexes. Consult with speech therapist to plan measures to promote independence and facilitate swallowing.
- ↓ environmental distractions, such as television or others' conversations. Fatigue affects ability to communicate; plan adequate sleep/rest.
- Communicate with patient as much as possible. General principles include facing patient and establishing eye contact, speaking slowly and clearly, giving patient time to process communication and give answer, keeping messages short and simple, staying with one clearly defined subject, avoiding questions with multiple choices and instead phrasing questions so that they can be answered "yes" or "no," and using same words each time when repeating a statement or question. If patient does not understand after repetition, try different words. Use gestures, facial expressions, and pantomime to supplement and reinforce message.
- When helping patients regain use of symbolic language, start with nouns first, and progress to more complex statements. For continuity, keep a record at the bedside of words to be used (eg, "pill" rather than "medication").
- Treat patient as an adult. It is not necessary to raise the volume of your voice unless patient is hard of hearing. Be respectful.
- When patients have difficulty expressing words or naming objects, encourage them to repeat words after you for practice in verbal expression. Be prepared for labile emotions because these patients become frustrated and emotional when faced with their impaired speech.
- Patients who have lost the ability to monitor their verbal output may not produce sensible language but may think they are making sense. Avoid labeling patient "belligerent" or "confused" when the problem is aphasia and frustration.
- Patients with nondominant (right) hemisphere damage often have no difficulty speaking; however, they may use excessive detail, give irrelevant information, and get off on a tangent. Bring patient back to the subject by saying "Let's go back to what we were talking about."
- Provide supportive and relaxed environment for patients unable to form words or sentences or speak clearly or appropriately. If patient makes an error, avoid criticism and use encouragement, eg, "That was a good try." Acknowledge frustration. To validate patient's message, repeat or rephrase it aloud.
- Ensure that call light is available and patient knows how to use it. If patient is unable to use call light, check frequently and anticipate needs to ensure safety and trust.

REFERENCES

American Heart Association: Guidelines for the management of patients with acute ischemic stroke, *Circulation* 90(3): 1588-1601, 1994.

Barch C: Stroke. In Swearingen PL, Keen JH (eds): *Manual of critical care nursing,* ed 3, St Louis, 1995, Mosby.

National Institute of Neurological Disorders and Stroke rt-PA Stroke Study Group: Tissue plasminogen activator for acute ischemic stroke, *N Engl J Med* 333(24): 1581-1587, 1995.

Pryse-Phillips W: Ticlopidine aspirin stroke study: outcome by vascular distribution of the qualifying event, *J Cerebrovasc Dis* 3(1): 49-56, 1993.

Shepard T, Fox S: Assessment and management of hypertension in the acute stroke patient, *J Neurosci Nurs* 28(1): 5-12, 1996.

US Department of Health and Human Services: Post-stroke rehabilitation, *Clin Pract Guidel* 16, May 1995.

Author: **Carol Barch**

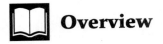 **Overview**

PATHOPHYSIOLOGY

Typically results from rupture of cerebral aneurysm or traumatic laceration of cerebral arterioles with severe head injury. Patients who survive initial effects, which include destruction of brain tissue by force of arterial blood, intracerebral hemorrhage, and sharply ↑ ICP with possible herniation of brain tissue, are also subject to numerous serious complications:

Cerebral Vasospasm: Occurs in up to 60% of patients with SAH; onset 4-14 days post-SAH; peaks at 7-10 days. The greater the volume of blood in the SAS and basal cisterns, the more pronounced the vasospasm. As clots begin to hemolyze, spasmogenic substances released that precipitate vasospasm.

Rebleeding: Risk greatest in patients with ruptured aneurysm. Usually occurs within first 48 h after initial incident, but may occur at any time within first 2 wks.

Communicating Hydrocephalus: Develops in ≈ 20% of patients. Blood in SAS and ventricles obstructs flow of CSF, causing ↑ in CSF pressure with concomitant ↓ in neurologic status.

Hypothalamic Dysfunction: Seen in ≈1/3 of hydrocephalus cases following SAH; may result from mechanical pressure on hypothalamus from a dilated third ventricle. Causes ↑ serum catecholamines and ↑ SNS activity.

Hyponatremia: Caused by cerebral salt-wasting syndrome, SIADH, or combination of factors influencing sodium and water metabolism. If not identified and corrected early, may lead to intracranial hypertension, cerebral ischemia, seizures, coma, and death.

HISTORY/RISK FACTORS

- Saccular or berry (congenital) aneurysm
- Septic, miliary, traumatic aneurysm
- Direct head injury (eg, high-impact vehicular collision)

CLINICAL PRESENTATION (immediately prior to rupture)

Headache, weakness, ptosis, visual disturbance

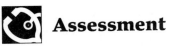 **Assessment**

PHYSICAL ASSESSMENT

Neuro: ↓ LOC, confusion, irritability, disorientation, hemisensory changes, hemiparesis/hemiplegia, worsening headache, pupillary changes, dysconjugate gaze, seizures

Pathologic Reflexes

Kernig's sign: Resistance to full leg extension at knee during hip flexion

Brudzinski's sign: Flexion of hip and knee with neck flexion

Resp: Irregular respiratory patterns (eg, Cheyne-Stokes, ataxic, apneustic, central neurogenic, hyperventilation)

CV: Bradycardia, ↑ SBP with widening pulse pressure associated with ↑ ICP

Hydrocephalus

Acute: Onset within 24 h; loss of pupillary reflexes; sudden onset of coma or persistent coma after initial SAH

Subacute: Onset within 1-7 days; gradual changes in LOC with confusion, drowsiness, lethargy, stupor

Chronic: Onset after 7 days; gradual changes in LOC and orientation with incontinence and impaired balance and gait; presence of frontal lobe reflexes (grasp and sucking), which are abnormal in adults

Hyponatremia: Anxiety, confusion, lethargy, coma, nausea, vomiting, abdominal pain, cold and clammy skin, generalized weakness, and lower extremity muscle cramps

Hypothalamic Dysfunction: Vomiting, glycosuria, proteinuria, hyponatremia. ↑ circulating catecholamines cause flushing, diaphoresis, pupillary dilatation, ↓ gastric motility, ↑ serum glucose, fever, hypertension, tachycardia, cardiac dysrhythmias, myocardial ischemia/infarction

VITAL SIGNS/HEMODYNAMICS

RR: Irregular, ↑ or ↓

HR: ↓ if ↑ ICP; ↑ if hypothalamic dysfunction

BP: ↑ as a result of catecholamine excess; widened pulse pressure suggests ↑ ICP

Temp: ↑ as a result of hypothalamic dysfunction or meningeal irritation

SVR: May be ↑ with catecholamine excess

ICP: ↑

CPP: ↓

ECG: Dysrhythmias; ischemic changes possible because of catecholamine excess r/t hypothalamic dysfunction

LABORATORY STUDIES

LP: Confirms presence of blood in CSF, which signals that SAH has occurred. Because CSF pressure may be as high as 250 mm H_2O, there is substantial risk of herniation and rebleeding. Therefore LP performed only when CT/MRI results nondiagnostic.

CSF Analysis: Will show ↑ protein and ↓ glucose; WBCs may be present.

ABGs: To detect hypoxemia and hypercapnia and guide respiratory therapy.

IMAGING

CT Scan: Identifies subarachnoid or intracerebral hemorrhage and size, site, and amount of bleeding. May reveal hydrocephalus.

Cerebral Angiography: Confirms diagnosis of ruptured aneurysm with SAH and determines accessibility of aneurysm and presence of hematoma, vasospasm, and hydrocephalus. Four-vessel study involving both carotids and vertebrals recommended because of 15%-20% chance of a second aneurysm.

Transcranial Doppler Ultrasonography: Evaluates blood flow through cerebral arteries and permits early detection of cerebral vasospasm.

Collaborative Management

Resp Support: To maintain airway and provide intubation and ventilation as necessary. Hypercapnia is a potent cerebral vasodilator that can ↑ ICP; hyperventilation therapy *via* mechanical ventilation may be necessary for $Paco_2$ >40-45 mm Hg.

Bed Rest with Activity Limitation: To help prevent stimulation and catecholamine release. Keep patient in quiet, calm environment with ↓ lights and noise level. Usually ADL completed by nursing staff. Passive ROM prescribed to prevent formation of thrombi, with subsequent pulmonary emboli.

ICP Monitoring: Uses variety of techniques (intraventricular cannula, subarachnoid screw, epidural or intraparenchymal fiberoptic sensor). Monitoring systems provide digital display of ICP, but CPP must be calculated. Maintain CPP between 60-80 mm Hg.

HOB Elevation: To help facilitate venous outflow from intracranial cavity and ↓ ICP. Angle of 15-45 degrees usually prescribed.

Fluid and Electrolyte Management: Fluids limited to 1500-1800 ml/24 h to prevent overhydration, with subsequent cerebral edema. Electrolytes replaced as indicated by clinical data, laboratory values. Hyponatremia treated based on assessment/identification of etiology. If cause is true hypovolemia (cerebral salt wasting), NS, PRBCs, and colloids recommended. If cause is dilutional hyponatremia (SIADH), free water restriction and sodium replacement recommended. Concurrent administration of diuretic (furosemide) and replacement of solute with 3% hypertonic saline may be prescribed.

Pharmacotherapy

Sedatives: Phenobarbital is the drug of choice to ↓ restlessness and irritability, which can ↑ BP and ICP.

Analgesics: Acetaminophen for mild pain, codeine sulfate for more severe pain. Codeine given in usual doses will not depress neurologic indicators, but it can cause constipation and thus is given with stool softeners to prevent straining.

Antipyretics: Acetaminophen used to control fever, which can ↑ cerebral metabolic activity. Chlorpromazine may be used to ↓ temp and control shivering. Aspirin avoided.

Corticosteroids: If ↑ ICP present, dexamethasone (Decadron) used for its antiinflammatory actions to relieve cerebral edema. Use is controversial.

Nimodipine and nicardipine: Calcium channel blockers that selectively dilate cerebral vessels.

Antihypertensives: If necessary to control hypertension in patients with ↑ ICP. Hydralazine hydrochloride (Apresoline), labetalol (Normodyne, Trandate), or sodium nitroprusside (Nipride) may be used in combination with a thiazide diuretic.

Osmotic diuretics: Mannitol (Osmitrol), urea (Ureaphil), others used to ↓ ICP and treat cerebral edema *via* diuresis. Potential for rebleeding caused by rapid removal of fluid from brain tissue and ↓ brain volume. Rebound ↑ in ICP possible ≈8-12 h after administration. Furosemide (Lasix) may be used to ↓ rebound effect of mannitol.

Triple H therapy: Investigational. Effective, but may precipitate ↑ in ICP. Careful monitoring of BP, CPP, neurologic status required.

Hypervolemia (saline, plasma protein fraction [Plasmanate], blood products): To ↑ circulating volume to reverse/prevent ischemia caused by vasospasm.

Hemodilution (albumin and crystalloid fluids): To ↓ blood viscosity and promote microvascular perfusion.

Hypertension (dobutamine [Dobutrex], phenylephrine [Neo-Synephrine], dopamine [Intropin], isoproterenol [Isuprel]): To ↑ BP, thereby ↑ CPP and preventing ischemia and infarction.

Shunt Placement for Hydrocephalus: To drain CSF, thereby preventing ventricular enlargement with compression of cerebral tissue and ↑ ICP. Complications include infection and malfunction.

Surgical Interventions: Considered for large intracranial clots that cause life-threatening intracranial shift; delayed with cerebral vasospasm until it subsides. Repair of cerebral aneurysm requires craniotomy with either an aneurysm clipping, ligation, or coagulation or an encasement of aneurysmal sac in surgical gauze.

PATIENT-FAMILY TEACHING

- Importance of avoiding activities that use isometric muscle contractions (pulling or pushing side rails, pushing against footboard)
- Importance of avoiding straining with bowel movements
- Rationale for exhaling through mouth when moving in bed or having bowel movement
- Rationale for avoiding coughing; importance of opening mouth when sneezing to minimize ↑ in ICP
- Measures to prevent constipation

Nursing Diagnoses/Interventions

Decreased adaptive capacity: Intracranial, r/t compromise of fluid dynamic mechanisms secondary to hemorrhage into SAS or cerebral vasospasm

Desired outcome: Patient exhibits adequate cerebral perfusion within 24-72 h of treatment: orientation × 3 (or consistent with baseline); equal and normoreactive pupils; BP wnl for patient; HR 60-100 bpm; RR 12-20 breaths/min with eupnea; bilaterally equal motor function with extremity strength and tone wnl for patient; ICP 0-15 mm Hg; CPP 60-80 mm Hg; and absence of headache, vomiting, and other indicators of ↑ ICP.

- Assess qh for ↑ ICP and herniation (altered mentation, ↑ BP with widening pulse pressure, irregular respirations, ↑ headache, pupillary changes).
- Assess for cerebral vasospasm: focal neurologic deficit with/without loss of consciousness or gradual onset of confusion and deteriorating LOC associated with focal motor deficits.
- Calculate CPP by means of the formula

$$CPP = MAP - ICP$$
$$\text{where } MAP = \frac{SBP + 2(DBP)}{3}$$

- Assess for ↑ ICP (ICP >15 mm Hg) or CPP <60 mm Hg.
- Assess for and treat conditions that can cause ↑ restlessness with concomitant ↑ ICP: distended bladder, constipation, hypoxemia, headache, fear, anxiety.
- Implement measures that help prevent ↑ ICP:
  Maintain complete bed rest.
  Keep HOB elevated 15-45 degrees.
  Avoid neck hyperflexion, hyperextension, or hyperrotation.
  Maintain quiet, relaxing environment.
  Minimize vigorous activity; assist with ADL.
  Maintain adequate ventilation to prevent cerebral hypoxia.
  Administer O_2 to maintain Sao_2 ≥0.94.
  Limit fluid intake to 1500-1800 ml/24 h or as otherwise prescribed.
  Monitor and record I&O.

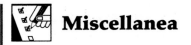 # Miscellanea

CONSULT MD FOR

- ICP >15 mm Hg or CPP <60 mm Hg
- Clinical indicators of ↑ ICP: altered mentation, ↑ BP with widening pulse pressure, irregular respirations, pupillary changes
- Clinical indicators of cerebral vasospasm: focal motor deficit with confusion, altered mentation, or loss of consciousness; ↑ headache with ↑ BP
- S&S of fluid overload, hyponatremia

RELATED TOPICS

- Alterations in consciousness
- Cerebral aneurysm
- Herniation syndromes
- Hypertensive crisis
- Hyponatremia
- Immobility, prolonged
- Increased intracranial pressure
- Intracranial surgery
- Mechanical ventilation
- Stroke: hemorrhagic
- Syndrome of inappropriate antidiuretic hormone
- Vasodilator therapy

ABBREVIATIONS

CPP: Cerebral perfusion pressure
PRBCs: Packed red blood cells
SAS: Subarachnoid space
SIADH: Syndrome of inappropriate antidiuretic hormone
SNS: Sympathetic nervous system

- Administer antihypertensives to prevent hypertension, but maintain CPP >60 mm Hg.
- If ↑ in ICP occurs suddenly, hyperinflate with a manual resuscitator at ≥50 breaths/min to ↓ $Paco_2$.
- If cerebral vasospasm occurs, administer prescribed medications (eg, mannitol, nitroprusside sodium, nimodipine) and IV fluids.
- If using hypervolemic-hemodilution therapy, observe for fluid overload: imbalanced I&O, crackles, respiratory distress, ↓ Hct, hyponatremia, JVD, peripheral edema, and ↑ CVP, RAP, and PAP.

Pain r/t headache, photophobia, and fever secondary to meningeal irritation

Desired outcome: Within 2 h of initiation of therapy, patient's subjective evaluation of discomfort improves as documented by pain scale.

- Devise pain scale with patient, rating discomfort from 0 (no pain) to 10.
- Monitor temp q2h and prn. Administer tepid baths or cooling blanket and antipyretics/antibiotics as needed.
- Avoid overstimulation, which may ↑ BP and aggravate patient's headache.
- Cluster patient care so that it is administered within a pattern that enables uninterrupted periods (at least 90 min) of rest.
- Organize visiting hours to ensure uninterrupted periods of rest.
- Darken room to minimize discomfort of photophobia. Provide blindfolds if darkening room not possible.
- Administer analgesics. Use pain scale to document degree of relief obtained.

REFERENCES

Bell TE et al: Transcranial Doppler: correlation of blood velocity measurement with clinical status in subarachnoid hemorrhage, *J Neurosci Nurs* 24(4): 215-219, 1992.

Mitchell PH: Neurological disorders. In Kinney M, Packa D, Dunbar S: *AACN's clinical reference for critical care nursing*, ed 3, St Louis, 1993, Mosby.

Sengupta R: The surgical management of the patient with subarachnoid haemorrhage, *Care Crit III* 10(5): 231-235, 1994.

Stowe AC: Cerebral aneurysm and subarachnoid hemorrhage. In Swearingen PL, Keen JH (eds): *Manual of critical care nursing*, ed 3, St Louis, 1995, Mosby.

Author: **Ann Coghlan Stowe**

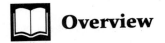 **Overview**

PATHOPHYSIOLOGY

Occurs when sustained HR >160 bpm or atrial rate >160 bpm without 1:1 conduction to ventricle. Several dysrhythmias included: A-tach, junctional tachycardia, A-flutter, A-fib.

INCIDENCE

Most common category of dysrhythmia in US.

HISTORY/RISK FACTORS

- CAD, electrolyte imbalance, hypovolemia, hypoxemia
- Hyperthyroidism, reentrant tachycardia or accessory conduction pathway, mitral valve prolapse
- Use of cocaine, other stimulant
- Cigarette smoking
- Suctioning of ET tube
- High-stress environment
- Heavy exercise
- Use of quinidine or digoxin; antidysrhythmic drug toxicity
- Malnutrition, anorexia, bulimia

CLINICAL PRESENTATION

Chest pain, SOB, dizziness, fainting, diaphoresis, nausea. May fatigue easily, feel heart "pounding" in chest, and appear distressed and pale.

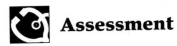 **Assessment**

PHYSICAL ASSESSMENT

Neuro: Altered LOC, syncope, weakness, fainting, vertigo, anxiety, restlessness
Resp: Dyspnea, SOB
CV: Chest pain, ST-segment depression on ECG, activity intolerance, hypotension

GI: Nausea, vomiting, heartburn-like pain
GU: ↓ UO
Integ: Diaphoresis, pallor, cyanosis

VITAL SIGNS/HEMODYNAMICS

RR: Nl or ↑
HR: ↑
BP: Nl, ↑, or ↓
Temp: Nl or ↑
CVP/PAWP: Nl, ↑, or ↓
CO: Nl or ↓
SVR: ↑
12/18-Lead ECG: Reflects change generated from more rapidly pacing site or multiple sites with atrial fibrillation.
A-tach: Regular rhythm; atrial rate 160-240 bpm; ventricular rate depends on AV conduction ratio. P waves difficult to identify because of rapid HR. QRS nl or widened if aberrant conduction or bundle branch block present.
Junctional tachycardia: Regular rhythm; pacemaker at AV node. Atrial rate cannot be determined because of P waves, which are hidden, inverted, out of sequence, or absent. Ventricular rate 100-250 bpm; QRS usually nl but may be widened if bundle branch block or accessory pathway present. PR interval cannot be determined.
A-flutter: Rhythm regular or irregular depending on AV conduction pattern. Atrial rate 240-350 bpm; ventricular rate depends on AV conduction. P waves saw-toothed or as "F" (flutter) waves. QRS nl or widened if aberrancy present. PR interval not measurable.
A-fib: Rhythm irregularly irregular. Atrial rate >350 bpm; ventricular rate variable and depends on chaotic AV conduction pattern. P waves appear as "f" (fibrillatory) waves. QRS nl, or wide if aberrancy or bundle branch block present. PR interval and P:QRS cannot be determined.

LABORATORY STUDIES

Serum Electrolytes: To identify values that may precipitate dysrhythmias. ↓ K^+ and Mg^{2+} may trigger SVT.

Therapeutic Antidysrhythmic Levels: Data necessary for rhythm control and drug toxicity prevention. Drugs used for hypertension, respiratory diseases, and other body system disorders may precipitate SVT.
Drug/Toxicology Screening: Identifies potential cause of SVT, eg, cocaine or amphetamine use.
ABGs: May reveal hypoxemia or pH abnormality that can interfere with electrolyte balance and cause dysrhythmias.

IMAGING

Chest X-ray: May reflect enlarged cardiac silhouette, indicative of heart disease.
Echocardiography: For noninvasive assessment of cardiac output, using ultrasound to evaluate ventricular pumping action. Includes estimation of ventricular EF.
Cardiac Catheterization: Assesses for CAD.

DIAGNOSTIC PROCEDURES

EP Study: Heart given pacing stimulus at various sites and varying voltages to determine point of origin for dysrhythmia, inducibility, effectiveness of drug therapy in dysrhythmia suppression.
Ambulatory/24-h Holter/Cardiac Event Monitoring: Identifies subtle or recurring dysrhythmias during which patient keeps ongoing written record of other symptoms.
Exercise Stress Testing: Used alone or in conjunction with 24-h Holter monitoring to detect various dysrhythmias and guide therapy. Test continues until patient reaches target HR or becomes symptomatic (eg, chest pain, dysrhythmias, abnormal BP, severe fatigue,) or has significant ECG changes from exercise stress.
Atrial Electrograms: Temporary epicardial pacing wires or special skin electrodes to record atria's electrical activity, including pacing and conduction.

Collaborative Management

GENERAL

Supplemental O$_2$: Promotes O$_2$ delivery to the tissues.

Continuous ECG Monitoring: Detects all dysrhythmias, onset and duration, and termination for intermittent dysrhythmias.

Management of Other Causes of Tachydysrhythmias: Eg, hypoxia, hypokalemia, hypomagnesemia, preexisting acidosis, hyperthermia, endocrine disorders (hyperthyroidism), drug overdose/toxicity.

Synchronized Cardioversion: For SVT that causes instability or severe symptoms of hypotension, chest pain, and generalized hypoxemia.

Cardiac Pacing: Rapid atrial or antitachycardia pacing initiated *via* transvenous wire or epicardial pacing wires (postcardiac surgery) to correct all types of SVT. Using pacemaker, operator exceeds patient's HR until capture attained, then slowly turns down HR. When successful, SVT pacing sites fail to override pacemaker, resulting in ↓ HR.

Spo$_2$: Detects ↓ O$_2$ saturation resulting from potentially lethal dysrhythmias.

Diet: Low-fat, low-cholesterol, ↓-caffeine diet for recurrent dysrhythmias.

CPR: Necessary for all pulseless rhythms that can result from deteriorating SVT, including PEA, VF, pulseless VT, and asystole.

PHARMACOTHERAPY

Lowest possible dose of antidysrhythmic that successfully terminates abnormal heart rhythm while avoiding drug toxicity, which can lead to lethal dysrhythmias. Goal of SVT management: ↓ HR sufficiently to allow ↑ time for ventricular filling to enable ↑ cardiac output.

β Blockers

Atenolol (Tenormin): 5 mg IV push at ≤1 mg/min. Wait 10 min. Repeat dose if needed.

Metoprolol (Lopressor): Initial dose 5 mg. Repeat 5 mg dose q2min for total of 15 mg.

Propranolol (Inderal): 1 mg IV push very slowly over 1 min, then assess response. May repeat up to total of 3 mg.

Calcium Blockers

Verapamil (Calan): 5 mg IV push very slowly over 2-3 min. Does not suppress accessory pathway conduction.

Diltiazem (Cardizem): 20 mg IV slow push over 2 min. May administer second dose of 25 mg in 15 min if ineffective. May administer additional doses (0.35 mg/kg) to control SVT. Follow with continuous IV infusion 5-15 mg/h for at least 24 h.

Other

Adenosine: For emergency management. Depresses AV node activity. Given 6 mg rapid IV push, followed immediately by 3-5 ml flush solution. May double dose to 12 mg and repeat × 2 if ineffective.

Digoxin: Slows conduction through AV node. Used in nonemergency management of A-fib with rapid ventricular response. *Loading dose:* total of 10 μg/kg divided into 4 doses over 24 h.

Procainamide: Class IA antidysrhythmic for VT and SVT. Give at 20-30 mg/min until one of the following occurs: dysrhythmia suppressed, BP ↓, QRS widens >50%, or total of 17 mg/kg given. *Maintenance infusion:* 1-4 mg/min.

SURGERY/THERAPEUTIC PROCEDURES

Implantable Cardioverter/Defibrillator: Instrument programmed to deliver synchronized cardioversion/defibrillation when the HR > programmed rate or manifests programmed abnormal ECG morphology. Newer devices also act as cardiac pacemakers.

Radiofrequency Catheter Ablation: Electrically generated heat stimulus applied to dysrhythmia's point of origin as determined by EP studies. Heat "burns" heart in a small, localized area, resulting in necrosis of abnormal tissue causing dysrhythmia.

Myocardial Revascularization: Done alone or in conjunction with EP mapping, with excision/cryoablation of dysrhythmia focus.

PATIENT-FAMILY TEACHING

- Importance of promptly reporting adverse symptoms
- Self-measuring of pulse rate/rhythm
- Causes of dysrhythmia; electrical devices used to treat it
- At-home dietary guidelines, especially regarding ↓ caffeine
- Importance of smoking cessation
- Relaxation techniques that help control environmental stress
- Altered sexuality if ICD in place
- Medications: purpose, dosage, schedule, precautions, drug-drug and food-drug interactions, and potential side effects
- Support groups

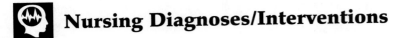

Nursing Diagnoses/Interventions

Decreased cardiac output r/t altered rate, rhythm, conduction; r/t negative inotropic cardiac changes secondary to cardiac disease

Desired outcome: Within 15 min of dysrhythmia onset, cardiac output adequate: BP $\geq$90/60 mm Hg, HR 60-100 bpm with NSR on ECG, PAP 20-30/8-15 mm Hg, PAWP 6-12 mm Hg, CVP 2-6 mm Hg, CO 4-7 L/min, CI 2.5-4.0 L/min/m^2, or all within 10% of baseline.

- Monitor continuous ECG, noting onset, duration, pattern, termination of dysrhythmias, and response to therapy.
- Monitor VS for baseline status and prn for changes in cardiac rhythm, including PAP, PAWP, and CVP if PA catheter in place.
- Document dysrhythmias *via* rhythm strips. Use 12/18-lead ECG to diagnose new, symptomatic dysrhythmias.

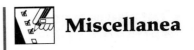

Miscellanea

CONSULT MD FOR
- Failure of dysrhythmia to respond to prescribed treatments
- Inappropriate "firing" of ICD device
- Failure to attain or exceeding of therapeutic antidysrhythmic drug level
- Worsening symptoms: chest pain; SOB; $\downarrow$ BP; altered mental status; Spo$_2$ <90%; $\uparrow$ PAP, PAWP, or CVP
- Possible complications: heart failure, cardiac arrest, hypoxemia, new or worsening dysrhythmias, antidysrhythmic drug toxicity

RELATED TOPICS
- Antidysrhythmic therapy
- Atrial fibrillation
- Coronary artery disease
- Drug overdose: amphetamines, cocaine, cyclic antidepressants, phencyclidines
- Heart failure, left ventricular
- Hypokalemia
- Hypomagnesemia

ABBREVIATIONS
EF: Ejection fraction
EP: Electrophysiologic
ICD: Implantable cardioverter/defibrillator
PEA: Pulseless electrical activity

- Note changes in Spo_2 with symptomatic dysrhythmias.
- Provide supplemental O_2 for symptomatic dysrhythmias.
- Monitor laboratory data to assess cause of dysrhythmias.
- Initiate ACLS algorithms or institutional protocols for emergency.
- ↓ as many environmental stressors as possible.
- Remain with patient if new dysrhythmias or deterioration occurs; treat as prescribed and monitor response.
- Administer medications that support cardiac output and BP if antidysrhythmics and cardioversion are ineffective.

REFERENCES

American Heart Association: *Textbook of advanced cardiac life support,* Dallas, 1994, The Association.

Dracup K: *Meltzer's intensive coronary care: a manual for nurses,* ed 5, Norwalk, Conn, 1995, Appleton & Lange.

Dziadulewicz L: The use of atrial electrograms in the diagnosis of supraventricular dysrhythmias: *AACN Clin Issues in Crit Care Nurs* 3(1): 203-208, 1992.

Futterman LG, Lemberg L: Radiofrequency catheter ablation for supraventricular tachycardias, *Am J Crit Care* 2(6): 500-505, 1993.

Goodrich CA: Management of tachyarrhythmias in the CCU: *Curr Issues Crit Care Nurs (Suppl):* 7-11, November 1995.

Jacobsen C: Arrhythmias and conduction disturbances. In Woods SL: *Cardiac nursing,* ed 3, Philadelphia, 1995, Lippincott.

Keen J, Baird M, Allen J: *Mosby's critical care and emergency drug reference,* ed 2, St Louis, 1996, Mosby.

Porterfield LM: The cutting edge in arrhythmias, *Crit Care Nurse (Suppl),* 1993.

Steuble BT: Dysrhythmias and conduction disturbances. In Swearingen PL, Keen JH (eds): *Manual of critical care nursing,* ed 3, St Louis, 1995, Mosby.

Authors: **Marianne Saunorus Baird and Barbara Tueller Steuble**

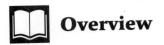 **Overview**

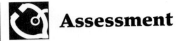 **Assessment**

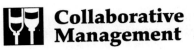 **Collaborative Management**

PATHOPHYSIOLOGY

Excessive release of ADH from the pituitary gland or ectopic ADH secretion from malignant tumors causing severe water retention that expands body fluid volume and dilutes serum Na^+, thereby ↓ serum osmolality. Glomerular filtration ↑ in response to fluid volume expansion, causing Na^+ loss in the urine. The ↓ serum osmolality causes water to move into the cells. The resultant water intoxication, cerebral edema, and profound hyponatremia may be life-threatening.

HISTORY/RISK FACTORS

- Cancer of the lung, pancreas, duodenum, prostate: can secrete a biologically active form of ADH
- Head trauma, brain tumor, hemorrhage, infection
- Positive pressure ventilation, physiologic stress, chronic metabolic illness, pulmonary disease
- Medications: chlorpropamide, IV cyclophosphamide, oxytocin, vasopressin

CLINICAL PRESENTATION

- Hyponatremia and hypoosmolality
- Inappropriately concentrated urine; inappropriate urine Na^+ level
- Neurologic symptoms caused by water movement into brain cells
- Weight gain without edema

PHYSICAL ASSESSMENT

Neuro: Fatigue, headache, ↓ LOC, confusion, seizures
CV: Nl or slightly ↑ BP
GI: Nausea, vomiting
GU: Nl to ↓ UO, urine specific gravity >1.020

VITAL SIGNS/HEMODYNAMICS

RR: Nl or slight ↑
HR: Nl or slight ↑
BP: Nl or slight ↑
Temp: Nl
CVP/PAWP: Nl or slight ↑

LABORATORY STUDIES

Serum Sodium Level: ↓ to <137 mEq/L.
Plasma Osmolality: ↓ to <275 mOsm/kg.
Urine Osmolality: ↑ disproportionately to plasma osmolality.
Urine Sodium Level: ↑ to >40 mEq/L.
Urine Specific Gravity: >1.030.
Plasma ADH Level: Elevated in conditions associated with ↑ production.

Fluid Restriction: Usually fluids limited to 1000 ml/day. Once serum Na^+ wnl, fluids may be ↑ to UO + insensible losses.
Isotonic (0.9%) or Hypertonic (3%) NaCl: For severe hyponatremia. May be given with IV furosemide (Lasix) or osmotic diuretics, such as mannitol, to promote water excretion.
Lithium or Demeclocycline (Declomycin): Inhibits action of ADH on distal renal tubules to promote water excretion.
Treatment of Underlying Cause: SIADH associated with surgery, trauma, or drugs usually temporary and self-limiting. If chronic, focus is on treating underlying cause, including surgery, radiation, or chemotherapy for cancer.

PATIENT-FAMILY TEACHING

- Reassurance that altered sensorium is temporary and will improve with treatment
- Necessity of water restriction

Nursing Diagnoses/Interventions

Altered protection r/t hyponatremia (serum sodium <120-125 mEq/L), induced alteration in neurologic function, or too rapid correction of hyponatremia

Desired outcomes: Within 24 h of treatment initiation, patient verbalizes orientation × 3. CVP, PAWP, BP wnl for patient. Serum Na$^+$ level ↑ to >125 mEq/L during first 48 h after treatment. Patient remains free of signs of physical injury caused by altered sensorium.

- Assess LOC, VS, hemodynamic measurements, and I&O qh; measure weight qd. Be alert to ↓ LOC; ↑ BP, CVP, PAWP; UO <0.5 mg/kg/h; and weight gain.
- Monitor electrolytes and other laboratory results. Be alert to ↓ serum Na$^+$ and plasma osmolality, ↑ urine osmolality, and ↑ urine Na$^+$.
- On average, Na$^+$ levels should not ↑ at a level >0.5 mEq/L/h because of risk of neurologic damage. Overall ↑ during first 24-48 h of treatment more important than hourly rate of ↑.
- Maintain fluid restriction. Do not keep water or ice chips at bedside. Ensure precise delivery of IV fluids by using a monitoring device.
- Elevate HOB 10-20 degrees to promote venous return and thus reduce ADH release. ↓ venous return is a stimulus to the release of ADH.
- Administer demeclocycline, lithium, and furosemide; carefully observe and document response.
- Administer hypertonic NaCl cautiously. Rate of administration usually is based on serial serum Na$^+$ levels. To minimize risk of hypernatremia, ensure that specimens for laboratory tests are drawn on time. Assess for intravascular fluid volume excess: ↑ BP, CVP, PAWP.
- Provide bedside care in a calm, unhurried manner to help minimize stress and pain, both of which ↑ ADH release.
- Keep side rails up and bed in lowest position with wheels locked.
- Use reality therapy, such as clocks, calendars, and familiar objects; keep these items at bedside within patient's visual field.
- If seizures anticipated, implement precautions and keep an appropriate size airway at bedside.
- Avoid giving hypotonic fluids, eg, medications in D$_5$W, tap water enemas.

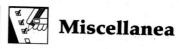 # Miscellanea

CONSULT MD FOR

- New onset S&S of water intoxication: ↓ LOC, ↑ BP, CVP >6 mm Hg, PAWP >12 mm Hg, weight gain, serum Na$^+$ <137 mEq/L, and plasma osmolality <275 mOsm/kg.
- S&S of intravascular fluid volume excess r/t treatment with isotonic, hypertonic NaCl: ↑ BP, CVP, PAWP.

RELATED TOPICS

- Head injury
- Hemodynamic monitoring
- Hyponatremia
- Increased intracranial pressure
- Mechanical ventilation

ABBREVIATION

ADH: Antidiuretic hormone

REFERENCES

Batcheller J: Syndrome of inappropriate antidiuretic hormone secretion, *Crit Care Nurs Clin North Am* 6(4): 687-692, 1994.

Horne MM: Endocrinologic dysfunctions. In Swearingen PL, Keen JH (eds): *Manual of critical care nursing,* ed 3, St Louis, 1995, Mosby.

Rose BD: *Clinical physiology of acid-base and electrolyte disorders,* ed 4, New York, 1994, McGraw-Hill.

Shuey KM: Heart, lung, and endocrine complications of solid tumors, *Semin Oncol Nurs* 10(3): 177-188, 1994.

Author: **Mima M. Horne**

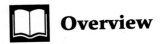 **Overview**

PATHOPHYSIOLOGY

Widespread nonspecific immune reaction. Insults from mechanical, ischemic, chemical, or microbial sources trigger immediate inflammatory and immune processes whose purpose is to protect the body and promote rapid healing. Vasodilatation, ↑ microvascular permeability, cellular activation and adhesion, and enhanced coagulation occur. In some instances regulatory mechanisms fail and uncontrolled systemic inflammation occurs. This leads to systemic vasodilatation, hypotension, generalized ↑ in vascular permeability, extravascular fluid sequestration, ↑ cellular aggregation with microvascular obstruction, and greatly accelerated coagulation. If allowed to progress, SIRS ultimately leads to MODS.

HISTORY/RISK FACTORS

- Burns, hemorrhage, infection, ischemia/reperfusion injury
- Pancreatitis, shock state, multisystem injury

CLINICAL PRESENTATION

Restlessness, confusion, ↓ LOC, fever, SOB, tachypnea, ↓ UO, hyperglycemia (early), hypoglycemia (late)

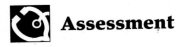 **Assessment**

PHYSICAL ASSESSMENT

Diagnosis based on the following laboratory and clinical findings: tachypnea (RR >20 breaths/min), hypocarbia (<32 torr), tachycardia (HR >90 bpm), temp >38° C or <36° C, WBCs >12,000 or <4000 μl, or >10% immature (band) forms (ACCP/SCCM, 1992). Clinical picture is one of a hyperdynamic circulatory state similar to sepsis, but without an identifiable source of infection.

Neuro: ↓ cerebral blood flow with CNS depression, stupor, coma

Resp: Hyperventilation to compensate for metabolic acidosis (early); later, crackles and respiratory depression/acidosis caused by CNS depression, ↑ lung water

GI: Hepatocellular dysfunction with resultant ↓ lactate clearance, metabolic acidosis

GU: ↓ renal perfusion, oliguria, anuria

VITAL SIGNS/HEMODYNAMICS

RR: ↑ >20 breaths/min

HR: ↑ >90 bpm

BP: ↓

Temp: ↑ >38° C or <36° C; fever (early), thermoregulatory failure and hypothermia (late)

CVP: ↓ initially caused by relative fluid deficit; later ↑ if heart failure present

PAP: ↓ initially; later ↑ caused by pulmonary vasoconstriction occurring with hypoxemia, pulmonary edema

PAWP: ↓ initially caused by relative fluid deficit; later ↑ if heart failure present

SVR: ↓ because of mediator-induced vasodilatation

CO/CI: Early ↑ as a result of ↓ SVR, SNS stimulation, which ↑ venous return, HR; later ↓ if heart failure present

CPP: ↓ as direct effect of chemical mediators and ↓ cerebral blood flow

LABORATORY STUDIES

CBC: WBCs usually ↑ early, with ↑ bands (left shift). Later, WBCs ↓ as a result of sequestration within organs and bone marrow exhaustion. Anemia, if present, contributes to hyperdynamic state and impaired tissue oxygenation.

Chemistries: Early ↑ in glucose results from gluconeogenesis; later ↓ results from hepatic failure. Venous lactate levels ↑ if tissue perfusion inadequate. Hepatic, renal, other organ failure reflected in electrolyte, enzyme abnormalities.

C&S: Blood, sputum, urine, surgical or other site; obtained if infection suspected.

ABGs: May show pH <7.35 and HCO₃⁻ <22 mm Hg because of metabolic acidosis. Also will reflect ventilatory status.

IMAGING

X-rays: Chest x-ray to check for pulmonary edema. Other x-rays as indicated according to underlying condition.

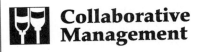 **Collaborative Management**

Oxygenation: Humidified O_2 for all patients; mechanical ventilation may be necessary if pulmonary edema, other ventilatory impairment present.

Fluids: Crystalloids, colloids administered to sustain adequate intravascular volume; hyperdynamic state supported until patient stabilized.

Hemodynamic/Flow Monitoring: To maximize Do_2, Vo_2, and CI. Goal: to maintain supradynamic values by adjusting fluids, inotropes, and vasopressors and ensuring adequacy of O_2-carrying capacity *via* optimal Hct and O_2 administration.

Urinary Drainage: To monitor hourly UO.

Pharmacotherapy

Antibiotics: Broad-spectrum antibiotics if infection suspected.

Analgesia, sedation: To relieve pain and agitation, which ↑ O_2 consumption.

Vasopressors (eg, dopamine, norepinephrine): For refractory hypotension. See Appendix for "Inotropic and Vasoactive Agents."

Nutritional Support: Enteral nutrition optimal, but often not possible. Short- and medium-chain fatty acids (absorbed more readily and metabolized more easily than long-chain fatty acids) given parenterally. Branched-chain amino acids, metabolized by muscle rather than the liver, may be used if there is evidence of hepatic failure.

PATIENT-FAMILY TEACHING

Purpose, anticipated sensations, expected results of all medical/nursing interventions

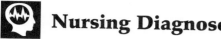

Nursing Diagnoses/Interventions

Fluid volume deficit r/t active loss from vascular compartment secondary to ↑ capillary permeability and shift of intravascular volume into interstitial spaces

Desired outcomes: Within 8 h of therapy initiation, patient normovolemic: peripheral pulses >2+ on 0-4+ scale, stable body weight, UO ≥0.5 ml/kg/h, SBP ≥90 mm Hg or wnl for patient, and absence of edema and adventitious lung sounds. PAWP 6-12 mm Hg, CO 4-7 L/min, and SVR 900-1200 dynes/sec/cm^{-5}.

- Assess fluid volume by monitoring BP, HR, and peripheral perfusion qh or more often if unstable. Continuous direct arterial pressure monitoring is optimal.
- During acute hypotension, position patient supine with legs elevated to optimize preload.
- Give crystalloids and colloids to maintain PAWP of 6-12 mm Hg or ≤18 mm Hg with LV failure. Assess PAWP and lung sounds frequently during fluid replacement to detect overload: crackles and ↑ PAWP. As indicated, administer PRBCs to ↑ O_2-carrying capacity of the blood.
- Monitor hemodynamic pressures and Svo_2 as available.
- In early stage, anticipate ↓ BP, PAWP and SVR; ↑ CO/CI. Give fluids, inotropes as necessary.
- In late stage, ↓ BP, ↑ PAWP, ↑ SVR, and ↓ CO/CI may occur. In general, use vasodilators if MAP >100 mm Hg or vasopressors if MAP <70 mm Hg. Fluids, inotropes, vasopressors, and vasodilators all may be necessary because of MODS and desensitization to endogenous catecholamines. Titrate carefully to optimize CI and maintain Svo_2 of 60%-80%.
- Weigh qd; monitor I&O every shift and UO qh, noting 24-h trends. Weight may ↑ despite actual fluid volume deficit as a result of shift of intravascular volume into interstitial spaces.
- Assess for interstitial edema as evidenced by pretibial, sacral, ankle, and hand edema, as well as lung crackles. Take measures to protect skin integrity.

Altered cerebral, renal, GI tissue perfusion r/t hypovolemia secondary to vasodilatation (early) or interrupted arterial/venous blood flow secondary to microcirculatory sludging (late)

Desired outcomes: Within 24 h of initiating therapy, patient has adequate perfusion: orientation × 3, peripheral pulses >2+ on 0-4+ scale, brisk capillary refill (<2 sec), UO ≥0.5 ml/kg/h, and ≥5 bowel sounds/min. BP 110-120/70-80 mm Hg (or wnl for patient), Svo_2 60%-80%, SVR 900-1200 dynes/sec/cm^{-5}, CO 4-7 L/min, and CI 2.5-4 L/min/m^2.

- Assess for ↓ cerebral perfusion: ↓ LOC, restlessness.
- Assess for ↓ renal perfusion: UO <0.5 ml/kg and ↑ BUN/creatinine and serum K^+ levels.
- Monitor BP continuously. ↓ SBP, nl or ↑ DBP, ↓ pulse pressures occur with ↓ perfusion.
- Assess for hypoperfusion: ↓ pulse amplitude, cool extremities, pallor or mottling, and delayed capillary refill.
- Monitor cellular O_2 consumption (Svo_2) as an indicator of tissue perfusion. With sepsis, cellular O_2 delivery ↓ as a result of precapillary vasoconstriction and thus cellular O_2 use ↓. This may result in abnormally high Svo_2.
- Treat underlying infection with appropriate antimicrobial therapy, being certain to administer precisely as scheduled to optimize bloodstream levels.
- Administer fluids, inotropes, and/or vasodilators or vasopressors to optimize SVR and CO/CI. Be aware that ↑ filling pressures may be necessary for optimal CO.
- Assess for ↓ splanchnic (visceral) circulation, including ↓/absent bowel sounds, ↑ amylase, ↑ liver enzymes, and ↓ platelet count.

Impaired gas exchange r/t alveolar-capillary membrane changes secondary to interstitial edema, alveolar destruction, and endotoxin release with activation of histamine and kinins

Desired outcome: Within 4 h of therapy initiation, patient's Pao_2 ≥80 mm Hg; $Paco_2$ ≤45 mm Hg; pH 7.35-7.45; and lungs clear.

- Administer supplemental O_2 to maximize O_2 available to tissues.
- If patient exhibits inadequate gas exchange (eg, Pao_2 <60 mm Hg on 100% oxygen *via* nonrebreathing mask), prepare for probability of ET intubation.
- Assess for/maintain patent airway by assisting with coughing or suctioning as necessary.
- Assess ABGs. Be alert to ↓ Pao_2, ↑ $Paco_2$, acidosis. Monitor for dyspnea, SOB, crackles, restlessness. Adjust supplemental O_2, ventilator settings as indicated.
- Closely monitor PAWP; keep as low as possible to avoid contributing to excess lung water. Be aware that a narrow range of optimal PAWP exists because of complex pathophysiology, including intravascular fluid volume deficit, ↑ capillary permeability, and possible LV failure.
- If patient is on mechanical ventilation, monitor for evidence of ARDS: ↑ peak inspiratory pressures (eg, ↓ lung compliance), Fio_2 >0.50, ↑ PEEP necessary to maintain adequate Pao_2, and diffuse bilateral pulmonary infiltrates ("white out") on chest x-ray.
- Turn q2h to maintain optimal V/Q ratios and prevent atelectasis.

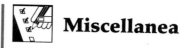

Miscellanea

CONSULT MD FOR
- S&S of inadequate tissue perfusion: altered mental status, restlessness; ↓ BP, peripheral pulses; UO <0.5 ml/kg/h × 2 h; Svo_2 <60% or >80%; ↓/absent bowel sounds
- S&S of complications: DIC, MODS, septic shock

RELATED TOPICS
- Disseminated intravascular coagulation
- Hemodynamic monitoring
- Mechanical ventilation
- Multiple organ dysfunction syndrome
- Shock, septic
- Vasopressor therapy

ABBREVIATIONS
Do_2: Oxygen delivery
FSPs: Fibrin split products
MODS: Multiple organ dysfunction syndrome
PRBCs: Packed red blood cells
SNS: Sympathetic nervous system
Svo_2: Mixed venous oxygen saturation
Vo_2: Oxygen consumption

REFERENCES
Ackerman M: The systemic inflammatory response, sepsis, and multiple organ dysfunction, *Crit Care Nurs Clin North Am* 6(2): 243-250, 1994.

American College of Chest Physicians/Society of Critical Care Medicine Consensus Conference Committee: Definitions for sepsis and organ failure and guidelines for the use of innovative therapies in sepsis, *Crit Care Med* 20(6): 864-874, 1992.

Hazinski MF: Mediator-specific therapies for the systemic inflammatory response syndrome, sepsis, severe sepsis, and septic shock, *Crit Care Nurs Clin North Am* 6(2): 309-319, 1994.

Lehmann S: Nutritional support in the hypermetabolic patient, *Crit Care Nurs Clin North Am* 5(1): 97-103, 1993.

Secor VH: The inflammatory/immune response in critical illness, *Crit Care Nurs Clin North Am* 6(2): 251-264, 1994.

Author: **Janet Hicks Keen**

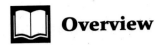 **Overview**

PATHOPHYSIOLOGY

Acute or chronic blood clotting disorder in which platelet aggregation causes ↓ overall platelet count as platelets "clump" together, forming microthrombi. Cause not believed to be mediated by inflammatory response. Both hemolysis and bleeding may result.

INCIDENCE

Occurs in 1 out of every 50,000 hospital admissions; more frequently in women than in men (3:2), most often in fourth decade of life.

HISTORY/RISK FACTORS

No known precipitating cause, but has been seen in conjunction with the following:
- Infections
- Collagen disorders
- Cancer
- Drug allergy
- Pregnancy
- AIDS
- Stress
- Polluted or "toxic" environment

CLINICAL PRESENTATION

Acute: Widespread clotting manifested by MODS, renal failure, GI infarction, heart block, MI, overt bleeding
Chronic: Remission/relapse pattern, in which patient is fatigued, activity intolerant, and has altered mental status and abdominal discomfort

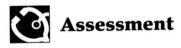 **Assessment**

PHYSICAL ASSESSMENT

Neuro: Confusion, loss of sensation in certain areas, headache, seizures, weakness, ↓ LOC
Resp: Dyspnea, SOB
ENT: Epistaxis, bleeding gums
CV: Chest discomfort, activity intolerance, ↓/absent peripheral pulses, heart failure, dysrhythmias
GI: Abdominal pain, nausea, vomiting, abdominal distention, GI bleeding
GU: Oliguria, anuria, hematuria
Integ: Pallor, cyanosis, skin necrosis, purpura

VITAL SIGNS/HEMODYNAMICS

RR: Nl or ↑
HR: ↑
BP: Nl or ↓

Temp: Nl or ↑
CVP/PAWP: Nl, ↑, or ↓
SVR: ↑
CO: Nl or ↓
12/18-Lead ECG: May reveal changes r/t myocardial ischemia (ST-segment depression), myocardial injury (ST-segment elevation), MI (Q wave). Tachycardia may ensue to promote oxygenation. PVCs, PACs, ventricular or atrial dysrhythmias signal myocardial hypoperfusion/hypoxemia.

LABORATORY STUDIES

Platelets: Severely ↓ (<50,000 μl) because of platelet aggregation.
LDH/Total Bilirubin: ↑ because of hemolysis.
Haptoglobin: ↓ (<5 mg/dl) because of reticuloendothelial system's removal of hemoglobin-haptoglobin complexes from the blood following hemolysis.
Coombs' Test: Negative; test r/o antigen-antibody reactions that may cause hemolytic anemia.
Blood Smear: Fragmented RBCs ("helmet cells") present.
Clotting Factors: ↑ FDPs/FSPs; PT and PTT nl.
Hgb/Hct/RBCs: ↓ because of hemolytic anemia.

IMAGING

Chest X-ray: May reveal enlarged cardiac silhouette of heart disease (more common with chronic TTP).
Arteriograms: To assess perfusion of various organs/systems.
Liver/Spleen Scans: May reveal disease or dysfunction of either organ, which could contribute to anemia.
CT Brain Scan: May reveal cerebral edema, thrombosis-related infarction, or hemorrhage.

DIAGNOSTIC PROCEDURE

Bone Marrow Aspiration: To confirm diagnosis of TTP. Reveals overproduction of precursors of RBCs, platelets, and WBCs.

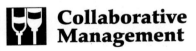 **Collaborative Management**

Treatments include a combination of therapies because of inability to identify cause of TTP.
Supplemental O₂: To support tissue oxygenation.
Plasma Exchange: 2-4 L exchanged over 5-10 days. Albumin, NS, or LR may be included in the exchange.
Transfusions/Blood Component Replacement: PRBCs necessary in management of anemia to ↑ O₂-carrying capacity of blood. Platelet transfusions ineffective as aggregation ensues, consuming new platelets and promoting vessel "clogging."
Volume Replacement: For hypovolemia and to prevent hypotension and shock. Also helps prevent deposition of hemolyzed RBCs and aggregated platelets in the microcirculation.
Spo₂: Detects ↓ O₂ saturation resulting from dysrhythmias.
Pharmacotherapy
Antiplatelet agents: Aspirin and dipyridamole most commonly used to inhibit aggregation and improve platelet survival time. Given in combination with plasma infusion.
Corticosteroids: Considered "mainstay" of TTP therapy; used in combination with other agents. ↑ survival rate noted when dextran and steroids combined. Only 10% of TTP patients respond to steroids alone.
Immunosuppressive agents: May be used to control vasculitis associated with TTP. Vincristine combined with plasma exchange has promoted long-lasting remission or possible cure in some patients.
γ Globulin: Neutralizes nl γ globulin and platelet aggregating factor in TTP. Use is controversial, since sepsis may result.
Splenectomy: Induces long-lasting remission in some patients as a single intervention. When combined with steroids, has yielded a 50% response rate. Also used with other pharmacologic therapies successfully.

PATIENT-FAMILY TEACHING

- S&S of bleeding, clotting, vessel occlusion, and shock
- Importance of avoiding trauma, including shaving with regular razors, using hard-bristled toothbrushes, participating in dangerous work/recreational activities
- Need to avoid vasoconstrictive agents, eg, caffeine, tobacco
- Medications: drug name, purpose, dosage, schedule, precautions, food-drug and drug-drug interactions, and potential side effects
- Purpose, expected results, anticipated sensations for all nursing/medical interventions
- Need for Medic-Alert bracelet; necessity of pneumococcal vaccination if splenectomy performed
- Local support groups

Nursing Diagnoses/Interventions

Altered protection r/t ↓ platelet count resulting in ↑ risk of bleeding and platelet aggregation with potential for clotting/blood vessel closure

Desired outcomes: Within 72 h of treatment onset, patient exhibits no clinical signs of new bleeding, bruising, or clotting/vessel occlusion. Secretions and excretions are negative for blood and VS are within 10% of nl for patient.

- Monitor for signs of bleeding: ↑ HR, ↑ RR, oozing from invasive sites, bleeding mucous membranes, hematuria, and GI bleeding.
- Monitor for signs of vessel occlusion that can lead to organ failure: ↓ peripheral pulses, ↓ UO, respiratory distress, chest pain, abdominal pain/distention, third spacing of body fluids.
- Avoid IM injections and all unnecessary venous and arterial punctures to minimize oozing from invasive sites.
- Monitor platelet counts, Hgb, and Hct qd for significant changes.
- Perform oral care using sponge-tipped applicator. Shave patient with electric razor and position carefully to avoid trauma.
- Assess for neurologic changes signaling stroke: altered mental status, sluggish or unequal pupils, seizures, weakness, paralysis, or changes in HR or RR.

Impaired gas exchange (or risk for same) r/t active loss of O_2-carrying RBCs secondary to bleeding, possible hemolysis, and vessel occlusion occurring with platelet aggregation

Desired outcome: Gas exchange remains adequate: HR 60-100 bpm, RR 12-20 breaths/min with eupnea, SBP >90 mm Hg, UO ≥0.5 ml/kg/h, PAP 20-30/8-15 mm Hg, PAWP 6-12 mm Hg, peripheral pulses ≥2+, NSR on ECG.

- Monitor ECG continuously for dysrhythmias, including ST-segment changes indicative of MI.
- Monitor SpO_2 continuously to assess O_2 delivery.
- Monitor hemodynamic parameters if available.
- Check quality of peripheral pulses at least qh.
- Administer supplemental O_2.
- Monitor I&O at least q2h.
- Note frequency and character of stools.
- Replace lost volume with plasma expanders or PRBCs as prescribed.
- Avoid platelet transfusions. Clotting/occlusion may accelerate as a result.
- Auscultate breath sounds qh for ↓ or adventitious sounds.
- Consider SvO_2 monitoring for complex hemodynamic therapy.

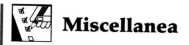 # Miscellanea

CONSULT MD FOR

- Platelet count <75,000 μl, uncontrolled bleeding
- Oliguria, anuria, hematuria
- Seizures; new onset weakness or paralysis
- Loss of peripheral pulses
- Progressive abdominal distention
- SvO_2 <60%, HR >140 bpm, RR >35 breaths/min, temp 38.8° C (102° F), chest pain
- Possible complications: renal failure, stroke, bowel infarction, GI bleeding, MODS, MI, liver failure, loss of limb/digits, pulmonary embolus

RELATED TOPICS

- Anemias
- HELLP syndrome
- Hemolytic crisis
- Idiopathic thrombocytopenic purpura
- Multiple organ dysfunction syndrome
- Myocardial infarction, acute
- Psychosocial needs, family/significant others
- Psychosocial needs, patient
- Pulmonary embolus, thrombotic
- Renal failure, acute
- Stroke: hemorrhagic and ischemic

ABBREVIATIONS

FDPs: Fibrin degradation products
FSPs: Fibrin split products
MODS: Multiple organ dysfunction syndrome
PRBCs: Packed red blood cells

REFERENCES

Baird M: Bleeding and thrombotic disorders. In Swearingen PL, Keen JH (eds): *Manual of critical care nursing,* ed 3, St Louis, Mosby, 1995.

Caswell DR: Thromboembolic phenomena, *Crit Care Nurs Clin North Am* 5(3): 489-497, 1993.

Kajs-Wyllie M: Thrombotic thrombocytopenic purpura: pathophysiology, treatment, and related nursing care, *Crit Care Nurse* 15(6): 44-52, 1995.

Kimbrell JD: Acquired coagulopathies, *Crit Care Nurs Clin North Am* 5(3): 453-458, 1993.

Secor VH: Mediators of coagulation and inflammation: relationship and clinical significance, *Crit Care Nurs Clin North Am* 5(3): 411-434, 1993.

Author: **Marianne Saunorus Baird**

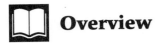 **Overview**

DESCRIPTION
The need for replacement of blood or blood products is r/t anemias, frank bleeding, covert bleeding, or any disorder that results in significantly ↓ Hct or Hgb.

HISTORY/RISK FACTORS
- Surgery, trauma
- DIC, bleeding/coagulation disorders, thrombocytopenia
- Chronic anemia, cancer, sickle cell disease, hemophilia

CLINICAL PRESENTATION
Variable, depending on underlying illness, extent of blood loss, ability to compensate for ↓ Hct and Hgb.
- Weakness, activity intolerance, fatigue, general malaise
- With failure of compensation: SOB, chest discomfort, hypotension, confusion, disorientation
- In extreme cases: total decompensation resulting in hemorrhagic shock leading to cardiac arrest

 Assessment

PHYSICAL ASSESSMENT
Varies with severity of anemia/blood loss
Neuro: Confusion, disorientation
Resp: SOB, dyspnea
CV: Chest pain, hypotension, tachycardia, dysrhythmias (PACs, PVCs, VT, SVT)
GI: ↓/absent bowel sounds, melena, hematemesis
GU: Oliguria, anuria, hematuria

VITAL SIGNS/HEMODYNAMICS
RR: ↑
HR: ↑
BP: ↑, ↓ with severe/acute blood loss, or nl
Temp: Nl or ↑
CVP/PAP: Nl; ↓ if acute blood loss occurs
CO: Nl; possible compensatory ↑ caused by ↑ HR, ↓ blood viscosity. ↓ if significant blood loss occurs.
SVR: Nl; slight ↓ caused by ↓ blood viscosity; ↑ if significant blood loss occurs.
ECG: Sinus tachycardia; possible ischemic changes if anemia severe.

LABORATORY STUDIES
Hct, Hgb: ↓; reflects bleeding or anemia.
CBC: Universally ↓ or elements of CBC ↓, depending on underlying disease.
Platelets: Possible ↓, depending on underlying disease.
Granulocytes: May be ↓ with oncologic disease.

IMAGING
Angiography: May be used to identify source of major bleeding.
CT Scan: May be used to identify areas of major bleeding or presence of tumors.

DIAGNOSTIC PROCEDURES
Bone Marrow Aspiration: To diagnose cause of persistent anemia or bleeding disorder.

Collaborative Management

Blood/Blood Products: Used to replace blood components necessary for oxygenation, hemostasis; for treatment of hypovolemic/hemorrhagic shock; or support of immune system.
Whole blood: 500 ml/U given over 2-4 h or more rapidly in life-threatening emergency.
PRBCs: 200-250 ml/U given for bleeding or anemia over 1-4 h or more rapidly in life-threatening emergency.
FFP: 200-250 ml/U thawed for 20 min then infused over ½-1 h or ½ h in emergencies; used for coagulopathy or to prevent clotting factor deficiency. Expands intravascular volume, but not used exclusively for this purpose because safer, less expensive products are available.
Platelets: 35-50 ml/U given direct IV push at 35-50 ml/min; may combine or pool several bags into one; given in multiple units to control bleeding caused by ↓ platelets.
Cryoprecipitate: 10-20 ml/U; may need 10-30 U infused at 1 U/min or 12-20 ml/min to control bleeding caused by coagulopathies.
Granulocytes: 300 ml/U infused over 1-2 h; administered slowly over first 5 min as a test dose. For immune system support when oncologic process has compromised granulocyte production.
Leukocyte-poor and washed, frozen RBCs: 250-300 ml/U given over 2 h or 1-2 h in emergencies for blood replacement in the immunocompromised.
Factor VIII concentrate: 10-20 ml/U; may need 10 U infused at 1 U/min. Given to control bleeding in hemophilia A or related coagulopathy.
Factor IX concentrate: 20-30 ml/U; may need >10 U infused at 1 U/min. Given to control bleeding in hemophilia B patients.
Volume expanders (albumin 5%, PPF): Infused at ≈ 1 ml/min or as rapidly as tolerated in shock states. Does not contain clotting factors.
BP Control *via* Crystalloids and Vasopressors: May be necessary for hypotension if BP does not recover with volume expansion alone.
Surgical Exploration: May be necessary to correct loss of integrity of blood vessels (eg, with blunt or penetrating trauma, recent surgery, invasive procedures).

PATIENT-FAMILY TEACHING
- Information regarding blood products from National Heart, Lung, and Blood Institute
- S&S of O₂ deficit for chronically anemic patients
- S&S of common and opportunistic infections for immunocompromised patients

Nursing Diagnoses/Interventions

Impaired gas exchange (or risk for same) r/t lack of O_2-carrying capacity of blood caused by hemorrhage

Desired outcomes: Within 1 h of treatment initiation, patient's gas exchange becomes adequate: $Pao_2 \geq 80$, $Paco_2$ 35-45 mm Hg, pH 7.35-7.45, RR 12-20 breaths/min with eupnea, Spo_2 >90%, HR 60-100 bpm, SBP $\geq$90 mm Hg, or all within 10% baseline.

- Assess respiratory status q15min until stable, then qh for $\geq$2 more h.
- Monitor O_2 saturation continuously *via* Spo_2.
- Monitor ABGs if S&S of hypoxemia present. Be alert to $\uparrow$ $Paco_2$, signaling hypoventilation.
- Assess for changes in sensorium (confusion, lethargy, somnolence), which may signal either inadequate cerebral oxygenation or CO_2 retention (respiratory insufficiency).
- Deliver O_2 within prescribed limits.

Altered cardiac, peripheral, cerebral, and GI tissue perfusion (or risk for same) r/t $\downarrow$ circulating blood volume secondary to hemorrhage

Desired outcome: Within 1 h of treatment completion, tissue perfusion is adequate: peripheral pulses >2+ on 0-4+ scale, brisk capillary refill (<2 sec), BP wnl for patient, CVP $\geq$5 cm H_2O or $\geq$2 mm Hg, PAWP 6-12 mm Hg, HR regular and <100 bpm, UO $\geq$0.5 ml/kg/h.

- Monitor ECG rhythm continuously when there is significant hemorrhage (>500 ml blood loss). Be alert for cardiac irritability (PACs, PVCs), tachycardias (PAT, SVT), and ischemic changes (ST-segment depression). Patients with preexisting CV disease are at $\uparrow$ risk for myocardial ischemia.
- Palpate peripheral pulses qh, noting pulse amplitude and regularity. Correlate pulse amplitude with ECG tracing.
- Monitor for chest discomfort, other symptoms suggesting myocardial ischemia. Correlate with ECG changes.
- Auscultate bowel sounds at least q4h. $\downarrow$/absent bowel sounds suggest GI ischemia, which can lead to bowel infarction.

Risk for injury r/t blood product administration

Desired outcome: Throughout transfusion and up to 8 h afterward, patient free of these S&S of blood transfusion reaction: fever, chills, flushing, rash, lesions; and has baseline RR, BP, HR.

- Check blood to be administered with another professional. Verify the following: patient's name and hospital number; blood unit number, expiration date, group, and type.
- When blood products are infusing, check VS q15min for the first h. Check patient frequently throughout first 15 min for S&S of acute hemolytic transfusion reaction: fever, chills, dyspnea, hypotension, flushing, tachycardia, back pain, hematuria, shock.
- Monitor for transfusion reactions throughout transfusion and during 8-h period afterward. In addition to acute intravascular hemolytic reactions, types of reactions are as follows:
  Acute extravascular hemolytic: Fever, $\uparrow$ bilirubin, $\downarrow$ Hct/Hgb; usually occurs within 8 h.
  Mild allergic: Rash, hives, pruritus within 1 h of starting transfusion.
  Anaphylactic: Dyspnea, SOB, bronchospasms, tachycardia, flushing, hypotension, shock within 30 min to 1 h of starting transfusion.
  Febrile: Fever, chills occurring within 4 h of starting transfusion.
  Hypervolemic: Dyspnea, tachycardia, basilar crackles, JVD, possible hypertension and headache within 1-2 h of starting transfusion.
  Septic: Fever, chills, tachycardia, hypotension, vomiting, shock, muscle pain, cardiac arrest within 5 min-4 h of starting transfusion.
- If a transfusion reaction occurs, implement the following:
  1. If transfusion in progress, stop the infusion *stat.*
  2. Maintain IV access with NS.
  3. Maintain BP with combination of volume infusion and vasoactive drugs, if indicated. Consult ACLS guidelines or unit protocol.
  4. Monitor HR and ECG for changes. Consult physician and treat symptomatic dysrhythmias as prescribed.
  5. Administer diuretics and fluids as prescribed.
  6. Obtain blood and urine specimens for transfusion workup per agency protocol.
  7. Perform blood cultures if patient exhibits S&S of sepsis.
- If intravascular hemolytic reaction confirmed, implement the following:
  1. Monitor coagulation studies, including PT, PTT, fibrinogen levels.
  2. Monitor renal status, noting BUN, creatinine, potassium, phosphate levels.
  3. Monitor laboratory values indicative of hemolysis: LDH, bilirubin, haptoglobin.

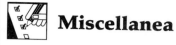

Miscellanea

CONSULT MD FOR
- S&S of any transfusion reaction
- Profound hypotension, uncontrolled bleeding, symptomatic cardiac dysrhythmias
- Persistent alteration in mental status, deterioration in ABGs, profound $\downarrow$ in O_2 saturation
- Difficulty breathing, fever, JVD

RELATED TOPICS
- Anemias
- Blood and blood products (see Appendix)
- Disseminated intravascular coagulation
- Hemolytic crisis
- Shock, hemorrhagic
- Vasopressor therapy

ABBREVIATIONS
FFP: Fresh frozen plasma
PPF: Plasma protein fraction
PRBCs: Packed red blood cells

REFERENCES
Baird M: Hematologic dysfunctions. In Swearingen PL, Keen JH (eds): *Manual of critical care nursing,* ed 3, St Louis, 1995, Mosby.

Menitove JE: Blood transfusions. In Bennett JC, Plum F (eds): *Cecil textbook of medicine,* ed 20, Philadelphia, 1996, Saunders.

Shuman M: Hemorrhagic disorders. In Bennett JC, Plum F (eds): *Cecil textbook of medicine,* ed 20, Philadelphia, 1996, Saunders.

Snyder EL: Transfusion reactions. In Hoffman R et al (eds): *Hematology: basic principles and practice,* New York, 1991, Churchill-Livingstone.

Tribett D: Hematological disorders. In Kinney M, Packa D, Dunbar S: *AACN's clinical reference for critical care,* ed 3, 1993, St Louis, Mosby.

Author: **Marianne Saunorus Baird**

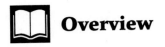 **Overview**

DESCRIPTION
Surgical approach to the pituitary gland. Treatment of choice for pituitary tumors of all types, with or without gland removal. Approximately 10%-25% of all intracranial tumors involve the pituitary gland. The procedure produces immediate results, has a low mortality rate, and can be effective in treating tumors resistant to radiation therapy.

HISTORY/RISK FACTORS
- Pituitary tumor (eg, adenoma)
- Neoplasia in pituitary region (eg, meningioma, optic nerve glioma)

CLINICAL PRESENTATION
Depends on location, tumor extent
Anterior Lobe: ACTH hypersecretion (Cushing's syndrome); ACTH suppression (Addison's disease); TSH stimulation (hyperthyroidism); TSH suppression (hypothyroidism). Other hormonal imbalances involve prolactin, FSH, LH, GH, MSH.
Posterior Lobe: ↑ ADH (SIADH); ↓ ADH (DI)
Pituitary Apoplexy (Acute Hemorrhage or Infarction of Pituitary Adenoma): Severe headache, visual disturbances, altered LOC

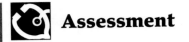 **Assessment**

PHYSICAL ASSESSMENT
Preop: Depends on tumor site
Neuro: Blurred vision, blindness, visual field disturbance, altered pupillary response, headache, eye pain
Other: Endocrine abnormalities associated with hypersecretion or hyposecretion of pituitary hormones
Postop: Depends on presence/absence of complications. *DI:* polyuria, ↓ urine specific gravity, thirst; *CSF leak:* persistent postnasal drip; *↑ ICP:* bradycardia, widening pulse pressure, altered LOC, change in motor function; *damage to cranial nerves:* diplopia, strabismus, ptosis; *optic nerve dysfunction:* partial or complete vision loss, visual field deficit; *hormonal deficiencies.*

LABORATORY STUDIES
Serum: Endocrine, electrolyte, osmolality profiles to identify hormonal and electrolyte imbalances: eg, with DI, ↑ Na^+ and ↑ osmolality present
Urine: 24-h collection; specific gravity, osmolality

IMAGING
Skull X-ray: To outline sella, identify abnormal vascular markings or calcifications
CT/MRI: To more precisely identify tumor type/extent
Cerebral Angiography: To r/o aneurysm, outline specific vascular changes

Collaborative Management

Transsphenoidal Hypophysectomy: To enter the sella turcica through the sphenoid process, the upper lip is elevated and an incision made in the gingiva above the maxilla. Because of the incision site, there is high risk for postop infection, particularly of the brain. To minimize this possibility, preop antibiotic nasal sprays are used; nasal packing impregnated with antibiotic ointment is kept in place for 24-72 h postop. *Complications:* DI, CSF leak, optic nerve dysfunction, carotid artery laceration, cranial nerve damage, hormonal deficiencies, and ↑ ICP resulting from edema or bleeding.

PATIENT-FAMILY TEACHING
- Purpose, expected results, anticipated sensations of transsphenoidal hypophysectomy.
- Necessity for lifetime exogenous hormone replacement if anterior posterior gland removed or damaged.
- If entire pituitary gland removed, S&S of hormone replacement excess or deficiency.
  Adrenal hormone excess: weight gain, moon face, easy bruising, fatigue, polyuria, polydipsia
  Adrenal hormone deficiency: weight loss, easy fatigability, abdominal pain, excess pigmentation
  Thyroid hormone excess: heat intolerance, irritability, tachycardia, weight loss, diaphoresis
  Thyroid hormone deficiency: bradycardia, cold intolerance, weight gain, slowed mentation
  Androgen replacement deficiency: some degree of sexual dysfunction, ranging from menstrual irregularities to infertility and impotence
- For patients with permanent need for hormone replacement, method for obtaining Medic-Alert bracelet and ID card outlining diagnosis and appropriate treatment in event of an emergency.

Nursing Diagnoses/Interventions

Decreased adaptive capacity: Intracranial, r/t interruption of blood flow secondary to cerebral edema or intracranial bleeding after transsphenoidal hypophysectomy

Desired outcome: Within 24 h after treatment initiation, patient has adequate intracranial adaptive capacity: ability to verbalize orientation × 3, RR 12-20 breaths/min with eupnea, equal and normoreactive pupils, and bilaterally equal motor strength and tone that are nl for patient.

- Elevate HOB 30 degrees to minimize ICP.
- Perform neurochecks at frequent intervals to assess for ↑ ICP. Be alert to restlessness, confusion, irritability, lethargy, irregularly irregular respiratory pattern, abnormal posturing, seizures, pupillary changes, bradycardia, widening pulse pressure.
- Teach patient to avoid coughing, sneezing, straining, bending, or other Valsalva-type activities because they can ↑ stress on operative site, ↑ ICP, and cause CSF leak. Explain that if coughing and sneezing are unavoidable, they should be done with mouth open to minimize ↑ in ICP. As appropriate, administer cathartics, stool softeners, or antiemetics to ↓ straining and nausea.
- If ↑ ICP develops, implement the following:
    Loosen constrictive objects around neck.
    If recently repositioned, return to original position.
    Maintain head in neutral position.
    Assess for factors contributing to ↑ ICP: distended bladder, fear, anxiety.
    Evaluate activities (eg, suctioning, bathing, dressing changes) that ↑ pressure; reorganize care plan accordingly.
    Hyperoxygenate before and after suctioning.

Risk for infection r/t inadequate primary defenses secondary to incisional opening into the sella turcica

Desired outcome: Patient infection free: orientation × 3 and absence of S&S of CSF leak or nuchal rigidity.

- Inspect nasal packing at frequent intervals for frank bleeding or evidence of CSF (nonsanguineous) leak. Collect and send all clear drainage for laboratory glucose analysis to determine if it is CSF. Glucose values of ≥30 mg/dl confirm CSF. Elevate HOB to minimize chance of bacterial migration to the brain.
- Be alert to S&S of infection, including ↑ temp, nuchal rigidity, and altered LOC.
- To prevent injury to operative site, which could lead to infection, teach patient to avoid brushing teeth until instructed to do so. Provide mouthwash and sponge-tipped applicators for oral hygiene.

Miscellanea

CONSULT MD FOR
- S&S of ↑ ICP
- S&S of suspected CSF leak or infection
- S&S of intracranial or other infection
- S&S of DI

RELATED TOPICS
- Adrenal insufficiency, acute
- Diabetes insipidus
- Intracranial surgery

ABBREVIATIONS
ACTH: Adrenocorticotropic hormone
ADH: Antidiuretic hormone
DI: Diabetes insipidus
FSH: Follicle-stimulating hormone
GH: Growth hormone
LH: Luteinizing hormone
MSH: Melanocyte-stimulating hormone
SIADH: Syndrome of inappropriate antidiuretic hormone
TSH: Thyroid-stimulating hormone

REFERENCES
Blisset PA: Pituitary tumor, hypophysectomy, and diabetes insipidus, *J Post Anesth Nurs* 7(3): 209, 1992.
Chipps E: Transsphenoidal surgery for pituitary tumors, *Crit Care Nurse* 12(1): 30-39, 1992.
Horne MM: Endocrinologic dysfunctions. In Swearingen PL, Keen JH (eds): *Manual of critical care nursing*, ed 3, St Louis, 1995, Mosby.
McEwen DR: Transsphenoidal adenomectomy *AORN J* 61(2): 321-336, 1995.

Author: **Mima M. Horne**

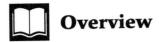 **Overview**

PATHOPHYSIOLOGY

Highly infectious disease spread by contact with respiratory droplets containing mycobacteria, generally the *Mycobacterium tuberculosis* bacillus. Most common transmission mode is inhalation of bacilli in airborne mucous droplets and, less frequently, ingestion or skin penetration. When infection occurs, lung parenchyma become inflamed. Eventually the area is walled off by fibrotic tissue, and the center becomes soft and cheesy in consistency, a process known as caseation. Of infected individuals, 90% do not progress to active disease.

HISTORY/RISK FACTORS

- Recent immigration from TB-endemic region: eg, Latin America, Asia, Africa, Caribbean
- Institutionalization: eg, prison, psychiatric facility
- Immunocompromise: eg, immunosuppressant therapy, HIV infection
- Advanced age
- Malnutrition, chronic illness
- IV drug use, alcoholism

CLINICAL PRESENTATION

Cough, afternoon temp elevation, night sweats, anorexia, weight loss

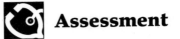 **Assessment**

PHYSICAL ASSESSMENT

It is important to assess whether patient exposed to a person with active TB. Also, patient's close contacts require identification so that they can undergo evaluation for infection.

Active Pulmonary Infection: Cough, usually productive for blood-tinged or rusty-colored sputum; ↓/adventitious breath sounds, including rhonchi, wheezing, dullness to percussion; possible cachexia attributable to malnutrition or underlying disease process; painful and enlarged lymph nodes.

VITAL SIGNS/HEMODYNAMICS

RR: ↑
HR: ↑
BP: Minimally affected
Temp: ↑
Hemodynamic Monitoring: Usually not indicated

LABORATORY STUDIES

Sputum Culture: To ascertain presence of *M. tuberculosis;* will not be positive during latency period; takes 8 wks postinfection to confirm. *M. bovis* and *M. avium* sometimes cause active pulmonary infection, usually in the immunocompromised.

Acid-Fast Stain: Positive for AFB if TB is active.

IMAGING

Chest X-ray: Will reveal calcification at original site, enlargement of hilar lymph nodes, parenchymal infiltrate, pleural effusion, cavitation.

DIAGNOSTIC PROCEDURES

Intradermal Injection of Antigen: Purified protein derivative (PPD); old tuberculin (OT). Considered positive when area of induration >10 mm present within 48-72 h after injection. Positive test indicates past infection and presence of antibodies; not definitive of active disease.

Gastric Washings: May reveal presence of tuberculosis bacilli secondary to swallowed sputum.

Collaborative Management

AFB Isolation: Until antimicrobial therapy is successful as indicated by absence of AFB in smears. Requires private room with special ventilation that dilutes and removes airborne contaminants and controls direction of air flow. High-efficiency particulate air filter masks designed to provide tight face seal and filter particles in the 1-5 micron range worn by all individuals entering the room and a regular mask worn by patient if it is necessary to leave the room.

Pharmacologic Agents: Resistance of *M. tuberculosis* to antimicrobial agents is a growing problem; therefore a combination of anti-infective agents used to prevent further resistance. The specific regimen depends on infection or disease stage, presence of extrapulmonary disease, and sensitivity to the chemotherapeutic agent. *Most common combination:* isoniazid and rifampin. Given for 6-12 mos. Other drugs, which may be added to this protocol if the organism shows resistance to first-line drugs, include ethambutol, pyrazinamide, streptomycin.

Surgery: Resection for persistent cavitary lesions; surgical intervention for massive hemoptysis, spontaneous pneumothorax, abscess drainage, other complications.

PATIENT-FAMILY TEACHING

- Pathophysiology of TB and mechanism by which it is spread.
- AFB isolation; rationale for posting AFB isolation/airborne precautions on door.
- Necessity of visitors wearing high-efficiency masks, including demonstration of their proper fit and use. Provide masks at doorway or other convenient place.
- Importance of covering mouth and nose with tissue when sneezing or coughing and disposing of used tissue in container suitable for biohazardous waste disposal.
- Importance of good hand washing technique to ↓ risk of ingesting the organism.
- Antituberculosis medications, including name, purpose, dosage, schedule, precautions, drug-drug and food-drug interactions, and potential side effects. Remind patient that medications are to be taken uninterruptedly for prescribed period of time.
- Importance of periodic reculturing of sputum.
- Arrangements with Community Health Department for follow up.

Nursing Diagnoses/Interventions

Ineffective airway clearance r/t presence of ↑ tracheobronchial secretions and ↓ ability to expectorate secondary to fatigue
Desired outcome: Within 24-48 h of treatment initiation, patient's airway free of excess secretions: presence of eupnea and absence of adventitious breath sounds and excessive coughing.
- Assess ability to clear secretions. Keep emergency suction equipment at bedside.
- Encourage oral fluid intake to help ↓ secretion viscosity.
- Encourage effective cough:
    Take several deep breaths.
    After last inhalation, cough 3-4 times on same exhalation until most of air expelled.
    Repeat several times until cough becomes productive.

Activity intolerance r/t fatigue, altered nutritional status, and fever
Desired outcome: Within 24-48 h of treatment initiation, patient verbalizes ↓ in fatigue and associated symptoms.
- ↓ metabolic demands for O₂ by limiting or pacing activities and procedures.
- Explain all procedures and offer support to minimize fear and anxiety, which can ↑ O₂ demands.
- Schedule rest times after meals to avoid competition for O₂ supply during digestion.
- Monitor Spo₂ during activity to evaluate limits of activity and recommend optimal positions for oxygenation.
- Assess temp q2-4h. Consult physician for ↑ in temp. Provide treatment as prescribed to ↓ temp and thus O₂ demands.
- Monitor nutritional intake and ensure adequate protein/calorie intake *via* oral, enteral, or parenteral feedings.

Miscellanea

CONSULT MD FOR
- Presence of AFB-positive smears after 2 wks of therapy. (AFB smears that are negative after 2 wks of therapy show successful initial therapy. Sputum will be checked at regular intervals to ensure compliance with regimen and detect resistant strains.)
- Persistence of cough after 1-2 wks of therapy.
- S&S of complications: significant hemoptysis, respiratory decompensation, pneumothorax.

RELATED TOPICS
- Recommendations for isolation precautions in hospitals (see Appendix)
- Nutritional support, parenteral
- Pneumothorax
- Respiratory failure, acute

ABBREVIATION
AFB: Acid-fast bacillus

REFERENCES
Cohen FL, Durham JD: *Tuberculosis: a sourcebook for nursing practice,* New York, 1995, Springer.
Grimes DE, Grimes RM: Tuberculosis: what nurses need to know to help control the epidemic, *Nurs Outlook* 43(4): 164-173, 1995.
Howard CA: Pulmonary tuberculosis. In Swearingen PL (ed): *Manual of medical-surgical nursing care,* ed 3, St Louis, 1994, Mosby.
LaRochelle DR, Carlson EVB: Protecting the provider from tuberculosis exposure, *Nurs Clin North Am* 30(1): 13-22, 1995.
Neville K et al: The third epidemic multidrug-resistant tuberculosis, *Chest* 105(1): 45-48, 1994.
Vesley DL: Respiratory protection devices, *Am J Infect Control* 23(2): 165-168, 1995.

Author: **Cheri A. Goll**

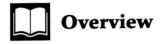 **Overview**

DESCRIPTION
Created when the bladder must be bypassed or removed, most commonly because of bladder cancer. Individuals with severe, non-malignant urinary problems also are candidates. Most urinary diversions are permanent, but reversal may be performed if condition changes. If an intestinal conduit is formed, fluid and electrolyte disorder and hyperchloremic metabolic acidosis may occur.

HISTORY/RISK FACTORS
- Bladder or other pelvic malignancies
- Radiation damage to bladder
- Vaginal fistula
- Neurogenic bladder
- Refractory urinary incontinence
- End-stage ureteral obstruction

CLINICAL PRESENTATION
Variable, according to underlying condition

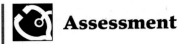 **Assessment**

PHYSICAL ASSESSMENT (postop)
Cutaneous Ureterostomy: Urine drainage *via* bilateral stomas and ureteral stents; light red for 24-48 h; >30 ml/h.
Intestinal (ileal) Conduit: Drainage *via* stoma and stents; light red with mucous threads for 24-48 h; >30 ml/h.
Continent Urinary Diversion/Reservoir: Drainage *via* catheter and stents; light red with mucous threads for 24-48 h; >30 ml/h. Continent urinary diversion with urethral anastomosis has a urethral catheter in place that drains urine.
   Kock urostomy: Usually has reservoir catheter; may have ureteral stents.
   Indiana (ileocecal) reservoir: Usually has ureteral stents exiting from stoma through which most of the urine drains; may have reservoir catheter exiting from a stab wound, which serves as an overflow catheter.
Stents: ↓ UO can signal anastomosis failure.
Stoma Drainage: ↓ urine can signal stomal stenosis.

Penrose Drains: Urine/lymph drainage, depending on placement. Light red in color for first 24-48 h.
Stomal Skin: Optimally, red and moist.
GI: Gastric tube; bowel sounds absent with gradual return in 24-48 h.
Fluid and Electrolytes: Optimally, wnl.

VITAL SIGNS/HEMODYNAMICS
Reflect underlying condition, level of hydration, presence/absence of infection.

LABORATORY STUDIES
Hgb/Hct: May be ↓ because of excessive blood loss during surgery.
Electrolytes/ABGs: Hypokalemia, hyperchloremic metabolic acidosis may result from use of intestine for conduit. Caused by anion gap created by loss of bicarbonate; more commonly occurs with use of jejunum segment.
Creatinine/BUN: To check renal functioning; BUN may be ↑ because of dehydration.
Urinalysis/Urine Culture: To check for UTI, other abnormalities.
Urinary pH: Needs to be acidic (≤6.0) to minimize risk of UTI.

Collaborative Management

SURGICAL PROCEDURES

Urinary stream may be diverted at multiple points: renal pelvis (pyelostomy or nephrostomy), ureter (ureterostomy), bladder (vesicostomy), or *via* intestinal conduit. Construction of intestinal (ileal) conduit is the most common type, resulting in a more nl urinary pattern.

Cutaneous Ureterostomy: Ureters resected from bladder and brought out through abdominal surface, either separately or with one attached to the other inside the body, resulting in only one abdominal stoma.

Intestinal (ileal) Conduit: 15-20 cm section of ileum resected from intestine to form urine passageway. Proximal end closed, and distal end brought out through abdomen, forming a stoma. Ureters are resected from bladder and anastomosed to ileal segment. Chronic diarrhea, dehydration, electrolyte disturbances are possible complications. Implications for specific intestinal segments:

Stomach tissue: Secretes H^+ and Cl^-, which can counteract hyperchloremic metabolic acidosis. Acidic medium ↓ risk of infection; does not produce as much mucus as intestinal sections.

Jejunum: High rate of hyperchloremia, hyperkalemia, hypokalemia, dehydration.

Ileum: When used with ileocecal valve, ↑ occurrence of diarrhea and steatorrhea.

Continent Urinary Diversion: Indiana reservoir and Kock continent urostomy most commonly performed. Indiana reservoir uses 15-18 cm of distal ileum and 20-24 cm of cecum sutured together to create a pouch or urine reservoir. An antireflux mechanism is established *via* ileocecal valve, which keeps urine in reservoir until a catheter is passed through skin-level stoma. Ureters attached at an angle to cecal wall, preventing urine reflux to the kidneys.

FLUID AND ELECTROLYTE MANAGEMENT

Total fluid intake should be 2-3 L/day unless restricted by heart failure or other underlying conditions. Potassium and other electrolytes replaced as necessary.

TREATMENT OF DIARRHEA

Psyllium, cholestyramine, loperamide as indicated.

PATIENT-FAMILY TEACHING

- S&S that necessitate medical intervention: fever, chills, nausea, vomiting, abdominal pain and distention, cloudy urine, incisional pain or redness, peristomal skin irritation, abnormal changes in stoma shape or color from nl bright and shiny red.
- Community resources, including local United Ostomy Association, American Cancer Society, and local ET nurse, if appropriate.
- Maintenance of fluid intake at ≥2-3 L/day to maintain adequate kidney function.
- Monitoring of urine pH, which is checked weekly and should remain at ≤6.0. Individuals with urinary diversions have a greater incidence of UTIs than the general public, so their urinary pH must be kept acidic. If >6.0, advise ↑ fluid intake and, with physician approval, ↑ vitamin C intake to 500-1000 mg/day, which promotes urine acidity.
- Care of stoma and application of urostomy appliances. Ensure proficiency in application technique before hospital discharge.
- Care of urostomy appliances. Teach proper cleansing to ↓ risk of bacterial growth, which would contaminate urine and ↑ risk of UTI.
- Importance of follow-up care with physician and ET nurse.

Nursing Diagnoses/Interventions

Altered protection r/t neurosensory, MS, and CV changes secondary to hyperchloremic metabolic acidosis with hypokalemia (can occur secondary to reabsorption of Na^+ and Cl^- from urine in the ileal segment, which results in compensatory loss of K^+ and HCO_3^-)

Desired outcome: Patient verbalizes orientation $\times$ 3 (wnl for patient) and remains free of injury caused by neurosensory, MS, and CV changes.

- For patients with ileal conduits, assess for indicators of hypokalemia and metabolic acidosis: nausea, irregular HR, and changes in LOC (from sleepy to combative) and muscle tone (convulsions to flaccidity).
- If patient is confused or exhibits signs of motor dysfunction, keep bed in lowest position and raise side rails.
- Encourage oral intake as directed, and assess need for IV fluids with K supplements.
- If patient is hypokalemic and allowed to eat, encourage foods high in K.
- Encourage ambulation by 2 or 3 days postop. Mobility helps prevent urinary stasis, which $\uparrow$ risk of electrolyte problems.

Impaired stomal tissue integrity (or risk of same) r/t altered circulation

Desired outcomes: Stoma is pink or bright red and shiny. The stoma of a cutaneous urostomy is raised, moist, and red.

- Inspect stoma at least q8h and as indicated. The stoma of an ileal conduit will be edematous and should be pink or red in color with a shiny appearance. If dusky or cyanotic, this signals insufficient blood supply and impending necrosis and must be reported to the surgeon *stat.*
- Also assess degree of swelling, and inform patient that stoma will shrink considerably over the first 6-8 wks and less significantly over the next year. For an ileal conduit, evaluate stomal height and plan care accordingly. The stoma formed by a cutaneous ureterostomy is usually raised during the first few wks after surgery, red in color, and moist.

Altered urinary elimination r/t postop use of ureteral stents, catheters, or drains and to urinary diversion surgery

Desired outcome: UO $\geq$ 30 ml/h; urine clear, straw-colored, and with characteristic odor.

- Monitor color, clarity, and volume of UO *via* stoma, stents, catheter.
- Monitor for S&S of anastomotic breakdown/intraabdominal urine leakage, which may occur with intestinal conduit or continent diversion: $\uparrow$UO from stoma or stents, flank pain, $\uparrow$ abdominal girth, $\uparrow$ drainage from Penrose drains.

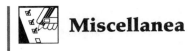 # Miscellanea

CONSULT MD FOR

- Complications: hyperchloremia, hyper/hypokalemia, metabolic acidosis, dehydration, chronic diarrhea, DVT, paralytic ileus
- S&S of infection: temp >38.33° C (101° F); erythema, tenderness, edema, purulent drainage from surgical site; cloudy urine; flank pain; chills
- S&S of postop hemorrhage: gross hematuria along with $\downarrow$BP, $\uparrow$HR, $\uparrow$RR

RELATED TOPICS

- Antimicrobial therapy
- Hypokalemia
- Hypovolemia
- Metabolic acidosis, acute and chronic
- Peritonitis
- Pyelonephritis, acute

ABBREVIATION

ET: Enterostomal therapy

- Monitor functioning of ureteral stents, which protrude from the stoma under the pouch. Amount produced by each is not important as long as each drains adequately and total drainage from all sources is ≥30 ml/h. Urine should be pink for the first 24-48 h and become straw-colored by 3 days postop. Absent/↓ amounts of urine may indicate a blocked stent or ureteral problems. If stent becomes blocked with mucus, this is not a problem as long as urine is draining adequately around the stent and output volume is adequate.
- Monitor functioning of stoma catheters. In continent urinary diversions, a catheter is placed in the reservoir to prevent distention and promote healing of suture lines. This new reservoir exudes large amounts of mucus, necessitating catheter irrigation with 30-50 ml of NS, which is instilled gently and allowed to empty *via* gravity. Expect output to include pink or light red urine with mucus and small clots for the first 24 h. Urine should become amber-colored with occasional clots in 3 postop days. Mucus production will continue but should ↓ in volume.
- Monitor drain functioning. Excessive lymph fluid and urine can be removed *via* these drains without putting pressure on suture lines. Drainage from Penrose drain may be light red to pink in color for the first 24 h and then lighten to amber color and ↓ in amount. In a continent urinary diversion, ↑ drainage after amounts have been low may signal reservoir leakage. Consult physician if this occurs.
- Monitor I&O, and record total UO from urinary diversion for the first 24 h postop. Differentiate and record separately amounts from all drains, stents, and catheters.
- Consult physician for total output <60 ml during a 2-h period, because this can signal ureteral obstruction, leak in the urinary diversion, or impending renal failure. Assess for other indicators of ureteral obstruction: flank pain, nausea, vomiting, anuria.
- To prevent urinary stasis, encourage intake of ≥2-3 L/day in nonrestricted patients.

Risk for infection r/t invasive surgical procedure and risk of ascending bacteriuria with urinary diversion

Desired outcome: Patient infection free: normothermia; WBCs ≤11,000 µl; absence of purulent drainage, erythema, puffiness, warmth, and tenderness along incision.

- Monitor temp q4h during the first 24-48 h postop. Be alert for temp 38.33° C (>101° F).
- Inspect the dressing frequently after surgery. Infection is most likely to be evident after the first 72 h. Assess for purulent drainage on the dressing. Change dressing when it becomes wet, using sterile technique. Use extra care to prevent drain disruption.
- Note condition of incision. Be alert to S&S of infection, including erythema, tenderness, local warmth, puffiness, purulent drainage.
- Monitor and record urine character at least q8h. Mucous particles are nl in urine with ileal conduits and continent urinary diversions. Cloudy urine can signal infection. Assess for other S&S of UTI: flank pain, chills, fever.
- Note stomal position relative to incision. If close together, apply the pouch first to avoid overlap of the pouch with the suture line. If necessary, cut the pouch down on one side, or place it at an angle to avoid contact with drainage, which may loosen the adhesive.
- Patients with cystectomies without anastomosis to the urethra may have an indwelling urethral catheter to drain serosanguineous fluid from the peritoneal cavity. Do not irrigate this catheter, because irrigation can result in peritonitis.

REFERENCES

Horne MM, Heitz UE, Swearingen PL: *Pocket guide to fluid, electrolytes, and acid-base balance*, ed 3, St Louis, 1996, Mosby.

Jansen PR: Urinary diversions. In Swearingen PL (ed): *Manual of medical-surgical nursing*, ed 3, St Louis, 1994, Mosby.

Lerner S, Skinner E, Skinner D: Radical cystectomy in regionally advanced bladder cancer, *Urol Clin North Am* 19(4): 713-723, 1992.

McGuire E: Fluid management by the urinary tract and vice versa, *J Urol* 154(2): 742-744, 1995.

Seigne J, McDougal W: Urinary diversion. *Surg Oncol Clin North Am* 3(2): 307-321, 1994.

Author: **Patricia R. Jansen**

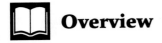 **Overview**

PATHOPHYSIOLOGY

Injuries to LUT, which includes ureters, urinary bladder, and urethra, have potential for lifelong complications or even death.

Ureteral Trauma: Lacerations most common at ureteropelvic junction, where upper ureter joins renal pelvis.

Bladder Trauma: Blunt blow all that is necessary to cause rupture.

Intraperitoneal rupture: Occurs at the dome, which is point of least resistance. Blood and urine may extravasate into peritoneal cavity.

Extraperitoneal rupture: Occurs most often with pelvic fractures. Bladder perforated at its base, leading to extravasation of blood and urine into space surrounding base.

Urethral Trauma: Less common in females than in males, whose urethra is 5 × longer.

INCIDENCE

Occurs in <1% of all trauma patients; blunt trauma most common cause.

HISTORY/RISK FACTORS

- Blunt injury with severe abdominal compression: vehicular collision, falls, sports-related injury, assaults
- Penetrating abdominal injury: stab and gunshot wounds
- Perineal trauma, straddle injuries, pelvic fractures, shearing forces
- Iatrogenic injuries: gynecologic, colonic, vascular surgery
- Failure to use safety devices (seat belt, air bag)
- Chronic illness
- Advanced age

CLINICAL PRESENTATION

Blood at urethral meatus, hematuria, possible flank or suprapubic pain, inability to void

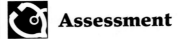 **Assessment**

PHYSICAL ASSESSMENT

Ureteral Trauma: Microscopic or gross hematuria. If ureter completely transected, nl urine from unaffected kidney may be voided. May exhibit urine at entrance or exit sites of penetrating wound. *Late signs:* fever, flank or abdominal discomfort.

Bladder Trauma: Suprapubic tenderness, inability to void spontaneously, gross hematuria. Perineal or scrotal edema and hematoma, abnormal position of prostate, abdominal distention, palpable suprapubic mass, palpable and overdistended bladder. *Late signs:* fever, abdominal discomfort.

Urethral Trauma: Urethral bleeding; prostate tenderness; microscopic or gross hematuria; genital pain, tenderness, bruising, discoloration; tracking of urine into tissues of thighs or abdominal wall.

VITAL SIGNS/HEMODYNAMICS

RR: ↑ with hemorrhage
HR: ↑ with hemorrhage
BP: ↓ with hemorrhage
Temp: ↑ with infection
PAWP/CVP: ↓ with hemorrhage
SVR: ↑ with hemorrhage; ↑ or ↓ with infection

IMAGING

Retrograde Urethrogram: Contrast material injected into urethra *via* small urinary catheter. X-ray outlines urethral size and shape. With urethral rupture, extravasation of contrast material occurs.

Cystogram: Bladder filled with 300 ml contrast material. X-rays determine if intra/extraperitoneal extravasation of contrast material occurs.

Excretory Urogram/IVP: Contrast material administered IV and filtered by kidneys before excretion through urinary tract. X-rays visualize nl or injured structures of KUB.

KUB Radiography: Evaluates position, size, structure, defects of kidney and LUT structures.

CT Scan: Reveals hematomas, renal lacerations, renal infarcts, urine extravasation.

MRI: Identifies subtle injuries, eg, posterior urethral trauma; enables estimation of injury length.

Collaborative Management

Pharmacotherapy

Antibiotics: For positive urine culture results, penetrating injuries, or peritonitis

Analgesics: IV morphine sulfate

Td immunization: Booster given if needed or hx unknown

Volume Resuscitation: For hemorrhagic shock

Blood/Urine Cultures: If infection suspected

Urinary Drainage: Suprapubic vs indwelling urethral catheter drainage controversial. Suprapubic catheters avoid complications of prolonged urethral catheterization and ↓ risk of urethral strictures. With urethral injury, suprapubic cystotomy necessary. If blood present at urethral meatus, catheterization contraindicated before urethrogram obtained. Internal ureteral catheters (stents) indicated for ureteral trauma to maintain ureteral alignment, ensure urinary drainage, and provide support during anastomosis.

Surgical Correction: Indicated for transected/torn ureter, bladder perforation, and injuries accompanied by rapidly expanding, pulsating hematomas. Urethral splinting and surgical reconstruction usually delayed for 3-6 mos to enable ↓ bruising and swelling.

PATIENT-FAMILY TEACHING

- Medications: drug name, purpose, dosage, schedule, precautions, food-drug and drug-drug interactions, potential side effects
- Purpose, expected results, anticipated sensations of all nursing/medical interventions
- Need for ↑ fluid intake
- Necessity to report ↑ blood in urine; urge but inability to void

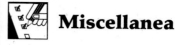

Nursing Diagnoses/Interventions

Altered urinary elimination r/t mechanical trauma secondary to injury to LUT structures and kidney

Desired outcome: Within 6 h after immediate trauma management, patient has UO of ≥0.5 ml/kg/h with no bladder distention.

- Encourage patient to void. If unable to void, assess need for catheterization or suprapubic drainage by palpating gently for a full bladder. Monitor for these signs of kidney or LUT trauma:
  - Urge but inability to void
  - Blood at urethral meatus
  - Difficult or unsuccessful urinary catheterization
  - Anuria after urinary catheterization
  - Hematuria
- Do not catheterize if there is blood at urethral meatus unless urethrogram has indicated it can be performed safely. Do not force catheter if resistance felt.
- Monitor serum BUN/creatinine. ↑ may reflect pending renal insufficiency. Nl BUN ≥20 mg/dl; nl creatinine ≤1.5 mg/dl.
- Document I&O qh. Assess patency of urinary collection system to determine if clots occluding system. If indicated, irrigate catheter according to agency policy.
- Sudden cessation of urine flow through collection system may signal catheter obstruction. If catheter irrigation does not resume urine drainage, consider changing urinary catheter.
- Ensure nephrostomy tube not occluded by patient's weight or external pressure. Irrigate *only* if prescribed and with ≤5 ml of fluid.
- Assess entrance site of nephrostomy tube for bleeding or urine leakage. Catheter blockage can cause sudden ↓ in UO. Consult physician if UO <0.5 ml/kg/h.
- Assess urine for color and presence/absence of clots. Expect hematuria for first 24-48 h after nephrostomy tube insertion.
- Ensure adequate hydration to enable clearing of contrast material after diagnostic testing.

Risk for infection r/t inadequate primary defenses and tissue destruction secondary to bacterial contamination of urinary tract with penetrating trauma, bladder rupture, or instrumentation

Desired outcome: Patient infection free: normothermia, WBCs ≤11,000 μl, and negative results of urine and wound drainage testing.

- Use aseptic technique when caring for urinary drainage systems. Maintain catheters and collection container at a level lower than bladder; keep drainage tubing unkinked.
- Record color, odor, and specific gravity of urine each shift. Culture urine specimen when infection suspected.
- Monitor WBC count qd and temp q4h for ↑.
- Assess for signs of peritonitis each shift: abdominal pain, abdominal distention with rigidity, nausea, vomiting, fever, malaise, and weakness.
- Assess catheter exit site for erythema, swelling, or drainage.
- Assess thigh, groin, and lower portion of abdomen for urinary extravasation: swelling, pain, mass(es), erythema, tracking of urine along fascial planes.
- Assess surgical incision for approximation of suture line and evidence of wound healing. Culture purulent or foul-smelling drainage.
- At least q8h assess skin at all catheter entrance sites for indicators of irritation: erythema, drainage, and swelling.
- Cleanse suprapubic catheter insertion site q8h with antimicrobial solution. Apply sterile gauze pads over site and tape securely with paper tape. Change dressings q24h or as soon as wet. If erythema and swelling occur as a result of maceration from contact with urine, consider use of a pectin wafer skin barrier.

Pain (acute tenderness in lower abdomen) r/t physical injury with LUT structural injury, procedures for urinary diversion, or surgical incisions

Desired outcomes: Within 2 h after giving analgesia, patient's subjective evaluation of discomfort improves, as documented by pain scale. Nonverbal indicators, such as grimacing, absent.

- Assess for pain at least q4h. Devise pain scale with patient. Be alert to shallow breathing in presence of abdominal pain, which can cause inadequate pulmonary excursion. Medicate promptly and document response to analgesia, using pain scale.
- Explain cause of pain.
- Assist into position of comfort. Often knee flexion relaxes lower abdominal muscles and helps ↓ discomfort.
- Implement nonpharmacologic measures for coping with pain: diversion, touch, conversation.

Miscellanea

CONSULT MD FOR

- Full bladder and inability to void
- New onset hematuria, frank bleeding, or blood at urethral meatus
- Anuria
- UO <0.5 ml/kg/h × 2
- Symptoms of peritonitis: abdominal rigidity and pain; fever
- Evidence of urinary extravasation: swelling, pain, mass(es), erythema, tracking of urine along fascial planes

RELATED TOPICS

- Renal injury
- Shock, hemorrhagic

ABBREVIATIONS

LUT: Lower urinary tract
Td: Combined tetanus diphtheria toxoid

REFERENCES

Levine E: Acute renal and urinary tract disease, *Radiol Clin North Am* 32(5): 989-1004, 1994.
Patterson BM: Pelvic ring injury and associated urologic trauma, *Semin Urol* 31(1): 25-33, 1995.
Ponce J, Lewis JV: Urethral injury associated with pelvic fractures, *J Tenn Med Assoc* 87(8): 335-336, 1994.
Sommers MS: Renal and lower urinary tract injury. In Swearingen PL, Keen JH (eds): *Manual of critical care nursing*, ed 3, St Louis, 1995, Mosby.

Author: **Marilyn Sawyer Sommers**

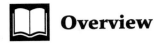 **Overview**

PATHOPHYSIOLOGY
Occurs when enterococci become resistant to the antibiotic vancomycin. Eradicating VRE colonization/infection is nearly impossible because VRE is also resistant to other antibiotics. Serious infections, including overwhelming septicemia leading to death, are possible because of ineffectiveness of traditional antimicrobial therapy.
Colonization: Presence of microorganisms that result from environmental contact (animate/inanimate).
Infection: Enterococci considered nl GI tract flora. Impaired defense mechanisms and disturbance of nl flora balance can result in infection at various sites.

INCIDENCE
Most often associated with ICUs in large or university hospitals.

HISTORY/RISK FACTORS
- Immunosuppression: eg, oncology, transplant
- Intraabdominal or cardiothoracic surgery
- Prolonged hospital stay
- Previous vancomycin/(multi)antimicrobial therapy
- Critical illness
- Exposure *via* health care environment and workers
- Indwelling urinary or vascular catheter

CLINICAL PRESENTATION
Colonization: No S&S of infection; laboratory-confirmed culture (stool, rectal swab, perineal area, axilla, umbilicus).
Infection: Laboratory-confirmed VRE culture isolated from specific body site. Likely sites include:
GI: Wound, fistula, abscess
GU: Catheter-associated UTI
CV: Coronary bypass surgery with purulent sternal wound; endocarditis valve vegetation (GI seeded)
Hemat: Septicemia

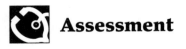 **Assessment**

PHYSICAL ASSESSMENT
Variable, depending on site of infection
Neuro: Confusion, change in LOC
GI: ↓/absent bowel sounds
Renal: Oliguria; cloudy, foul-smelling urine

Integ: Incision or open wound with erythema, edema, tenderness, pain, warmth, dryness, irritation, drainage

VITAL SIGNS/HEMODYNAMICS
Variable, according to underlying condition and site of infection
RR: ↑
HR: ↑
BP: Nl or ↓ if septicemic
Temp: ↑
CVP/PAWP: Often ↓ from insensible fluid loss or SIRS
CO: Early ↑; later ↓ if septicemic
SVR/MAP: ↓ if septicemic
ECG: Nl or sinus tachycardia

LABORATORY STUDIES
C&S Panel of Suspected Site: Vancomycin resistance is at level 8 MIC (level at which specific antibiotic is effective). A culture result does not always indicate infection; it may indicate colonization of the organism.
WBCs: ↑ in immature neutrophils (left shift).

IMAGING
X-ray: To r/o masses, abscess, collections of purulent material.
CT Scan: To r/o abscess.

DIAGNOSTIC PROCEDURE
Needle Aspiration: Of fluid collection, abscess; may be CT-directed. Aspirate sent for culture.

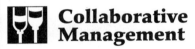 **Collaborative Management**

VRE-related policies/procedures are based on facility's epidemiologic data, scientific literature, and published guidelines. If uncertain of any aspect, check with infection control practitioner. Best preventative measure for transmission of VRE and most organisms is thorough hand washing. In addition, practice CDC Standard Precautions, including aseptic technique and appropriate stool and wound drainage precautions at all times for all patients.

VRE-SPECIFIC MEASURES
Cleaning and Disinfecting: Of patient care area and equipment.
Institutional Policy for VRE Colonization/Infection: Usually CDC Transmission-Based (Contact) Precautions. See "Recommendations for Isolation Precautions in Hospitals" in Appendix.
Infection Control: Multidisciplinary, institution-wide committee, which may include staff

of quality assurance/improvement, infection control, clinical patient care, education, environmental service, safety, employee health, microbiology, and information systems, as well as physicians and administrators.
Monitoring Incidence: Usually *via* microbiology lab and infection control department. Should include computer or manual system of flagging/tracking readmissions of VRE colonized/infected patients.

VANCOMYCIN USE
VRE coincides with ↑ incidence of enterococcal resistance to penicillin and aminoglycosides. General guidelines include limiting use to the following situations:
Serious Infections: Those caused by β-lactamase–resistant microorganisms.
Infections Caused by Gram-Positive Microorganisms: In patients with serious allergies to β-lactamase antimicrobials.

SITUATIONS IN WHICH VANCOMYCIN MAY BE INAPPROPRIATE
Routine Surgical Prophylaxis: Unless life-threatening allergy to β-lactamase.
Single Positive Blood Culture: For coagulase-negative *Staphylococcus,* a frequent skin contaminant, if other blood cultures taken during same time frame are negative.

PREVENTION OF SPREAD OF VANCOMYCIN RESISTANCE
Careful Prescription of Vancomycin: According to current CDC guidelines.
Education of Providers: Regarding vancomycin resistance.
Verification by Qualified Laboratory: Of exact organism and resistance (can easily be misidentified).
Timely Reporting: To physicians, infection control practitioners, and patient care units.
Ongoing Adherence to Standard Infection Control Practices

SURGERY
I&D: To open and drain wound to clean out purulent material.
Surgical Repair/Flap: Débridement, possibly with free-flap graft.

COMMUNITY REFERRAL
- Local and state health departments consulted when developing discharge plan for VRE-infected/colonized patients to nursing homes, other hospitals, or home health care. This plan should be part of a larger strategy for handling patient with resolving infection/colonization with antimicrobial-resistant microorganisms.
- CDC telephone: 404-639-6413

Nursing Diagnoses/Interventions

Risk for infection r/t inadequate primary defenses secondary to interruption in skin integrity; presence of invasive lines, drains, or catheters; and immunocompromised status
Desired outcomes: Patient infection free: normothermia, WBCs <11,000 μl, negative culture results, no clinical indicators of infection. There is no evidence of colonization/infection with VRE by cross-contamination from personnel or environment.

- Compliance with precautions is essential, since prevention and control of nosocomial transmission is more likely to succeed if VRE is confined to a few patients.
- Place patient in private room or in room with another patient with VRE.
- Wear clean, nonsterile gloves when entering patient's room. VRE can contaminate environment extensively. Change gloves after contact with stool or other drainage/secretions that could contain high concentrations of VRE. Wash hands after removing gloves and before donning new gloves.
- Use clean, nonsterile gown when entering patient's room if substantial contact is expected with patient or patient's secretions/drainage. Incontinence, ileostomy/colostomy, diarrhea, wound drainage not contained by dressing, are factors that ↑ risk of VRE contact.
- Remove gloves and gown before leaving room. Immediately wash hands (contamination or glove leaks can occur) with antiseptic soap (eg, chlorhexidine gluconate, iodine, PCMX, triclosan) or waterless antiseptic agent.
- Do not recontact environmental surfaces (eg, doorknob) after removing barriers.
- Dedicate noncritical items (eg, stethoscope) to VRE patient's room, or clean/disinfect before reuse.
- Screen roommates for VRE (*via* stool or rectal swab cultures).
- Discontinue contact isolation precautions at direction of institutional policy or infection control.

Social isolation r/t altered health status, inability to engage in satisfying personal relationships, altered mental status, or altered physical appearance
Desired outcome: Within 24 h of informing patient of resistant organism or implementing isolation precautions, patient demonstrates interaction and communication with others.

- Determine and when possible correct factors contributing to social isolation:
  Restriction of visitors and visitors' use of special precautions
  Absence of/inadequate support system
  Inability to communicate (eg, mask use, door closed)
  Physical changes that affect self-concept (drainage, foul smell)
  Denial or withdrawal
- Recognize patients at higher risk for social isolation: elders, disabled, chronically ill, economically disadvantaged, those with cultural or language barriers.

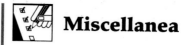 # Miscellanea

CONSULT MD FOR

- VRE-positive culture results
- New-onset symptoms of infection: erythema, tenderness, induration, purulent drainage, temp >38.33° C (101° F), WBCs >11,000 μl
- Early symptoms of septicemia: flushed skin, tachycardia, fever, bounding pulse, ↑ CO with ↓ SVR

RELATED TOPICS

- Antimicrobial therapy
- Enterocutaneous fistulas
- Methicillin-resistant *Staphylococcus aureus*
- Multiple organ dysfunction syndrome
- Pneumonia, hospital-associated and immunocompromised
- Shock, septic
- Systemic inflammatory response syndrome

ABBREVIATIONS

MIC: Minimum inhibitory concentration
SIRS: Systemic inflammatory response syndrome

REFERENCES

Bisno AL: Molecular aspects of bacterial colonization, *Infect Control Hosp Epidemiol* 16(11): 648-657, 1995.

Jackson MM: Infection prevention and control. In Swearingen PL, Keen JH (eds): *Manual of critical care nursing*, ed 3, St Louis, 1995, Mosby.

Jarvis WR: The epidemiology of colonization, *Infect Control Hosp Epidemiol* 17(1): 47-52, 1996.

US Department of Health and Human Resources/Centers for Disease Control: Recommendations for preventing the spread of vancomycin resistance: recommendations of the hospital infection control practices advisory committee (HICPAC), *MMWR, Sept 1995.*

Author: **Janice Speas**

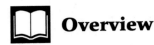 **Overview**

DESCRIPTION

Used to ↓ BP in hypertension or hypertensive crisis and to ↓ myocardial workload/O₂ consumption during heart failure, MI, and cardiogenic shock. Vasodilators cause blood vessels to dilate, resulting in ↓ arterial pressure, which assists the failing heart to eject blood into aorta. For treatment of hypertension, BP ↓; with heart failure, BP may ↑ as a result of ↑ CO/ventricular ejection.

INCIDENCE

>63 million Americans are hypertensive; 1% of this group experience hypertensive crisis.

HISTORY

- Heart failure, hypertension, hypertensive crisis, CAD, MI, angina
- Pulmonary embolism, pulmonary hypertension, pulmonary edema
- ASD, VSD, TIAs
- Peripheral vascular disease
- Aortic stenosis, aortic regurgitation, aortic aneurysm
- ↑ BP as a secondary problem to renal and endocrine disorders, pregnancy, drug-induced disorders, coarctation of aorta

RISK FACTORS

Vary with cause. If diuretic therapy unable to manage heart failure or ↑ BP effectively, vasodilators are the next treatment option. IV vasodilators used when immediate intervention necessary.

CLINICAL PRESENTATION (for patients requiring vasodilator therapy)

Cardiac Patients: Chest pain, SOB, activity intolerance
Hypertensive Patients: Headache, dizziness, fainting, fatigue, blurred vision
Hypertensive Crisis: Loss of vision, focal deficits, stupor, coma

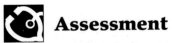 **Assessment**

(for patients requiring vasodilator therapy)

PHYSICAL ASSESSMENT

Findings vary with underlying disorder; when vasodilator therapy effective, many adverse symptoms should resolve.

Neuro: Confusion, restlessness, headache, visual disturbances
Resp: Crackles, dyspnea
CV: S₃ or summation gallop, pulsus alternans, JVD, tachycardia, dysrhythmias, fatigue
GI: Abdominal tenderness, nausea, vomiting, anorexia
GU: ↓ UO, possible hematuria or nocturia

VITAL SIGNS/HEMODYNAMICS

RR: ↑
HR: ↑
BP: ↓ with heart disease; ↑ with hypertension
Temp: Nl
CVP/PAWP: ↑ with heart failure and severely ↑ BP
CO: ↓
SVR: ↑
ECG: For patients with underlying CV disease or longstanding untreated hypertension, myocardial ischemia (depressed ST segments, inverted T waves) may be present. LV hypertrophy may be reflected by ↑ voltage in V₅-V₆.

LABORATORY STUDIES

Urinalysis: If ↑ BP or chronic heart failure has caused renal impairment, specific gravity may be low (<1.010) and proteinuria may be present.
Chemistries: If heart disease or hypertension is affecting kidneys, serum creatinine may be >1.3 mg/dl, BUN may be >20 mg/dl.
CBC: May reveal ↓ Hgb/Hct if dilutional anemia present.
ABGs: May signal hypoxemia (Pao₂ <80 mm Hg) if heart is failing.
Liver Enzymes (AST, ALT): If right side of heart is failing, hepatic veins may be congested, resulting in ↑ enzymes.

IMAGING

Chest X-ray: May reveal enlarged cardiac silhouette indicative of heart failure.
Echocardiography: Identifies LV hypertrophy with or without dilatation.
MUGA Scan: Evaluates LV function and detects aneurysms, wall motion abnormalities, and intracardiac shunting.
Angiography: May identify structural problems with the vasculature, eg, aortic aneurysm, or adrenal tumors.

DIAGNOSTIC PROCEDURE

Eye Assessment: For patients with visual disturbances with severely ↑ BP. Funduscopic evaluation of retina may reveal hemorrhage, fluffy cotton exudates, or vessel thickening, which can lead to severe visual impairment.

Collaborative Management

Supplemental O₂: To ↑ O₂ delivery to the tissues.
Hemodynamic Monitoring: To help guide fluid management, vasodilator therapy, and use of other vasoactive/inotropic drugs.
Fluid Restriction: Careful fluid management initiated to enable adequate filling of dilated vasculature while avoiding fluid overload.
Spo₂: For continuous monitoring of O₂ saturation.
ABGs: To assess for V/Q mismatching that may ensue with dilatation of the pulmonary vasculature.
Pharmacotherapy
Nitroprusside (Nipride): Dilates systemic arteries more than veins; used for hypertensive crisis to ↓ BP. Also used in combination with positive inotropic agents to ↓ afterload and ↑ CO/BP in LV failure. *Dosage range:* 0.5-8.0 μg/kg/min *via* continuous infusion, titrated to BP response.
Morphine: Dilates veins more than systemic arteries; used to ↓ preload in heart failure patients to ↑ or optimize pumping action of the heart. Relieves pulmonary edema. *Dosage range:* 2-5 mg IV push in incremental doses, titrated to BP response.
NTG: Dilates coronary arteries; dilates systemic veins more than arteries. Used to ↓ preload and ↑ coronary perfusion in heart failure. *Dosage range:* 5 μg/min to start, up to 200 μg/min. Not recommended as primary therapy for hypertension.
Hydralazine (Apresoline): Dilates systemic arteries more than veins; used for management of hypertension (adjunctive only for hypertensive crisis). Not recommended for treatment of heart failure; may aggravate angina. *Dosage range:* 10-20 mg IV bolus. May repeat to ↓ BP.
Labetalol (Normodyne): For management of severe hypertension and hypertensive crisis as primary therapy. Not recommended for heart failure. *Dosage range:* 20-80 mg IV push slowly, followed by IV infusion of 2 mg/min to total an additional 50-200 mg.
Amrinone (Inocor): Used to dilate arteries and veins to ↓ myocardial workload in heart failure management. Combination positive inotrope and vasodilator. *Dosage range:* 2-20 μg/kg/min following loading dose of .05 mg/kg over 10 min.
Milrinone (Primacor): Used to dilate arteries and veins to ↓ myocardial workload in heart failure management; combination positive inotrope and vasodilator. *Dosage range:* 0.375-0.75 μg/kg/min (average 0.5 μg/kg/min) following loading dose of 0.75 mg/kg over 2 min.

Nursing Diagnoses/Interventions

Altered cardiopulmonary, cerebral, GI, and renal tissue perfusion r/t ↓ arterial blood flow secondary to vasoconstriction that occurs with disturbance in autoregulation of BP

Desired outcome: Tissue perfusion corrected within 4 h of treatment onset: BP 100-160/60-100 mm Hg (or within 10% baseline); MAP 70-100 mm Hg; pupils equal and reactive to light; strength, sensation, and movement of extremities nl and bilaterally equal; UO >0.5 ml/kg/h; stable weight; breath sounds clear with RR 12-20 breaths/min; heart sounds S_1 and S_2 nl with HR 60-100 bpm. Within 48 h: BP <140/90 mm Hg, CO 5-7 L/min (CI 2.0-4.0 L/min/m^2), SVR 900-1400 dynes/sec/cm^{-5}, no chest pain, no headache.

- Monitor BP q1-5min (with MAP) during initial titration of IV drugs. As patient stabilizes, monitor BP q15min × 4, then at least qh. Be alert to sudden ↑ or ↓ in BP.
- Compare invasive arterial line BP to noninvasive BP reading. Document return to flow readings to validate accuracy of BP measurements. Compare to PA pressures, if available.
- Assess neurologic status at least qh until BP within acceptable range for patient; then check status at least q4h.
- Measure UO qh. Maintain careful I&O.
- Consider fluid restriction if renal impairment is suggested by BUN >20 mg or serum creatinine ≥1.5 mg/dl.
- If aortic aneurysm suspected, monitor pulses at least qh until stable, then q4h. Measure BP bilaterally in these patients.
- If aortic dissection suspected, be alert to any change in color, capillary refill, and temp of each extremity.
- Strive to relieve headache or chest discomfort with vasodilators. Be aware, though, that NTG relieves chest pain but may cause headache. Relief of angina is the goal, with headache an acceptable side effect.

Impaired gas exchange (or risk for same) r/t alveolar-capillary membrane changes secondary to heart failure

Desired outcome: Within 4 h of treatment initiation, patient has improved gas exchange: PaO_2 >80 mm Hg, $PaCO_2$ 35-45 mm Hg, HCO_3^- 22-26 mEq/L, pH 7.35-7.45, RR 12-20 breaths/min with eupnea, and absence of crackles.

- Monitor RR q1-2h. Be alert to RR >30 breaths/min with irregular rhythm or cough.
- Auscultate breath sounds, noting presence of crackles, wheezes, other adventitious sounds.
- Provide supplemental O_2 as indicated.
- Monitor SpO_2 for values <90%.
- Assess ABG findings. Note changes in response to supplemental O_2 or with treatment of altered hemodynamics.
- Place in high-Fowler's or semi-Fowler's position to maximize chest excursion and venous pooling (↓ preload occurs with pooling).

Miscellanea

CONSULT MD FOR
- Inability to control BP, profound dyspnea, chest pain, progressive abdominal distension, loss of peripheral pulses, uncontrollable headache, O_2 saturation <90%
- Possible complications: hypoxemia, MI, stroke, hypotension

RELATED TOPICS
- Aortic aneurysm/dissection
- Heart failure, right and left ventricular
- Hypertensive crisis
- Multiple organ dysfunction syndrome
- Myocardial infarction, acute
- Renal failure, acute

ABBREVIATIONS
ASD: Atrial septal defect
VSD: Ventral septal defect

REFERENCES
American Heart Association: *1993 heart and stroke facts statistics,* Publication No 55-0502, Dallas, 1993, The Association.

American Heart Association: *Textbook of advanced cardiac life support,* Dallas, 1994, The Association.

Baas LS: Hypertensive crisis. In Swearingen PL, Keen JH (eds): *Manual of critical care nursing,* ed 3, St Louis, 1995, Mosby.

Keen J, Baird M, Allen J: *Mosby's critical care and emergency drug reference,* ed 2, St Louis, 1996, Mosby.

Kinney M, Packa D, Dunbar S: *AACN's clinical reference for critical care nursing,* ed 3, St Louis, 1993, Mosby.

Steuble BT: Congestive heart failure/pulmonary edema. In Swearingen PL, Keen JH (eds): *Manual of critical care nursing,* ed 3, St Louis, 1995, Mosby.

Author: **Marianne Saunorus Baird**

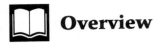 **Overview**

DESCRIPTION

For management of hypotension and shock states to ↑ size of vasculature, resulting in ↓ systemic pressure. Used with fluid therapy to ↑ BP in hypotension; may be particularly useful in vasodilated states, including anaphylactic, neurogenic, and septic shock.

HISTORY (for predisposition to shock state)
- Wound infection, insect bite
- IV contrast (dye)
- Spinal anesthesia
- Spinal cord injury
- Sepsis, bacteremia
- Surgery, trauma
- MI, CAD, rheumatic heart disease
- Immunosuppression, splenectomy
- Addison's disease, myxedema coma
- IV drug use

CLINICAL PRESENTATION (of patient in need of vasopressor therapy)
- May appear anxious, nervous, restless, possibly disoriented with tachypnea or respiratory distress; may have chest discomfort and feeling of impending doom.
- Unconsciousness in some patients
- If vasodilated, skin warm and moist
- If vasoconstricted, skin cool/clammy

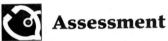 **Assessment**

(of patient progressing into shock state)

PHYSICAL ASSESSMENT
Neuro: Confusion, syncope, lightheadedness
Resp: Tachypnea, dyspnea, to acute respiratory distress (anaphylaxis); crackles (heart failure)
CV: Tachycardia, possible dysrhythmias; pulses may be ↓; hypotension; possible palpitations
GI: ↓/absent bowel sounds, nausea, vomiting
GU: ↓ UO
Integ: Varies with type of shock and other underlying conditions

VITAL SIGNS/HEMODYNAMICS
RR: ↑ early; ↓ late
HR: ↑ early; ↓ late
BP: ↓
Temp: Nl, subnormal, or ↑

ECG: May exhibit ST-segment depression caused by myocardial ischemia. SVT may be present to compensate for underlying perfusion/oxygenation deficit.

LABORATORY STUDIES
CBC with Differential: May reflect blood loss r/t hemorrhage or ↑ WBCs reflective of infectious process.
C&S of Suspect Infectious Sites: To identify source(s) of infection.
ABGs: May reflect metabolic acidosis caused by lactate accumulation during low perfusion states.
BUN/Creatinine: ↑ reflects ↓ renal perfusion.
Clotting Studies: May show ↑ PT, ↑ PTT, ↑ bleeding time, ↑ FDPs, ↓ platelets, which signal development of DIC resulting from shock state.
Liver Studies: AST, ALT, and LDH may be ↑ from liver ischemia caused by hypotension.

IMAGING
Chest X-ray, CT Scan of Chest/Abdomen: May reveal site of injury or disease process in lungs, heart, chest, or abdominal cavity(ies).
Spinal X-ray/CT Scan: If SCI suspected, may reveal site/extent of injury.
Echocardiogram: May reveal impairment of ventricular pumping action or structural abnormalities of the heart.
Angiography: May identify source of bleeding, vascular abnormalities.

DIAGNOSTIC PROCEDURE
Hemodynamic Monitoring: To guide fluid and vasopressor therapies and assist in diagnosing etiology of shock state/hypotension.

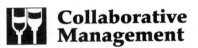 **Collaborative Management**

Varies, depending on type of shock or underlying disease process causing hypotension.
Supplemental O$_2$: Assists with delivery of O$_2$ to the tissues.
Spo$_2$: Monitors O$_2$ saturation and detects deficits/changes.
Fluid Resuscitation: Includes crystalloids and colloids to hydrate cells and retain fluids within the vasculature (↑ BP).
MAST: Will ↑ SVR *via* compression of blood vessels in lower extremities, optimally resulting in ↑ BP. Use is controversial.
ECG Monitoring: To detect cardiac dysrhythmias.

Hemodynamic Monitoring: For assessment of CO, PAP, SVR. Svo$_2$ monitoring *via* specialized catheter.
Correction of Acidosis: NaHCO$_3$ given IV push; guided by serial ABGs.
Pharmacotherapy
Norepinephrine (Levophed): Dose range is 2-12 μg/min IV infusion. Not indicated when hypotension is secondary to loss of intravascular volume (eg, bleeding, dehydration) unless aggressive rehydration/volume resuscitation is in progress. A very potent vasoconstrictor which, if misused, can cause severe peripheral tissue ischemia and necrosis. Titrate drug to BP response.
Dopamine (Intropin): Dose range for BP support is 3-10 μg/kg/min IV to ↑ pumping action of the heart. 11-20 μg/kg/min causes vasoconstriction while still allowing some effect of ↑ cardiac pumping action. Effects of doses <2 μg/kg/min cause dilatation of renal and mesenteric vessels *only* and should not have any effect on BP. Titrate drug to BP response.
Epinephrine (Adrenalin): Given IV push in ≥1 mg doses ≈ q3min in cardiac arrest/resuscitation situations. Average infusion dose range for BP support is 1-4 μg/min to ↑ pumping action of the heart. Infusion dose range for vasoconstriction (to ↓ size of blood vessels) is 4-12 μg/min. Titrate drug to BP response.
Phenylephrine (Neo-Synephrine): Average *initial* dose range for IV infusion is 100-180 μg/min; *maintenance* is 40-60 μg/min. Drug is a potent vasoconstrictor that should be used with aggressive fluid replacement therapy. Titrate to ↑ BP.
Methoxamine HCl (Vasoxyl): Older drug rarely used except when others have failed to ↑ BP. Average IV infusion dose is 5 μg/min, titrated to ↑ BP. Use with aggressive fluid therapy.

PATIENT-FAMILY TEACHING
- Purpose for hemodynamic monitoring, IV fluid administration, ECG, and O$_2$ delivery
- If anaphylactic shock experienced, information regarding how to identify and avoid antigen in future
- Support groups if trauma has resulted in loss of any bodily functions
- Purpose, expected results, anticipated sensations for nursing/medical interventions
- Medications: drug name, purpose, dosage, schedule, precautions, drug-drug and food-drug interventions, and potential side effects

Nursing Diagnoses/Interventions

Altered cardiopulmonary, cerebral, GI, and renal tissue perfusion r/t ↓ arterial blood flow secondary to shock/hypotension

Desired outcome: Tissue perfusion corrected within 4 h of treatment onset: HR 60-100 bpm, SBP >90 mm Hg, MAP >60 mm Hg, CVP 4-6 mm Hg, PAP 20-30/8-14 mm Hg, PAWP 6-12 mm Hg, SVR 900-1200 dynes/sec/cm^{-5}, peripheral pulses ≥2+ on 0-4+ scale, UO ≥0.5 ml/kg/h, and NSR on ECG.

- Assess for hypoxia, including confusion, agitation, restlessness, and irritability.
- Ensure patent airway *via* proper positioning of neck and frequent assessment of WOB and need for suctioning, as appropriate.
- Provide appropriate O_2 therapy, including mechanical ventilation, if indicated. Mechanical ventilation promotes oxygenation, ↓ $Paco_2$ to help relieve acidosis, and ↓ WOB.
- Monitor ABG values, paying particular attention to pH, $Paco_2$, and HCO_3^-. Low pH (<7.30), high $Paco_2$ (>45 mm Hg), or low HCO_3^- (<22 mEq/L) may signal deteriorating respiratory status and/or onset of lactic acidosis caused by hypoperfusion.
- Consider checking serum lactate level if ABGs continue to reflect acidosis despite aggressive fluid management, vasopressor infusions, and O_2 therapy/mechanical ventilation.

Miscellanea

CONSULT MD FOR

- Inability to control BP, profound dyspnea, chest pain, progressive abdominal distension, loss of bowel sounds, loss of peripheral pulses
- O_2 saturation <90%, UO <0.5 ml/kg/h for 2 consecutive h, temp >38.6° C (101.5° F)
- Inability to tolerate food or nutritional support for >24 h
- Possible complications: ARF, bowel ischemia or infarction, paralytic ileus, hypoxemia, peripheral ischemia, peripheral tissue anoxia resulting in loss of digits/limbs, MODS

RELATED TOPICS

- Anaphylaxis
- Hemodynamic monitoring
- Shock, cardiogenic
- Shock, hemorrhagic
- Shock, neurogenic
- Shock, septic

ABBREVIATIONS

FDPs: Fibrin degradation products
MODS: Multiple organ dysfunction syndrome

REFERENCES

American Heart Association: *Textbook of advanced cardiac life support,* Dallas, 1994, The Association.

Baas LS, Meissner JE: Cardiovascular care. In *Illustrated manual of nursing practice,* ed 2, Springhouse, Pa, 1994, Springhouse.

Keen J, Baird M, Allen J: *Mosby's critical care and emergency drug reference,* ed 2, St Louis, 1996, Mosby.

Kinney M, Packa D, Dunbar S: *AACN's clinical reference for critical care nursing,* ed 3, St Louis, 1993, Mosby.

Lasater M: Combining vasoactive infusions for maximal cardiac performance in the postoperative period, *Crit Care Nurs Q* 16(2): 11-16, 1993.

Author: **Marianne Saunorus Baird**

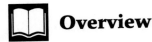 **Overview**

DESCRIPTION

Mechanical device used as a temporary measure to support massive LV and/or RV dysfunction by promoting rest and healing of damaged myocardium. VAD provides conduit that diverts blood from ventricle to an artificial pump and back to pulmonary or peripheral circulation. Recovery time, if achievable, ranges from 2-10 days.

Complications: Coagulopathy, bleeding, embolization, infection, sepsis, RV failure (with left-sided heart assist only), and renal failure.

HISTORY/RISK FACTORS

Indicated for individuals with the following:

- Acute ventricular dysfunction
- Shock after cardiotomy, angioplasty, or MI
- Cardiac arrest
- Massive pulmonary embolism
- Inability to wean from cardiopulmonary bypass

CLINICAL PRESENTATION

Pre-VAD

- Severe LV failure or cardiogenic shock: dyspnea at rest, extreme weakness, ↓ mental acuity, lethargy.
- Possible pallor, diaphoresis, cyanosis.
- Symptoms of biventricular failure: dyspnea, weakness, pallor; possible chest pain and diaphoresis.

Post-VAD

- Patient sedated, immobile.
- With thoracic approach, sternum is open for the cannulae, vasoactive drips, mechanical ventilation.

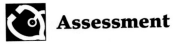 **Assessment**

PHYSICAL ASSESSMENT

Neuro: Agitation, restlessness, lethargy, confusion, unresponsiveness caused by ↓ cerebral perfusion

Resp: Hyperventilation, orthopnea, dyspnea at rest, crackles

CV: Pulses weak and often irregular, pulsus alternans, S_3 or S_4 sounds

GU: Oliguria

Integ: Cold, clammy, mottled skin

VITAL SIGNS/HEMODYNAMICS

RR: ↑

HR: ↑

BP: ↓ with narrow pulse pressure

Temp: Nl or ↓

RAP: ↑

PAP: ↑

PAWP: ↑

SVR: >1200/dynes/sec/cm^{-5}

CO: <4 L/min

CI: <1.5 L/min/m^2

Svo$_2$: <50%

ECG: Dysrhythmias may occur because of infarction, injury to areas of the conduction system or myocardium, or electrolyte imbalance. ST-segment change may denote ischemia or injury patterns.

Collaborative Management

VAD: LV assistance provided *via* either percutaneous cannulation of femoral artery or direct cannulation of atrium and ascending aorta, whereas a right VAD is used in right atrium and main pulmonary artery. In RV and LV failure, biventricular assistance is available. As condition improves, the goal is gradual weaning from device by ↓ flow rate.

IABP: Often used to ↓ afterload and promote pulsatile flow.

Prevention of Decannulation: *Via* pain control and sedation to maintain proper placement.

Pharmacotherapy

Positive inotropes, diuretics, afterload reduction: As needed, for medical treatment of underlying condition.

Paralytic agents: Sometimes used to prevent movement that might cause decannulation. These measures also will ↓ activity and thus ↓ tissue O_2 needs.

Dextran, heparin: For anticoagulation to prevent thrombi from forming on VAD.

Acid suppression therapy: Eg, with antacids, H_2 blockers. Usually prescribed to prevent GI bleeding.

Supplemental O$_2$: Humidified O_2 and mechanical ventilation often necessary to optimize tissue oxygenation.

PATIENT-FAMILY TEACHING

- Purpose, expected results, anticipated sensations of VAD insertion.
- Explanation that patient will be sedated and kept comfortable. Medical immobilization device for patient safety may be necessary.

If Femoral Incision Used

- Need to keep affected leg straight, as indicated, and remain on complete bed rest.
- Passive foot exercises without hip flexion.
- Importance of notifying staff member if pain, numbness, or tingling occurs in involved leg.

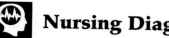

Nursing Diagnoses/Interventions

Altered protection r/t risk of bleeding secondary to therapeutic anticoagulation and effects of cardiopulmonary bypass, IABP, or VAD on blood components
Desired outcome: Throughout hospitalization, patient has no symptoms of internal or external bleeding: secretions and excretions negative for blood, chest-tube drainage within acceptable amounts (<100 ml/h), absence of ecchymoses and abdominal or back pain.
- Monitor Hct qd.
- Test gastric drainage and stool for blood qd.
- Monitor daily clotting studies (PT, PTT), platelets, and ACT. Desired range depends on whether patient is receiving anticoagulants. Anticoagulation with VAD in place is desirable but may not be feasible if patient is bleeding actively from surgical site.
- Inspect all drainage for evidence of bleeding.
- Administer coagulation factors as prescribed: platelets, FFP, cryoprecipitate, vitamin K, protamine sulfate, aminocaproic acid.
- Test gastric pH prn; administer acid suppression therapy to maintain pH >5.0.

Risk for disuse syndrome r/t imposed restrictions against movement secondary to presence of VAD or debilitated state
Desired outcome: Patient maintains baseline ROM without evidence of muscle atrophy or contracture formation.
- Patient can be turned gently from side to side if appropriate when VAD is in place. Do this q2h, observing VAD cannulas closely to ensure that tension is not placed on them during repositioning.
- Provide passive ROM to extremities qid.

Decreased cardiac output (or risk for same) r/t altered preload and negative inotropic changes secondary to ↓ RV contraction occurring with left-sided assist device
Note: This is a complication of the left-sided assist device, particularly when the outflow cannula is located in left ventricle. When left ventricle is decompressed, septal wall motion is diminished, thereby ↓ RV contraction. Patients with pulmonary hypertension or impaired RV function from AMI or cardiopulmonary bypass are especially prone to this problem.
Desired outcome: Within 24 h of this diagnosis, cardiac output is adequate: measured CO 4-7 L/min, RAP 4-6 mm Hg, PVR 60-100 dynes/sec/cm^{-5}, and LAP ≥10 mm Hg.
- Monitor for ↓ CO with associated ↑ in RAP and PVR, which are diagnostic of the complication just described.
- Ensure that patient attains prescribed IV fluid intake to maintain minimal LAP of 10 mm Hg. An adequate preload is necessary to prevent a vacuum effect from the device, which would aggravate this problem.

Miscellanea

CONSULT MD FOR
- Stool or gastric drainage positive for occult blood
- PT, PTT, ACT, INR ↑ above desired range
- Platelets <100,000 μl
- Left VAD impairment of RV contractility: ↓ CO with ↑ RAP, PVR
- UO <0.5 ml/kg/h × 2 h

RELATED TOPICS
- Cardiac transplantation: preoperative
- Cardiomyopathy
- Heart failure, left ventricular and right ventricular
- Pulmonary embolus, thrombotic
- Shock, cardiogenic

ABBREVIATIONS
FFP: Fresh frozen plasma
IABP: Intraaortic balloon pump

REFERENCES
Brannon P, Towner S: Ventricular failure: new therapy using the mechanical assist device, *Crit Care Nurse* 6(2): 70-84, 1986.
Coombs M: Ventricular assist devices for the failing heart: a nursing focus, *Intensive and Crit Care Nurs* 9(1): 17-23, 1993.
Ley J: Myocardial depression after cardiac surgery: pharmacologic and mechanical support, *AACN Clin Issues in Crit Care Nurs* 4(2): 301-306, 1993.
Vaca KS, Lohmann DP, Moroney DA: Current status and future trends of mechanical circulatory support, *Crit Care Nurs Clin North Am* 7(2): 249-259, 1995.

Author: **Cheryl L. Bittel**

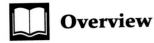 **Overview**

PATHOPHYSIOLOGY
Cardiac dysrhythmia during which multiple ventricular ectopic pacing sites fire so rapidly that heart quivering occurs, resulting in loss of all ventricular pumping action. Cardiac arrest requires immediate defibrillation to stabilize the heart's electrical potential.

INCIDENCE
Most common dysrhythmia causing cardiac arrest/sudden cardiac death

HISTORY/RISK FACTORS
- CAD, AMI, angina
- Electrolyte imbalances, hypoxemia
- Cocaine use
- Electric shock from AC current
- Antidysrhythmic drug toxicity, especially quinidine, procainamide, disopyramide
- Malnutrition
- Risk factors for CAD: eg, cigarette smoking, DM
- Unusual stress in patients with hx of CAD

CLINICAL PRESENTATION
Immediate cardiac arrest/sudden death manifested by pulselessness and apnea

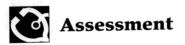 **Assessment**

PHYSICAL ASSESSMENT
Neuro: Unconsciousness, unresponsive to painful stimuli
Resp: Apnea, absent breath sounds
CV: Pulselessness, absent heart tones
GI: Possible vomiting, incontinence
GU: Possible incontinence
Integ: Cold, clammy, cyanotic, or greyish skin

VITAL SIGNS/HEMODYNAMICS
RR: Absent
HR: Absent
BP: Absent
Temp: Nl or ↓
CVP/PAWP: ↓ or absent
SVR: ↓
CO: Absent
12/18-Lead ECG: Reflects rhythm generated from multiple, chaotic ventricular pacing sites. Rhythm irregular with inability to determine atrial rate; ventricular rate >360/min of chaotic "quivering;" absence of P waves, QRS complexes replaced by fibrillatory waves; P: QRS relationship unable to be determined.

LABORATORY STUDIES
Serum Electrolytes: To identify values, eg, ↓ K^+ and Mg^{2+}, that may precipitate dysrhythmias.
Antidysrhythmic Drug Levels: Key in rhythm control and prevention of drug toxicity. Levels of medications used for hypertension, respiratory diseases, or other disorders also may precipitate VF. Medications used to treat PVCs sometimes precipitate VT or VF when PVCs are controlled.
Drug/Toxicology Screening: For amphetamines, cocaine, and other street drugs; may reveal possible cause for VF.
ABGs: May reflect hypoxemia or pH abnormality that can interfere with electrolyte balance.

IMAGING
Chest X-ray: May reflect enlarged cardiac silhouette indicative of heart disease. Also used to evaluate ET tube placement if used during resuscitation.
Echocardiography: To evaluate cardiac structural anomalies and ventricular pumping action after stabilization.
Cardiac Catheterization: To assess for CAD either before event or after stabilization.

DIAGNOSTIC PROCEDURES
EP Study: Pacing stimulus given at varying sites and voltages; useful for diagnosing potential for future episodes of VT and VF.

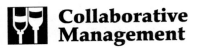 **Collaborative Management**

GENERAL
Immediate Defibrillation: At 200 watt/sec.
- If unsuccessful, shock at 300 watt/sec.
- If unsuccessful, shock at 360 watt/sec.
- After three shocks, assess rhythm, check pulse, and begin CPR.
  If no defibrillator available initially, continue CPR until defibrillator available. When defibrillator arrives, and following initial three shocks, shock at 360 watt/sec ≈ q3min.
Oxygenation: ET intubation and bag-valve-tube ventilation with 100% O_2 if rhythm not immediately restored.

PHARMACOTHERAPY
ACUTE
Epinephrine: ≥1 mg IV push given ≈ q3min throughout resuscitation.
Lidocaine: 1.0-1.5 mg/kg given IV push q3-5min up to maximum of 3 mg/kg administered.
Bretylium: If lidocaine ineffective. Given 5 mg/kg IV push. If ineffective, 5 min later, 10 mg/kg given IV push.
Procainamide: If bretylium ineffective. Given at 30 mg/min IV infusion, up to maximum of 17/kg IV push.
MgSO₄: 1-2 g IV infusion or slow IV push given in torsades de pointes, suspected hypomagnesemic state, or refractory VF.
PREVENTIVE/ADJUNCTIVE
β Blockers (ie, propranolol, metoprolol): May be given IV push during resuscitation if other medications fail or PO to help prevent further occurrences of VF. Effective in VF prevention for patient with AMI.
Class IA Antidysrhythmics (quinidine, procainamide, disopyramide): Avoided for maintenance therapy, since they ↓ VF threshhold.
Sotalol, Amiodarone: May be used to prevent/treat VF if K^+ level nl. Hypokalemia promotes VF when these medications used.

SURGERY
ICD: Programmed to deliver synchronized cardioversion or defibrillation when patient's HR > programmed rate or manifests programmed abnormal ECG morphology. Newer devices also act as cardiac pacemakers.
LV Aneurysmectomy and Infarctectomy: Excision of possible focal spots of ventricular dysrhythmias.
Stellate Ganglionectomy and Block: Alters electrical stability of the myocardium and predisposition to ventricular dysrhythmias.
Myocardial Revascularization: For patients with CAD to ↑ perfusion to all heart areas. Ischemia may trigger ventricular dysrhythmias.

PATIENT-FAMILY TEACHING
- Importance of reporting all adverse symptoms promptly
- Discussion of VF in relation to cause, medications, electrical devices used to treat it, expected results, and anticipated sensations
- Importance and purpose of smoking cessation
- Support groups
- Alteration in sexuality if ICD placed

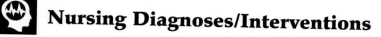 **Nursing Diagnoses/Interventions**

Decreased cardiac output r/t cardiac arrest secondary to altered rate, rhythm, conduction, and negative inotropic effects of VF
Desired outcomes: Within 15 min of VF onset, patient converted to a rhythm with adequate cardiac output: all stated parameters returned to within 10% of baseline *or* SBP >90 mm Hg, HR 60-100 bpm, NSR on ECG, PAP 20-30/8-15 mm Hg, PAWP 6-12 mm Hg, CVP 2-6 mm Hg, CO 4-7 L/min, CI 2.5-4.0 L/min/m^2.

- Defibrillate and continue treatment according to agency protocol or ACLS guidelines.
- Perform CPR according to BLS guidelines.
- Monitor ECG continuously during and following resuscitation, noting onset, duration, pattern, and termination of dysrhythmias, including response to antidysrhythmics.
- Monitor VS at least q5min during immediate postresuscitation period.
- Save rhythm strips for documentation of VF.
- Use 12/18-lead ECG to diagnose new, symptomatic dysrhythmias.
- Monitor SpO$_2$ continuously, noting changes with dysrhythmias.
- Monitor laboratory data closely for ↓ Mg^{2+} and K$^+$ values.
- Reduce as many environmental stressors as possible.
- Remain with patient if new dysrhythmias or deterioration occurs. Monitor response to treatments.
- Provide supplemental O$_2$ for symptomatic dysrhythmias.

Altered cerebral, renal, peripheral, and cardiopulmonary tissue perfusion r/t interrupted arterial blood flow to vital organs secondary to inadequate arterial pressure
Desired outcomes: Within 24 h of resuscitation, patient has adequate tissue perfusion: all vital parameters returned to within 10% of baseline *or* HR 60-100 bpm, SBP >90 mm Hg, RR 12-20 breaths/min, UO ≥0.5 ml/kg/h, oriented × 3, peripheral pulses ≥2+ on 0-4+ scale, brisk capillary refill (<2 sec), skin warm and dry.

- Check neurologic status q1-2h to assess cerebral perfusion.
- Monitor I&O qh to assess renal perfusion.
- Monitor ABGs as needed/prescribed to check pH for normalization postcode.
- Check serum lactate level to monitor for improvement of perfusion/tissue oxygenation.
- Monitor peripheral pulses, capillary refill, and skin q2h.
- Titrate vasoactive drugs, if needed, to maintain SBP >90 mm Hg.

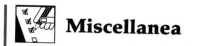 **Miscellanea**

CONSULT MD FOR
- Recurrent VF with cardiac arrest
- Failure of dysrhythmia to respond to prescribed treatments
- Inappropriate "firing" of ICD device
- Failure to attain or exceeding of therapeutic antidysrhythmic drug level
- Chest pain, SOB, ↓ BP, altered mental status before/after resuscitation
- SpO$_2$ <90%
- ↑ PAP, CVP, PAWP before/after resuscitation
- Possible complications: hypoxemia, MODS, heart failure, renal failure, stroke, antidysrhythmic drug toxicity, refractory VF

RELATED TOPICS
- Antidysrhythmic therapy
- Coronary artery disease
- Heart failure, left
- Hypokalemia
- Hypomagnesemia
- Implantable cardioverter/defibrillator
- Myocardial infarction, acute
- Drug overdose: amphetamines, cocaine

ABBREVIATIONS
BLS: Basic life support
EP: Electrophysiologic
ICD: Implantable cardioverter/defibrillator
MODS: Multiple organ dysfunction syndrome

REFERENCES
American Heart Association: *Textbook of advanced cardiac life support,* Dallas, 1994, The Association.
Darling EJ: Overview of cardiac electrophysiological testing, *Crit Care Nurs Clin North Am* 6(1): 1-14, 1994.
Dracup K: *Meltzer's intensive coronary care: a manual for nurses,* ed 5, Norwalk, Conn, 1995, Appleton & Lange.
Jacobsen C: Arrhythmias and conduction disturbances. In Woods SL: *Cardiac nursing,* ed 3, Philadelphia, 1995, Lippincott.
Keen J, Baird M, Allen J: *Mosby's critical care and emergency drug reference,* ed 2, St Louis, 1996, Mosby.
Morton PG: Update on new antidysrhythmic drugs, *Crit Care Nurs Clin North Am* 6(1): 69-84, 1994.
Porterfield LM: The cutting edge in arrhythmias, *Crit Care Nurse (Suppl):* June 1993.
Steuble BT: Dysrhythmias and conduction disturbances. In Swearingen PL, Keen JH (eds): *Manual of critical care nursing,* ed 3, St Louis, 1995, Mosby.
Witherell CL: Cardiac rhythm control devices, *Crit Care Nurs Clin North Am* 6(1): 85-102, 1994.

Authors: **Marianne Saunorus Baird and Barbara Tueller Steuble**

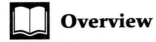 **Overview**

PATHOPHYSIOLOGY

Cardiac dysrhythmia in which the pacing site is located on the ventricle and HR >100 bpm and usually <150 bpm. Symptomatic VT must be treated *stat* as it can deteriorate into a pulseless rhythm, necessitating CPR with management identical to VF.

HISTORY/RISK FACTORS

- CAD (and its risk factors), AMI
- Unusual stress in patients with hx of CAD
- Electrolyte imbalances, hypoxemia
- Cocaine, amphetamine use
- Antidysrhythmic drug toxicity (especially quinidine, procainamide, disopyramide)
- Anorexia, bulimia, malnutrition

CLINICAL PRESENTATION

- Symptoms of low CO and perfusion deficits: altered mental status, activity intolerance, hypotension, chest pain, oliguria
- SOB, dizziness, fainting, diaphoresis, nausea, easy fatigability, sensation of heart "pounding" in chest, distressed appearance, pallor

 Assessment

PHYSICAL ASSESSMENT

Neuro: Altered LOC, syncope, weakness, fainting, vertigo, anxiety, restlessness
Resp: Dyspnea, SOB
CV: Activity intolerance, hypotension, possible CV collapse
GI: Nausea, vomiting, heartburn-like pain
GU: ↓ UO
Integ: Diaphoresis, pallor, cyanosis

VITAL SIGNS/HEMODYNAMICS

RR: Nl or ↑
HR: ↑ apical; radial may be ↓
BP: Nl or ↓
Temp: Nl
CVP/PAWP: Nl or ↓
SVR: ↑
CO: ↓
12/18-Lead ECG: Rhythm generated from a ventricular pacing site regular to slightly irregular; atrial rate indeterminable; ventricular rate usually 150-250 bpm but may be as low as 100 bpm; P waves usually not visible; QRS complex bizarre with wide appearance (>0.12 sec); PR interval and P:QRS cannot be determined.
Ambulatory Monitoring/24-h Holter/Cardiac Event Recording: Identifies subtle or periodic dysrhythmias with patient keeping ongoing record of symptoms.

LABORATORY STUDIES

Serum Electrolytes: To identify abnormal values (eg, ↓ K^+, Mg^{2+}) that may precipitate VT.
Therapeutic Drug Levels: Monitoring antidysrhythmic drug levels key in controlling rhythm and preventing toxicity.
Drug/Toxicology Screening: For amphetamines, cocaine, and other stimulants that cause VT.
ABGs: May reflect hypoxemia or pH abnormality that can interfere with electrolyte balance.

IMAGING

Chest X-ray: May reflect enlarged silhouette of heart disease.
Echocardiography: To evaluate ventricular pumping action, including estimation of ventricular EF.
Cardiac Catheterization: Assesses if patient has CAD.

DIAGNOSTIC PROCEDURES

EP Study: Pacing stimulus given at varying sites and voltages to determine point of origin, inducibility, effectiveness of drug therapy in suppressing VT.

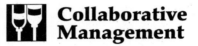 **Collaborative Management**

GENERAL

Supplemental O_2: To support oxygenation of the tissues.
Cardiac Monitoring: To detect all dysrhythmias, observing onset, duration, termination of intermittent dysrhythmias.
Management of Other Causes of Tachydysrhythmias: Eg, hypoxia, hypokalemia, hypomagnesemia, preexisting acidosis, endocrine disorders (hyperthyroidism), or drug overdose/toxicity.
Synchronized Cardioversion: To convert VT, using ACLS guidelines.
Defibrillation: To convert pulseless VT to rhythm that generates a pulse, following ACLS guidelines.
Cardiac Antitachycardia Pacing: Operator of pulse generator exceeds patient's HR using pacemaker until capture attained and then slowly ↓ HR.
Spo₂: Detects ↓ O_2 saturation caused by potentially lethal dysrhythmias; assesses for hypoxia.

PHARMACOTHERAPY

To avoid drug toxicity, dysrhythmias treated with lowest possible dose that successfully terminates abnormal rhythm. Goal: to convert pacing site to atrial site, ideally SA node, to enable most effective cardiac cycle.

Class I Antidysrhythmic Drugs: ↓ ventricular automaticity, ↓ ventricular conduction velocity, delay ventricular repolarization, and ↑ conduction through AV node.
Lidocaine: Drug of choice for VT. Given 1.0-1.5 mg/kg IV push initially, followed by 0.5-0.75 mg/kg IV q5-10min to a maximal dose of 3 mg/kg. Initial loading followed by a 1-4 mg/min IV infusion.
Procainamide: Second choice for VT. Given 20-30 mg/min to a maximal total dose of 17 mg/kg for rhythm conversion. Dosage stopped if QRS widens >50% or hypotension occurs. Initial loading dose followed by 1-4 mg/min IV infusion.
Others: Quinidine, mexiletine, disopyramide.
Class III antidysrhythmic drugs: ↑ action potential and refractory period of Purkinje fibers, ↑ VF threshold, restore injured myocardial cell electrophysiology toward nl, and suppress reentrant dysrhythmias.
Bretylium: Third choice for VT. Given 5-10 mg/kg over 8-10 min to a maximal total dose of 30 mg/kg over 24 h. Initial loading followed by a 1-4 mg/min IV infusion.
Others: Amiodarone, sotalol.

SURGERY/OTHER PROCEDURES

ICD: Programmed to deliver synchronized cardioversion or defibrillation when HR > programmed rate or abnormal ECG morphology present. Newer devices also act as cardiac pacemakers.
Myocardial Revascularization: Excision or cryoablation of dysrhythmia focus.
LV Aneurysmectomy/Infarctectomy: Excision of focal points of ventricular dysrhythmias.
Encircling Ventriculotomy: Excision of diseased portion of ventricle without compromising myocardial blood supply.
Stellate Ganglionectomy and Block: Alters electrical stability of myocardium and predisposition to ventricular dysrhythmias.
Radiofrequency Catheter Ablation: Electrically generated heat stimulus applied to specific point of origin of dysrhythmia (determined by EP studies); results in necrosis of abnormal tissue generating dysrhythmia.

PATIENT-FAMILY TEACHING

- Importance of promptly reporting chest pain, lightheadedness, SOB, activity intolerance, syncope
- Self-measuring of pulse rate/rhythm
- Causes of VT; pacing devices used during/after hospitalization
- Medications: purpose, dosage, schedule, precautions, drug-drug and food-drug interactions, and potential side effects
- Support group information
- Potential for altered sexuality if patient has an ICD

Nursing Diagnoses/Interventions

Decreased cardiac output r/t altered rate, rhythm, conduction; r/t negative inotropic cardiac changes secondary to cardiac disease

Desired outcome: Within 15 min of dysrhythmia onset, cardiac output adequate: BP $\geq$90/60 mm Hg, HR 60-100 bpm with NSR on ECG, PAP 20-30/8-15 mm Hg, PAWP 6-12 mm Hg, CVP 2-6 mm Hg, CO 4-7 L/min, CI 2.5-4.0 L/min/m^2, or all within 10% baseline parameters.

- Monitor continuous ECG, noting onset, duration, pattern, and termination of dysrhythmias, including response to antidysrhythmics.
- Monitor VS at least q5min throughout dysrhythmia if patient unstable.
- Document dysrhythmias *via* rhythm strips.
- Note changes in SpO$_2$ with symptomatic dysrhythmias.
- Manage life-threatening dysrhythmias using ACLS/institutional guidelines.
- Provide supplemental O$_2$ for symptomatic dysrhythmias.
- Monitor lab values, noting K$^+$ and Mg^{2+} carefully.
- Reduce as many environmental stressors as possible.
- Administer medications that support CO and BP if antidysrhythmics or cardioversion ineffective.
- Remain with patient if new dysrhythmias or deterioration occur; monitor response to treatments.

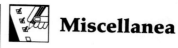

Miscellanea

CONSULT MD FOR
- Failure of dysrhythmia to respond to treatments
- Inappropriate "firing" of ICD device
- Failure to attain/exceeding of therapeutic antidysrhythmic drug level
- Chest pain, SOB, $\downarrow$ BP, altered mental status
- SpO$_2$ <90%; $\uparrow$ PAP, CVP, PAWP
- Possible complications: hypoxemia, cardiac arrest, heart failure, new or worsened dysrhythmias, antidysrhythmic drug toxicity, stroke

RELATED TOPICS
- Antidysrhythmic therapy
- Coronary artery disease
- Drug overdose: amphetamine
- Drug overdose: cocaine
- Hypokalemia
- Hypomagnesemia
- Myocardial infarction, acute
- Ventricular fibrillation

ABBREVIATIONS
EF: Ejection fraction
EP: Electrophysiology
ICD: Implantable cardioverter/defibrillator

REFERENCES
American Heart Association: *Textbook of advanced cardiac life support,* Dallas, 1994, The Association.

Darling EJ: Overview of cardiac electrophysiological testing, *Crit Care Nurs Clin North Am* 6(1): 1-14, 1994.

Dracup K: *Meltzer's intensive coronary care: a manual for nurses,* ed 5, Norwalk, Conn, 1995, Appleton & Lange.

Finkelmeier BA: Ablative therapy in the treatment of tachyarrhythmias, *Crit Care Nurs Clin North Am* 6(1): 103-110, 1994.

Goodrich CA: Management of tachyarrhythmias in the CCU: *Curr Issues Crit Care Nurs (Suppl):* 7-11, 1995.

Jacobsen C: Arrhythmias and conduction disturbances. In Woods SL: *Cardiac nursing,* ed 3, Philadelphia, 1995, Lippincott.

Keen J, Baird M, Allen J: *Mosby's critical care and emergency drug reference,* ed 2, St Louis, 1996, Mosby.

Moser DK, Woo MA: Recurrent ventricular tachycardia, *Crit Care Nurs Clin North Am* 6(1): 15-26, 1994.

Porterfield LM: The cutting edge in arrhythmias, *Crit Care Nurse (Suppl):* June 1993.

Authors: **Marianne Saunorus Baird and Barbara Tueller Steuble**

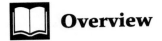 **Overview**

PATHOPHYSIOLOGY

A wound is disruption of tissue integrity caused by trauma, surgery, or underlying medical disorder. Clean, surgical, or traumatic wounds whose edges are closed with sutures, clips, or sterile tape strips are referred to as wounds closed by primary intention.

HISTORY/RISK FACTORS (for impaired healing)

- Obesity
- Advanced age
- Diabetes mellitus
- GI, digestive disorders
- Malignancy
- Undernourishment
- Corticosteroid therapy
- Immunosuppression, chemotherapy, radiation therapy
- Impaired perfusion to wound site

CLINICAL PRESENTATION

Impaired healing may manifest as dehiscence, evisceration, infection, or delayed healing.

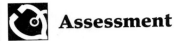 **Assessment**

PHYSICAL ASSESSMENT
Optimal Healing

- Initially, incision line warm, well approximated, reddened, indurated, and tender.
- After 1 or 2 days: no drainage from incision line.
- After 7-9 days: formation of healing ridge, a palpable accumulation of scar tissue.

Impaired Healing

- Lack of adequate inflammatory response: absence of initial warmth, induration and inflammation that persist or occur after fifth postinjury day.
- Continued drainage from incision line 2 days after injury (when no drain present).
- Absence of healing ridge by ninth day.
- Presence of purulent exudate.

VITAL SIGNS/HEMODYNAMICS

RR: NI; ↑ with infection
HR: NI; ↑ with infection
BP: NI
Temp: NI; ↑ with infection or inflammatory response
CVP/PAWP: NI
CO: NI; may be ↑ with infection or inflammatory response
SVR: NI; may be ↓ with infection or inflammatory response

LABORATORY STUDIES

WBCs with Differential: ↑ with left shift for infection.
Gram's Stain: If infection suspected, aids in selection of preliminary antibiotics.
C&S: Determines optimal antibiotic according to sensitivities of specific organism. Infection signaled by ≥10^5 organisms per gram of tissue or ≥4 organisms.

Collaborative Management

Sterile Dressing: Protects wound from external contamination/ trauma; may provide pressure. Usually, surgeon removes initial dressing.
Nutrition: Regular diet promotes positive nitrogen balance for optimal wound healing. Enteral supplements, tube feedings, or PN may be necessary for malnourished patients or those with GI dysfunction.
Multivitamins, Especially C: Promote tissue healing.
Minerals, Especially Zinc and Iron: Prescribed, depending on serum levels, to promote healing.
I&D: To drain pus when infection present and localized. Allows healing by secondary intention. Wound may be irrigated with antimicrobials.
Pharmacotherapy
Insulin: Controls glucose levels in individuals with DM, since ↑ blood glucose interferes with tissue healing.
Local or systemic antibiotics: Used prophylactically and when infection present.

PATIENT-FAMILY TEACHING

- Wound care procedure, purpose, expected results, anticipated sensations
- Signs of infection, impaired healing
- Medications: drug name, purpose, dosage, schedule, precautions, food-drug and drug-drug interactions, potential side effects

Nursing Diagnoses/Interventions

Impaired tissue integrity: Wound, r/t altered circulation, infection, metabolic disorders (eg, DM), alterations in fluid volume and nutrition, and medical therapy (chemotherapy, radiation therapy, steroid administration)

Desired outcome: Patient exhibits the following signs of wound healing: well-approximated wound edges; good initial postinjury inflammatory response (erythema, warmth, induration, pain); no inflammatory response after fifth day postinjury; no drainage (without drain present) 48 h after closure; healing ridge present by 7-9 days postop.

- Assess wound for indications of impaired healing: absence of healing ridge, presence of drainage or purulent exudate, delayed or prolonged inflammatory response. Monitor VS for signs of infection: ↑ temp and HR. Document findings.
- Follow proper infection-control techniques when changing dressings. If a drain is present, keep it sterile, maintain patency, and handle it gently to prevent dislodging it. If wound care will be necessary after hospital discharge, teach dressing change procedure to patient and significant others.
- For persons with DM, perform serial monitoring of blood glucose and administer insulin to keep glucose level <200 mg/dl.
- Explain that deep breathing promotes oxygenation, which enhances wound healing. If indicated, provide incentive spirometry at least qid. Stress importance of position changes and activity as tolerated to promote ventilation. Splint incision as needed.
- Monitor perfusion status by checking BP, HR, capillary refill in tissue adjacent to incision, moisture of mucous membranes, skin turgor, volume and specific gravity of urine, and I&O.
- For nonrestricted patients, ensure fluid intake of at least 2-3 L/day.
- Encourage ambulation or ROM exercises as allowed to promote circulation to wound.
- To promote positive nitrogen balance, which enhances wound healing, provide a diet with adequate protein, vitamin C, and calories. Encourage between-meal supplements. If patient complains of feeling full with three meals a day, give more frequent small feedings.

Miscellanea

CONSULT MD FOR
- Signs of impaired wound healing
- Inflammation that persists/occurs after fifth day
- Persistent drainage from incision line after 48 h
- Presence of purulent exudate
- ↑ WBC with left shift
- Positive wound C&S

RELATED TOPICS
- Antimicrobial therapy
- Nutrition, enteral and parenteral
- Shock, septic
- Wounds healing by secondary intention

ABBREVIATION
PN: Parenteral nutrition

REFERENCES
Krasner D: The ABCs of wound care dressings, *Ostomy/Wound Management* 39(8): 66-72, 1993.

Stotts NA, Wipke-Tevis D: Co-factors in impaired wound healing, *Ostomy/Wound Management* 42(2): 44-56, 1996.

Stotts NA: Determination of bacterial burden in wounds, *Adv Wound Care* 8(4): 28-52, 1995.

Stotts NA: Wound and skin care. In Swearingen PL, Keen JH (eds): *Manual of critical care nursing,* ed 3, St Louis, 1995, Mosby.

Author: **Nancy Stotts**

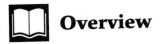 **Overview**

PATHOPHYSIOLOGY
Involves wounds with tissue loss or heavy contamination that form granulation tissue and contract in order to heal. Most often, healing impairment caused by infection or impaired perfusion, oxygenation, and nutrition.

HISTORY/RISK FACTORS (for impaired healing)
- Obesity
- Advanced age
- Diabetes mellitus
- GI, digestive disorders
- Malignancy
- Undernourishment
- Corticosteroid therapy
- Immunosuppression, chemotherapy, radiation therapy
- Impaired perfusion to wound site

CLINICAL PRESENTATION
Initially, wound edges inflamed, indurated, and tender.

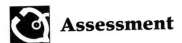 **Assessment**

PHYSICAL ASSESSMENT
Optimal Healing: At first, granulation tissue on wound floor and walls is pink, progressing to deeper pink and then to beefy red; it should be moist. As healing occurs, wound edges become pink, angle between surrounding tissue and wound becomes less acute, and wound contraction occurs. Occasionally a wound has a tract or sinus that gradually ↓ in size as healing occurs. Time frame for healing depends on wound size/location and physical/psychologic status.
Impaired Healing: Exudate appears on wound floor and walls and does not abate as healing progresses. It is important to note exudate distribution, color, odor, volume, and adherence. Assess surrounding skin for tissue damage: disruption, discoloration, and ↑ pain. When drain in place, evaluate drainage volume, color, and odor.

VITAL SIGNS/HEMODYNAMICS
RR: Nl; ↑ with infection
HR: Nl; ↑ with infection

Temp: Nl; ↑ with infection or inflammatory response
CVP/PAWP: Nl
CO: Nl; may be ↑ with infection or inflammatory response
SVR: Nl; may be ↓ with infection or inflammatory response

LABORATORY STUDIES
CBC with WBC Differential: To assess Hct and possible infection. Watch for ↑ WBC and shift to left, which indicates infection. Monitor lymphocyte count; ≤1800 µl may be a sign of malnutrition. For optimal healing, Hct should be >20 g/dl.
Gram's Stain: If infection suspected, aids in selection of preliminary antibiotics.
C&S: Determines optimal antibiotic according to sensitivities of specific organism. Infection present when there are ≥10^5 organisms per gram of tissue or ≥4 organisms.

IMAGING
Ultrasound, Sonogram, or Sinogram: To determine wound size, especially when abscesses or tracts suspected.

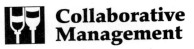 **Collaborative Management**

PHARMACOTHERAPY
Insulin: Controls glucose levels in individuals with DM, since ↑ blood glucose interferes with tissue healing.
Local or Systemic Antibiotics: Used prophylactically and when infection present.
Multivitamins, Especially C: Promote tissue healing.
Minerals, Especially Zinc and Iron: Prescribed, depending on serum levels, to promote healing.
Débriding Enzymes: Soften and remove necrotic tissue, eg, collagenase (Santyl).
Absorbent Agents: Remove contaminants and excess exudate, eg, dextran beads or paste (Envisan) or polymer flakes (Bard Absorption Dressing).

DRESSINGS
Provide débridement, keep healthy wound tissue moist, provide antiseptic agents.
Moist Gauze With or Without Antiseptic: Insert and remove while moist. Provides means for topical antiinfective agent; good débridement; not painful; inexpensive. If excessively wet, can cause tissue maceration.

Impregnated (Xeroform, Vaseline gauze): Provides topical antiseptic; keeps tissue hydrated; minimal pain with removal.
Transparent (eg, OpSite, Tegaderm, Bioclusive): Prevents wound fluid loss; protects from external contamination, friction, and fluid loss; minimal pain with removal. May withdraw excess exudate and reseal dressing; presence of exudate may erroneously suggest infection.
Hydrocolloid (eg, Duoderm, Cutinova): Protects wound; provides autolytic débridement; easy to apply; minimizes pain.
Hydrogel (Hypergel, FLEXDERM): Protects wound; absorbent; autolytic; débrides; can administer topical drugs.
Foam (Lyofoam, NU-DERM, Allevyin): Insulates wound; provides padding; easy to apply.
Alginate (eg, Sorbsan, Kaltostat): Absorbs drainage; fills dead space; minimal pain; requires secondary dressing.

HYDROTHERAPY
Softens and removes debris mechanically.

WOUND IRRIGATION WITH OR WITHOUT ANTIINFECTIVE AGENTS
Dislodges and removes bacteria and loosens necrotic tissue, foreign bodies, and exudate.

DRAIN(S)
Remove excess tissue fluid or purulent drainage.

SURGICAL INTERVENTIONS
Débridement: Removes dead tissue and ↓ debris and fibrotic tissue.
Skin Graft: Provides wound coverage if necessary.
Tissue Flaps: Fill tissue defects and provide wound closure.

NUTRITION
Regular diet promotes positive nitrogen balance for optimal wound healing. Enteral supplements, tube feedings, PN may be necessary for malnourished patients or those with GI dysfunction.

PATIENT-FAMILY TEACHING
- Wound care procedure, expected results, anticipated sensations
- Signs of infection, impaired healing
- Medications: drug name, purpose, dosage, schedule, precautions, food-drug and drug-drug interactions, potential side effects

Nursing Diagnoses/Interventions

Impaired tissue integrity: Wound, r/t infection, metabolic disorders (eg, DM), medical therapy (eg, chemotherapy, radiation therapy), altered perfusion, immunosuppression, malnutrition
Desired outcomes: Wound exhibits signs of healing: initially, postinjury wound edges inflamed, indurated, tender; with epithelialization, edges pink within 1 wk of injury; granulation tissue develops (identified by pink tissue that becomes beefy red) within 1 wk of injury. There is no odor, exudate, or necrotic tissue. Patient or significant other successfully demonstrates wound care procedure before hospital discharge.

- Monitor for impaired healing: ↓ inflammatory response postinjury or response that lasts >5 days; epithelialization slowed or mechanically disrupted and noncontinuous around wound; granulation tissue remaining pale or excessively dry or moist; presence of odor, exudate, and/or necrotic tissue.
- Apply prescribed dressing. Insert dressing into all tracts to promote gradual closure of those areas. Ensure good hand washing before/after dressing changes; dispose of contaminated dressings appropriately.
- When drain used, maintain its patency and prevent kinking of tubing; secure tubing to prevent drain from becoming dislodged. Use aseptic technique when caring for drains.
- To help prevent contamination, cleanse skin surrounding wound with a mild disinfectant, eg, soap and water. Do not use friction with cleansing if tissue is friable.
- If irrigation prescribed to ↓ contaminants, provide a large volume of irrigant with high-pressure irrigation, using a 35-ml syringe and 18-gauge needle. If tissue is friable or wound is over a major organ or blood vessel, use extreme caution with irrigation pressure.
- Topically applied antiinfective agents, eg, neomycin and iodophors, are absorbed by wound and can produce systemic side effects. When these agents are used, be alert to toxicity to wound cells, nephrotoxicity, acidosis.
- When an absorbent dressing (eg, Debrisan, Bard Absorption Dressing) is prescribed, remove it with high-pressure irrigation. If agent removed with a 4×4 or surgical sponge, friction will disrupt capillary budding and delay healing.
- When topical enzymes prescribed, use on necrotic tissue only and follow package directions carefully. Be aware that agents such as povidone-iodine deactivate enzymes. Protect surrounding undamaged skin with zinc oxide or aluminum hydroxide paste.

Miscellanea

CONSULT MD FOR
- Signs of impaired wound healing: persistent exudate, exudate that is ↑ or has foul odor, presence of necrotic tissue, pale granulation tissue, no ↓ in wound size
- ↑ WBCs with left shift
- Positive wound C&S

RELATED TOPICS
- Antimicrobial therapy
- Enterocutaneous fistulas
- Methicillin-resistant *Staphylococcus aureus*
- Nutritional support, enteral and parenteral
- Shock, septic
- Vancomycin-resistant enterococci
- Wounds healing by primary intention

ABBREVIATION
PN: Parenteral nutrition

REFERENCES
Krasner D: The ABCs of wound care dressings, *Ostomy/Wound Management* 39(8): 66-72, 1993.
Stotts NA, Wipke-Tevis D: Co-factors in impaired wound healing, *Ostomy/Wound Management* 42(2): 44-56, 1996.
Stotts NA: Determination of bacterial burden in wounds, *Adv Wound Care* 8(4): 28-52, 1995.
Stotts NA: Wound and skin care. In Swearingen PL, Keen JH: *Manual of critical care nursing*, ed 3, St Louis, 1995, Mosby.

Author: **Nancy Stotts**

Conversions and Calculations

CONVERSIONS
Volume
5 ml = 1 teaspoon (tsp)

15 ml = 1 tablespoon (T)

30 ml = 1 ounce (oz) = 2 T

500 ml = 1 pint (pt)

1000 ml = 1 quart (qt)

Length
2.5 centimeters (cm) = 1 inch

Pressure
1 mm Hg = 1.36 cm H_2O

Weight
1 kilogram (kg) = 2.2 pounds (lb)

1 gram (g) = 1000 milligrams (mg)

1 mg = 1000 micrograms (μg)

1 grain (gr) = 60 mg

$\frac{1}{100}$ gr = 0.6 mg

$\frac{1}{150}$ gr = 0.4 mg

Centigrade (C)/Fahrenheit (F)
$°C = (F - 32) \times \frac{5}{9}$

$°F = (C \times \frac{9}{5}) + 32$

CRITICAL CARE CALCULATIONS
Drug Concentration
mg/ml = drug in solution (mg)/volume of solution (ml)

μg/ml = mg/ml $\times$ 1000

Delivery Rate
ml/min = ml/hr $\div$ 60 min/hr

$$\mu g/kg/min = \frac{\mu g/ml \times ml/min}{weight\ (kg)}$$

$$ml/hr = \frac{\mu g/kg/min\ prescribed \times kg \times 60\ min/hr}{\mu g/ml\ of\ solution}$$

Rule of 15
Use for drugs that are dosed in μg/kg/min.

   Patient weight (kg) $\times$ 15 = mg of drug to add to 250 cc.

   Set flow rate to deliver desired dose as follows:

      1 μg/kg/min = 1 microgtt/min (1 ml/hr)

      2 μg/kg/min = 2 microgtt/min (2 ml/hr)

From Keen JH, Baird MS, Allen JH: *Mosby's critical care and emergency drug reference,* ed 2, St Louis, 1996, Mosby.

APPENDIX B

Hemodynamic Values and Calculation Formulas

Cardiac output (CO)	$\dfrac{O_2 \text{ consumption}}{A\text{-}Vo_2 \text{ difference}}$	4-7 L/min
Cardiac index (CI)	$\dfrac{CO}{\text{Body surface area (BSA)}}$	2.5-4 L/min/m^2
Stroke volume (SV)	$\dfrac{CO}{HR} \times 1000$	55-100 ml/beat
Arterial oxygen content (Cao$_2$)	$(Hgb \times 1.34) \times Sao_2$	18-20 ml/vol%
Venous oxygen content (Cvo$_2$)	$(Hgb \times 1.34) \times Svo_2$	15.5 ml/vol%
Oxygen delivery (Do$_2$)	$Cao_2 \times CO \times 10$	800-1000 ml/min
Arteriovenous oxygen content difference (C[a-v]o$_2$)	$Cao_2 - Cvo_2$	4-6 ml/vol%
Oxygen consumption (Vo$_2$)	$CO \times 10 \times C(a\text{-}v)o_2$	200-250 ml/min
Systemic vascular resistance (SVR)	$\dfrac{MAP - RAP}{CO} \times 80$	900-1200 dynes/sec/cm^{-5}
Pulmonary vascular resistance (PVR)	$\dfrac{PAM - PAWP}{CO} \times 80$	60-100 dynes/sec/cm^{-5}
Left ventricular stroke work index (LVSWI)	$SVI \times (MAP - PAWP) \times 0.136$	40-75 g/m^{2}beat
Mean arterial pressure (MAP)	$\dfrac{\text{Systolic BP} + 2(\text{Diastolic BP})}{3}$	70-105 mm Hg
Mean pulmonary artery pressure (MPAP, PAM)	$\dfrac{PAS + 2(PAD)}{3}$	10-15 mm Hg
Mixed venous oxygen saturation (Svo$_2$)	$(CO \times Cao_2 \times 10) - Vo_2$	60%-80%
Central venous pressure (CVP)		2-6 mm Hg
Right atrial pressure (RAP)		4-6 mm Hg
Left atrial pressure (LAP)		8-12 mm Hg
Right ventricular pressure (RVP)		25/0-5 mm Hg
Pulmonary artery pressure (PAP)		20-30/8-15 mm Hg
Pulmonary artery wedge pressure (PAWP)		6-12 mm Hg

From Keen JH, Baird MS, Allen JH: *Mosby's critical care and emergency drug reference,* ed 2, St Louis, 1996, Mosby.

National Institutes of Health Stroke Scale

			Baseline	30 min	1 h	2 h	24 h	48 h	7-10 days
1.a. Level of consciousness (LOC)	Alert	0							
	Drowsy	1							
	Stuporous	2							
	Coma	3							
1.b. LOC questions	Answers both correctly	0							
	Answers one correctly	1							
	Incorrect	2							
1.c. LOC commands	Obeys both correctly	0							
	Obeys one correctly	1							
	Incorrect	2							
2. Best gaze	Normal	0							
	Partial gaze palsy	1							
	Forced deviation	2							
3. Best visual	No visual loss	0							
	Partial hemianopia	1							
	Complete hemianopia	2							
	Bilateral hemianopia	3							
4. Facial palsy	Normal	0							
	Minor	1							
	Partial	2							
	Complete	3							
5. Best motor arm	No drift	0							
	Drift	1							
	Can't resist gravity	2							
	No effort against gravity	3							
	No movement	4							
6. Other arm	For brainstem stroke (Use same scale as above)	0-4							
7. Best motor leg	No drift	0							
	Drift	1							
	Can't resist gravity	2							
	No effort against gravity	3							
	No movement	4							
8. Other leg	For brainstem stroke (Use same scale as above)	0-4							
9. Limb ataxia	Absent	0							
	Present in upper or lower	1							
	Present in both	2							
10. Sensory	Normal	0							
	Partial loss	1							
	Dense loss	2							
11. Neglect	No neglect	0							
	Partial neglect	1							
	Complete neglect	2							
12. Dysarthria	Normal articulation	0							
	Mild to moderate dysarthria	1							
	Near unintelligible or worse	2							
13. Best language	No aphasia	0							
	Mild to moderate aphasia	1							
	Severe aphasia	2							
	Mute	3							

Continued

			Baseline	30 min	1 h	2 h	24 h	48 h	7-10 days
14. Change from previous examination	Same Better Worse	S B W							
15. Change from baseline	Same Better Worse	S B W							

From National High Blood Pressure Education Program, National Institutes of Health, and National Heart, Lung, and Blood Institute: NIH Pub No 93-1088, January 1993.

APPENDIX D

Glasgow Coma Scale

Parameter	Patient Response	Score
Best eye opening response (record "C" if eyes closed due to swelling)	Spontaneously	4
	To speech	3
	To pain	2
	No response	1
Best motor response (record best upper limb response to painful stimuli)	Obeys verbal command	6
	Localizes pain	5
	Flexion—withdrawal	4
	Flexion—abnormal	3
	Extension—abnormal	2
	No response	1
Best verbal response (record "E" if ET tube is in place or "T" if tracheostomy tube is in place)	Conversation—oriented $\times$ 3	5
	Conversation—confused	4
	Speech—inappropriate	3
	Sounds—incomprehensible	2
	No response	1

Total Score	Interpretation
15	Normal
13-15	Minor head injury
9-12	Moderate head injury
3-8	Severe head injury
$\leq$7	Coma
3	Deep coma or brain death

Mini Mental Status Examination

1. What is the year, season, date, day, month (5 points)
2. Where are we: state, county, town, hospital, room (5 points)
3. Name three objects (3)
4. Count backward by sevens (eg, 100, 93, 86, 79, 72) (5 points)
5. Repeat same three objects from number 3 above (3 points)
6. Name a pencil and watch (2 points)
7. Follow a three-step command (3 points)
8. Write a sentence (1 point)
9. Follow the command "close your eyes" (1 point)
10. Copy a design (eg, two hexagons) (1 point)

APPENDIX F

Cognitive Recognition Scale

Level	Response	Goal/Intervention

I
II
III
	None
	Generalized
	Localized
		Goal: Provide sensory input to elicit responses of ↑ quality, frequency, duration, and variety.
		Intervention: Give brief but frequent stimulation sessions, and present stimuli in an organized manner, focusing on one sensory channel at a time, eg:
		   Visual: Intermittent television, family pictures, bright objects.
		   Auditory: Tape recordings of family or favorite song, talking to patient, intermittent TV or radio.
		   Olfactory: Favorite perfume, shaving lotion, coffee, lemon, orange.
		   Cutaneous: Touch or rub skin with different textures such as velvet, ice bag, warm cloth.
		   Movement: Turn, ROM exercises, up in chair.
		   Oral: Oral care, lemon swabs, ice, sugar on tongue, peppermint, chocolate.

IV	Confused, agitated	*Goal:* ↓ agitation and ↑ awareness of environment. This stage usually lasts 2-4 wks.
		Interventions: Remove offending devices (eg, NG tube, restraints) if possible.
		   Do not demand patient follow-through with task.
		   Provide human contact unless this increases agitation.
		   Provide a quiet, controlled environment.
		   Use a calm, soft voice and manner around patient.

V
VI
	Confused, inappropriate
	Confused, appropriate
		Goal: ↓ confusion and incorporate improved cognitive abilities into functional activity.
		Interventions: Begin each interaction with introduction, orientation, and interaction purpose.
		   List and number daily activity in the sequence in which it will be done throughout the day.
		   Maintain a consistent environment.
		   Provide memory aids (eg, calendar, clock).
		   Use gentle repetition, which aids learning.
		   Provide supervision and structure.
		   Reorient as needed.

VII
VIII
	Automatic, appropriate
	Purposeful
		Goal: Integrate ↑ cognitive function into functional community activities with minimal structuring.
		Interventions: Enable practicing of activities.
		   Reduce supervision and environmental structure.
		   Help patient plan adaptation of ADL and home living skills to home environment.

Data from Rancho Los Amigos Hospital, Inc, Levels of Cognitive Functioning (scale based on behavioral descriptions or responses to stimuli). From Swift CM: Neurologic disorders. In Swearingen PL (ed): *Manual of medical-surgical nursing care,* ed 3, St Louis, 1994, Mosby.

Cranial Nerves: Functions and Dysfunctions

Cranial Nerve	Type	Functions	Dysfunctions
I Olfactory	Sensory	Smell	Anosmia

II Optic	Sensory	Sight
		  Visual acuity
		  Visual fields
			Blindness
			Visual field deficits

III Oculomotor	Motor	Pupillary constriction Elevation of upper eyelid Extraocular movements	Ptosis, diplopia, pupillary dilatation, strabismus
IV Trochlear	Motor	Downward and inward movement of eye	Eye will not move down or out
V Trigeminal	Sensory and motor	*Motor:* Temporal and masseter muscles (jaw clenching and lateral movement for mastication) *Sensory:* Facial, scalp, anterior two thirds of tongue, lips, teeth, proprioception for mastication, corneal reflex	Paresis or paralysis of muscles of mastication, decreased facial sensation Loss of corneal reflex
VI Abducens	Motor	Lateral eye movement	Eye will not move laterally
VII Facial	Sensory and motor	*Sensory:* Taste in anterior two thirds of tongue, proprioception for face and scalp *Motor:* Facial expression, lacrimal and salivary glands	Loss of taste in anterior two thirds of tongue Paresis or paralysis of facial muscles, facial droop, loss of secretion of submandibular, sublingual, and lacrimal glands
VIII Acoustic	Sensory	*Cochlear division:* Hearing *Vestibular division:* Balance	Tinnitus, deafness . Vertigo, nystagmus
IX Glossopharyngeal	Sensory and motor	*Sensory:* Taste in posterior one third of tongue; pain, touch, heat, cold in tongue, tonsils, soft palate, and pharynx *Motor:* Elevation of the soft palate, movement of pharynx, secretion and vasodilatation of parotid glands for saliva; gag reflex	Loss of taste, pain, touch, heat, and cold in posterior one third of tongue, tonsils, and soft palate. Paresis or paralysis of soft palate and pharynx, dysphagia, dysarthria, hoarseness, loss of gag reflex
X Vagus	Sensory and motor	*Sensory:* Muscles of pharynx, larynx, esophagus, and thoracic and abdominal viscera; external ear, mucous membranes of larynx, trachea, esophagus, thoracic and abdominal viscera; lungs (stretch receptors), aortic bodies (chemoreceptors), respiratory/GI tract (pain receptors) *Motor:* Muscles of pharynx, larynx, esophagus, thoracic and abdominal viscera; respiratory/GI tract (smooth muscle), pacemaker and cardiac atrial muscle	Similar to dysfunction of glossopharyngeal Loss of gag reflex and difficulty swallowing
XI Spinal accessory	Motor	Sternocleidomastoid and trapezius muscles	Paresis or paralysis of sternocleidomastoid and trapezius muscles Inability to turn head or shrug shoulders
XII Hypoglossal	Motor	Tongue movement	Paresis or paralysis of the tongue

From Swearingen PL, Keen JH (eds): *Manual of critical care nursing,* ed 3, St Louis, 1995, Mosby.

APPENDIX H
Respiratory Patterns

Type	Waveform	Characteristics	Possible Clinical Condition
Eupnea		Nl rate and rhythm for adults and teenagers (12-20 breaths/min)	Nl pattern while awake
Bradypnea		Decreased rate (<12 breaths/min); regular rhythm	Nl sleep pattern; opiate or alcohol use, tumor, metabolic disorder
Tachypnea		Rapid rate (>20 breaths/min); hypoventilation or hyperventilation	Fever, restrictive respiratory disorders, pulmonary emboli
Hyperpnea		Depth of respirations > nl	Meeting increased metabolic demand (eg, sepsis, MODS, SIRS, and exercise)
Apnea		Cessation of breathing; may be intermittent	Intermittent with CNS disturbances or drug intoxication; obstructed airway; respiratory arrest if it persists
Kussmaul's		Deep, rapid (>20 breaths/min), sighing, labored	Renal failure, DKA, sepsis, shock
Cheyne-Stokes		Alternating patterns of apnea (10-20 sec) with periods of deep and rapid breathing; lesions located bilaterally and deep within cerebral hemispheres	Heart failure, opiate or hypnotic overdose, thyrotoxicosis, dissecting aneurysm, subarachnoid hemorrhage, ↑ ICP, aortic valve disorders; may be nl in elders during sleep
Central neurogenic hyperventilation		Rapid (>20 breaths/min), deep, regular; lesions of midbrain or upper pons thought to be source of pattern	Primary injury (ischemia, infarction, space-occupying lesion); secondary injury (↑ ICP, metabolic disorders, drug overdose)

From Swearingen PL, Keen JH (eds): *Manual of critical care nursing,* ed 3, St Louis, 1995, Mosby.

APPENDIX I

Blood and Blood Products

Product	Approximate Volume	Indications	Precautions/Comments
Whole blood (WB)	500-510 ml (450 WB; 50-60 anticoagulants)	Acute, severe blood loss; hypovolemic shock; ↑ both red cell mass and plasma	Must be ABO and Rh compatible. Do not mix with dextrose solutions; always prime tubing with NS. Observe for dyspnea, orthopnea, cyanosis, and anxiety as signs of circulatory overload; monitor VS.
PRBCs	250 ml	↑ RBC mass and O_2-carrying capacity of the blood	Must be ABO and Rh compatible. Leukocyte-depleted RBCs may be used to reduce the risk of antibody formation and nonhemolytic reactions. Irradiated RBCs may be used to prevent graft-vs-host disease in immunocompromised patients. PRBCs have less volume than WB, which reduces the risk of fluid overload.
FFP	250 ml	Treatment of choice for combined coagulation factor deficiencies and factor V and XI deficiencies; alternate treatment for factor VII, VIII, IX, and X deficiencies when concentrates are not available	Must be ABO compatible; supplies clotting factors. Usual dosage is 10-15 ml/kg body weight; transfuse within 24 h of thawing. Do not use if patient needs volume expansion only.
Random donor platelet concentrate	50 ml (usual adult dose is 5-6 U)	Treatment of choice for thrombocytopenia; also used for leukemia and hypoplastic anemia	Usual dosage is 0.1 U/kg body weight to ↑ platelet count to 25,000/μl; administer as rapidly as tolerated. ABO compatibility is preferable. Effectiveness is reduced by fever, sepsis, and splenomegaly. Febrile reactions are common. Use special platelet tubing and filter. Special filters are available for removing leukocytes and thus reducing the risk of alloimmunization to human leukocyte antigen (HLA). Platelets must be infused within 4 h of initiation.
Platelet concentrate by platelet pheresis (single donor platelets)	200 ml (may vary)	Treatment for thrombocytopenia that is refractory to random donor platelets	Involves removing donor's venous blood, removing platelets by differential centrifuge, and returning blood to donor. Approximately 3-4 L of whole blood is processed to obtain a therapeutic dose of platelets. May use special donors who are HLA matched to patient.
Cryoprecipitate (factor VIII)	10-25 ml	Routine treatment for hemophilia (factor VII deficiency) and fibrinogen deficiency (factor XIII deficiency)	Made from FFP; infuse immediately upon thawing.
AHG (factor VIII) concentrates	20 ml	Alternative treatment for hemophilia A	Allergic and febrile reactions occur frequently. Administer by syringe or component drip set. Can store at refrigerator temperature, making it convenient for hemophiliacs during travel.
Factor II, VII, IX, X concentrate	20 ml	Treatment of choice for hemophilia B and factor IX deficiencies	Can precipitate clotting. Allergic and febrile reactions occur occasionally. Contraindicated in liver disease.
Albumin*	50 or 250 ml	Hypovolemic shock, hypoalbuminemia, protein replacement for burn patients	Osmotically equal to 5 × its volume of plasma. Used as a volume expander in conjunction with crystalloids. Also used in hypoalbuminemic states. Commercially available.
PPF*	250 ml (83% albumin with some α- and β-globulins)	Volume expansion	Commercially available; expensive. Certain lots reported to have caused hypotension, possibly r/t vasoactive amines used in preparation.
Granulocyte transfusion (collected from a single apheresis donor)	200 ml (may vary)	Leukemia with granulocytopenia r/t treatment	Uncommon treatment; febrile and allergic symptoms are common. Must be ABO compatible.

From Steuble BT: Hematological disorders. In Swearingen PL (ed): *Pocket guide to medical-surgical nursing*, ed 2, St Louis, 1996, Mosby.

*No risk of disease transmission.

Note: When administering blood products, it is important to recognize that delivery of most blood products carries some risk (eg, transmission of HIV, HBV, HCV, CMV, and human T-cell lymphotrophic virus, type I [HTLV-1]).

Note: DNA recombinant technology may reduce complications from factor concentrates.

Types and Characteristics of Viral Hepatitis

	Hepatitis A Virus (HAV)	Hepatitis B Virus (HBV)	Hepatitis C Virus (HCV)	Hepatitis D Virus (HDV)	Hepatitis E Virus (HEV)
Likely modes of transmission	Fecal-oral; food-borne most common; parenteral transmission rare; most infectious 2 wks before symptoms appear	Contact with blood or serum; sexual contact; perinatal transmission; often transmitted by chronic carriers; most infectious before symptoms appear and for 4-6 mos after acute infection	Contact with blood or serum; perinatal transmission rare unless mother is HIV infected; often transmitted by chronic carriers; most infectious 1-2 wks before symptoms appear and throughout acute infection	Similar to HBV; can cause infection only if individual already has HBV; blood infectious throughout HDV infection	Fecal-oral; food-borne; water-borne
Population most often affected	Children; individuals living in or traveling to areas with poor sanitation	Injecting drug users; health care and public safety workers exposed to blood; clients and staff of institutions for the developmentally disabled; homosexual men; men and women with multiple heterosexual partners; young children of infected mothers; recipients of certain blood products; hemodialysis patients	Injecting drug users; individuals who received blood products before 1991; potential risk to health care and public safety workers exposed to blood	Injecting drug users; hemophiliacs; recipients of multiple blood transfusions (infects only individuals who already have HBV)	People living in or traveling to parts of Asia, Africa, or Mexico where sanitation is poor
Incubation	2-6 wks	6 wks-6 mos	18-180 days	Varies; not well established	
Serum markers of acute infection	Antibody to HAV (anti-HAV); IgG-class antibody to HAV (IgG anti-HAV) indicates immunity	HBsAg; HBeAG; IgM-class antibody to HBcAg (IgM anti-HBc)	Only test available is antibody to HCV (anti-HCV), which detects chronic but not acute cases	Antibody to HDV (anti-HDV)	
Measures for reducing exposure	Hand washing; good personal hygiene; sanitation; appropriate infection control measures (see Appendix N)	Hand washing; good personal hygiene; appropriate infection control measures (see Appendix N); autoclaving of all nondisposable items; careful handling of needles and sharps; ensuring that needles are not reused and are discarded carefully in special containers	As for HBV	As for HBV	As for HAV
Prophylaxis	Sanitation measures; immunization; immunoglobulin within 1-2 wks after exposure	Screening of donated blood; protective devices for providers and immunization for all health care workers who come in contact with blood, as well as for risk groups noted above; use of condoms; HBIG for known exposure to HBsAg-contaminated material; also, CDC recommends routine immunization of all children	Screening of donated blood; protective devices for health care providers; no vaccine exists for HCV	Immunization against HBV	Effectiveness of immunoglobulin manufactured in the United States is not known

Continued

	Hepatitis A Virus (HAV)	Hepatitis B Virus (HBV)	Hepatitis C Virus (HCV)	Hepatitis D Virus (HDV)	Hepatitis E Virus (HEV)
Comments	Symptoms usually mild; rarely causes fulminant hepatic failure	HBsAg persists in carrier state; chronic hepatitis may develop; fulminant hepatic failure may result	Carrier state and chronic hepatitis may develop; fulminant hepatic failure may result	Increased risk of serious complications (including fulminant hepatic failure) and death; carrier state and chronic hepatitis may develop	Disease is not endemic in the United States or western Europe

From Keen JH: Gastrointestinal disorders. In Swearingen, PL (ed): *Pocket guide to medical-surgical nursing*, ed 2, 1996, Mosby.
HBcAg, hepatitis B core antigen; *HBeAg*, *hepatitis B early antigen; HBIG*, hepatitis B immunoglobulin; *HBsAg*, hepatitis B surface antigen; *IgG*, immunoglobulin G; *IgM*, immunoglobulin M.

Specialized Administration Routes Used in Critical Care

ROUTE	MANAGEMENT

ROUTE

Endotracheal (ET)

When IV access not available, selected emergency medications (eg, epinephrine, lidocaine, atropine) can be administered endotracheally; dose usually 2-2.5 times recommended IV dose.

Intraosseous (IO)

During emergencies in children <6 yrs, catheter may be placed into proximal tibia to administer drugs/fluids; blood products, isotonic fluids, medications may be administered IO; used for temporary access only.

Intraperitoneal (IP)

Medications, especially antibiotics, sometimes added to peritoneal dialysate or lavage; medications have local/systemic effects, depending on absorption; local instillation of antibiotics reduces intraperitoneal bacteria

Gastric feeding tube (G-tube)

Route used for patients with functioning GI tracts/swallowing impairment; G-tube usually placed previously for enteral feeding or gastric decompression

MANAGEMENT

- For adults, dilute drug in 10 ml 0.9% NaCl or sterile water. Use smaller volume (eg, 1-2 ml) for children.
- Place sterile catheter just past tip of ET tube; quickly spray medication into tube.
- Follow with 3-4 rapid insufflations to aerosolize medication.

- Using sterile technique, insert standard 16- to 18-gauge hypodermic, spinal, or bone marrow needle into anterior surface of tibia.
- Confirm placement by aspiration of bone marrow, freely flowing IV solution without evidence of infiltration.
- Secure firmly with sterile dressing; tape to prevent dislodgment.
- Monitor for extravasation, patency.
- Flush with dilute heparin or saline to prevent clotting.
- Dilute hypertonic/alkaline solutions before administration.

- Use sterile technique when adding medications to fluid for peritoneal lavage/dialysis.
- Confirm compatibility before adding multiple medications.
- Systemic absorption of aminoglycoside antibiotics may depress respiration, especially if patient has recently received NMBAs.

- Verify presence of GI activity (eg, bowel sounds), tube placement before medication administration.
- Use commercial liquid preparations when possible. If liquid is not available, many standard tablets can be crushed and mixed with water for administration. NEVER CRUSH TIME-RELEASED, LIQUID-FILLED, OR ENTERIC COATED PREPARATIONS. When in doubt, consult pharmacist.
- Use only commercially prepared liquid preparations with small-bore feeding tubes. Suspensions of crushed tablets may obstruct tube.

Continued

- Flush tube thoroughly before and after medication administration.
- Hyperosmolar liquids such as KCl, sorbitol, may cause gastric irritation, diarrhea. Dilute with water before administration.
- Administer multiple medications separately, flushing after each, to avoid incompatibilities.
- If suction prescribed, do not reconnect for 1-2 h after medication administration.
- Feedings may affect the absorption of some drugs (eg, phenytoin, warfarin, carbamazepine). Avoid resuming feedings for 1-2 h if absorption could be affected.

From Keen JH, Baird MS, Allen JH: *Mosby's critical care and emergency drug reference;* ed 2, St Louis, 1996, Mosby.

APPENDIX L

Equianalgesic Doses of Opioid Analgesics

Class/Name	Route	Equianalgesic Dose (Mg)*	Average Duration (Hr)
Morphine-like Agonists			
Codeine	IM, SC	75†	3
	PO	130†	3
Hydromorphone (Dilaudid)	IM, SC	1.5	4
	PO	7.5	4
Levorphanol (Levo-Dromoran)	IM, SC	2.0	6
	PO	4.0	6
Morphine	IM, SC	10	4
	PO	30-60	
Oxycodone (Percodan)	PO	30†	4
Hydrocodone (Cortab, Vicodin)	PO	30†	4
Oxymorphone (Numorphan)	IM, SC	1.0-1.5	4
	rectal	10	4
Meperidine-like Agonists			
Fentanyl (Sublimaze)	IV, IM, SC, TD	0.1-0.2	1‡
Meperidine (Demerol)	IM, SC	100	3
	PO	300†	3
Methadone-like Agonists			
Methadone (Dolophine)	IM, SC	10	6
	PO	20	6
Propoxyphene (Darvon)	PO	130-250†	4
Mixed Agonist-Antagonists§			
Buprenorphine (Buprenex)	IM	0.3-0.4	4
Butorphanol (Stadol)	IM, SC	2.0	3
Nalbuphine (Nubain)	IM, SC	10	4
Pentazocine (Talwin)	IM	60	3
	PO	150†	3

Adapted from Koda-Kimble MA et al: *Applied therapeutics: the clinical use of drugs*, ed 5, Vancouver, Wash, 1992, *Applied therapeutics and acute pain management: operative and medical procedures and trauma, clinical practice guideline*, AH CPR Pub No 92-0032, Agency for Health Care Policy and Research, Public Health Service, Rockville, Md, 1992, US Department of Health and Human Services.

*Recommended starting dose; actual dose must be titrated to patient response.

†Starting doses lower (codeine 30 mg, oxycodone 6 mg, meperidine 50 mg, propoxyphene 65-130 mg, pentazocine 50 mg).

‡Respiratory depressant effects persist longer than analgesic effects.

§Mixed agonist/antagonist analgesics may precipitate withdrawal in opioid-dependent patients.

APPENDIX M

Acute Hypersensitivity (Allergic) Reactions

CLINICAL PRESENTATION

Symptoms generally start within 30 min of exposure, almost always within 2 h; if not treated, may lead to death by asphyxia, CV collapse. "Late-phase" reactions may occur; patient appears to be recovered, but 6-8 h later anaphylaxis recurs.

System	Manifestations
Integ	Pruritus, urticaria, erythema, angioedema
GI	Nausea, abdominal pain, vomiting, diarrhea
Resp	Chest tightness, stridor, bronchospasm
CV	Hypotension, tachycardia, dysrhythmias

MANAGEMENT

1. Discontinue suspected drug.
2. Airway: Establish/maintain patency.
3. O_2: Administer at 6-10 L/min or as indicated by clinical condition.
4. Epinephrine: Causes bronchodilation, increases BP; administer SC/IM adults: 1:1000, 0.3-0.5 mg.
5. IV fluids: Establish IV access; administer crystalloids for hypotension; use vasopressors (eg, norepinephrine) for hypotension unresponsive to fluid therapy.
6. Diphenhydramine: Blocks H_1 receptors; administer IV; IM route may be used if CV status stable; adults: 10-50 mg, may repeat. Combination therapy with H_2 antagonists (eg, cimetidine) may benefit patients with allergic skin disorders who do not respond adequately to H_1 receptor blockade.
7. Hydrocortisone sodium succinate: Blocks late phase reaction; adults: $\geq$100 mg IV, up to 2g; follow with 100 mg IV q2-4h; convert to PO therapy when possible, continue for 1-3 days.
8. Aminophylline: Sometimes used for severe or refractory bronchospasm.

From Keen JH, Baird MS, Allen JH: *Mosby's critical care and emergency drug reference,* ed 2, St Louis, 1996, Mosby.

Recommendations for Isolation Precautions in Hospitals (CDC, 1996)

	Standard Precautions	Transmission-based Precautions: Airborne	Transmission-based Precautions: Droplet	Transmission-based Precautions: Contact
When to use	All patients	Use in addition to Standard Precautions for patients known to be or suspected of being infected with microorganisms transmitted by airborne droplet nuclei (≤5 microns) of evaporated droplets containing microorganisms that can remain suspended in the air and can be widely dispersed by air currents	Use in addition to Standard Precautions for patient known to be or suspected of being infected with microorganisms transmitted by droplets (>5 microns) that can be generated during coughing, sneezing, talking, or performance of procedures	Use in addition to Standard Precautions for specified patients known to be or suspected of being infected or colonized with epidemiologically important microorganisms that can be transmitted by direct contact with patient, such as occurs during patient care activities, or by indirect contact, such as touching surfaces or equipment in patient's environment
Hand washing	Wash hands after touching blood, body fluids, secretions, execretions, and contaminated items, regardless of whether gloves are worn; wash hands immediately after gloves are removed, between patient contacts, and to prevent transfer of microorganisms to other patients or environments; use plain (nonantimicrobial) soap for routine hand washing			Wash hands with an antimicrobial agent or a waterless antiseptic agent
Gloves	Wear nonsterile gloves when touching blood, body fluids, secretions, excretions, and contaminated items; put on clean gloves just before touching mucous membranes and nonintact skin; remove gloves promptly after use, before touching noncontaminated items, environmental surfaces, and before going to another patient; wash hands immediately to avoid transfer of microorganisms to other patients or environment			In addition to glove use as described in Standard Precautions, wear gloves when entering the room. During patient care, change gloves after contact with infective material (eg, fecal material or wound drainage). After glove removal and hand washing, do not touch items in room.

Continued

	Standard Precautions	Transmission-based Precautions: Airborne	Transmission-based Precautions: Droplet	Transmission-based Precautions: Contact
Mask, eye protection, face shield	Wear mask and eye protection or face shield to protect mucous membranes of eyes, nose, and mouth during procedures and patient care activities likely to generate splashes or sprays	Wear respiratory protection when entering room of patient known to have or suspected of having tuberculosis (a type of particulate respirator is recommended) Do not enter room of patient known to have or suspected of having measles (rubeola) or varicella (chickenpox) if susceptible to these infections	Wear a mask when working within 3 ft of patient	
Gown	Wear clean, nonsterile gown to protect skin and prevent soiling of clothing during procedures and patient care activities likely to generate splashes or sprays of blood, body fluids, secretions, or excretions, or to cause soiling of clothing; remove gown promptly when tasks are completed; wash hands			Wear clean, nonsterile gown when entering room if substantial contact is anticipated with patient, surfaces, or items in environment; wear gown when entering room if patient is incontinent, has diarrhea, an ileostomy, colostomy, or uncontained wound drainage; remove gown carefully when tasks are completed; wash hands
Patient care equipment	Handle used patient care equipment in manner that prevents skin and mucous membrane exposures, contamination of clothing, and environmental soiling			When possible, dedicate use of noncritical patient care equipment to a single patient to avoid sharing between patients; if common equipment or items must be shared, adequately clean and disinfect them between uses
Linen	Handle, transport, and process used linen in manner that prevents skin and mucous membrane exposure, contamination of clothing, and environmental soiling			
Patient placement	Place patient who contaminates environment or who does not (or cannot) assist in maintaining appropriate hygiene or environmental control in private room, if possible; consult infection control professionals for other alternatives	Place patient in private room that has (1) monitored negative air pressure in relation to surrounding areas, (2) 6-12 air exchanges per hour, and (3) appropriate discharge of air outdoors or monitored high-efficiency filtration of room air before air is circulated to other areas of the hospital; keep room door closed when patient is in room	Place patient in private room; when a private room is not available, cohort* infected patients or maintain spatial separation of at least 3 ft between infected patient and other patients and visitors; consult infection control professional for other alternatives	Place patient in private room; when a private room is not available, cohort* infected patients; consult infection control professionals for selection of suitable roommates or other alternatives

*Cohorting is a term used when patients share a room if infected by the same microorganism, provided they are not infected with other potentially transmissible microorganisms and the likelihood of reinfection with the same organism is minimal. Cohorting is used when there is a shortage of private rooms and may be useful during outbreaks.

Continued

	Standard Precautions	Transmission-based Precautions: Airborne	Transmission-based Precautions: Droplet	Transmission-based Precautions: Contact
Patient placement—cont'd		When a private room is not available, patient may be placed in room with another patient who has an active infection with the same microorganism; consult infection control professionals for alternatives		
Patient transport		Limit movement and transport of patient from room to essential purposes only; if transport or movement is necessary, minimize patient dispersal of droplet nuclei by placing surgical mask on patient, if possible	Limit movement and transport of patient from room to essential purposes only; if transport or movement is necessary, minimize patient dispersal of droplets by masking patient, if possible	Limit movement and transport of patient from room to essential purposes only; if transport is necessary, ensure that precautions are maintained to minimize contamination of environmental surfaces or equipment
Environmental control	Ensure that hospital has adequate procedures for routine care, cleaning, and disinfection of environment and patient care items			Ensure that patient care items, bedside equipment, and frequently touched surfaces receive daily cleaning
Occupational Safety and Health Administration (OSHA) bloodborne pathogens standard (1991)	Take care to prevent injuries when using needles, scalpels, and other sharp instruments or devices; when handling sharp instruments after procedures; when cleaning used instruments; and when disposing of used needles Never recap used needles or otherwise manipulate them using both hands, or use any other technique that involves directing the point of a needle toward any part of the body Use either one-handed "scoop" technique or mechanical device designed for holding needle sheath if recapping is required by procedure Do not remove used needles from disposable syringes by hand; do not bend, break, or manipulate used needles by hand Place used sharps in appropriate puncture-resistant containers located as close as practical to location of use Use mouthpieces, resuscitation bags, or other ventilation devices as an alternative to mouth-to-mouth resuscitation methods in areas where need is predictable			

Adapted from Garner JS: CDC guideline for isolation precautions in hospitals, *Infect Control Hosp Epidemiol* 17:53-80, 1996.

REFERENCES

Bennett JV, Brachman PS (eds): *Hospital infections*. ed 4, Boston, 1996, Little, Brown.

Centers for Disease Control and Prevention: Guidelines for isolation precautions in hospitals, *Infect Control Hosp Epidemiol:* 17:53-80, 1996.

Centers for Disease Control: Guideline for isolation precautions in hospitals, *Infect Control* 4:245-325, 1983.

Department of Labor, Occupational Safety and Health Administration: Occupational exposure to bloodborne pathogens: final rule, 29 CFR part 1910:1030, *Federal Register* 56:64003-64182, Dec 6, 1991.

Jackson MM: Infection prevention and control, *Crit Care Nurs Clin North Am* 4(3):401-409, 1992.

Jackson MM, Lynch P: Developing a numeric scale to assess health-care worker risk for bloodborne pathogen exposure, *Am J Infect Control* 23:13-21, 1995.

Mayhall CG (ed): *Hospital epidemiology and infection control;* Baltimore, 1996, Williams & Wilkins.

Pugliese G, Lynch P, Jackson MM, editors: *Universal Precautions: policies, procedures, and resources,* Chicago, 1990, American Hospital Publishing.

Wenzel RP: *Prevention and control of nosocomial infections,* ed 2, Baltimore, 1993, Williams & Wilkins.

Author: **Marguerite McMillan Jackson**

APPENDIX O
Glossary

Anion gap Reflects unmeasurable anions present in plasma. Calculated as follows: anion gap = $Na^+ - (Cl^- + HCO_3^-)$. Nl anion gap = 12 (± 2) mEq/L.

Asterixis Hand-flapping tremor elicited by arm extension and wrist dorsiflexion. Often accompanies metabolic disorders; seen with hepatic encephalopathy.

Babinski's reflex When firmly stroking the lateral aspect of the sole of the foot, the big toe dorsiflexes while the other toes fan and extend. Presence of this reflex is nl in infants. It is abnormal in children and adults, in whom it is a sign of motor nerve dysfunction.

Battle's sign Ecchymosis of the mastoid process behind the ear; associated with fracture of the middle fossa of the base of the skull.

Beck's triad Distended neck veins, hypotension, muffled heart sounds. Associated with cardiac tamponade.

Brudzinski's sign Involuntary flexion of arms, hips, and knees when neck is flexed. Diagnostic of meningitis.

Chvostek's sign Facial muscle spasm in response to tapping on the facial nerve just in front of the ear. A sign of tetany in hypocalcemia.

Cullen's sign Bluish discoloration around the umbilicus; may be present with intraperitoneal bleeding from the liver or spleen.

Cushing's triad Bradycardia, ↑ SBP, and widened pulse pressure. A late sign of mechanical brainstem compression or other severe brainstem dysfunction.

Decerebrate posturing Extension and internal rotation of the arms, leg extension, and plantar flexion of the feet. Usually seen in comatose patient with low-level brainstem compression.

Decorticate posturing Flexion of the arms at the elbows and wrists with potential leg flexion. Usually seen in comatose patient with mesencephalic brain lesion.

Grey Turner's sign Bluish discoloration of the flank; a signal of retroperitoneal bleeding from the pancreas, duodenum, vena cava, aorta, or kidneys.

Halo sign Yellowing ring that appears around blood drainage from the nose or ear. A sign of CSF leakage.

Hepatojugular reflux ↑ pressure in the internal jugular vein when pressure is applied over the abdominal RUQ for 30-60 seconds. ↑ jugular vein pressure is manifested by a sustained jugular distention or rise of ≥1 cm of jugular venous fluid. This sign is diagnostic of RV heart failure.

Janeway lesions Painless, small, hemorrhagic lesions found on the fingers, toes, nose, or earlobes. A classic finding with infective endocarditis.

Kehr's sign Left shoulder pain caused by diaphragmatic irritation usually as a result of splenic bleeding.

Kernig's sign Pain in lower back and resistance to leg extension when the thigh is flexed on the abdomen. Usually diagnostic of meningitis.

Kussmaul's sign ↑ in JVD on deep inspiration; associated with RV heart failure, constrictive pericarditis, or mediastinal tumor.

Nuchal rigidity (stiff neck sign) Pain and resistance to neck motion when the examiner flexes patient's neck and attempts to make the chin touch the sternum. Seen with meningitis.

Oculocephalic response/reflex Also called "doll's eye reflex." Inability of the eyes to lag behind head movement or return to midline when the patient's head is moved quickly from one side to the other. Signal of a lesion on the ipsilateral side at brainstem level.

Oculovestibular response/reflex Also known as "ice water coloric." Usually performed by a physician. After first ensuring an intact tympanic membrane, a small amount (20-50 ml) of ice water is injected into the external auditory canal. Nl response is a rapid, nystagmus-like deviation toward the ear being irrigated, signaling brainstem integrity. Abnormal response, signaling a brainstem lesion, is dysconjugate eye movement. No response is a sign of minimal or no brainstem function.

Osler's nodes Painful, red, subcutaneous nodules found on finger pads or on the feet, probably caused by microemboli. A classic finding with infective endocarditis.

Pulsus alternans A pulse that alternates between weak and strong beats in the same cycle; a sign of LV heart failure.

Pulsus paradoxus Abnormal ↓ (≥10 mm Hg) in SBP and pulse wave amplitude during inspiration. May be a sign of cardiac tamponade, pericarditis, lung disease, or heart failure. Also known as *paradoxical pulse.*

Splinter hemorrhages Small red streaks on distal third of fingernails or toenails. A classic finding with infective endocarditis.

Starling's law of the heart Contractility is determined by the length of the fibers in the wall of the myocardium. Greater volume ↑ the length of the fibers and hence ↑ the strength of contraction. The patient should have enough fluid volume to stretch the fibers, but not so much of a stretch that contractility and cardiac output are ↓.

Summation gallop Presence of S_4 and S_3, which combine to form a single loud sound during mid-diastole; often associated with a rapid HR in patients with LV heart failure.

Abbreviations

α   Alpha
β   Beta
ε   Epsilon
γ   Gamma
ω   Omega
AAL   Anterior axillary line
ABA   American Burn Association
ABG   Arterial blood gas
ac   Before meals
ACE   Angiotensin-converting enzyme
ACh   Acetylcholine
AChR   Acetylcholine receptor
ACI   Acute cerebral infarct
ACLS   Advanced cardiac life support
ACT   Activated clotting time
ACTH   Adrenocorticotropic hormone
AD   Autonomic dysreflexia
ADA   American Diabetes Association; American Dietetic Association
ADH   Antidiuretic hormone
ADL   Activities of daily living
AFB   Acid-fast bacillus
A-fib   Atrial fibrillation
A-flutter   Atrial flutter
AHA   American Heart Association
AIDS   Acquired immunodeficiency syndrome
ALG   Antilymphocyte globulin
ALP   Alkaline phosphatase
ALS   Amyotrophic lateral sclerosis
ALT   Alanine aminotransferase
AMI   Acute myocardial infarct
ANS   Autonomic nervous system
A-P   Anterior-posterior
ARDS   Adult respiratory distress syndrome
ARF   Acute respiratory failure, acute renal failure
ASA   Acetylsalicylic acid (aspirin)
ASD   Atrial septal defect
AST   Aspartate aminotransferase
A-tach   Atrial tachycardia
ATGAM   Antithymocyte gamma globulin
ATN   Acute tubular necrosis
ATP   Adenosine triphosphate
AV   Atrioventricular; arteriovenous
AV$_{DO_2}$ Arterial venous difference in oxygen
AVM   Arteriovenous malformation
bid   Twice a day
BLS   Basic life support
BMI   Body mass index
BP   Blood pressure
bpm   Beats per minute
BSA   Body surface area
BUN   Blood urea nitrogen
C   Cervical; Centigrade
C3   Third component of complement
Ca/C^{2+}   Calcium; free ionized calcium
CABG   Coronary artery bypass grafting
CAD   Coronary artery disease
CAPD   Continuous ambulatory peritoneal dialysis
CAVH   Continuous arteriovenous hemofiltration

C(a- v)o$_2$ Arterial-venous oxygen content difference
CBC   Complete blood cell count
CCU   Coronary care unit
CDC   Centers for Disease Control
CI   Cardiac index
CK-MB   Creatinine kinase-myocardial band
Cl/Cl$^-$ Chloride/chloride ion
cm   Centimeter
CMV   Cytomegalovirus; controlled mechanical ventilation
CNS   Central nervous system
CO   Cardiac output; carbon monoxide
CO$_2$ Carbon dioxide
COPD   Chronic obstructive pulmonary disease
CPAP   Continuous positive airway pressure
CPK   Creatinine phosphokinase
CPP   Cerebral perfusion pressure; coronary perfusion pressure
CPR   Cardiopulmonary resuscitation
CRF   Chronic renal failure
C&S   Culture and sensitivity
CSF   Cerebrospinal fluid
C-spine   Cervical spine
CT   Computerized (axial) tomography
CV   Cardiovascular
CVA   Cerebrovascular accident, costovertebral angle
CVC   Central venous catheter
CVP   Central venous pressure
CVVH   Continuous venovenous hemofiltration
D$_5$NS   5% dextrose in normal saline
D$_5$W   5% dextrose in water
D$_{50}$ 50% dextrose
DBP   Diastolic blood pressure
DI   Diabetes insipidus
DIC   Disseminated intravascular coagulation
DKA   Diabetic ketoacidosis
dl   Deciliter
DM   Diabetes mellitus
Do$_2$ Oxygen delivery
DPL   Diagnostic peritoneal lavage
DTR   Deep tendon reflex
DTs   Delirium tremens
DVT   Deep vein thrombosis
EACA   ε-aminocaproic acid
ECF   Extracellular fluid
ECG   Electrocardiogram
EDV   End-diastolic volume
EEG   Electroencephalogram
EF   Ejection fraction
eg   For example
EMG   Electromyography
EMS   Emergency Medical Services
ENT   Ear, nose, and throat
EP   Electrophysiologic
ERCP   Endoscopic retrocholangiopancreatography
ESR   Erythrocyte sedimentation rate
ESRD   End-stage renal disease
ET   Endotracheal; enterostomal therapy
ET$_{CO_2}$ Endotracheal carbon dioxide

ETOH   Ethanol
F   Fahrenheit, French
FBS   Fasting blood sugar
FDA   Federal Drug Administration
FDP   Fibrin degradation product
FEV   Forced expiratory volume
FFP   Fresh frozen plasma
FHF   Fulminant hepatic failure
Fio$_2$ Fraction of inspired oxygen
FRC   Functional residual capacity
FRF   Filtration replacement fluid
FSH   Follicle-stimulating hormone
FSP   Fibrin split product
FTI   Free thyroxine index
g   Gram
G6PD   Glucose-6-phosphate dehydrogenase
GABA   γ-aminobutyric acid
GBS   Guillain-Barré syndrome
GFR   Glomerular filtration rate
GH   Growth hormone
GI   Gastrointestinal
GOT   Glutamic oxaloacetic transaminase
GU   Genitourinary
h   Hour
H$_1$ Histamine-1
H$_2$ Histamine-2
H$_2$CO$_3$ Carbonic acid
HAV   Hepatitis A virus
HBIG   Hepatitis B immunoglobulin
HBV   Hepatitis B virus
HCl   Hydrochloric acid
HCO$_3^-$ Bicarbonate
Hct   Hematocrit
HCV   Hepatitis C virus
HDV   Hepatitis D virus
HELLP   Hemolysis, elevated liver enzymes, low platelet count
HEV   Hepatitis E virus
Hgb   Hemoglobin
HHNS   Hyperosmolar hyperglycemic nonketotic syndrome
HI   Head injury
HIT   Heparin-induced thrombocytopenia
HIV   Human immunodeficiency virus
HLA   Human leukocyte antigen
HOB   Head of bed
HOCA   High-osmolality contrast agent
HOCM   Hypertrophic obstructive cardiomyopathy
HR   Heart rate
hs   Hour of sleep (at bedtime)
HVWP   Hepatic venous wedge pressure
hx   History
IABP   Intraaortic balloon pump
ICA   Internal carotid artery
ICD   Implantable cardioverter/defibrillator
ICF   Intracellular fluid
ICH   Intracranial hematoma
ICP   Intracranial pressure
↑ICP   Increased intracranial pressure
ICS   Intercostal space
ICU   Intensive care unit

I&D Incision and drainage
IDDM Insulin-dependent diabetes mellitus
IE Infective endocarditis
I/E Inspiration to expiration
IgA Immunoglobulin A
IgE Immunoglobulin E
IgG Immunoglobulin G
IgM Immunoglobulin M
IL Interleukin
IM Intramuscular
INR Internal normalized ratio
Integ Integumentary
I&O Intake and output
IPD Intermittent peritoneal dialysis; intracranial pressure dynamics
IPPB Intermittent positive pressure breathing
IRV Inverse-ratio ventilation
ITP Idiopathic thrombocytopenic purpura
IU International unit
IV Intravenous
IVC Inferior vena cava
IVP Intravenous pyelogram
JVD Jugular venous distention
K/K$^+$ Potassium/potassium ion
KCl Potassium chloride
kg Kilogram
KUB Kidney, ureter, bladder
KVO Keep vein open
L Liter; lumbar
LA Left atrial
LAP Left atrial pressure
lb Pound
L&D Labor and delivery
LDH Lactate dehydrogenase; also abbreviated LD
LGIB Lower gastrointestinal bleeding
LGL Lown-Ganong-Levine
LH Luteinizing hormone
LLQ Left lower quadrant
LOC Level of consciousness
LOCA Low-osmolality contrast agent
LP Lumbar puncture
LR Lactated Ringer's
LSB Left sternal border
L-spine Lumbar spine
LUQ Left upper quadrant
LUT Lower urinary tract
LV Left ventricular
LVEDP Left ventricular end-diastolic pressure
LVEDV Left ventricular end-diastolic volume
LVEF Left ventricular ejection fraction
LVH Left ventricular hypertrophy
MAL Midaxillary line
MAO Monoamine oxidase
MAP Mean arterial pressure
MAST Military antishock trousers
MB Myocardial band
MCA Middle cerebral artery
MCL Modified chest lead; midclavicular line
MCV Mean corpuscular volume
MD Medical doctor
mEq Milliequivalent
mg Milligram
MG Myasthenia gravis
Mg/Mg^{2+} Magnesium/magnesium ion
MgSO$_4$ Magnesium sulfate
MI Myocardial infarction
MIC Minimum inhibitory concentration
min Minute

ml Milliliter
mm Hg Millimeters of mercury
mmol Millimole
mo Month
MODS Multiple organ dysfunction syndrome
mOsm Milliosmole
MPAP Mean pulmonary artery pressure; also abbreviated PAM
MRA Magnetic resonance arteriogram
MRI Magnetic resonance imaging
MRSA Methicillin-resistant *Staphylococcus aureus*
MS Multiple sclerosis; musculoskeletal
MSAP Mean systolic arterial pressure
MSH Melanocyte-stimulating hormone
MUGA scan Multiple-gated acquisition scan
μg Microgram
μl Microliter
μm Micrometer
μm^3 Cubic micrometer
N Nitrogen
Na/Na$^+$ Sodium/sodium ion
NaCl Sodium chloride
NaHCO$_3$ Sodium bicarbonate
NCV Nerve conduction velocity
Neuro Neurovascular
ng Nanogram
NG Nasogastric
NH$_3$ Ammonia
NH$_4^+$ Ammonium
NIDDM Non-insulin-dependent diabetes mellitus
NIH National Institutes of Health
nl Normal
NMBA Neuromuscular blocking agent
NPO Nothing by mouth
NREM Non-REM
NS Normal saline
NSAID Nonsteroidal antiinflammatory drug
NSR Normal sinus rhythm
NTG Nitroglycerin
O$_2$ Oxygen
OR Operating room
OT Occupational therapist
OTC Over-the-counter
PA Pulmonary artery
P (A-a)O$_2$ Alveolar-arterial oxygen tension difference
PAC Premature atrial complexes
Paco$_2$ Partial pressure of dissolved carbon dioxide in arterial blood
PADP Pulmonary artery diastolic pressure
PAo$_2$ Partial pressure of alveolar oxygen
Pao$_2$ Partial pressure of dissolved oxygen in arterial blood
PAP Pulmonary artery pressure
PAS Pulmonary artery systolic
PASG Pneumatic antishock garment
PAT Paroxysmal atrial tachycardia
PAWP Pulmonary artery wedge pressure
PBV Percutaneous balloon valvuloplasty
pc After meals
PCA Patient-controlled analgesia
PD Peritoneal dialysis
PE Pulmonary embolus
PEA Pulseless electrical activity
PEEP Positive end-expiratory pressure
PEG Percutaneous endoscopic gastrostomy
PET Positron emission tomography

pH Hydrogen ion concentration
PJC Premature junctional complexes
PMI Point of maximal impulse
PN Parenteral nutrition
PO By mouth
PO$_4$/PO$_4^{3-}$ Phosphorus/phosphate ion
PPF Plasma protein fraction
PPN Peripheral parenteral nutrition
PRBCs Packed red blood cells
prn As needed
PT Physical therapist; prothrombin time
PTCA Percutaneous transluminal coronary angioplasty
PTH Parathyroid hormone
PTT Partial thromboplastin time
PTU Propylthiouracil
PVC Premature ventricular complexes, peripheral venous catheter
PVD Peripheral vascular disease
PVR Pulmonary vascular resistance
q Every
qd Every day
qh Every hour
qid Four times a day
RA Rheumatoid arthritis; right atrial
RAP Right atrial pressure
RBC Red blood cell
RBF Renal blood flow
RDA Recommended dietary allowance
REM Rapid eye movement
Resp Respiratory
RLQ Right lower quadrant
r/o Rule out
ROM Range of motion
RPE Rate(d) perceived exertion
RQ Respiratory quotient
RR Respiratory rate
RRT Renal replacement therapy
RSB Right sternal border
r/t Related to
RUQ Right upper quadrant
RV Right ventricular
RVEDP Right ventricular end-diastolic pressure
RVP Right ventricular pressure
SA Status asthmaticus
SAH Subarachnoid hemorrhage
Sao$_2$ Saturation of hemoglobin by oxygen
SAS Subarachnoid space
S-B Sengstaken-Blakemore
SBP Systolic blood pressure
SC Subcutaneous
SCI Spinal cord injury
sec Second
SGOT Serum glutamic oxaloacetic-acid-transaminase
SGPT Serum glutamic pyruvic transaminase
SIADH Syndrome of inappropriate antidiuretic hormone
SIRS Systemic inflammatory response syndrome
SL Sublingual
SLE Systemic lupus erythematosus
SNS Sympathetic nervous system
SOB Shortness of breath
SPECT Single photon emission computed tomography
Spo$_2$ Peripheral arterial oxygen saturation
S&S Signs and symptoms

stat Immediately
Svo₂ Mixed venous oxygen saturation
SVR Systemic vascular resistance
SVT Supraventricular tachycardia
T Thoracic
T₃ Triiodothyronine
T₄ Thyroxine
TB Tuberculosis
TBSA Total body surface area
TD Transdermal
Td Combined tetanus diphtheria toxoid
Temp Temperature
TENS Transcutaneous electrical nerve stimulation
TIA Transient ischemic attack
tid Three times a day
TIPS Transjugular intrahepatic portosystemic shunt
TKO To keep open

TPN Total parenteral nutrition
TRH Thyrotropin-releasing hormone
TSF Triceps skinfold thickness
TSH Thyroid-stimulating hormone
T-spine Thoracic spine
TTP Thrombotic thrombocytopenic purpura
TUR Transurethral resection
U Unit
UA Urinalysis
UGI Upper gastrointestinal
UGIB Upper gastrointestinal bleeding
UO Urinary output
URI Upper respiratory infection
UTI Urinary tract infection
UV Ultraviolet
VAD Venous access device; ventricular assist device
VC Vital capacity
VEDP Ventricular end-diastolic pressure

VEDV Ventricular end-diastolic volume
VF Ventricular fibrillation
VMA Vanillamandelic acid
Vo₂ Oxygen consumption
V/Q Ventilation/perfusion
VRE Vancomycin-resistant enterococci
VS Vital signs
VSD Ventricular septal defect
VT Ventricular tachycardia
VWf Von Willebrand's factor
WBC White blood cell
WHO World Health Organization
wk Week
wnl Within normal limits
WOB Work of breathing
WPW Wolff-Parkinson-White
↓ Decrease
↑ Increase
× Times

INDEX